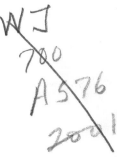

E. Nieschlag, H. M. Behre (Eds.)

ANDROLOGY
**Male Reproductive Health
and Dysfunction**

2nd Edition

Springer

Berlin
Heidelberg
New York
Barcelona
Hong Kong
London
Milan
Paris
Singapore
Tokyo

E. Nieschlag · H. M. Behre (Eds.)

ANDROLOGY

2nd Edition **Male Reproductive Health and Dysfunction**

Contributors

H. van Ahlen, M. Brinkworth
T. G. Cooper, C. De Geyter, M. De Geyter
K. Demmer, U. H. Engelmann, P. Gassner
J. Gromoll, D. J. Handelsman, L. Hertle, A. Holstein
A. Kamischke, S. Kliesch, U. A. Knuth, E. Leifke
A. Lerchl, D. Meschede, F. A. Muthny, S. Nieschlag
F. Oberpenning, R. Oberpenning, C.-J. Partsch
C. Rolf, H.P.G. Schneider, U. Schwarzer
M. Simoni, G. F. Weinbauer, C.-H. Yeung

With 172 Figures and 43 Tables

 Springer

Nieschlag, Eberhard, Prof. Dr. med., FRCP
Institute of Reproductive Medicine
of the University
Domagkstr. 11
D-48129 Münster, Germany
Tel.: +49-251/835 60 97
Fax: +49-251/835 60 93
Email: Nieschl@uni-muenster.de

Behre, Hermann M., Prof. Dr. med.
Andrology Unit
Department of Urology of the University
Magdeburger Str. 16
D-06097 Halle
Tel.: +49-345/557 14 46
Fax: +49-345/557 17 83
Email: Hermann.Behre@medizin.uni-halle.de

Assistant Editor
Nieschlag, Susan, M. A.
Institute of Reproductive Medicine
of the University
Domagkstr. 11
D-48129 Münster, Germany

ISBN 3-540-67224-9
Springer-Verlag Berlin Heidelberg New York

CIP data applied for

Die Deutsche Bibliothek – CIP-Einheitsaufnahme
Andrology: male reproductive health and dysfunction;
with 43 tables / E. Nieschlag; H. M. Behre (ed.). Contributors
H. van Ahlen ... –
2. ed. – Berlin; Heidelberg; New York; Barcelona; Hong Kong;
London; Milan; Paris; Singapore; Tokyo: Springer, 2000
   Dt. Ausg. u. d. T.: Andrologie
   ISBN 3-540-67224-9

Springer-Verlag Berlin Heidelberg New York a member of
BertelsmannSpringer Science + Business Media GmbH
© Springer-Verlag Berlin Heidelberg 2001
Printed in Germany

The use of general descriptive names, registered names, trade-
marks, etc. in this publication does not imply, even in the
absence of a specific statement, that such names are exempt
from the relevant protective laws and regulations and therefore
free for general use.

Product liability: The publishers cannot guarantee the accuracy of any information about dosage and application contained in this book. In every individual case the user must
check such information by consulting the relevant literature.

Cover design: E. Kirchner, Heidelberg
Typesetting: Data conversion by B. Wieland, Heidelberg
Printing and bookbinding: Stürtz AG, Würzburg

SPIN 10758477   22/3130 – 5 4 3 2 1 0
Printed on acid-free paper

Preface to the 2nd Edition

Andrology, as the science of male reproductive function and dysfunction, has experienced exceptional progress in recent years. Especially clinical applications of molecular biology and molecular genetics to male infertility and hypogonadism, the "invention" of intracytoplasmic sperm injection (ICSI) as a treatment of male infertility and the introduction of effective oral medication for erectile dysfunction can be considered major breakthroughs. The magnitude of these developments, along with many others, prompted this second edition of *Andrology: Male Reproductive Health and Dysfunction.*

As in the first edition, the textbook follows the principles of evidence-based medicine and provides a firm scientific basis for clinical andrology. As before, we consider andrology as part of the comprehensive field of reproductive medicine, but we are convinced that it can coexist alongside gynecology only when it qualifies as a scientific and clinical field in its own right. For this reason this textbook seeks to strengthen andrology as a field, along with acting as a source of information.

All chapters have been throughly revised and extended; some were completely rewritten. Among the new features: the diagnostic sections reflect the newest WHO guidelines on semen analysis (1999); the sections on testicular biopsy were enlarged by a contribution from Prof. A.F. Holstein (Hamburg); the pathophysiological basis of numerous disease entities is explained by insights newly gained from molecular biology and molecular genetics;. ICSI treatment and its genetic ramifications are thoroughly discussed; other therapeutic methods, especially the treatment of varicocele, have been brought up to date. Without disregarding the art of exact diagnosis, medical treatment of erectile dysfuntion is covered in detail. Because of increasing interest, the chapters on male contraception and the aging male have been expanded. As in the earlier edition, a chapter on the ethical aspects of reproductive medicine completes the picture. The layout of the first edition, with typographical features designed for the reader's orientation, has been maintained and is supplemented with color illustrations and figures, contributing to a lively presentation.

In order to provide a uniform work, we selected authors who are either past or currently colleagues at the Institute of Reproductive Medicine at the University of Münster or who work at collaborating centers. The interest shared by the authors contributed to a uniform presentation of andrology and prompted reviewers of the first edition to speak of a "Münster school of andrology". The editors are grateful to all contributors for their excellent cooperation. As before, Susan Nieschlag M.A., as assistant editor, contributed a high degree of professionalism and tireless effort to this second edition. The word processing skills of Angelika Schick, Barbara Bahnes and Maria Schalkowski, secretaries at the Institute, deserve special mention. Particular thanks go to Dr. Trevor Cooper and Dr. Andrea Wagenfeld for their punctilious and professional review of all manuscripts. Finally, we are grateful to Dr. Udo Lindner, Dr. Annette Zimpelmann, Bernd Wieland and Axel Treiber of Springer Verlag for their enthusiastic support of the present volume. They encouraged our input, which was rewarded by speedy production of the volume.

Many suggestions for the second edition were provided by reviewers and readers, and we gratefully incorporated their ideas. This dialogue was particularly helpful and we would like to repeat our earlier request for critical suggestions. We hope that the reader will again use this volume to his own advantage and to that of his patients.

Eberhard Nieschlag, Hermann M. Behre
Münster, Spring 2000

Preface to the 1st Edition

The present volume sets forth the basic principles and the clinical practice of andrology as the science of male reproductive health and dysfunction.

This book is to be viewed against the background of the development of reproductive medicine and andrology at our center in Münster, Germany. Following the establishment of the Clinical Research Group for Reproductive Medicine by the Max Planck Society in 1980, which was succeeded by the Institute of Reproductive Medicine at the Westphalian Wilhelms University in Münster in 1989, a center of andrological research and patient care developed, based on close cooperation between basic scientists and physicians. This close cooperation between basic research and clinical practice aims to apply scientific methods to explore the reproductive functions of the male and to harness them for mankind, both in positive and negative terms. The combination of research and patient care necessitates close contact between university clinics and institutes, in particular, the Woman's Hospital, Department of Urology, Institute of Human Genetics, Institute for Clinical Radiology, Institute for Medical Microbiology, and Institute for Medical Psychology. In addition, the Institute of Reproductive Medicine participates in the network of the WHO Collaborating Centers (since 1987) and the Training Centers for Clinical Andrology of the European Academy of Andrology (since 1994).

Over the course of time we have accumulated experience in patient care and have developed clinical principles which have been published in numerous articles, reviews, and book chapters. We consider the time ripe to present our experience and our view of andrology in a textbook.

In order to present a unified volume we chose our authors either from past or present coworkers of the Institute of Reproductive Medicine or from cooperating institutions. Past or present coworkers include Dr. Martin Brinkworth, Dr. M. Angelines Castel, Dr. Trevor G. Cooper, Dr. Jörg Gromoll, Dr. Axel Kamischke, Dr. Eckhard Leifke, Priv.-Doz. Dr. Alexander Lerchl, Dr. Carl-Joachim Partsch, Dr. Claus Rolf, Dr. Manuela Simoni, Priv.-Doz. Dr. Gerhard F. Weinbauer, and Dr. Ching-Hei Yeung as well as Priv.-Doz. Dr. Christian De Geyter, Dr. Maria De Geyter, Dr. Sabine Kliesch, Priv.-Doz. Dr. Ulrich A. Knuth, and Dr. Dieter Meschede. Prof. David J. Handelsman spent a 9-month sabbatical at our Institute while the book was being written. Intensive cooperation with the Woman's Hospital under the directorship of Prof. Dr. Hermann P. G. Schneider is of essential importance for patient care. We are closely connected to the University Urology Clinic, and this cooperation is reflected in the authorship of Prof. Dr. Lothar Hertle, Priv.-Doz. Dr. Hermann van Ahlen, and Dr. Frank Oberpenning. Our patients receive psychological counselling from Prof. Dr. F. M. Muthny, and Dr. Regina Oberpenning, of the Institute of Medical Psychology. Prof Dr. Klaus Demmer, a native of Münster, has advised the Institute on ethical questions for many years. Susan Nieschlag, M. A., serves as the Institute's editor and has contributed editorial input for this volume as well. She has translated some chapters in their entirety and language-edited all others. We hope that the intellectual background shared by the authors will help to present a unified picture of andrology in this book.

We thank all authors for their speedy cooperation. Strict adherence to deadlines contributed to the volume's unified appearance and to its timeliness. The Institute's secretaries, Kerstin Neuhaus and Angelika Düthmann deserve a great measure of thanks for word processing. Thanks too go to members of the Springer Publishing House, Dr. Carol Bacchus, Marga Botsch and Bernd Reichenthaler, who were responsible for the book's appearance and prompt handling.

We hope that the reader will use this volume to his own advantage and to that of his patients. We are grateful for all comments and criticism.

E. Nieschlag, H. M. Behre
Münster, November 1996

Contents

7 Diseases of the Hypothalamus and the Pituitary Gland
H. M. Behre · E. Nieschlag · D. Meschede
C. J. Partsch

8 Disorders at the Testicular Level
E. Nieschlag · H. M. Behre
D. Meschede · A. Kamischke

11 Disorders of Androgen Target Organs
D. Meschede · H. M. Behre · E. Nieschlag

12 Testicular Dysfunction in Systemic Diseases
D. J. Handelsman

13 Environmental Influences on Male Reproductive Health
M. H. Brinkworth · D. J. Handelsman

---

17 Assisted Fertilization

C. De Geyter · M. De Geyter
D. Meschede · H. M. Behre

---

18 Cryopreservation of Human Semen

S. Kliesch · A. Kamischke · E. Nieschlag

---

19 The Psychology of Fertility Disorders

R. Oberpenning · F. Oberpenning · F. A. Muthny

22 Ethical Aspects of Reproductive Medicine
K. DEMMER

List of Contributors

Behre, Hermann M., Prof. Dr. med.
Andrology Unit
Department of Urology of the University
Magdeburger Str. 16
D-06097 Halle, Germany

Brinkworth, Martin, Ph. D.
Department of Biomedical Sciences
University of Bradford
Bradford BD7 1DP, United Kingdom

Cooper, Trevor G., Ph. D.
Institute of Reproductive Medicine of the University
Domagkstr. 11
D-48129 Münster, Germany

De Geyter, Christian, Priv.-Doz. Dr. med.
Women's Hospital of the University
Schanzenstr. 46
CH-4031 Basel, Switzerland

De Geyter, Maria, Dr. rer. nat.
Women's Hospital of the University
Schanzenstr. 46
CH-4031 Basel, Switzerland

Demmer, Klaus, Prof. Dr. theol.
Pontifica Universitá Gregoriana
Via della Pace 20
I-00186 Roma, Italy

Engelmann, Udo H., Prof. Dr. med.
Urological Hospital of the University
Joseph-Stelzmann-Str. 9
D-50931 Köln, Germany

Gassner, Paul, Dr. rer. nat.
Institute of Reproductive Medicine of the University
Domagkstr. 11
D-48129 Münster, Germany

Gromoll, Jörg, Priv.-Doz. Dr. rer. nat.
Institute of Reproductive Medicine of the University
Domagkstr. 11
D-48129 Münster, Germany

Handelsman, David. J., Prof. MB BS, FRACP, Ph. D.
ANZAC Research Institute
Department of Andrology
Concord Hospital, Dept. of Medicine
University of Sydney
Sydney, NSW 2006, Australia

Hertle, Lothar, Prof. Dr. med.
Urological Hospital of the University
Albert-Schweitzer-Str. 33
D-48129 Münster, Germany

Holstein, Adolf, Prof. Dr. med.
Anatomical Institute
of the University Hospital Eppendorf
Martinistr. 52
D-20246 Hamburg, Germany

Kamischke, Axel, Dr. med.
Institute of Reproductive Medicine of the University
Domagkstr. 11
D-48129 Münster, Germany

Kliesch, Sabine, Dr. med.
Urological Hospital of the University
Albert-Schweitzer-Str. 33
D-48129 Münster, Germany

Kopfensteiner, Thomas, Prof. Dr.
Kenrick Seminary
St. Louis, Missouri, USA

Knuth, Ulrich A., Priv.-Doz. Dr. med.
Gemeinschaftspraxis Bohnet & Knuth
Schomburgstr. 120
D-22767 Hamburg, Germany

Leifke, Eckehard, Dr. med.
Medical University Hannover
Dept. of Endocrinology
Konstanty-Gutschow-Str. 8
D-30625 Hannover, Germany

Lerchl, Alexander, Priv.-Doz. Dr. rer. nat.
Institute of Reproductive Medicine of the University
Domagkstr. 11
D-48129 Münster, Germany

Meschede, Dieter, Dr. med.
Institute of Human Genetics of the University
Vesaliusweg 12–14
D-48129 Münster, Germany

Muthny, Fritz A., Prof. Dr. Dr.
Institute of Medical Psychology of the University
Von-Esmarch-Str. 56
D-48129 Münster, Germany

Nieschlag, Eberhard, Prof. Dr. med., FRCP
Institute of Reproductive Medicine of the University
Domagkstr. 11
D-48129 Münster, Germany

Nieschlag, Susan, M. A.
Institute of Reproductive Medicine of the University
Domagkstr. 11
D-48129 Münster, Germany

Oberpenning, Frank, Dr. med.
Urological Hospital of the University
Albert-Schweitzer-Str. 33
D-48129 Münster, Germany

Oberpenning, Regina, Dr. rer. medic., Dipl.-Psych.
Institute of Reproductive Medicine of the University
Domagkstr. 11
D-48129 Münster, Germany

Partsch, Carl-Joachim, Dr. med.
Children's Hospital of the University
Schwanenweg 20
D-24105 Kiel, Germany

Rolf, Claus, Dr. med.
Institute of Reproductive Medicine of the University
Domagkstr. 11
D-48129 Münster, Germany

Schneider, H. P. G., Prof. Dr.
University Women's Hospital
Albert-Schweitzer-Str. 33
D-48129 Münster, Germany

Schwarzer, U., Dr. med.
Urological Hospital of the University
Joseph-Stelzmann-Str. 9
D-50931 Köln, Germany

Simoni, Manuela, Prof., M. D., Ph. D.
Institute of Reproductive Medicine of the University
Domagkstr. 11
D-48129 Münster, Germany

van Ahlen, Hermann, Prof. Dr. med.
Urological Hospital of the University
Klinikum Osnabrück GmbH
Postfach 3806
D-49028 Osnabrück, Germany

Weinbauer, Gerhard F., Prof. Dr. phil.
Institute of Reproductive Medicine of the University
Domagkstr. 11
D-48129 Münster, Germany

Yeung, Ching-Hei, Dr. Ph. D.
Institute of Reproductive Medicine of the University
Domagkstr. 11
D-48129 Münster, Germany

CHAPTER 1

Scope and Goals of Andrology

E. NIESCHLAG

1.1   Definition of Andrology

"Andrology is defined as the branches of science and medicine dealing with reproductive functions of the male under physiological and pathological conditions" (Statutes of the European Academy of Andrology, 1992).

If this definition were to be interpreted in the context of sociobiology, considering reproduction the central task of life to which the entire organism is devoted (e. g. Dawkins 1994), andrology would be a broad field. Generally and also for the purpose of this book, andrology is considered the science and practice of dealing with male reproductive functions and their disturbances in the strict sense.

The central topics of andrology:
- Infertility,
- Hypogonadism
  (with and without desired paternity),
- Male contraception,
- Erectile dysfunction and
- Male senescence.

Generally and following the definition of WHO, andrology deals with **male reproductive health**.

1.2   Andrology, Gynecology, Reproductive Medicine: Reproductive Health

Every layman knows that a man and a woman are necessary to produce offspring. However, a barren couple does not necessarily know whether the affliction lies on the male or the female or both sides. Therefore, it would be sensible for the couples to turn to a physician in a discipline dealing holistically with problems of infertility.

No matter how logical this concept may appear to the patients, medicine has barely offered appropriate solutions. Most often the individual partners of a barren couple continue to consult physicians of different disciplines in order to be diagnosed and treated. For the woman it is relatively easy to find a competent physician, since **gynecology** is a traditional field of medicine and amply represented.

It is much more difficult for the afflicted male. If he suspects problems of infertility on his part, he does not know immediately to whom he should turn. One third first consults the primary health care physician or family practitioner, one quarter turns to (his wife's) gynecologist and the remaining patients consult urologists (and in Germany also dermatologists) (Bruckert 1991) and perhaps endocrinologists. As a firm discipline of medicine andrology is established in very few countries. Only in France and Italy is andrology a speciality, practiced there, however, within the frame of endocrinology. In addition, andrology is a speciality in Egypt and Indonesia. In other countries andrology is not a discipline that the patient may identify. In Germany, in addition to urologists, endocrinologists, and gynecologists, dermatologists see infertile patients as an anachronism from the times when male infertility was predominantly caused by venereal deseases – as it is now still the case in Subsaharan Africa. The goal of improved medical training in the field of male reproductive health (Cummins and Jequier 1999) has been taken up by the European Academy of Andrology (EAA) which has established over 15 centers in Europe (EAA 1999).

From the point of view of the afflicted couple, a specialized interdisciplinary field of **reproductive medicine** would seem to offer a solution (Fig. 1.1) (Nieschlag 1986). A few such services are in fact available at universities or in individual practices. It is, however, seldom that both partners of an infertile couple are cared for by one person; usually an interdisciplinary team consisting of an andrologist and a gynecologist working together represent reproductive medicine.

The *World Health Organization (WHO)* considers the couple as a single entity in its definition of "reproductive health", which it defines as freedom from disease and disturbances of reproductive functions, both in the male and in the female. As part of its concept of reproductive health the WHO postulates that reproduction should take place in an environment of physical, mental and social well-being. In addition, in its demand for self determination of the number of children by the couple, it assumes that both partners have free access to reliable contraceptive methods. In its research programme on human reproduction the WHO devotes itself to problems both in the female and in the male (WHO 1994–1998). Whereas in previous years the investigation of female reproductive functions stood in the foreground, more recently studies on male fertility have been given equal weight. On an international level initial efforts towards an interdisciplinary field of **reproductive medicine** are being made.

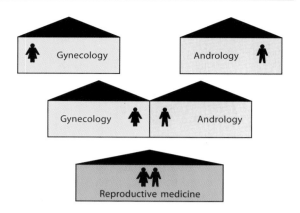

Fig. 1.1. Symbolic representation of various ways in which men and woman or the couple seeking offspring may be cared for

As desirable as care for the infertile couple by only one attending physician may appear, it should not be overlooked that, apart from the initial consultation and those eventually occurring during the course of treatment, the actual investigations of husband and wife do not necessarily proceed in synchrony. Only when techniques of assisted fertilisation, which, however, are still only appropriate for selected couples, are applied is closest cooperation mandatory. Moreover, andrology covers certain aspects of male reproductive functions which can be treated largely without recourse to the partner, e. g. **replacement therapy in hypogonadism, delayed pubertal development, erectile dysfunction, contraception** and **male senescence.** For this reason, **in addition to gynecology,** the part of reproductive medicine dealing with the male, i. e. **andrology,** is indispensable. Moreover, the field of reproductive gynecology is so comprehensive that it cannot adequately deal with problems of the male as well. At present the development of **gynecology and andrology** as separate fields seems to offer the most advantages, not forgetting, however, that both fields should **cooperate most closely** in the care of the infertile couple, e. g. within the framework of a center for reproductive medicine. When treatment consists of assisted reproduction, German guidelines (Bundesärztekammer 1998) require that one of a minimum of three physicians must be an andrologist. For practical purposes this means that an andrologist must be part of every center of reproductive medicine.

1.3 Infertility, Subfertility, Sterility, Fecundity: Definition of Terms

When speaking of disturbed fertility, certain concepts must be introduced and defined. It must also be taken into consideration that terminology may change over time.

Fertility refers to the capability to conceive or induce a pregnancy. **Fecundity** refers to the probability of producing a live birth arising from a given menstrual cycle.

Infertility is the term used when a couple fails to induce a pregnancy within one year of regular unprotected intercourse. **Primary infertility** defines the condition when no pregnancy at all has been achieved, and **secondary infertility** means no further pregnancies have occurred. The term infertile can be applied to both men and women.

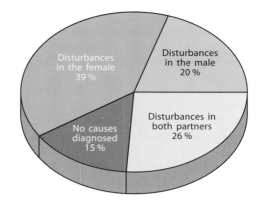

Fig. 1.2. Distribution of causes of involuntary childlessness between men and women (WHO 1987)

In addition to infertility the term **sterility** is also used. Historically, it is an even older term. However, **infertility** is the more general term which may also include sterility (Templeton 1992). "Infertility" is doubtless the most accurate description for childlessness. "Sterility", on the other hand, is a term with additional meanings as well (e. g. in the context of hygiene). "Infertility" also has the advantage of making less of a value judgement and avoids terminological ambiguity, for infertility and sterility are not separable nosological entities. The change in usage is reflected by the fact that up to 1982 the database Medline used "**sterility**"; since then "**infertility**" has been in use as a headline word (National Library of Medicine 1993).

One objection to general use of the concept of "infertility" as opposed to "fertility" is that what is meant may actually be **subfertility**, as basically, the ability to sire or conceive may actually exist, e. g. with another partner. However, here too it is difficult to delineate sharply between definitions.

For these reasons in this volume we use the term **infertility** to refer to disturbed fertility in general and we speak of it when, within one year of regular, unprotected intercourse, no pregnancy occurs. One can discriminate between primary and secondary infertility, depending on whether a pregnancy has once been induced or not.

1.4 The Infertile Couple as Target Patients

Even if medical care of the female suffering from disturbed fertility is much better organized than that of the man, an analysis of the distribution of causes of disturbed fertility shows that in up to half of the couples wishing offspring the male may be implicated (Fig. 1.2). Disturbances in fertility may remain latent for years and only become evident when a couple develops a firm desire for a child. It is of particular importance that the

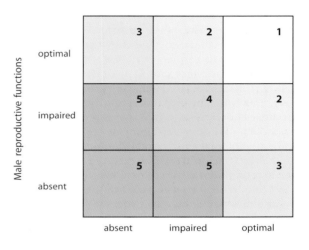

Female reproductive functions

Fig. 1.3. Interdependence of male and female reproductive functions. Couples from *group 1*, with both partners having optimal reproductive functions, will not consult a physician because of childlessness. The suboptimal functions of one partner in couples of *group 2* will probably be compensated for by the optimal functions of the other partner. These couples are probably more prevalent in the general population than their representation in fertility clinics may suggest. In couples of *group 3* treatment will be concentrated only on one partner and treatment by only either gynecologist or andrologist will suffice. Both partners of *groups 4 and 5* require treatment. Therapeutic success i. e. pregnancy will be achieved more rapidly the more intensive and coordinated medical care is. Precisely these couples benefit most from treatment in a center for reproductive medicine where physicians have both gynecological and andrological training

suboptimal reproductive capacities of one partner may become evident because of the infertility of the other partner. This demonstrates the **interdependence of male and female reproductive functions,** as shown schematically in Fig. 1.3.

In order to evaluate the effects of limited reproductive functions it is important to know the **time span** within which a "normal" couple of group 1 (Fig. 1.3) will conceive. If a young couple of group 1 plans a pregnancy it will occur within 3 months in 75 % of couples (Falk and Kaufmann 1950). In unselected women attending the delivery ward of a larger German municipal hospital 70 % conceived within the first 6 months and 90 % conceived within the first 12 months of unprotected intercourse (Knuth and Mühlenstedt 1991).

However, this rate decreases steadily with the **age of the female partner.** In women older than 25 years pregnancy occurs in 80 % of couples only within 20–28 months (Bender 1953). In women whose husbands are azoospermic and who submitted to donor insemination, a rapid decline of fecundity could be found after the age of 30 (Van Noord-Zaadstra et al. 1991).

Moreover, the frequency of coitus plays an important role. When both semen parameters and female factors are normal, the interval to conception decreases with the frequency of coitus as long as sperm production is not exhausted. Partners complaining of involuntary childlessness of more than 12 months' duration and in whom andrological factors have been excluded achieve a maximum conception rate when coitus takes place 3–4 times per week (McLeod et al. 1955). When sperm production is limited, however, this direct relationship is no longer valid.

Also the **timing of coitus** is of great importance. Most conceptions occur on the day of ovulation and the two preceding days, few conceptions, if intercourse takes place on days 3–5 before ovulation, but no conceptions after the day of ovulation (Wilcox et al. 1995).

It follows that **younger couples** should be examined only after they have tried to found a family for at least one year. Should the **woman** be **over 30 years,** investigations may be initiated earlier. In industrialized nations married childless couples tend to belong to the latter group as the average age at marriage is increasing. Whereas in Germany it was 23.7 for women and 25.9 for men in 1990, by 1997 it had increased to 27.9 for women and 30.4 for men. However, in the meantime 30 % of all German children are born out of wedlock so that the age at marriage no longer corresponds to the age at which parenthood is to be realized. The age of the couples visiting the fertility clinic rises correspondingly. Thus the average age of the female partner at her first visit of our center in 1985 was 30.1±4.2 years (mean±SD) and 33.4±4.9 year in 1999, and her partner's age was 32.9±5.0 and 33.8±5.5 years. In the USA it was 20.1 and 24.5 years for women and 22.5 and 26.7 for men in 1956

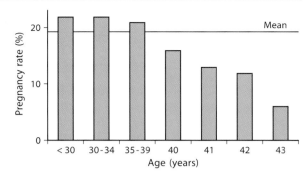

Fig. 1.4. Pregnancy rate per follicle puncture in 12,150 IVF cycles in relation to the age of the women (Deutsches IVF-Register 1998)

and 1994 respectively. As the reproductive functions in men of good health remain intact to an advanced age, from a physiological point of view increasing age of the male partner alone does not warrant premature medical intervention (see Chap. 21).

The interdependencies of male and female reproductive functions described above should provide reason enough to examine both partners simultaneously in the event of involuntary childlessness. Both partners should be examined with the same degree of thoroughness. Good medical practice requires a full anamnesis, careful physical examination followed by all necessary technical and laboratory investigations.

The entity represented by the couple with disturbed fertility must not be ignored. For this reason, although this volume deals primarily with andrology, it also provides an overview of diagnosis and therapy of female infertility (see Chap. 14).

1.5 Prevalence of Infertility

Information on the prevalence of infertility indicates great variability and only few reliable data are available (review in Schmidt and Münster 1995; Templeton 1992). Infertility shows considerable geographic variation; according to WHO primary infertility is lowest in the Middle East and highest in Central Africa (Farley and Belsey 1988). No absolutely firm data are available for **Germany.** Estimations assumed a prevalence of (primary and secondary) infertility **of up to 15 % and more** of all couples of reproductive age (Bruckert 1991; Juul et al. 1999). There are marked regional variations within Europe and even between East and West Germany (Juul et al. 1999). Conversely, little change has occurred in the "time-to-pregnancy" curves which have been constructed over centuries (Fig. 1.5). This applies particularly to the decreasing ability of the oocyte to be fertilized, as results from assisted reproduction show (Fig. 1.4). Whether the incidence of infertility is increasing is not com-

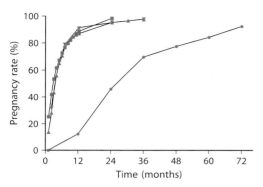

Fig. 1.5. Cumulative pregnancy rates of different normal populations in different epochs. Stolwijk et al. (1996) investigated Canadian church registers from the 17th and 18th centuries, Tietze et al. (1950) analyzed a population in New York and Knuth at al. (1991) interviewed mothers of newborns in a maternity ward in Germany. For comparison, pregnancy rates of untreated couples with sperm surface antibodies in seminal plasma are shown (Abshagen et al. 1998)

■ Stolwijk et al., 1996
n = 18970 from 1664 to 1772

▼ Tietze et al., 1950
n = 1727

▲ Knuth et al., 1991
n = 474

● Abshagen et al., 1998
n = 61

pletely clear. The proportion of couples seeking medical treatment for infertility is estimated at 4–17 %. Ultimately 3–4 % of all couples remain involuntarily childless at the end of their reproductive life phase (Templeton 1992).

As male causes for infertility are found in half of involuntarily childless couples, it must be assumed that **about 7 % of all men** are confronted with the problem of disturbed fertility in the course of their lives. This means that the prevalence of infertility in men clearly exceeds that of diabetes mellitus (types I and II), which is often considered almost endemic.

The incidence of individual disturbances of fertility will be dealt with in connection with the diseases discussed in the following chapters.

1.6 Evidence-Based Andrology

There are many reasons why andrology has not developed into an independent specialized medical discipline. One important reason may be that, until recently, diagnostic and therapeutic measures had not reached a critical mass great enough to justify establishment of an independent field. It is a fact that research efforts investigating the physiology and pathology of male reproductive functions were not undertaken systematically before the 1960s and pathophysiological concepts explaining individual diseases only gradually emerged. One factor contributing to the situation was also that andrological diagnostic techniques lacked standardisation and tended to produce vague diagnoses. At least 30 % of cases of disturbed male fertility still remain etiologically unclear and are referred to as **idiopathic infertility** (see Chaps. 5 and 16).

These shortcomings, characterizing andrology as well as other specialities, often meant that the physician's personal authority and experience tended to become the dominating factor in management decisions. The situation makes it tempting for some physicians to apply innumerable empirical therapeutic procedures whose effectiveness remain uncertain. Many errors in judgement – not only in andrology – can be attributed to this attraction to meddlesome but unproven treatments.

With the advance of basic research and scientific thinking in andrology, the dilemma became obvious to those actively practicing clinical andrology and a "**new andrology**" operating on scientific thinking and rationally based medical practice was called for. "**Evidence-based andrology**" developed simultaneously with the beginnings of "**evidence-based medicine**", which is increasingly becoming a pervasive force in all fields of medicine. It marks a gradual shift of paradigm in clinical medicine.

> The term "evidence-based medicine" signifies that clinical decisions must be based on results from controlled clinical studies and applied statistics and not rely predominantly on intuition, empiricism and traditional protocols (Evidence-Based Medicine Working Group 1992; Antes 1998).

Whereas they remained rare in the 60s, today **controlled, prospective, randomized and, if possible, double-blind clinical studies** are the accepted standard for evaluating the effectiveness of a diagnostic or therapeutic measure. No medication, no interventional measure nor any diagnostic test should be incorporated into clinical practice if its effectiveness has not been proven by appropriate controlled studies. (There will, of course, be exceptions to this, as e. g. hormonal replacement therapy for which the physiological hormone levels in serum represent the target parameters.) While the clinical andrologist found it particularly difficult to incorporate this **shift of paradigm into the decision-making pro-**

cess, the exponential increase in clinical studies concerning infertility treatment over the past decade shows that this concept is finally becoming established in andrology as well (Vandekerckhove et al. 1993).

The details of carrying out **controlled clinical studies** cannot be dealt with here. The most important elements are the studies' design and statistical evaluation. Over and beyond the problems generally caused by performing controlled studies in other fields of medicine, studies on infertility treatment face the particular difficulty that not **one** patient is being dealt with, a **second** participant must not only fulfill strict inclusion criteria, but is in fact the person in whom the end-point, pregnancy, occurs. The fact that pregnancy rates are naturally relatively low and that therefore large numbers of patients must be followed over prolonged periods of time creates special problems in controlled clinical studies on infertility treatment.

"Evidence-based medicine" also subjects **pathophysiological concepts**, on which diagnosis and therapeutic measures are based, to **critical examination** and assumes that not all pathophysiological concepts must be correct **a priori**. This is supported by experience from basic research showing that errors do in fact occur, that research results may be translated prematurely into clinical strategies, thus giving rise to conceptual "short circuits". Examples of this are demonstrated by the various ill-founded treatments of idiopathic male infertility (see Chap. 16). Evidence-based medicine demands that translation of a scientific concept into a clinical strategy be provable by rational means and that it stand up under conditions of a controlled clinical study. The goal of this volume is to follow the precepts of evidence-based medicine to the extent possible and thus it is justified to apply the term evidence-based andrology to the message of this book.

One of the important components of evidence-based andrology is **standardised diagnostics**, making results within one laboratory as well as between laboratories comparable. In this respect the "*WHO Laboratory Manual for the Examination of Human Semen and Sperm-Cervical Mucus Interaction*" (1st edition 1980, 4th edition 1999) was a pioneer work. It was intended to provide the basis for all andrological laboratory diagnosis. Notwithstanding that Chapter 6 of the present volume briefly describes semen analysis as a laboratory technique, the WHO Manual must be considered as an **appendix to this volume**. The methodology described provides the basis for both internal and external quality control in the andrology laboratory which even today remains in its beginning stages. It is to be hoped that other areas of andrological diagnostics will be standardized to further buttress evidence-based andrology.

While it is desirable that andrology increasingly be given a firm scientific base and that diagnostic and therapeutic measures be tested by their results, it must not

be forgotten that **the patient or couple** requiring care remains the **center point of medical attention**. This includes providing time for extensive counselling, for clarifying physical and pathological facts, for explaining diagnostic findings and therapeutic measures, for answering questions concerning sexuality, for exploring the importance of a child to each partner and to the couple. The patient must be convinced by practice that precisely these aspects are of greatest importance to the physician, whereas scientific validity of his management must be the unspoken precondition of professional expertise underlying patient-doctor interaction.

The **placebo-effect of medical advice and attention** must never be underestimated. This assumes that the **placebo be defined** as a measure lacking a specific effect, but which will nevertheless have a significantly greater influence on the desired outcome than no measure at all (Gotzsche 1994). It must be stressed that the placebo so defined has no negative connotation, of which it is often accused. The meaningfulness of such a placebo-effect becomes clear from results of a controlled study on therapy for varicocele: patients subjected to surgical or angiographic intervention showed the same pregnancy rates as those only counselled and examined at regular intervals (Nieschlag et al. 1998).

> Knowing the placebo-effect of medical attention and applying it in treatment strategies is just as much a part of evidence-based andrology as its scientific basis.

When judging the success of therapy it should also be considered that infertility does not represent an absolute diagnosis, but that factors related to time may play an important role. In the course of time pregnancies may

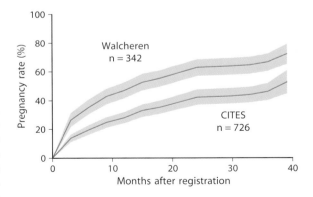

Fig. 1.6. Cumulative pregnancy rates in two populations of diagnosed, but untreated couples in centers of primary care (Walcheren) and of tertiary care (Canadian Infertility Therapy Evaluation Study CITES). Only pregnancies resulting in live births were computed. (From Snick et al. 1997)

occur spontaneously, without any medical intervention. When couples on the Dutch island of Walcheren consulting a primary care center for infertility were left "untreated", after 2 years the spontaneous pregnancy rate was 40 % (Snick et al. 1997). When patients at a tertiary fertility center were treated similarly, after the 2-year observation period the pregnancy rate was 20 % (Canadian Infertility Therapy Evaluation Study; Collins et al. 1995) (Fig. 1.6). The figures show that the selection of couples plays an important role and that even at a specialized center spontaneous pregnancies occur. Such occurrences must be taken into consideration when judging therapeutic measures; they are the basis for models predicting the chances for pregnancies (Collins et al. 1995).

1.7 Male Contribution to Contraception

Providing male contraceptive methods is one of the **tasks of andrology.** Here the question arises whether the andrologist (or the specialist for reproductive medicine) is not at odds with himself if, on the one hand, he treats disturbed fertility and contributes to increasing birthrates, and on the other hand, provides contraceptive methods, thus influencing birthrates negatively.

The **apparent contradiction** is easily resolved as it is a matter of two sides of the same coin. Once the reproductive system has been understood, it can be influenced both positively and negatively. Andrology and reproductive medicine **do not in the first instance** concern themselves with the **politics of population control.** Rather they are primarily directed towards the individual and strive to help the individual couple to improve its affected reproductive functions, or to control them if they are not required. In this fashion reproductive medicine should help to reduce the suffering experienced by the couple wanting a child, while simultaneously creating the prerequisites allowing the couple to freely determine the size of its family. Finally, creating the medical preconditions also provides the means of curbing the world's overpopulation as a byproduct of care for the individual patients and their voluntary rights to reproductive freedom and family planning. As male contraceptive methods in particular are lacking, research leading to the development of such methods appears strongly needed.

Reproduction can be considered as compensation for death. If medical progress allows increasing numbers of people to reach reproductive age, and if, during periods of increasing birthrates the date of death continues to be pushed forward thus leading to overpopulation, then medicine must also provide contraceptive methods in order to maintain or restore a balance between reproduction and death. Andrology must contribute to this goal.

1.8 References

Abshagen K, Behre HM, Cooper TG, Nieschlag E (1998) Influence of sperm surface antibodies on spontaneous pregnancy rates. Fertil Steril 70: 355–356

Antes G (1998) Evidence based medicine. Internist 39:899–908

Bender S (1953) End results in treatment of primary sterility. Fertil Steril 4:34–40

Bruckert E (1991) How frequent is unintentional childlessness in Germany? Androl 23:245–250

Bundesärztekammer (1998) Richtlinien zur assistierten Reproduktion. Dtsch Ärztebl 95:C2230–C2235

Collins JA, Burrows EA, Willian AR (1995) The prognosis for live birth among untreated infertile couples. Fertil Steril 64:22–28

Cummins J, Jequier A (1999) Gazing into the crystal ball: future diagnosis and management in andrology. In: Glover TD, Barratt CLR (eds) Male fertility and infertility. Cambridge University Press, Cambridge, pp 248–266

Dawkins R (1994) The selfish gene, 2nd edn. Oxford University Press, Oxford

Deutsches IVF-Register (DIR) (1998) Bad Segeberg

European Academy of Andrology (EAA) Handbook 1999. Int J Androl 22 [Suppl] 1

Evidence-Based Medicine Working Group (1992) Evidence-based medicine: a new approach to teaching the practice of medicine. JAMA 17:2420–2425

Falk HC, Kaufmann SA (1950) What constitutes a normal semen? Fertil Steril 1:489–496

Farley TMM, Belsey FH (1988) The prevalance and aetiology of infertility. In: Biological Components of Fertility. The Proceedings of the African Population Conference, Dakar, Senegal, November 1988. International Union for the Scientific Study of Population, Liège, Belgium, vol 1, pp 2.1.15–2.1.30

Gotzsche PC (1994) Is there logic in the placebo? Lancet 344:925–926

Juul S, Karmaus W, Olsen J and The European Infertility and Subfecundity Study Group (1999) Regional differences in waiting time to pregnancy: pregnancy-based surveys from Denmark, France, Germany, Italy and Sweden. Hum Reprod 14:1250–1254

Kamischke A, Nieschlag E (1999) Analysis of medical treatment of male infertility. Hum Reprod 14 [Suppl 1]:1–23

Knuth UA, Mühlenstedt D (1991) Kinderwunschdauer, kontrazeptives Verhalten und Rate vorausgegangener Infertilitätsbehandlung. Geburtsh Frauenheilkd 51:1

McLeod J, Gold RZ, McLane CM (1955) Correlation of the male and female factors in human infertility. Fertil Steril 6:112–120

National Library of Medicine (1993) Medical subject headings: annotated alphabetical list 1994. National Institutes of Health, Bethesda MD

Nieschlag E (1986) Perspektiven der Reproduktionsmedizin. Hautarzt 37:190–197

Nieschlag E, Hertle L, Fischedick A, Abshagen K, Behre HM (1998) Update on treatment of varicocele: counselling as effective as occlusion of the vena spermatica. Hum Reprod 13:2147–2150

Schmidt L, Münster K (1995) Infertility, involuntary infecundity, and the seeking of medical advice in industrialized countries 1970–1992: a review of concepts, measurements and results. Hum Reprod 10:1407–1418

Schneider HPG (1994) Einführung in die Thematik der Infertilität und Sterilität. In: Krebs D, Schneider HPG (eds) Endokrinologie und Reproduktionsmedizin III. Klinik der Frauenheilkunde und Geburtshilfe, vol 3. Urban and Schwarzenberg, Munich, pp 89–92

Snick HKA, Snick TS, Evers JLH, Collins JA (1997) The spontaneous pregnancy prognosis in untreated subfertile couples: the Walcheren primary care study. Hum Reprod 12:1582–1588

Stolwijk AM, Straatman H, Zielhuis GA, Jongbloet PH (1996) Seasonal variation in the time to pregnancy: avoiding bias by using the date of onset. Epidemiology 7:156–160

Templeton AA (1992) The epidemiology of infertility. In: Templeton AA, Drife JO (eds) Infertility. Springer, London, pp 23–32

Tietze C, Guttmacher AF, Rubin S (1950) Time required for conception in 1727 planned pregnancies. Fertil Steril 1:338–346

Vandekerckhove P, O'Donavan PA, Lilford RJ, Harada TW (1993) Infertility treatment: from cookery to science. The epidemiology of randomized controlled trials. Br J Obstret Gynaecol 10:1005–1036

van Noord-Zaadstra BM, Looman CWN, Alsbach H, Habbema JDF, te Velde ER, Karbaat J (1991) Delaying childbearing: effect of age on fecundity and outcome of pregancy. Br Med J 302:1361–1365

Wilcox AJ, Weinberg CR, Baird D (1995) Timing of sexual intercourse in relation to ovulation: effects on the probability of conception, survival of the pregnancy, and sex of the baby. N Engl J Med 333:1517–1521

WHO Task Force on the Diagnosis and Treatment of Infertility (1987) Towards more objectivity in diagnosis and management of male infertility. Int J Androl [Suppl] 7

WHO (1999) Laboratory manual for the examination of human semen and sperm-cervical mucus interaction, 4th edn. Cambridge University Press, Cambridge

WHO Special Programme of Research, Development and Research Training in Human Reproduction (1994–1998) Challenges in reproductive health research. Biennial Reports. WHO, Geneva

Comparative Biology of Reproduction

A. LERCHL

In this chapter, some of the basic principles of reproduction are discussed without trying to give a complete overview. Instead, some examples are presented which represent common principles of reproduction. In addition, some aspects of human reproduction are described in order to highlight interesting species differences.

2.1 The "Invention" of Sexuality

It is general knowledge that the information about the structure and function of an organism is located in its genetic make-up which is transferred to the next generation. In the most simple cases (e.g., the division of unicellular organisms), the genetic information is duplicated and each new individual inherits one copy of the genetic code, ideally identical to the master-copy. This is the simplest form of genetic replication. Furthermore, there is no need for a partner, an important precondition for populating new territories. The big disadvantage of this principle, however, lies in the genetic identity of preceding and subsequent generations. There is no "backup copy" of the genetic information and any mutation is also copied.

Sexual reproduction is completely different and the enormous possibilities afforded by combining genes from different individuals provide the key to the diversity of life on earth. A unicellular organism is only able to transfer its own genes (Fig. 2.1). Under normal circumstances, this means error-free copies of the DNA or the RNA: the genetic information coding for the descendents is not different from that of the parent. Sexual reproduction, on the other hand, requires the division of the chromosomes in order to produce haploid gametes. This process is the main function of gametogenesis. As a consequence, the genetic information of the gametes is different from that of the somatic cells (Fig. 2.1). In the example shown, with only two chromosome pairs, there are four possible chromosomal combinations of the chromosomes in the gametes (2^2). In humans (22 autosomal chromosomes and the sex chromosomes X and Y), there are more than 8 million possibilities for the distribution of chromosomes in the gametes (2^{23}).

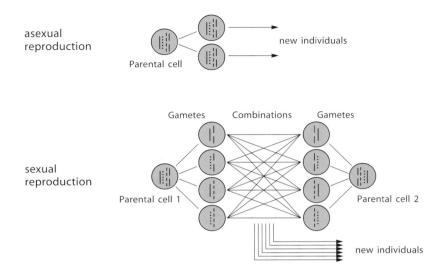

Fig. 2.1. Representation of the main advantage of sexual reproduction. Whereas asexual reproduction always leads to an identical replication of the genome, sexual reproduction implies a new combination of chromosomes with each new generation. During meiosis, each parental chromosome has a 50 % chance of getting into a gamete. The same happens in the other sex so that the genes are thoroughly mixed in each individual of the new generation. With 2 chromosomes, as in this example, a maximum number of 16 combinations ($2^2 \times 2^2$) is possible. In humans, there are more than 70×10^{12} possible combinations ($2^{23} \times 2^{23}$)

Because sexual reproduction requires two partners, the possibilities of chromosomal combinations are further increased. Thus, for human reproduction, a theoretical spectrum of 70×10^{12} possibilities for chromosomal combinations shows that it is indeed quite unlikely to identify two humans with the same genetic make-up, with monozygotic twins being the exception.

This presumably well-explored field still holds surprises in store: a Chilean desert rat was discovered to have a quadruple set of chromosomes but appeared perfectly normal, in contrast to established opinion that multiples of single chromosomes cause severe damage (Gallards et al. 1999). The mechanism of cell division in this rodent species, especially during meiosis, remains unclear.

In addition to the aforementioned mechanisms, other processes such as "crossing-over" of chromosomes during meiosis lead to an even more complex distribution pattern of genes in the new generation.

During evolution, sexual reproduction has been, and still is, an extremely powerful principle. Jacob, one of the founders of molecular biology states: "The two most important inventions [of evolution] are sexuality and death" (Jacob 1970). Thus, the great advantage of sexual reproduction over asexual reproduction is the genetic diversity that results.

From quite another point of view, sexuality may play an equally decisive role. Long-lived organisms, especially all vertebrates, are under constant attack from bacteria, viruses, fungi and parasites which are characterized by short-lived generations and whose strongest weapon is thus genetic variability. At some point in the course of time the appropriate key to the immune system of the potential victim will be found and the victim will be attacked or destroyed. Such variability can only be opposed by the host's genetic complexity created by sexual (re)combination of genes arising with every new generation (Wickler and Seibt 1998). The genes of the major histo-compatability complex (MHC) clearly demonstrate this phenomenon: they possess the highest variability of all known genes and are of utmost importance for the immune response. Precisely these genes and their sexual recombination guarantee maximum immunological individuality. Following conception, that set of female chromosomes most similar to that of the sperm's MHC genes is rejected as a polar body. This selection guarantees the embryo the highest immunological protection possible.

2.1.1 Sex and Hermaphroditism

The most important implication of sexuality is the need for a partner of the opposite sex. However, this clear-cut distinction between two sexes is not at all the norm. There are many examples of intermediate stages that have arisen during evolution, sometimes with rather bizarre consequences.

Snails are widely known as being true hermaphrodites, having both female and male sex organs. For reproduction, however, they depend on a partner. This is different from the situation in animals that normally reproduce sexually but if there is no partner available, they may also reproduce by auto-fertilization. In general, parasites have developed some of the most interesting and complex methods of reproduction, involving sexual and non-sexual pathways.

In a few species of fish and snails, the same individual belongs first to one sex, then to the other (sequential hermaphrodites). In some, the animals are initially females and then males (protogyn) while in others, the opposite sequence exists (protandric). However, this sequence is not always determined by time: colonies of protandric anemone fish have only one functioning α-male and one functioning α-female while all other members of the colony are infertile. If the female is removed from the colony, however, the male becomes a functioning female, and another member of the colony, formerly infertile, becomes the α-male.

Frogs are often examples of the more bizarre categories of reproductive strategies. The water frog *Rana esculenta* is not a distinct species, but a hybrid between *Rana ridibunda* and *Rana lessonae*. It is assumed that during the last ice age, the separation of a population formerly genetically identical, led to the formation of two new species. However, these two species are still able to interbreed and produce fertile descendants, termed *Rana esculenta*. These animals, in turn, are in fact unique in the way they reproduce. When *Rana esculenta* is cross-bred with one of its parental species, only *Rana esculenta* frogs are produced and no intermediate forms, as expected. The explanation for this odd result is truly fascinating: during gametogenesis in *Rana esculenta*, a complete set of chromosomes, one genome, is eliminated; thus the genetic contribution of one parental species is erased (Ohtani 1993; Fig. 2.2). Therefore, frogs of the species *R. esculenta* are usually associated with their "parent" species, with the combination *R. esculenta* and *R. lessonae* being most frequent (Uzzell et al. 1980). This rare kind of reproduction is called hybridogenesis (sometimes, the term "sexual parasite" is used). Apart from the frog species mentioned, it is also found in some carps.

There exists an even more complex kind of reproduction in frogs in relation to hybridogenesis. In a certain species, there exist obviously only males. The animals live in forests near Fontainebleau (France). They are triploid with one chromosome set of *Rana ridibunda* and two sets of *Rana lessonae* chromosomes (RLL). Cross-breeding these males with females having RL- or RR-chromosomes always results in male RLL frogs because only diploid LL-sperm are produced. As in other

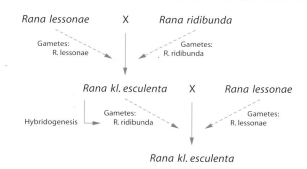

Fig. 2.2. The reproduction of the water frog *Rana kl. esculenta*. The abbreviation "kl" stands for "klepton" (Greek: thief) because *Rana esculenta* behaves in fact like a thief. The "species" *Rana kl. esculenta* is a hybrid between *Rana lessonae* and *Rana ridibunda*. In the populations of *Rana kl. esculenta* and *Rana lessonae*, the most common combination of these water frog species, *Rana kl. esculenta* depends on *Rana lessonae* as the sexual partner. However, the genome of *Rana lessonae* is then eliminated during spermatogenesis (hybridogenesis) so that only *Rana kl. esculenta* is produced

water frogs, complete elimination of a genome during spermatogenesis plays a crucial role. Although most of the underlying mechanisms are not yet understood, they seem to take place before meiosis. Because of differences in the centromeres, the targeted chromosomes seem to be excluded from cell division (Graf and Polls-Pelaz 1989).

There are many other examples of the complexity of reproduction. Although we usually think in terms of sexual reproduction, this is indeed a limited view. During evolution, many different pathways for the transportation of genetic information into the next generation have been developed, all for the sake of preventing extinction.

2.1.2 Competition, Attractiveness, and Sexual Dimorphism

Apart from the instinct of self-preservation, the propagation of its own genome is characteristic of all organisms. The transmission of genes, the basic principle of evolution, is only efficient for a life form if this transmission is as successful as possible. Thus, a high reproduction rate is an important part of its genetic fitness, which is a measure of the ability of a species to survive. In order to reach the goal of high individual reproduction rates, competition between individuals of the same sex is crucial. A vast number of competition strategies has been developed during evolution on all levels of sensory perception, e. g., bird songs, scent marking, bright colors etc. These characteristics serve to impress the possible partner of the opposite sex while the competitor is defeated. Consequently, such signs tend to be amplified during evolution; colors get brighter, songs louder, and scents stronger. It is most important to note, however, that the prime goal of competition is not to prevent the competitor completely from reproduction: most of such fights are rather harmless, thus protecting the propagation of the species.

Often, it is quite clear in which way the partner is to be impressed. For instance, well-designed nests directly guarantee a better survival of the offspring than those built in a sloppy manner. Thus, architects of such homes are likely to be rewarded with breeding success and thus transmitting their genes. Also, presentation of attributes not directly associated with breeding success results in higher reproduction rates, e.g. bright colors of feathers, ruffling, or the typical imposing behavior of certain bird species, are meant to convince the partner of the presentor's attractiveness. There is no direct connection between these signs and reproductive success or fitness. Rather, the effect on the partner is assumed to be an indirect one, such as "Choose me, and your kids are going to be just as gorgeous as I am!"

The following studies prove that greater attractiveness has physiological advantages: female grey tree frogs (*Hyala versicolor*) choose their partners according to call duration. Breeding experiments showed markedly improved larval and juvenile development of offspring of frogs with protracted calls (Welch et al. 1998). Female zebra finches choose their mates according to certain external characteristics which can easily be manipulated in experimental settings. Males with red bands on their legs are considered more attractive than those with green bands. The yolk of offspring of attractive males contains more testosterone than that of less attractive males, causing juvenile birds to demand food more frequently, to mature better and, in turn, have better chances when competing for females (Gil et al. 1999). Both studies support the "good gene hypothesis" according to which greater attractiveness goes hand in hand with improved genetic make-up.

During evolution, a separation has developed between the roles of males and females in respect to care of the offspring, which is often directly correlated with the differential display of competition. It is a general rule that the more different the roles for raising offspring, the larger is the difference between the sexes (sexual dimorphism). The explanation for this fact is difference in energy invested in rearing. Thus the sex not investing in rearing can invest more in sexual display. In many bird species, for example, males and females invest approximately the same energy, while in mammals, usually females carry the burden.

In this context it is interesting to consider how sexual dimorphism and role division in caretaking affect lifespan. Studies on various primate species have produced astonishing results (Allman et al. 1998). In most primates the female carries the burden of child rearing and the males are more or less uninvolved. Only in a few species (*Aotus, Callicebus*) are roles reversed, with the female caring only for feeding, while all other tasks are performed by the male. The lifespan shows distinct differences: fathers who are involved in caretaking live relatively longer than those unconcerned with offspring. In the course of evolution the sex rearing offspring has obviously acquired a better constitution and thus a longer lifespan. Contrary to common belief, the male hormone, testosterone, does not have any general life-shortening effect, as was shown in historical comparisons of the lifespan of eunuchoidal and intact singers (Nieschlag et al. 1993).

2.1.3 Reproductive Strategies

A frequently asked question addresses the pronounced difference between the numbers of sperm and oocytes that is found in most animal species. The answer lies in the different strategies used by females and males to reach maximal reproductive success. While the female strategy aims for large oocytes, which have a high probability of being fertilised and of surviving, the males try to produce a large number of very small gametes to increase the possibility that at least one reaches its target. Both strategies are divergent, thus, there is always a trend for an even more pronounced difference in size (anisogamy).

A large number of possibilities exist to increase the success of sperm. A high production rate, for example, is useful if the sperm have to compete with those from competitors, as in polyandric primates. Here, the females are often almost flooded by sperm from the many copulations with different males. Another, quite extreme example in this respect is seen in whales (*Eubalaena australis*). Likewise polyandric, many males try to copulate with one female, resulting in impressively large testes of about 3 meters in length at a weight of approximately 500 kilograms. Completely different is the way that some insects try to increase their reproductive success. Unlike vertebrates, insects must obey energetic limitations preventing them from producing sperm in excess. Consequently, the aim is that the sperm of the copulating male are the only ones in the female. The fruitfly *Drosphila bifurca* produces extremely large sperm with a length of approximately 6 centimetres, thus 20 times larger than the size of the fly (Pitnick et al. 1995). These results are being discussed as a possibility of having a one-to-one ratio of fertilizable eggs to fertilizing sperm. It appears also possible that these sperm, purely because of their size, prevent other sperm from entering the female tract after another successful copulation.

Sperm production is not determined solely by genetic factors, but may also depend on social factors. The development of male larval moths depends on the number of same-sex individuals in their vicinity. In the presence of many potential competitors the testes and ejaculate parameters increase while the thorax and rump remain comparatively small; a smaller number of competitors causes the opposite effect. Presumably the number of competitors results in a strategy that is best-suited for the individuals, favoring high sperm production and greater motility in the face of great competition.

There are many different possibilities for sexual associations between females and males. The most simple is monogamy, resulting in very stable, often life-long, relationships. If one partner dies, the surviving animal will often not begin a new relationship. In polygamous societies, one male has access to many females (harem), and no other fertile male is tolerated. Before other young males can become potent competitors, they are expelled from the group.

Some somatic characteristics are related to the type of reproductive strategy, especially in primates (Potts and Short 1999). For example, male gorillas which are polygamous are much larger and stronger than females, resulting in an advantage to the biggest males when males are competing for access to females, thus favoring even larger and stronger males during the process of evolution. On the other hand, the males' testes are quite small, and the relative content of deformed sperm in the ejaculate is quite high. Female gorillas show no sign of ovulation.

This scenario is completely different in the chimpanzee. Although the males are considerably larger than the females, this difference plays no decisive role for reproductive success of males since during estrous many males copulate with one female. On the other hand, the chimpanzees' testes are quite large and their ejaculates contain comparatively few deformed sperm; the females' estrous is presented to the males by enlarged and red labia. These differences between the two primate species are caused by their different reproductive strategies: male gorillas must defeat their competitors to reach the top position and to be the only reproducing male. This explains the advantage of large body size. On the other hand, these winners only very rarely have sexual intercourse since females are in estrous only every 4 years or so. Thus, there is no real need for large testes and high sperm production. In the chimpanzee, however, many males may have intercourse with the females in estrous. In this polyandric system, selective pressure exists for high sperm production, resulting in large testes. Likewise, selective pressure results in a better quality of sperm. In other words, this kind of sexual partnership leads to intravaginal male competition (Smith 1984).

Humans tend also to show sexual dimorphism with men being some 10 to 15 % taller than women. Men's testes are quite small, compared with our ape relatives, while the ejaculates contain a comparatively high number of malformed sperm. There is no visible sign of ovulation in women, and intercourse does not happen exclusively during the fertile phase of the cycle. On the other hand, humans have two very pronounced secondary sex characteristics, namely large breasts and a large penis. This combination led Potts and Short (1999) to speculate that humans belong to a category of polygamous primates with a special kind of partnership, called "serial monogamy". Could this be a suitable explanation for high divorce rates?

In fact, humans are not at all monogamous (Fig. 2.3). Rather, social and cultural developments and conventions have led to the present form of society in which monogamous relations are preferred. Polygamy and especially polyandry are stigmatized. It is, furthermore, interesting to observe that the difference in age between men and women at the time of marriage is higher when

Fig. 2.3. Monogamy is obviously not a typical characteristic for human populations. Looking at ethnic groups before they have been influenced by modern civilization, monogamous relations are not at all the norm (upper figure). Furthermore, there is no clear difference between women and men (lower figure). Redrawn from Short (1994)

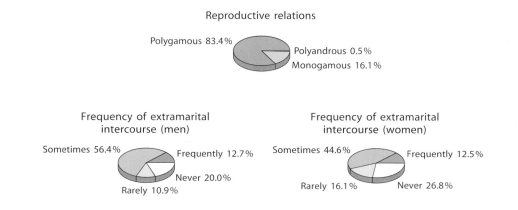

Reproductive relations

Polygamous 83.4%
Polyandrous 0.5%
Monogamous 16.1%

Frequency of extramarital intercourse (men)

Sometimes 56.4%
Frequently 12.7%
Never 20.0%
Rarely 10.9%

Frequency of extramarital intercourse (women)

Sometimes 44.6%
Frequently 12.5%
Rarely 16.1%
Never 26.8%

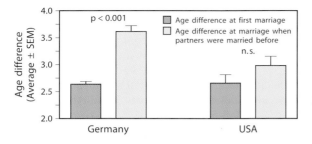

Fig. 2.4. At the time of marriage men are, on average, several years older than women. This age-difference becomes even more pronounced if both partners have been married before. Data from the German Federal Bureau for Statistics (1988) and Schoen et al. (1985)

the partners have been married before (Fig. 2.4). This fact seems to support the view of serial monogamy since even old men are fertile (see Chap. 21).

2.1.4 Sex Ratio at Birth

According to Mendel's laws, one would expect a 1:1 ratio of females and males at birth. However, a mean ratio of 1:1 is an exception rather than the rule and has provoked a great deal of investigation and speculation. In this section, only the sex ratio at birth is discussed; those events taking place after birth are dealt with in the section "infanticide" (2.5.2).

Some exotic exceptions exist with respect to the normal way the sex of offspring is determined, which is by sex chromosomes. In voles, the sex of the descendants is determined in a quasi-autosomal way, with dominant and recessive inheritance (Fregda 1994). In some mouse strains, a significant deviation from the 1:1 ratio may be the result of inbreeding (Beamer and Whitten 1991). The normal ratio of close to 1:1 is believed to be changed by environmental factors, e.g., availability of food. Thus, a

higher number of females may be advantageous in times of restricted energy supply (Trivers and Willard 1973). The underlying mechanism may be either a sex-selective intrauterine death, or a neglect of the males *post partum*. So what is the advantage of producing more females during hard times? Based on observations in polygamous rodents, it is speculated that the reproductive success of weak (underfed) females is optimized if they produce more females, which are not so dependent on strength and physical fitness as males. On the other hand, the reproductive success of a healthy and well-fed animal will be increased by producing more healthy males which, in turn, may defeat competitors because of their condition. Thus, the benefit of shifting the sex-ratio shows up only in the second generation but it works, which is the reason why it has arisen during evolution.

In human populations, the average sex ratio is shifted by between 1 and 3 % towards boys. At first sight, this difference appears to be without significance, especially when looking at an individual family. However, this sex ratio is not constant and is subject to cultural and increasingly to socioeconomic influences and changes.

The sex ratio in Germany throughout the last century is illustrated in Fig. 2.5. It can clearly be seen that both World Wars had tremendous impact on the sex ratio at birth, a phenomenon known also for other countries. Before considering the specific reasons for the observed changes, one may ask why a ratio different from the theoretical 1:1 distribution actually exists. One obvious reason could be an unequal distribution of X- and Y-bear-

Fig. 2.5. Fluctuations of the sex ratio at birth in Germany from 1872 to 1998. The influence of the two wars is clearly seen. No data are available for 1940–1945

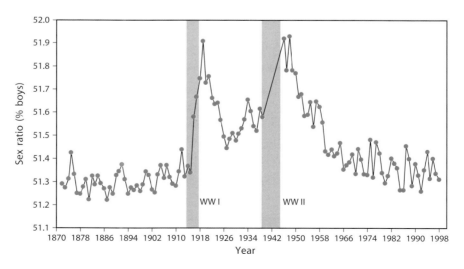

ing spermatozoa. This is, however, not the case. The vast majority of investigations addressing this topic were unable to identify any marked deviation from 50 % of each sex (Goldman et al. 1993; Lobel et al. 1993). Thus, either the underlying reasons must be found on the female side or the functions of the X- and Y-bearing sperm are subject to influence. In fact, the sex ratio at birth is considerably influenced by the time of conception (James 1980). More boys are born when the time of conception is early or late during the days of possible fertilization of the menstrual cycle. In the middle of these days, thus close to the LH peak, the proportion of girls born 9 months later is significantly higher than 50 %. This observation could be the explanation for the relative changes during war since the frequency of intercourse is known to be much higher before combat duties or during short home leaves, thus leading to an increased proportion of early fertilizations, resulting in a higher frequency of male births.

If one looks at the sex ratio of fraternal twins, it becomes also clear that ovulation plays a crucial role. A random distribution would result in approximately the same numbers of twins with the same sex as those with a different sex. However, there are actually significantly more twins of the same sex, even when taking into account the slightly higher proportion of boys at birth (James 1979, 1980). Similarly interesting is the observation that the duration of a twin pregnancy depends on the sex of the children. If no boy is present, the pregnancy is some 2 weeks longer compared with pregnancies with one or two boys, likewise supporting the idea that the time of conception has an influence (Chen et al. 1993; James 1994). Finally, the relative proportion of females is higher after assisted fertilization, compared with the normal population, also indicating an endocrine component on the female side (Guerrero 1974; Orlebeke et al. 1993).

Of course, the sex of the offspring is determined by whether the spermatozoon is carrying the X- or the Y-chromosome. Thus, the question remains what makes the difference? It is not yet clear whether a sex-specific spontaneous abortion rate is in fact responsible (Bartels 1990; James 1980). Other possibilities include different fertilization rates of X- and Y-spermatozoa and the ability of the oocytes to select spermatozoa, possibly influenced by hormones.

In mammals external temperature during sperm maturation may influence the sex of offspring. In bats and rats high temperatures are accompanied by more male offspring, while relatively low temperatures favor the birth of female offspring. In humans a similar situation may exist (Lerchl 1999). Interestingly, after relatively high temperatures occurring 10 – 11 months prior to birth more boys were born, a result indicating effects of temperature during spermatogenesis. It is, however, unclear what is responsible for these results.

2.2 Population Dynamics

As previously mentioned, the most important process during evolution is the transmission of the genome to the next generation. However, this whole process is doomed to failure if too few of the next generation survive. Sooner or later, the species would be extinct. This trivial fact has played a central role in evolution; by several mechanisms, the survival rate was optimised. The most extreme forms are called r-strategies and K-strategies, respectively. Both terms stem from the formula for the growth of populations:

$$\frac{dN}{dt} = r \cdot \left(\frac{K-N}{K}\right) \cdot N$$

where dN/dt is the growth rate of the population, expressed as new individuals (dN) per time unit (dt), often expressed as per cent growth rate. It is a function of two variables, the reproduction rate r and a variable K, representing the maximum capacity of the environment for individuals of the particular species. If K is unlimited, the term

$$\frac{K-N}{K} = 1,$$

is equal to 1, thus the growth of the population is merely a function of the present size (N) and the reproduction rate r, which means a pure, exponential growth rate. Such a theoretical growth rate would only be possible, though, if there were no enemies, no shortage of food were present, and no other effects existed as a result of the growing population, respectively. Organisms possessing a high reproduction rate under ideal conditions are called r-strategists (Fig. 2.6a). As soon as there is an opportunity, they reproduce very quickly, which is a particular advantage when new territories are to be colonized or in areas that exist only for a short time. Typical representatives of r-strategists are rodents and bacteria. Of course, there are no pure r-strategists since their own reproduction would lead to an increased population, itself representing a factor that eventually becomes limiting.

K-strategists, on the other hand, try to occupy a territory with limited resources by filling it over a comparatively long period of time, but aiming at relatively constant population densities. To this end, high reproduction rates are not needed but it is important that the descendants occupy their place successfully. Cactuses, most primate species, and cave-dwelling animals are typical representatives.

At present, there is no estimate of K for the human population (Fig. 2.6b). In this context it is interesting to note that the growth rate changed rather suddenly

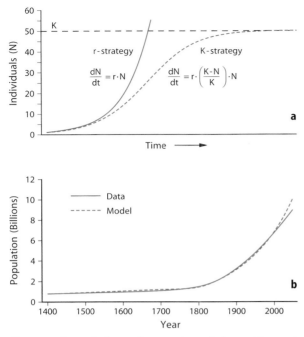

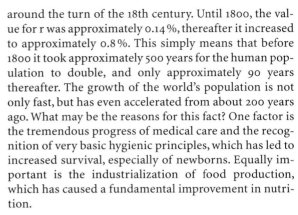

around the turn of the 18th century. Until 1800, the value for r was approximately 0.14%, thereafter it increased to approximately 0.8%. This simply means that before 1800 it took approximately 500 years for the human population to double, and only approximately 90 years thereafter. The growth of the world's population is not only fast, but has even accelerated from about 200 years ago. What may be the reasons for this fact? One factor is the tremendous progress of medical care and the recognition of very basic hygienic principles, which has led to increased survival, especially of newborns. Equally important is the industrialization of food production, which has caused a fundamental improvement in nutrition.

2.3 Seasonal Reproduction

Seasons are a great problem for most life forms on earth since the survival of offspring is a function of temperature, rain, and availability of food. All of these annual

Fig. 2.6. a Theoretical growth rates of populations with r- and K-strategies (K=50). Whereas r-strategists aim at occupying the territory by high reproduction rates, the K-strategists try to reach the same goal but with slower reproduction rates. **b** Growth rate of the human population. The original data (World Bank 1984) are shown, together with a mathematical simulation demonstrating an average increase of 0.14% per year until 1800 and growth rate of 0.8% thereafter. It is interesting to note the sudden increase in growth rate after 1800

Fig. 2.7. Changes of body weight, fur color, reproductive state and other parameters in male Djungarian hamsters (*Phodopus sungorus*) kept under natural photoperiods throughout the year. These animals show very pronounced changes in these features, making them ideal models for studies addressing photoperiodic influences on reproduction

▼

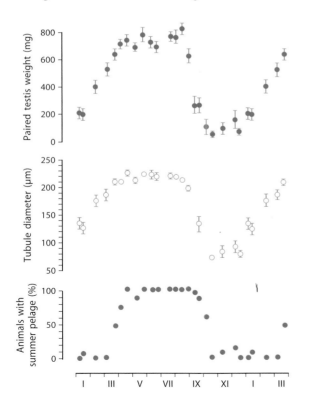

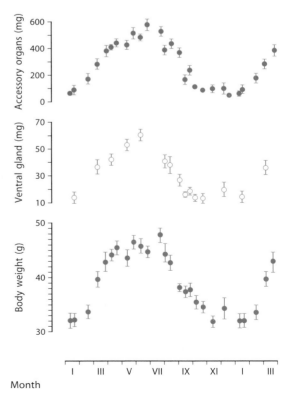

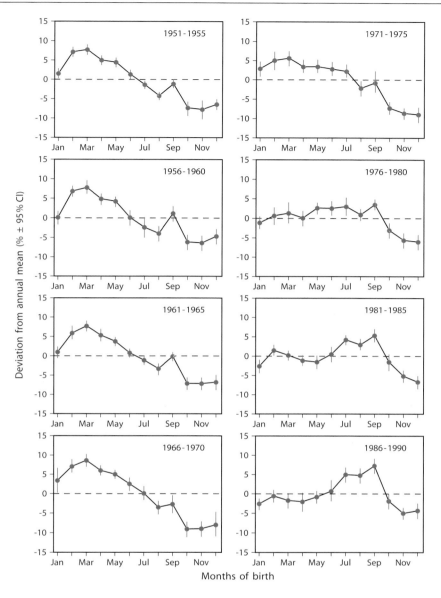

Fig. 2.8. Changes in the seasonal variation of birth rates in Germany from 1951 to 1990. Until about the mid 1970's, most births took place during the first half of the year. Later on, this annual variation shifted by approximately 6 months (Lerchl et al. 1993)

changes are caused by changes of the daylength (photoperiod) which is, in turn, a consequence of the earth's angle of inclination. During evolution, a number of adaptations have been developed to handle this problem, the most important being seasonal reproduction. This means that the time of the year in which animals reproduce is limited to a few weeks or months. In most cases, the prime goal is to deliver the offspring during the most favourable time of the year (spring or early summer) and to avoid birth during autumn or winter, thus increasing the survival rate. Due to the different durations of pregnancies, the season of highest sexual activity differs between animal species. For instance, the rutting season of sheep is during autumn or early winter, while rodents with a relatively short gestation, reproduce mainly during the spring and summer.

Instead of relying on temperatures or rain, mammals use the photoperiod itself for precisely synchronizing their sexual activity with the appropriate time of the year. This is done by translating the photoperiod into an endocrine signal, the synthesis duration of the pineal hormone melatonin. In virtually all vertebrates investigated so far, the duration of melatonin synthesis during the night reflects the photoperiod. The longer the length of the day in summer, the shorter the melatonin synthesis duration, the shorter the day length, the longer the melatonin synthesis. Although many of the features of melatonin synthesis and its impact on reproduction still have to be clarified, this hormone plays the crucial role in photoperiodism in vertebrates.

The fact that seasonal reproduction is controlled by the photoperiod has an important practical consequence: it is relatively easy to simulate seasonal reproduction in the laboratory by simply changing the photoperiod. Thus, animals responding to photoperiod manipulations can be transferred easily into a state of gonadal quiescence that can be manipulated, e. g. by hormones. Thus, there is no need for invasive interventions to reach the same goal, for example by hypophysectomy or by administration of GnRH antagonists. A very suitable animal model for such studies is the Djungarian hamster (*Phodopus sungorus*). Its reactions to changes of the photoperiod are drastic indeed (Fig. 2.7) and it is thus quite easy to study extremely different physiological situations in animals by simply exposing them to different light regimens. It is of particular importance that the release of FSH and LH, the key hormones of the pituitary for reproduction, cease almost completely under short-day type photoperiods. Using this animal model it was possible to demonstrate the relative importance of FSH for spermatogenesis (Niklowitz et al. 1989).

What of humans, who are fertile throughout all seasons? Are we completely non-seasonal? The answer is "no" since in almost all countries studied so far, clear deviations from a random monthly distribution of births have been identified (Roenneberg and Aschoff 1990). In Germany, such seasonal variations have also been found (Fig. 2.8; Lerchl et al. 1993). However, these variations are not stable over time and secular trends in the last few decades have led to a picture that is quite different from the situation before. Beginning around the mid-1970's, the seasonality of human reproduction has undergone a phase-shift of six months, a fact for which an explanation is still lacking. It is quite unlikely, though, that the introduction of oral contraceptives and the consequent drop in birth rates is responsible since both events took place well before the shift occurred. Instead, it is speculated that the biological influences formerly dominating seasonality were replaced by social ones. This assumption is related to the fact that humans are more and more isolated from climatic influences, mostly living in air-conditioned or heated environments all day long. However, definite proof for this theory is still lacking.

2.4 Pheromones

In many animal species, reproductive processes are influenced by pheromones, especially by those transmitting information about the reproductive state of the individual and those evoking specific physiological or behavioural adjustments. Often, these substances are released in urine or faeces, explaining the evident interest of many animals in these excretions. Pheromone research is notoriously difficult for two reasons: first, the substances are chemically often rather exotic and present in very complex "cocktails"; secondly, compared with animals, our sense of smell is almost completely lacking.

Among the substances acting as pheromones are derivatives of cholesterol: androsterone is especially well-characterized. This resembles testosterone and is produced by male animals and men. When applied to sows as spray, it induces "lordosis", the willingness for copulation, an important effect for artificial insemination in pigs. Exactly the same substance, androsterone, is produced by the truffle. Therefore, sows are perfectly qualified to search for truffles because they expect a buried boar when smelling the mushroom. The biological reason behind this odd coincidence is probably the reproduction of the fungus whose spores are distributed by being eaten and excreted.

Pheromones may also be used as tools of deceit for the sake of an individual's reproductive success. During the reproductive season, thousands of males and females of a certain viper species assemble in a small area. Interestingly, every seventh male or so wears the phenomenal dress of females, thus being pushed by a number of other males. Thus, these individuals are hindered from fertilising females, the duty finally being performed by the deceiver.

In salmon, pheromones also play a crucial role. It was unclear for a long time how the animals manage to find the place where they were born after they have grown up in the open sea. It is now known that this phenomenon is due to some kind of pheromonal imprinting such that the adult salmon knows where it has to go because of the unique "smell" of the river in which it was born.

There has been much speculation about whether there may be a function of pheromones in humans, especially with respect to sexuality. Some facts do speak in favour of this assumption, for example the existence of the vomeronasal organ, which responds to pheromones, at least in electrophysiological experiments (Monti-Bloch and Grosser 1991). Presumably, this organ plays a role in transmission of olfactory signals not perceived consciously. Another phenomenon could be the synchronization of menstrual cycles of women living together for extended periods of time. It has been speculated that pheromones may be the synchronizing factor, however, this subject is still a matter of intense discussion (Weller and Weller 1993; Wilson 1992).

2.5 Social Factors

Reproduction is not only demanding for the individual, but is also a demanding event for the population, especially in populations with a well-developed social structure. Some of the resulting consequences are easily understood, others appear quite strange. One of the most widespread misunderstandings is that individuals do everything for the sake of their own species ("altruism"). There is no true altruism, although such behavior may sometimes appear to play a role in complex social structures. The main force during evolution is still genetic egoism. Even in insects living in large colonies with only one fertile queen, each individual is somehow involved in the transmission of "its own" genome. Some examples may illustrate the importance of social factors for reproductive processes.

2.5.1 Rank and Reproduction

It is common knowledge that social status has an impact on reproductive success, even if this is not scientifically proven for all cases. The most simple situation is where only one fertile male is on top of a hierarchy, e. g., as in populations of lions, gorillas or others with a pronounced "harem" character. Here, the only fertile male is also the only possible procreator. This situation becomes more difficult if more than one fertile male is present, as in many associations of primates. There are many observations in wild animals as well as laboratory-based studies indicating a higher copulation rate in high-ranking males and females, as compared with the members of the same species at lower social positions (D'Amato 1988; Dewsbury 1982). The question arises as to whether this fact automatically leads to higher reproductive success in terms of a better probability of transmitting the α-male's genome. This is not necessarily the case: modern DNA fingerprinting analysis in rhesus monkeys has revealed that the α-male is not at all the only male actually reproducing (Nurnberg et al. 1993).

This is obviously true not only for animals. Although in humans the social system is totally different, it is quite interesting to note that approximately 18 % of men who have accepted paternity turned out to be definitively not the father as shown by DNA fingerprinting; likewise, the proportion of "wrong" fathers is comparatively similar in Yanoama indians and in men from central USA (approximately 10 %; Forsyth 1987). Hence, one has to accept that progress in culture does not necessarily imply the loss of basic biological processes.

Yet another question is whether the social status of the parents has any positive effect on the reproductive success of the descendants. The answer is yes. Both the status of the father but more especially the rank of the mother can have beneficial effects on the survival of the offspring (Packer et al. 1995; Vessey et al. 1989). This advantage leads, in turn, to a better chance of reaching high social positions, thus ultimately resulting in "clans" as in many primate species. One may think about parallels in human populations, for instance the caste systems of India, or the aristocratic systems in Europe.

2.5.2 Infanticide

To kill ones own offspring appears to be an absurd action since such an act is an obvious violation of the prime aim of life, the transmission of one's own genome. However, it is generally more efficient to produce descendants that can provide the next generation than to waste energy for those that are unable to do so. Thus, it is sometimes beneficial to rear one strong young than to take care of two that become comparatively weak as adults, being finally defeated by competitors. Most of those infanticides happen by neglect, so that one or more of a litter starve to death, particularly during periods of food shortage. In birds, this behavior is quite common. Under adverse circumstances, the young hatching late are smaller than their litter mates, grow even more slowly due to less effective access to food, and finally die.

In primates, probably in lions as well, active infanticide has been observed. In the langur *Presbytis entellus,* infanticide always takes place when a new male assumes the α-position of the group. Because these males only have a limited period to maintain their position before another candidate defeats them, and because the females are not fertile as long as they are rearing young, infanticide gives the new α-male the chance of transmitting its own genes as the female is receptive to male advances immediately after loss of her offspring. In apes, infanticide has been reported for chimpanzees and gorillas. The infanticide in gorillas is correlated, at least in most cases, with a change in alliance of the female to the killing male. In chimpanzees, the situation is far more complex. Here, attacks from females are also known, which are characterized by cannibalism and planned strategies against certain members of the group. The dramatic events concerning infanticide are well-documented in the reports of Jane Goodall (1991) for chimpanzees and by Dian Fossey (1992) for gorillas.

Another way of reducing litter size is known as siblicide, the killing of members of one's own litter. Examples are again found in birds (e. g., in some species of hawks and heron) where the chicks get rid of their siblings by direct killing, preventing them from getting food, or by simply throwing them out of the nest. The strongest survives. The young of some shark species may suffer the same fate even before they are born. The stronger sibling kills and eats the weaker one while still inside the mother. Yet another example is the spotted hyena, which normally produces twins. Immediately after birth, a life-and-death struggle starts between the siblings which already have well-developed and sharp teeth and fully-opened eyes, both features being very unusual even in carnivores. Furthermore, young female hyenas are extremely androgenized during pregnancy by high levels of testosterone. Most interesting, though, is the fact that the fight between the siblings ends in death for one if they have the same sex. In opposite-sex twins, both animals usually survive (Frank et al. 1991). It is speculated that only same-sex litter mates may eventually become competitors as adults, so that the killing of siblings of the other sex has no particular advantage.

In humans, infanticides are unfortunately also reality, not because of biological reasons but because of economic and social reasons. It is true in many countries on earth: to have a boy means prosperity, a girl stands for financial disaster. Therefore, boys are highly preferred to girls, in particular in rural regions because a boy means another worker. Additionally, only boys are believed to be able to perform certain religious ceremonies for their deceased relatives, for example in some Indian societies. Finally, boys somehow represent an old-age pension while girls are integrated into their husband's families after marriage. It is therefore logical that such couples may be willing to take action in whatever respect to prevent the birth of girls, or to ensure the birth of boys. As a consequence of this desire, the ratio of girls to boys is increasingly imbalanced. For instance, an increased sex-ratio from 51.2 % boys to 53.2 % in 1990 has been observed in China. This shift will lead to a shortage of women, resulting in approximately 1 million fewer women of marriageable age than men in 2010. Although it is theoretically possible that these girls have not been officially registered by the parents, there are several reports of infanticides in China (Coale and Banister 1994; Tuljapurkar and Feldman 1995).

In the last few years, modern analytical methods have been used for determination of the foetal sex, and consequently the sex-selective abortion rate has increased. As an example, Booth et al. (1994) reported a significant effect in the Punjab (India). In this investigation, there was a shift from 7 % more boys than girls in 1982 to 32 % more boys in 1993. Moreover, whereas approximately 14 % of women delivering a boy had performed prenatal sex-determination, this applied to only 2 % of mothers delivering a girl. Even in these 2 %, however, the girls had either been incorrectly identified as boys or they had a male twin. The conclusion from this study is quite clear: sex-selective abortions are performed to the detriment of girls, the ultimate form of sexual discrimination. It follows that the sex of a child would be better determined even before implantation. Although this request is understandable from a physician's point of view, one must keep in mind that such manipulations will have a large impact on the whole social structure of a community (Park and Cho 1995; Tuljapurkar and Feldman 1995).

2.6 Outlook

During the process of evolution, mankind has increased its cognitive and analytical abilities far above the level of other animals, and the transmission of cultural information to the next generation is ever increasing. Nevertheless, humans are not purely rational; we do have our genetic roots, which should not be ignored. Rather, we should try to understand them. The main power for evolution has been, and will be, the struggle for survival of the individual and consequently of a species. These strategies are imprinted in our genes and even if we do not use all of them, they are still present. Sometimes, remnants may emerge. We stand to learn a considerable amount from observing our ancestors closely and thereby our own genetic roots.

The "head of Janus" is our ever-increasing knowledge about principles of reproduction. We may influence reproduction, in humans and in animals, either in a "bad" or in a "good" direction, both terms being not biological categories, but ethical and moral.

This is the major problem of modern reproductive biology and reproductive medicine. Due to the latest developments of techniques in the field of molecular biology and other areas, we are able to perform artificial inseminations, we are able to determine and to influence the sex of an individual and we will soon, in theory, be even able to treat diseases on the genetic level inside the stem cells. Furthermore, the somatic consequences of inherited diseases, e. g., the lack of seminal ducts, may be by-passed by assisted fertilization (see Chap. 17) while the genes for this disease are still transmitted even if they are recessive. The consequences, in terms of genetic, ethical, and legal aspects, are currently being discussed by politicians, physicians, scientists, and lawyers all over the world. When taking these points into consideration, one has to accept that there is both a need for risk estimation as well as a need for a thorough understanding of the biological principles of reproduction.

2.7 References

Allman G, Rosin A, Kumar R, Hasenstaub A (1998) Parenting and survival in anthropoid primates: caretakers live longer. Proc Natl Acad Sci USA 95:6866–6869

Bartels I, Hansmann I, Eiben B (1990) Excess of females in chromosomally normal spontaneous abortuses. Am J Med Genet 35:297–298

Beamer WG, Whitten WK (1991) Do histocompatibility genes influence sex ratio (% males)? Reprod Fertil Dev 3:267–276

Booth BE, Verma M, Beri RS (1994) Fetal sex determination in infants in Punjab, India: correlations and implications. Br Med J 309:1259–1261

Chen SJ, Vohr BR, Oh W (1993) Effects of birth order, gender, and intrauterine growth retardation on the outcome of very low birth weight in twins. J Pediatr 123:132–136

Coale AJ, Banister J (1994) Five decades of missing females in China. Demography 31:459–479

D'Amato FR (1988) Effects of male social status on reproductive success and on behavior in *mice (Mus musculus)*. J Comp Psychol 102:146–151

Dewsbury DA (1982) Dominance rank, copulatory behavior, and differential reproduction. Q Rev Biol 57:135–159

Forsyth A (1986) A natural history of sex. Kindler, Munich

Fossey D (1983) Gorillas in the mist. Houghton Mifflin, Boston

Frank LG, Glickman SE, Licht P (1991) Fatal sibling aggression, precocial development, and androgens in neonatal spotted hyenas. Science 252:702–704

Fregda K (1994) Bizarre mammalian sex-determining mechanisms. In: Short RV, Balaban E (eds) The differences between the sexes. Cambridge University Press, Cambridge, pp 419–431

Gallardo MH, Bickham GW, Honeycutt RL, Ojeda RA, Köhler N (1999) Karyotyping: a mammal with tetraploidy. Nature 401:341

Gil D, Graves J, Hazon N, Wells A (1999) Male attractiveness and different testosterone investment in zebra finch eggs. Science 286:126–128

Goldman AS, Fomina Z, Knights PA, Hill CJ, Walker AP, Hulten MA (1993) Analysis of the primary sex ratio, sex chromosome aneuploidy and diploidy in human sperm using dual-colour fluorescence in situ hybridisation. Eur J Hum Genet 1:325–334

Goodall J (1990) Through a window. Thirty years with the chimpanzees of Gombe. Weidenfels and Nicolson, London

Graf JD, Polls-Pelaz M (1989) Cytogenetic analysis of spermatogenesis in unisexual allotriploid males from a *Rana lessonae – Rana kl. esculenta* mixed population. In: Hallyday T, Baker J, Hosie L (eds) First World Congress of Herpetology, Canterbury

Guerrero R (1974) Association of the type and time of insemination within the menstrual cycle with the human sex ratio at birth. N Engl J Med 291:1056–1059

Harlap S (1979) Gender of infants conceived on different days of the menstrual cycle. N Engl J Med 300:1445–1448

Jacob F (1970) La logique du vivant: une historie de l'hérédité. Gallimard, Paris

James WH (1979) Is Weinberg's differential rule valid? Acta Genet Med Gemellol Roma 28:69–71

James WH (1980) Time of fertilization and sex of infants. Lancet i:1124–1126

James WH (1994) Cycle day of insemination, sex ratio of offspring and duration of gestation. Ann Hum Biol 21:263–266

Lerchl A, Simoni M, Nieschlag E (1993) Changes in seasonality of birth rates in Germany from 1951 to 1990. Naturwissenschaften 80:516–518

Lerchl A (1999) Sex ratios and environmental temperatures. Naturwissenschaften 86:340–342

Lobel SM, Pomponio RJ, Mutter GL (1993) The sex ratio of normal and manipulated human sperm quantitated by the polymerase chain reaction. Fertil Steril 59:387–392

Monti-Bloch L, Grosser BI (1991) Effect of putative pheromones on the electrical activity of the human vomeronasal organ and olfactory epithelium. J Steroid Biochem Mol Biol 39:573–582

Nieschlag E, Nieschlag S, Behre HM (1993) Lifespan and testosterone. Nature 366:215

Niklowitz P, Khan S, Bergmann M, Hoffmann K, Nieschlag E (1989) Differential effects of follicle-stimulating hormone and luteinizing hormone on Leydig cell function and restoration of spermatogenesis in hypophysectomized and photoinhibited Djungarian hamsters, *Phodopus sungorus*. Biol Reprod 39:489–498

Nurnberg P, Berard JD, Bercovitch F, Epplen JT, Schmidtke J, Krawczak M (1993) Oligonucleotide fingerprinting of free-ranging and captive rhesus macaques from Cayo Santiago: paternity assignment and comparison of heterozygosity. EXS 67:445–451

Ohtani H (1993) Mechanism of chromosome elimination in the hybridogenetic spermatogenesis of allotriploid males between Japanese and European water frogs. Chromosoma 102:158–162

Orlebeke JF, Boomsma DJ, Eriksson AW (1993) Epidemiological and birth weight characteristics of triplets: a study from the Dutch twin register. Eur J Obstet Gynecol Reprod Biol 50:87–93

Packer C, Collins DA, Sindimwo A, Goodall J (1995) Reproductive constraints on aggressive competition in female baboons. Nature 373:60–63

Park CB, Cho NH (1995) Consequences of son preference in a low-fertility society: imbalance of the sex ratio at birth in Korea. Popul Dev Rev 21:59–84

Pitnick S, Spicer GS, Markow TA (1995) How long is a giant sperm? Nature 375:109

Potts M, Short R (1999) Ever since Adam and Eve: the evolution of human sexuality. Cambridge University Press, Cambridge

Roenneberg T, Aschoff J (1990) Annual rhythm of human reproduction: I. Biology, sociology, or both? J Biol Rhythms 5:195–216

Schoen R, Urton W, Woodrow K, Baj J (1985) Marriage and divorce in twentieth century America cohorts. Demography 22:101–114

Short RV (1994) A man's a man for a' that. In: Short RV, Balaban E (eds) The differences between the sexes. Cambridge University Press, Cambridge, pp 451–456

Smith RL (1984) Human sperm competition. In: Smith RL (ed) Sperm competition and the evolution of animal mating systems. Academic Press, London, pp 601–659

Statistisches Bundesamt of Germany (1988) Statistisches Jahrbuch 1988

Trivers RL, Willard DE (1973) Natural selection of parental ability to vary the sex ratio of offspring. Science 179:90–92

Tuljapurkar S, Li N, Feldman MW (1995) High sex ratios in China's future. Science 267:874–876

Uzzell T, Hotz H, Berger L (1980) Genome exclusion in gametogenesis by an interspecific Rana hybrid: evidence from electrophoresis of individual oocytes. J Exp Zool 214:251–259

Vessey SH, Meikle DB, Drickamer LC (1989) Demographic and descriptive studies at La Parguera, Puerto Rico. P R Health Sci J 8:121–127

Welch AM, Semlitisch RD, Gerhardt HC (1998) Call duration as an indicator of genetic quality in male gray tree frogs. Science 280:1928–1930

Weller L, Weller A (1993) Human menstrual synchrony: a critical assessment. Neurosci Biobehav Rev 17:427–439

Wickler W, Seibt U (1998) Männlich-Weiblich? Ein Naturgesetz und seine Folgen. Spektrum, Heidelberg

Wilson HC (1992) A critical review of menstrual synchrony research. Psychoneuroendocrinology 17:565–591

World Bank (1984) World Development Report 11:113–138

Chapter 3

Physiology of Testicular Function

3

G. F. Weinbauer · J. Gromoll · M. Simoni · E. Nieschlag

> The testis fulfills two essential functions: production and maturation of the male gametes and synthesis and secretion of the sexual hormones.

This chapter presents the physiological basis for the comprehension of the dual function of the male gonad. Unless otherwise noted the situation in the human is described. Data obtained exclusively in experimental animals will be presented when the corresponding human mechanism is not known or cannot be clarified for ethical reasons. The description of the anatomical organization of the testis and of the physiological basis of germ cell maturation are directed towards the situation in the human testis and provides the basis for understanding the endocrine and paracrine regulation of testicular function. The following sections then include the functional description of the hypothalamo-pituitary-testicular axis, a classical endocrine system, and the local regulation of testicular function, important for the fine tuning of germ cell maturation. The final section provides a comprehensive account of the synthesis and biological actions of androgens.

3.1 Functional Organization of the Testis

The testes produce the male **gametes** and the male sexual hormones (**androgens**). The term **spermatogenesis** describes and includes all the processes involved in the production of gametes, whereas **steroidogenesis** refers to the enzymatic reactions leading to the production of male steroid hormones. Spermatogenesis and steroidogenesis take place in two compartments morphologically and functionally distinguishable from each other. These are the tubular compartment, consisting of the seminiferous tubules (**tubuli seminiferi**) and the interstitial compartment (**interstitium**) between the seminiferous tubules (Figs. 3.1–3.3). Although anatomically separate, both compartments are closely connected with each other. For quantitatively and qualitatively normal production of sperm the integrity of both compartments is necessary. The function of the testis and there-

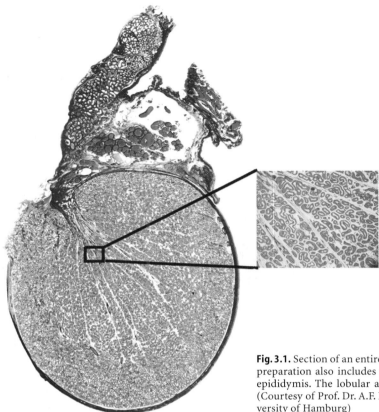

Fig. 3.1. Section of an entire human testis cut transversally. The preparation also includes parts of the efferent ducts and the epididymis. The lobular architecture of the testis is evident. (Courtesy of Prof. Dr. A.F. Holstein, Institute of Anatomy, University of Hamburg)

by also the function of its compartments are primarily influenced by structures of the hypothalamus and the pituitary gland (**endocrine regulation**). In addition, **local control mechanisms (paracrine and autocrine factors)** play an important role in the regulation of testicular function.

3.1.1 Interstitial Compartment

The most important cells of this compartment are the Leydig cells. These cells are the source of testicular testosterone. Aside from Leydig cells, the interstitial compartment also contains immune cells, blood and lymph vessels, nerves, fibroblasts and loose connective tissue. In experimental animals this compartment comprises about 2.6% of the total testicular volume. In the human testis the interstitial compartment represents about 12–15% of the total testicular volume, 10–20% of which is occupied by **Leydig cells**. Human testes contain approximately 200×10^6 Leydig cells (Petersen et al. 1996).

3.1.1.1 Leydig Cells

These cells were first described in 1850 by Franz Leydig (1821–1908). Leydig cells produce and secrete the most important male sexual hormone, **testosterone**. From the morphological point of view two types of Leydig cells can be distinguished: immature and adult Leydig cells (Teerds 1996).

Adult Leydig cells are rich in smooth endoplasmic reticulum and mitochondria with tubular cristae. These physiological characteristics are typical for steroid-producing cells and are very similar to those found in other steroidogenic cells, such as those in the adrenal gland and in the ovary. Other important cytoplasmic components are lipofuscin granules, the final product of endocytosis and lyosomal degradation, and lipid droplets, in which the preliminary stages of testosterone synthesis take place. Special formations, called Reinke's crystals, are often found in the Leydig cells. These are probably subunits of globular proteins whose functional meaning is not known. The proliferation rate of the Leydig cells in the adult testis is rather low and is influenced by LH. In the adult testis, Leydig cells develop from mesenchymal cells and from fibroblast-like cells in the interstitium. The differentiation of these cells into Leydig

Fig. 3.2. Histology of human seminiferous tubule. Arrowhead denotes a degenerating germ cell. Elimination of testicular cells occurs mainly through apoptosis. 5 μm section of tissue fixed in Bouin's solution, embedded in paraffin and stained with hematoxylin. These preparations are suited for histological diagnosis and for the application of immunocytochemistry and in-situ-hybridisation

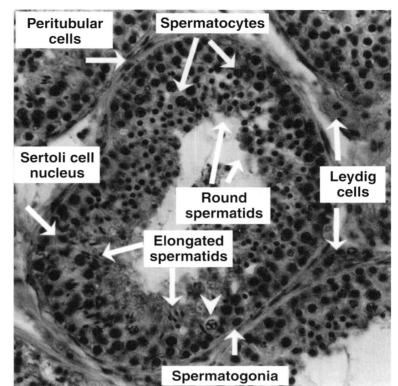

Fig. 3.3. Histology of human seminiferous tubule. Semithin (1.0 μm) section of tissue fixed in glutaraldehyde/osmium-tetroxide, embedded in epoxy resin and stained with toluidine. These preparations are particularly suited for the detailed analysis of specific cellular structures. Note the tubular wall that is composed of several layers of cells. *RB* Residual body, *ES* Elongated spermatids, *ELS* Elongating spermatids, *RS* Round spermatids, *SPZ* Spermatocytes, *SPG* Spermatogonia, *SZ* Sertoli cells, *PTZ* peritubular cells. *Asterisks* denote lipid droplets and lipofuscin deposits in Sertoli cells, *large white triangles* denote the basal lamina, *small white triangles* denote peritubular cell layers and *black triangles* denote the nuclei of peritubular cells

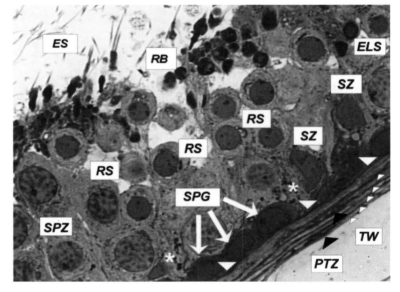

cells is induced by LH (Chemes 1996). In the fetal testis, mesenchymal cells differentiate into Leydig cells when exposed to hCG. Whether Leydig cells also derive from testicular macrophages or neuronal cells is not clarified as yet (Holstein 1999).

3.1.1.2 Macrophages and Lymphocytes

Besides Leydig cells, the interstitial compartment also contains cells belonging to the immune system: **macrophages** and **lymphocytes**. For every 10–50 Leydig cells one macrophage is to be found. The macrophages probably influence the function of the Leydig cells, in particular their proliferation, differentiation and steroid production, through the secretion of cytokines. Macrophages secrete stimulators and inhibitors of steroidogenesis (Hutson 1998). In mice lacking the colony-stimulating factor 1 (CSF-1) macrophages are not present (Cohen et al. 1997). Interestingly, testosterone production is markedly reduced but is restored following administration of CSF-1. The immunological meaning of these cells for testicular physiology will be discussed under Sect. 3.5.

3.1.2 Tubular Compartment

Spermatogenesis takes place in the tubular compartment. This compartment represents about 60–80 % of the total testicular volume. It contains the germ cells and two different types of somatic cells, the **peritubular cells** and the **Sertoli cells**. The testis is divided by septa of connective tissue into about 250–300 lobules (Fig. 3.1), each one containing 1–3 highly convoluted seminiferous tubules. Overall, the human testis contains about 600 seminiferous tubules. The length of individual seminiferous tubules is about 30–80 cm. Considering an average number of about 600 seminiferous tubules per testis and an average length of the tubuli seminiferi of about 60 cm each, the total length of the tubuli seminiferi is about 360 m per testis, i. e. 720 m of seminiferous epithelium per man.

3.1.2.1 Peritubular Cells

The seminiferous tubules are covered by a **lamina propria**, which consists of a **basal membrane**, a layer of collagen and the **peritubular cells (myofibroblasts)**. Myofibroblasts are poorly differentiated myocytes with the capacity of spontaneous contraction. These cells are stratified around the tubulus and form up to 6 concentric layers that are separated by collagen layers (Fig. 3.3). These characteristics differentiate the human testicle from the majority of the other mammals, whose seminiferous tubules are surrounded only by 2–4 layers of myofibroblasts. Peritubular cells produce several factors that are involved in cellular contractility: **panactin, desmin, gelsolin, smooth muscle myosin** and **actin** (Holstein et al. 1996). These cells also secrete extracellular matrix and factors typically expressed by connective tissue cells: vimentin and fibroblast protein. Rat studies showed that periodical contractions occur in the peritubular cells leading to a **peristaltic contraction** of the seminiferous tubules (Harris and Nicholson 1998). It is believed that mature sperm are transported towards the exit of the seminiferous tubules by contraction of these cells. Potential regulators of cell contractions are **oxytocin**, oxytocin-like substances, **prostaglandins** and an-

drogenic steroids. **Endothelins**, endothelin converting enzymes and endothelin receptors influence peritubular cell properties in animal models (Tripiciano et al. 1998). Human peritubular cells express endothelin receptors (Ergün et al. 1998). However, the relevance of these factors for myoid cell activity under in-vivo conditions is not entirely clear.

In the prepubertal testis myofibroblasts do not contain actin (Schlatt et al. 1993). However, testosterone induces production of actins and thereby the contractility of the tubular cells. Thus, testosterone is an important physiological differentiation factor for the myofibroblasts of the testis. Disturbances of testicular function and decreased or absent spermatogenic activity are associated with a thickening of the layer of collagen fibres and of the material present between the peritubular cells. When this is the case, the tubular wall becomes **fibrotic** or – based on the histological appearance – **hyalinized**. Experimentally induced hypogonadism in non-human primate models provokes a dramatic thickening of the tubular wall but is entirely reversible upon cessation of treatments (Weinbauer et al. 1987). The decrease of testicular volume involves folding of the wall along the length of the tubuli seminiferi, thereby causing an enlargement of the tubular diameter. This becomes particularly evident when fluid is injected into regressed seminiferous tubules. Tubular diameter increases and tubular wall thickness decreases (Schlatt et al. 1999).

3.1.2.2 Sertoli Cells

Sertoli cells are somatic cells located within the germinal epithelium. In adulthood these cells are mitotically inactive. They are named after Enrico Sertoli (1842–1910), the Italian scientist who first described these cells in 1865 and, due to their prominent cytoplasmatic projections and ramifications called them "cellulae ramificate". These cells are located on the basal membrane and extend to the lumen of the tubulus seminiferous and, in a broad sense, can be considered as the **supporting structure of the germinal epithelium**. Along the cell body, extending over the entire height of the germinal epithelium, all morphological and physiological differentiation and maturation of the germinal cell up to the mature sperm take place. Special ectoplasmic structures sustain alignment and orientation of the sperm during differentiation. About 35–40 % of the volume of the germinal epithelium is represented by Sertoli cells. The intact testis with complete spermatogenesis contains $800–1200 \times 10^6$ Sertoli cells (Petersen et al. 1996; Zhengwei et al. 1998a).

Sertoli cells synthesize and secrete a large variety of factors: proteins, cytokines, growth factors, opioids, steroids, prostaglandins, modulators of cell division etc. The morphology of Sertoli cells is strictly related to their various physiological functions. Cytoplasm contains endoplasmic reticulum both of the smooth (**steroid synthesis**) and rough type (**protein synthesis**), a prominent Golgi apparatus (**elaboration and transport of secretory products**), lysosomal granules (**phagocytosis**) as well as microtubuli and intermediate filaments (**adapation of the cell** shape during the different phases of germ cell maturation). It is generally assumed that Sertoli cells coordinate the spermatogenic process topographically and functionally. On the other hand, more recent data support the contention that germ cells control Sertoli cell functions. Data from experiments on heterologous germ cell transplantation (Clouthier et al. 1996) underscore this view. At least the time pattern of germ cell transitions and development during the spermatogenic cycle seem to be autonomous. One spermatogenic cycle lasts about 8 days in mice and 12–13 days in rats. Notably, the cycle duration of rat germ cells transplanted into mouse testis remained 12–13 days and that of the host germ cells was maintained at 8 days (Franca et al. 1998).

Another important function of Sertoli cells is that they are responsible for final **testicular volume** and **sperm production** in the adult. Each individual Sertoli cell is in morphological and functional contact with a defined number of sperm. The number of sperm per Sertoli cell depends on the species. In men we observe about 10 germ cells or 1.5 spermatozoa per each Sertoli cell (Zhengwei et al. 1998a). In comparison, every macaque monkey Sertoli cell is associated with 22 germ cells and 2.7 sperm (Zhengwei et al. 1997; 1998b). This suggests that within a certain species a higher number of Sertoli cells results in a greater production of sperm, assuming that all the Sertoli cells are functioning normally.

Which factors stimulate the type of proliferation of Sertoli cells and thereby the testicular volume in the adult? Stereological investigations suggest that the number of Sertoli cells in men increases until the 15th year of life. In the prepubertal Java and Rhesus monkey Sertoli cells exhibit little mitotic activity; however, their proliferative activity can be clearly stimulated experimentally with trophic factors such as androgens and follicle-stimulating hormone (Schlatt et al. 1995). Both Sertoli cell number and expression of markers of cell division are stimulated by these hormones. The division of Sertoli cells ends when the first germ cells undergo meiotic division. At this point Sertoli cells have built **tight junctions** between each other, the so-called **blood testis barrier** (see Sect. 3.5). Defects during pubertal Sertoli cell differentiation can be associated with alterations of spermatogenesis in the adult testis (Steger et al. 1999a). In the rat, the experimental prolongation of the division phase of Sertoli cells, produced for example by a deprivation of thyroid hormones, results in an increase of testicular weight and sperm production by about 80%. On the other hand, the decrease of Sertoli cell numbers such as that produced by an antimitotic substance leads to a reduction of testicular volume and sperm production. Patients with Laron dwarfism suffer from a disturbance of thyroid function and often have testicles larger than normal (Hoffmann et al. 1991).

Through the production and secretion of tubular fluid Sertoli cells create and maintain the patency of the **tubulus lumen** (Griswold and Russell 1999). More than 90% of Sertoli cell fluid is secreted in the tubular lumen. Special structural elements of the blood testis barrier prevent reabsorption of the secreted fluid, resulting in pressure that maintains the patency of the lumen. Sperm are transported in the tubular fluid, the composition of which is known in detail only in the rat (Setchell 1999). Unlike blood, the tubular fluid contains a higher concentration of potassium ions and a lower concentration of sodium ions. Other constituents are bicarbonate, magnesium and chloride ions, inositol, glucose, carnitine, glycero-phosphorylcholine, amino acids and several proteins (Cooper et al. 1992). Therefore, the germ cells are immersed in a fluid of **unique composition**.

The basolateral aspect of neighboring Sertoli cells comprises membrane specializations forming a band sealing the cells to each other and obliterating the intracellular space (occluding tight junctions). The physiological function of the blood testis barrier has been proven in experiments showing that dyes or lanthanum applied outside the barrier could diffuse only up to the tight junctions without reaching the lumen of the seminiferous tubules. The establishment of a functional blood testis barrier depends on the maturity of Sertoli cells and can be perturbed in cases of spermatogenic dysfunction (Caviccia et al. 1996). The closure of the blood testis barrier coincides with the beginning of the first meiosis in the germinal cells (preleptotene, zygotene) and with the arrest of proliferation of Sertoli cells. Through the blood testis barrier the seminiferous epithelium is divided in two regions which are anatomically and functionally completely different from each other. Early germ cells are located in the basal region and the later stages of maturing germ cells in the adluminal region. During their development germ cells are displaced from the **basal** to the **adluminal compartment**. This is accomplished by a synchronized dissolution and reassembly of the tight junctions above and below the migrating germ cells.

Two important functions are postulated for the blood testis barrier: the physical isolation of haploid and thereby antigenic germ cells to prevent recognition by the immune system (prevention of autoimmune orchitis, see Sect. 3.5) and the preparation of a special milieu for the meiotic process and sperm development. Human Sertoli cells express connexin-34 at the sites of cellular contact (Steger et al. 1999b). This protein is not produced in spermatogenic stages II and III when primary spermatocytes are transferred from the basal to the adluminal compartment. In certain seasonal breeders the opening and closure of the barrier depends much more on the activity of the Sertoli cells than on the developmental phase of the germinal epithelium. The constitution of the blood testis barrier and its selectivity in excluding certain molecules means that the cells localized in the adluminal compartment have no direct access to metabolites deriving from the periphery or from the interstitium. Therefore, these cells are completely dependent on Sertoli cells for their maintenance. This "nourishing function" could be exercised through different mechanisms: selective transport and transcytosis as well as synthesis and vectorial secretion.

3.1.2.3 Germinal Cells

Spermatogenesis starts with the division of stem cells and ends with the formation of mature **sperm** (Fig. 3.4). The various germ cells are arranged in typical cellular associations within the seminiferous tubules known as spermatogenic stages (Fig. 3.5). The entire spermatogenic process can be divided into three phases:

- Mitotic proliferation and differentiation of diploid germ cells (spermatogonia),
- Meiotic division of tetraploid germ cells (spermatocytes),
- Transformation of haploid germ cells (spermatids) into sperm (**spermiogenesis**).

Spermatogonia lie at the base of the seminiferous epithelium and are classified as type A and type B spermatogonia. Two types of A spermatogonia can be distin-

guished, originally from a cytological and now also from a physiological point of view: the Ad (dark) spermatogonia and the Ap (pale) spermatogonia. The Ad spermatogonia do not show any proliferating activity under normal circumstances (Schlatt and Weinbauer 1994) and should be considered the stem cells of spermatogenesis. These germ cells, however, undergo mitosis when the overall spermatogonial population is drastically reduced, for example due to radiation (de Rooij 1998; Meistrich and van Beek 1993). In contrast, the Ap spermatogonia divide and differentiate into two B spermatogonia (Sharpe 1994). From B spermatogonia the preleptotene spermatocytes are derived directly before the beginning of the meiotic division. The latter germ cells commence DNA synthesis. Mother and daughter cells remain in close contact with each other through intercellular bridges (Alastalo et al. 1998). This "clonal" mode of germ cell development is possibly the basis and at the same time probably the prerequisite for the coordinated maturation of gametes in the seminiferous epithelium.

Tetraploid germ cells are known as **spermatocytes** and go through the different phases of the meiotic division (Fig. 3.5). The pachytene phase is characterized by intensive RNA synthesis. **Haploid germ cells**, the spermatids, result from the meiotic division. The meiotic process is a critical event in gametogenesis, during which recombination of genetic material, reduction of chromosome number and development of spermatids

Fig. 3.4. Schematic representation of human gametogenesis. For the sake of clarity, complete development of only one spermatogonium is shown. The developmental process from spermatogonium to sperm takes at least 64 days. The human testis contains about 1 billion sperm. Since the human seminiferous epithelium contains only one generation of B-type spermatogonia, the final germ cell number produced depends on the production of A-type spermatogonia. *Ad* A-dark spermatogonium, *Ap* A-pale spermatogonium, *B* B spermatogonium, *SC1* primary spermatocyte, *SC2* secondary spermatocyte, *RS* round spermatid, *ES* elongated spermatid

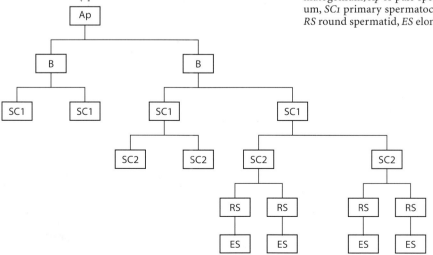

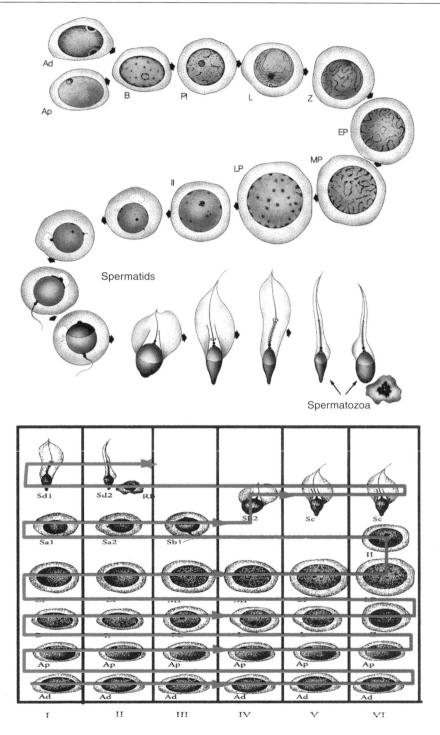

Fig. 3.5. Representation of the development of the different germ cells and their arrangement in specific stages of spermatogenesis of the human testis. A tubular cross-section contains typical germ cell associations that are denoted as stages of spermatogenesis. The 6 stages (I–VI) in the human last altogether 16 days. Since a spermatogonium has to pass through minimally 4 cell layers (red line), the complete duration of spermatogenesis in men is at least 64 days. *Ad* A-dark spermatogonium, *Ap* A-pale spermatogonium, *B* B spermatogonium, *Pl* preleptotene spermatocytes, *L* leptotene spermatocytes, *EP* early pachytene spermatocytes, *MP* mid pachytene spermatocytes, *LP* late pachytene spermatocytes, *II* 2nd meiotic division, *RB* residual body, *Sa1–Sd2* developmental stages of spermatid maturation

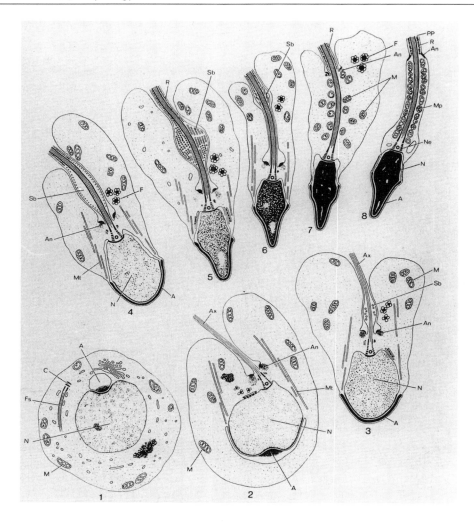

Fig. 3.6. Schematic representation of the differentiation of human spermatids (Holstein and Roosen-Runge 1981). *1* Golgi phase, *2–4* cap phase, *5–6* acrosome phase, *7–8* maturation phase. *A* acrosome, *An* annulus, *Ax* axoneme, *C* centriole, *F* flower-like structures, *Fs* flagellar substructures, *M* mitochondria, *Mp* middle piece, *Mt* manchette, *Ne* neck, *N* nucleus, *PP* principal piece, *R* ring fibers, *Sb* spindle-shaped body

have to be accomplished. Secondary spermatocytes are derived from the first meiotic divison. These germ cells contain a haploid chromosomal set in duplicate form. During the second meiotic division spermatocytes are divided into the haploid spermatids. The prophase of the first meiosis lasts 1–3 weeks, whereas the other phases of the first meiosis and the entire second meiosis are concluded within 1–2 days.

Spermatids are derived from the second meiotic division and are round mitotically inactive cells which undergo a remarkable and complicated transformation leading to the final production of differentiated elongated spermatids and sperm (Fig. 3.6). These processes include condensation and structural shaping of the cell nucleus, the formation of a **flagellum** and the expulsion of a large part of cytoplasm. The overall process is called **spermiogenesis** and, from a qualitative point of view, is identical in all species. It is useful to divide spermiogenesis into 4 phases: Golgi, cap, acrosomal and maturation phases.

During the **Golgi phase** acrosomal bubbles and craniocaudal symmetry appear. In the **cap phase** the spermatids become elongated and the acrosome develops, covering the cranial half to two-thirds of the spermatid. During the fertilization process enzymes are released by the acrosome, allowing the sperm to penetrate the egg (see Chap. 4).

In the **acrosomal phase** the cell nucleus becomes further condensed and elongation of the cell continues. During condensation the majority of histones are lost and gene transcription stops. Nuclear chromatin is now extremely condensed, implying that the proteins necessary for spermiogenesis have to be transcribed before this timepoint and justifying the finding of RNA species with very long half-life and RNA binding proteins (Venables and Eperon 1999). This is the case for transition proteins (Steger 1999) and protamines (Saunders et al. 1996). The mRNA translational control mechanisms are just being unravelled and RNA-binding proteins seem to play an important role. The **flagellum** is now mature.

The principal event during the **maturation phase** of the spermatids is the extrusion of the rest of the cytoplasm as the so-called **residual body**. Residual bodies are phagocytosed by Sertoli cells and have a regulatory role. Elongated spermatids and their residual bodies influence the secretory function of Sertoli cells (production of tubular fluid, inhibin, androgen-binding protein and interleukin-1 and 6) (Stephan et al. 1997). In parallel with degradation of the residual bodies, a new spermatogenic cycle begins.

The release of sperm into the tubular lumen is designated as **spermiation**. This event is influenced by plasminogen activators and possibly also by thimet oligopeptidases (Pineau et al. 1999). This process can be particularly affected by hormonal modifications, temperature and toxins. The reasons for this sensitivity are, however, not yet known. Sperm that are not released are phagocytosed by Sertoli cells. Round and elongated spermatids already contain all the information necessary for fertilization; since introduction of intracytoplasmatic injection of testicular sperm and even round spermatids it has become possible to induce pregnancies successfully (see Chap. 4 for details).

3.1.2.4 Kinetics of Spermatogenesis

The complex process of division and differentiation of germ cells follows a precise pattern. All germ cells pass through several stages characterized by particular **cellular associations**. Recognizing that acrosome development is stage-dependent was crucial for the understanding of germ cell maturation. The **number of stages of spermatogenesis** differs depending on the species. While spermatogenesis encompasses 14 stages (I-XIV) in the rat and 12 stages (I-XII) in macaque monkeys; spermatogenesis in man develops through 6 stages (I-VI). The succession of all stages along time is called the **spermatogenic cycle.**

> The duration of the spermatogenic cycle depends on the animal species and lasts between 8–17 days. **One human spermatogenic cycle requires 16 days.**

For the development and differentiaton of an A spermatogonium into a mature sperm at least four spermatogenic cycles are necessary. It can be deduced that the **overall duration of spermatogenesis** is calculated as 51–53 days in the rat, 37–43 days in different monkey species and at least 64 days in man (Weinbauer and Nieschlag 1999). Investigations carried out in the sixties led to the conclusion that the duration of spermatogenesis is genetically determined, does not vary througout life and cannot be influenced experimentally. However, many indirect experimental findings oppose this hypothesis. For example, the first spermatogenic cycle during puberty proceeds faster than in the adult age. It has also been demonstrated in the rat that the duration of germ cell maturation can actually be manipulated by exogenous factors (Rosiepen et al. 1995). In contrast, endocrine factors do not alter the duration of spermatogenic cycles (Aslam et al. 1999).

The spermatogenetic stages are precisely **ordered**, not only in **time** but also in **space**. In the rat, serial transversal sections through the seminiferous tubules show that stage I is always followed by stage II, stage III always by stage IV and so on. This is known as the **spermatogenic wave**. Since each section contains only a certain stage, it is concluded that in the rat the topography of the spermatogenic stages follows a longitudinal pattern. In contrast, in the entire human testis and in several parts of the testis of different monkeys each section shows different stages simultaneously. Quantitative analysis of the germ cell population has demonstrated that the distribution of spermatogenic stages in these species does not follow an irregular pattern, as originally supposed. The association of stages in the same transverse section becomes understandable when a **helical pattern** is considered. In other words, several helices are spaced apart with spermatogonia at their basis and elongated spermatids at their apical part (Schulze and Rehder 1984, Fig. 3.7). If the scroll of the helix is very narrow, several stages can be seen in each horizontal section and vice versa. In this way, the longitudinal pattern of spermatogenic stages can be reconciled with helices also situated quite far away from each other but with very short scrolls. Other investigations of human spermatogenesis confirmed the principle of helical patterns but not the presence of a complete spermatogenic wave, i.e. the complete succession of all stages (Johnson 1994; Johnson et al. 1996). At the most, 2–4 consecutive stages could be found on serial sections. The topographical distribution of the stages could be reproduced by assigning random numbers. This led to the postulate that the arrangement of the human spermatogenic stages along the seminiferous tubule is random.

Besides the duration of spermatogenesis and the spatial pattern of spermatogenic stages, human spermatogenesis shows another peculiarity: in absolute terms, the number of Sertoli cells in the rat is about twice as high

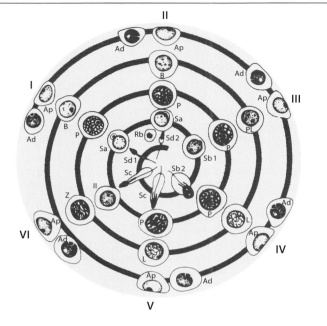

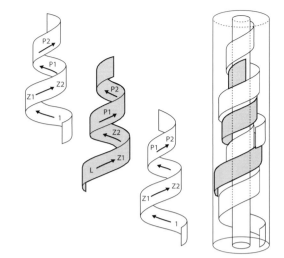

Abb 3.7. The six stages of human spermatogenesis are arranged in a helical manner in cross-sectioned seminiferous tubules. The analysis of 3-dimensional reconstructions from small segments of seminiferous tubules showed the helical arrangement of the spermatogenic stages. The diameter of the helix decreases towards the lumen and several spirals are overlapping in a concentric pattern (Schulze and Rehder 1984; Kerr 1992). Subsequent investigation by others has challenged this view (Johnson 1994; Johnson et al. 1996)

Fig. 3.8. Hormonal regulation of the testicular function and effects of androgens. Key hormones are luteinizing hormone (LH) and follicle-stimulating hormone (FSH), synthesized and secreted under hypothalamic control of gonadotropin-releasing hormone (GnRH). Leydig cells are located between the seminiferous tubules and synthesize and secrete testosterone under the control of LH. Testosterone stimulates the maturation of germ cells in seminiferous tubules. FSH acts directly on the seminiferous tubules. In the germinal epithelium only Sertoli cells possess receptors for testosterone and FSH. It is therefore believed that the trophic effects of testosterone/FSH on gametogenesis are mediated via somatic Sertoli cells. The testis and the hypothalamo-pituitary system communicate through steroids and protein hormones. Testosterone inhibits the secretion of GnRH and gonadotropins. Inhibin B and follistatin suppress selectively the release of FSH from the pituitary gland, while activin stimulates this process. Beside the effects on gametogenesis, testosterone plays an important role in hair growth, bone metabolism, muscle mass and distribution, secondary sexual characteristics and function of the male reproductive organs

as in men. Therefore, the density of germ cells in the human testis is comparably low. Similarly, the number of sperm per Sertoli cell is also very low in men. These factors and the low number of 1.5 sperm/Sertoli cells on average result in relatively low sperm production. When expressed in millions of sperm per g/testicle in 24 hours, the rat has values of 10–24, non-human primates values of 4–5 and men values of 3–7. To account for this lower germ cell production, pronounced germ cell loss has been implicated. Earlier work suggested that about 50 % of germ cells are lost during the meiotic divisions (Johnson 1995). However, more recent studies using contemporary stereological approaches failed to detect meiotic germ cell losses in nonhuman primates (Zhengwei et al. 1997; 1998b) or in men (Zhengwei et al. 1998a).

> Primate sperm production is controlled through the number of spermatogonia entering meiosis.

3.1.2.5 Apoptosis and Spermatogenesis

Programmed cell death (**apoptosis**) comprises a coordinated sequence of signalling cascades leading to **cell suicide**. Unlike necrosis, this form of cell death occurs under physiological conditions (spontaneous apoptosis) but can also be induced by exposure to toxicants, disturbances of the endocrine milieu, etc. In the human testis spermatogonia, spermatocytes and spermatids undergoing apoptosis have been detected (Brinkworth et al. 1997). Ethnic differences in the incidence of testicular apoptosis have been suggested (Sinha Hikim and Swerdloff 1999). Blockade of apoptotic events in the mouse model leads to accumulation of spermatogonia and infertility. Quantitative studies also revealed that in

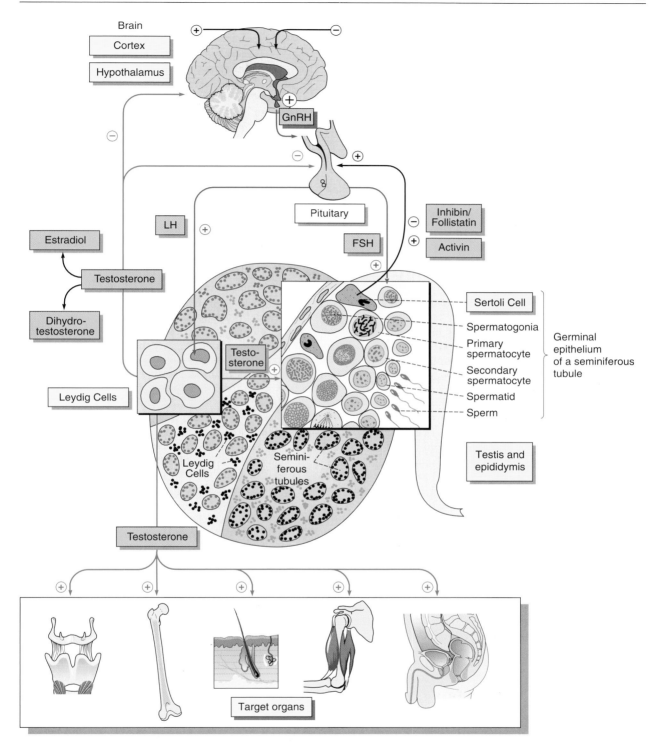

Brain

Cortex

Hypothalamus

GnRH

Pituitary

LH

FSH

Inhibin/
Follistatin

Activin

Estradiol

Testosterone

Dihydro-
testosterone

Testo-
sterone

Sertoli Cell

Spermatogonia

Primary
spermatocyte

Secondary
spermatocyte

Spermatid

Sperm

Germinal
epithelium
of a seminiferous
tubule

Leydig Cells

Leydig
Cells

Semini-
ferous
tubules

Testis and
epididymis

Testosterone

Target organs

the intact germinal epithelium primarily spermatogonia and early spermatocytes undergo apoptosis (Krishnamurthy et al. 1998). Hence, **apoptosis is a physiological and necessary event during spermatogenesis.**

3.2 Hormonal Control of Testicular Function

The endocrine regulation of testicular function, i.e. the production of sperm and of androgens is well investigated. Understanding the hormonal interactions has important clinical consequences, presented in the following paragraphs. Fig. 3.8 offers an overview of the systems involved, of the endocrine factors and of their physiological effects.

3.2.1 Functional Organization of the Hypothalamo-Pituitary System

The **gonadotropins luteinizing hormone (LH) and follicle-stimulating hormone (FSH)** are produced and secreted by the gonadotropic cells of the anterior pituitary. Their designation is derived from the function exerted in females. In males, they control steroidogenesis and gametogenesis in the testis (Weinbauer and Nieschlag 1998). The pituitary gland is the central structure controlling gonadal function and is, in turn, regulated by the hypothalamic **gonadotropin-releasing hormone (GnRH)**. Since GnRH secretion is pulsatile, gonadotropin release also occurs in discrete peaks, more evident in the case of LH, due to its shorter half-life in circulation compared to FSH. The pituitary function is also under the control of gonadal steroids and peptides that influence its activity both directly and through the hypothalamus (Fig. 3.8). Due to their very strict anatomical and functional connections, hypothalamus and pituitary gland have to be considered as an unique functional unit.

The hypothalamus is the rostral extension of the brain stem reticular formation. It contains, among others, the cellular bodies of neurons that project their axon terminals toward the median eminence (ME), a specialized region of the floor of the third ventricle from which the pituitary stalk originates. The **hypothalamus** is classically subdivided into three longitudinal zones, periventricular, medial and lateral, the latter functioning as the connecting area between limbic and brain stem regions, whereas the former two contain most of the nuclei controlling neuroendocrine and visceral functions. The ME is the ventral bulge of the hypothalamus and is the site where the axon terminals of the neurosecretory neurons make contact with the capillary plexus, giving rise to the hypophyseal portal circulation. The nerve terminals form buttons on the capillaries and release the neurohormones into the portal blood by diffusion through the basal membrane. The ME is outside the blood-brain barrier and thereby freely accessible to the regulatory influences of hormones and substances present in the systemic circulation and mediating the release of neurohormones in portal blood. The blood supply of the ME is provided by the superior hypophyseal arteries. The long portal hypophyseal vessels originate from the confluence of capillary loops which supply the anterior pituitary gland with the highest blood flow of any organ in the body. In humans, the perikarya of neurons stained positive for GnRH are especially found in the ventral part of the mediobasal hypothalamus, between the third ventricle and the ME, scattered throughout the periventricular infundibular region.

The **pituitary gland** lies in the sella turcica, beneath hypothalamus and optic chiasm, covered with the sellar diaphragm. Thus, pituitary tumors can result in visual impairment by exerting pressure on the optical nerves. Gonadotropic cells are localized in the adenohypophysis, the most ventral part of the gland, of ectodermic origin from Rathke's pouch. The **adenohypophysis** consists of the anterior lobe (or pars distalis, the anatomically and functionally most important part), the pars intermedia and pars tuberalis.

The pars distalis is of pivotal importance for pituitary function. Gonadotropin-producing cells constitute approximately 15% of the adenohypophyseal cell population, are scattered in the posteromedial portion of the pars distalis and are basophilic and PAS-positive. Although the secretion of LH and FSH can be partially dissociated under certain circumstances, the same cell type is believed to secrete both gonadotropins. About 80% of the gonadotropic cells in men contain both LH and FSH (Schlatt et al. 1991). The cells have a very well developed RER, a large Golgi complex and are rich in secretory granules. In normal men, the pituitary contains approximately 700 IU of LH and 200 IU of FSH. Following gonadectomy or in primary hypogonadism the cells become vacuolated and large (castration cells). Finally, pituitary gonadotropes are often found in close connection with prolactin cells, suggesting a paracrine interaction between the two cell types.

3.2.2 GnRH

3.2.2.1 Structure

GnRH is a decapeptide produced in the GnRH neurons of the hypothalamus. Unique among neurons producing hypothalamic neurohormones, they originate from olfactory neurones and during embryonic development migrate toward the basal forebrain along branches of the terminal and vomeronasal nerves, across the nasal septum. This neuronal migration is guided by an N-CAM (neural adhesion molecule) (Schwanzel-Fukuda et al. 1999). N-CAM is not present in GnRH neurons but in neurons that connect the olfactory epithelium and the forebrain. These GnRH containing cells migrate along the cells expressing N-CAM. In about 10% of patients with Kallman syndrome and anosmia due to a hypoplasia of the bulbus olfactorius, mutations or deletions of the Kal-1 gene on the X chromosome were detected. This gene encodes for anosmin-1 which is produced in the bulbus and in other tissues, and which is transiently expressed as an extracellular matrix and basal membrane protein during organogenesis. The precise pathogenesis of the Kallmann syndrome is not yet fully understood. However, the lack of anosmin-1 might interfere with the migration or the differentiation of olfactory neurons (Hardelin et al. 1999). These findings explain why the olfactory capacity is compromised in these partients.

In primates, the main locations of GnRH neurons are the medio-basal hypothalamus and the arcuate nucleus, but they are found also in the anterior hypothalamus, preoptic area, septum and other parts of the forebrain. GnRH neurons are synaptically connected with terminals stained positive for pro-opiomelanocortin-related peptides and enzymes involved in the metabolism of catecholamines and γ-aminobutyric acid (GABA). Furthermore, GnRH-positive neurons of the nucleus arcuatus are connected to neuropeptide Y (NPY) neurons in the preoptical area and in the eminentia mediana. All these substances are known to influence GnRH secretion (Evans 1999; Li et al. 1999).

GnRH is produced by successive cleavage stages from a longer precursor, called preproGnRH, transported along the axons to the ME and there released into portal blood. The structure of the decapeptide, of its precursor and of the GnRH gene is reported in Fig. 3.9. Besides the "classical" GnRH, two further GnRH molecules were discovered in animal species and in men (Fernald and White 1999) but the physiological role of these new GnRH variants is currently unknown. Phylogenetically GnRH is a rather ancient hormone, highly conserved among different species with 80% sequence identity between mammals and fish. In the precursor with a length of 92 amino acids, GnRH is preceded by a signal peptide consisting of 24 amino acids, and followed by a stretch of 56 amino acids forming the GnRH-associated peptide (GAP). PreproGnRH is processed in the rough endoplasmic reticulum and in the Golgi complex, the first step being the removal of the signal peptide and the cyclization of the aminoterminal Gln residue to pyroGlu. At the junction between GnRH and GAP a Gly-Lys-Arg sequence provides a processing signal important for the cleavage of GAP and C-terminal amidation of the last Pro residue. Mature GnRH is therefore a single chain decapeptide cyclized at the N-terminus and amidated at the C-terminus and assumes a folded conformation as the result of a β-II type bend involving the central Tyr-

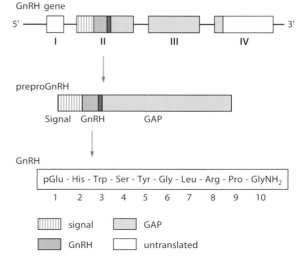

Fig. 3.9. Gonadotropin-releasing hormone (GnRH) is a decapeptide produced by the hypothalamus. It originates from cleavage of preproGnRH, containing a signal peptide. Moreover, the tripeptide Gly-Lys-Arg is necessary to process correctly the final GnRH and the GnRH-associated-peptide (GAP). The GnRH gene has 4 exons and 3 introns. Exon 2 encodes the signal peptide, GnRH and the first part of GAP. Exon 1 and the largest part of exon 4 are not translated

Gly-Leu-Arg residues that brings the N- and C termini in close proximity (Seeburg et al. 1989).

GnRH has a very short half-life (<10 min) and is mostly retained and degraded in the pituitary gland immediately after secretion by several peptidase systems. Deciphering the GnRH sequence earned A. Schally the 1977 Nobel prize, and enabled the development of analogs with agonistic or antagonistic properties (Weinbauer and Nieschlag 1992). As the generation of synthetic analogs of GnRH has shown, the amino acids in position 6–10 are important for high affinity binding of the neuropeptide, whereas positions 1–3 are critical for biological activity and positions 5–6 and 9–10 are involved in enzymatic degradation (Karten et al. 1986). The discovery of the amino acid sequence of GnRH permitted the design of GnRH analogs exerting agonistic or antagonistic action relative to the endogenous GnRH (Weinbauer and Nieschlag 1998).

GnRH and GAP coexist in the GnRH neurons and are cosecreted in portal blood. The physiological role of GAP in the human, however, is unclear to date. A very important function of GAP is related to the correct processing and folding of the mature hormone, in analogy to the role of C-peptide in insulin formation. This is suggested by the fact that the genetic defect of the **hpg** mouse, a model for human hypogonadotropic hypogonadism, is a large deletion in the gene involving GAP but leaving untouched the sequence coding for GnRH (Sher-

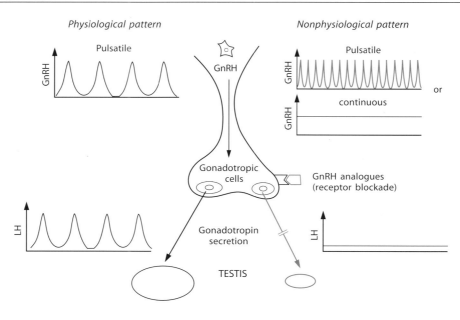

Fig. 3.10. Importance of the pulsatile pattern of GnRH secretion for gonadotropin secretion and testicular function. Unphysiologically high GnRH pulse frequencies or continuous administration of GnRH inhibit gonadotropin secretion and testicular function (*red*). Similarly, blockade of GnRH receptors by means of GnRH analogs results in suppression of testicular function

wood et al. 1993). Yet no mutations in the GAP or GnRH genes causing the pathophysiological picture of hypogonadotropic hypogonadism have been identified so far.

The gene encoding GnRH is localized at the chromosomal site 8p21-p11.2 and consists of 4 exons and 3 introns (Fig. 3.9) Exon 2 encodes the signal peptide, GnRH and the first portion of GAP. Exon 1 and most parts of exon 4 remain untranslated. The 5' flanking region contains conventional sequences with promoter activity (TATA and CAAT boxes) and consensus sequences for several transcription factors. Interestingly, it also includes an estrogen response element and the estrogen receptor can bind to the 5' flanking region of the GnRH gene (Sherwood et al. 1993). In all species studied so far, no estrogen or progesterone receptors could be detected in the GnRH neurons but only in those cells in close vicinity that express galanin, GABA or glutamate. These findings raise the possibility that gonadal hormones influence GnRH secretion via paracrine mechanisms (McEwen and Alves 1999).

3.2.2.2 Secretion of GnRH

GnRH is released into the portal blood in discrete pulses. Although this event cannot be directly demonstrated in vivo, all the experimental data accumulated up to now demonstrate that each LH peak is induced by a GnRH pulse. It is the frequency of GnRH pulses and the amplitude of its secretory episodes that determine the type of LH and FSH secretion from the pituitary gland (Fig. 3.10). GnRH is the sole releasing factor for both gonadotropins, but modulating its frequency results in

preferential release of LH or FSH (Hayes and Crowley 1998).

It is not yet clear what determines the pulsatile nature of GnRH secretion. It has been shown that isolated immortalized GnRH neurons have a spontaneous pulsatile secretory activity in vitro, but it is also possible that the pulse generator in vivo is influenced by noradrenergic stimuli such as galanin and nitric oxide. The pulse generator is under the continuous tonic inhibition of peripheral steroids and, e.g. gonadectomy results in an immediate increase of frequency and amplitude of gonadotropin secretion. Thus, in the absence of steroids the pulse generator becomes free-running (Lopez et al. 1998).

In man, the major hormone controlling GnRH secretion is testosterone, which inhibits gonadotropin secretion via negative feedback both at the hypothalamic and pituitary level (Fig. 3.8). Testosterone can act as such or after metabolism to DHT or estradiol. The effects of testosterone and its metabolites appear to vary depending on the experimental model but, in general, we can assume that both T and DHT act mainly at the hypothalamic level by decreasing the frequency of GnRH pulsatility, whereas estrogens depress gonadotropin secretion by reducing the amplitude of LH and FSH peaks at the pituitary level (Hayes and Crowley 1998). Progesterone inhibits gonadotropin release but the site of progesterone action in the brain remains unclear. The negative feedback action of androgens and progestins is most important for the development of a male fertility control regimen (Weinbauer and Nieschlag 1998 and Chap. 20).

A regulatory role of gonadotropins on GnRH (short feedback) has been repeatedly postulated but data obtained in sheep have shown that the GnRH discharge into the portal blood is not altered by the administration of GnRH agonists or antagonists, thereby excluding direct control of the pituitary on the hypothalamus. Among the neurotransmitters and neuromodulators that might influence GnRH secretion, the noradrenergic system and NPY show stimulatory activity, whereas interleukin-1, dopaminergic, serotoninergic and GABA-ergic systems are inhibitory. Opioid peptides seem to modulate the negative feedback of gonadal steroids. Finally, leptin has been shown to stimulate gonadotropin secretion. Leptin is produced by the fat cells of the body and influences the interactions concerning the control of body mass and gonadotropin secretion. This effect is partially mediated by the hypothalamus and NPY and POMC containing neurons with numerous receptors for leptin (Baskin et al. 1999).

3.2.2.3 Mechanism of GnRH Action

GnRH acts through interaction with a **specific receptor**. The GnRH receptor belongs to a family of G-coupled receptors linked by the typical seven-membrane domain structure (Fang et al. 1995). This group also encompasses the receptors for LH, FSH and TSH. With 328 amino acids, it is the smallest G protein-coupled receptor known up to now and possesses a rather short extracellular domain (Fig. 3.11). The intracellular C-terminus is practically absent and the signal transduction is probably carried out by the intracytoplasmic loops connecting the seven membrane spanning segments, especially the third one which is unusually long. The receptor contains two glycosylation sites, projecting into the extracellular space, of uncertain function.

The conformation of the binding site is unknown. The gene encoding the human GnRH receptor includes three exons separated by two introns. The 5' flanking region contains multiple TATA transcription initiation sites and several cis-acting regulatory sequences which confer responsiveness to cAMP, glucocorticoids, progesterone, thyroxin, PEA-3, AP-1, AP-2 and Pit-1-sensitive sequences. GnRH is specifically expressed in the gonadotropic cells within the pituitary. An orphan receptor, steroidogenic factor 1(SF-1) is involved in the expression of human GnRH (Ngan et al. 1999). Transcription factors such as SF-1, Pit-1 and Pro-Pit-1 are generally needed for

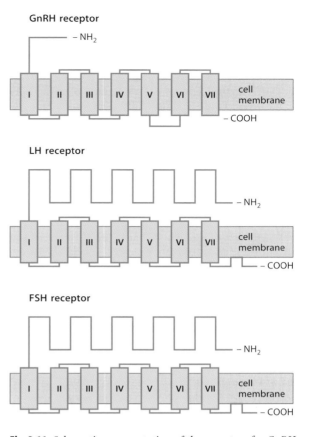

Fig. 3.11. Schematic representation of the receptors for GnRH (upper panel), LH (middle panel) and FSH (bottom panel). These receptors belong to the family of G protein-coupled receptors. They possess an extracellular domain, a transmembrane domain with 7 membrane spanning segments and an intracellular domain. The GnRH receptor is characterized by a very short extracellular domain and practically no intracellular domain. On the contrary, the extracellular domain is very large in the gonadotropin receptors, where it plays a crucial role in hormone binding. The intracellular domain is important for signal transduction

the development and maturation of the hypothalamo-hypophyseal-gonadal axis. SF-1-deficient mice and patients bearing a mutation in the Pro-Pit-1 gene exhibit pronounced alterations of gonadotropin secretion. Recently, a second GnRH receptor gene was identified, the role of which is yet unknown (Millar et al. 1999).

Following GnRH-receptor interaction, a **hormone receptor complex** is formed. This results in the interaction with Gq protein, hydrolysis of phosphoinositide and production of diacylglycerol and inositol trisphosphate, which leads to calcium mobilization from the intracellular stores and influx of extracellular calcium into the cell. Diacylglycerol and calcium then activate protein kinase C (PKC), inducing protein phosphorylation and further activation of calcium channels. The increase in intracellular calcium results in prompt gonadotropin release by exocytosis and, with time, more sustained gonadotropin synthesis and secretion. Thereafter, the hormone-receptor complex is internalized by endocytosis and undergoes degradation in lysosomes.

GnRH is capable of **modulating number and activity** of its own **receptors** and the effects depend on the secretory pattern and dose of neurohormone. The receptor expression is higher when GnRH is given in a pulsatile manner and the withdrawal of GnRH during the interpulse intervals leads to increase of GnRH binding sites just before the next pulse occurs (self priming). Conversely, continuous exposure to GnRH results in an initial rise in response followed by desensitization. This property of the GnRH receptor is exploited in therapy with GnRH agonists that, owing to their prolonged and sustained stimulatory activity, cause slow receptor desensitization and decrease of gonadotropin secretion. The molecular mechanism of receptor desensitization is not completely understood. Owing to the lack of an intracellular domain, GnRH agonists cannot induce phosphorylation and rapid desensitization of the receptor.

3.2.3 Gonadotropins

3.2.3.1 Structure

LH and FSH are **glycoprotein hormones** secreted by the pituitary gland that control development, maturation and function of the gonad. Like the related thyroid stimulating hormone (TSH) and human chorionic gonadotropin (hCG), they consist of two polypeptide chains, α and β, bearing carbohydrate moieties N-linked to asparagine (Asn) residues. The α subunit is common to all members of the glycoprotein hormone family, whereas the β subunit, although structurally very similar, differs in each hormone and confers specificity of action.

The subunits are encoded by separate genes localized on different chromosomes but structurally related (Gharib et al. 1990). The gene encoding for the α subunit is composed of four exons and three introns, whereas the β genes consist of three exons separated by two introns. The FSH β gene is located on chromosome 11 and differs from the other glycoprotein hormone β subunit genes in possessing a rather long 3' untranslated region probably involved in RNA stability. The LH β gene belongs to an extraordinary complex cluster of genes also including at least seven nonallelic hCGβ-like genes arranged in tandem on chromosome 19. The regulation of gene expression of LH and FSH has been extensively studied in experimental animals, expecially in rodents, and involves a complex interplay between hypothalamic GnRH and gonadal steroids and peptides acting at the hypothalamic and pituitary level.

The common α subunit contains two glycosylation sites, at position 52 and 78. The glycosylation sites of FSH ß are 7 and 24, whereas LH is glycosylated only at position 30. In mammals the α subunit is also produced by the placenta and, conversely, the pituitary gland has been shown to contain and secrete trace amounts of hCG. α and β subunits are non-covalently linked and the probable tertiary structure of pituitary gonadotropins can be approximated and deduced by analogy with its cognate hCG, whose crystal structure has been resolved recently (Lapthorn et al. 1994). The two gonadotropin subunits α and β have a similar Y-shaped structure, with three disulphide bonds forming a cysteine knot, a structural motif also found in some growth factors. A peculiar feature is represented by a segment of the β subunit which wraps around the α subunit like a seatbelt, stabilizing the heterodimer with an internal disulphide bond.

LH and hCGβ subunits are structurally very simular and, in fact, LH and hCG act on the same receptor. A peculiar feature of hCGβ is a carboxyl-terminal extension containing four O-linked sugar residues that remarkably reduces the rate of metabolism and increases the half-life of the hormone. This peculiarity of hCGß has been recently exploited for the production of a synthetic gonadotropin hybrid containing a similar C-terminal extension in the ß subunit which resulted in a conspicuous increase of the gonadotropin half-life. A prolongation of the half-life of hCG was achieved by producing a chimera containing fusioned α and β chains (Boime and Ben-Menahed 1999).

The oligosaccharide structure consists of a central mannose core, bound to an Asn residue through two residues of N-acetyl-glucosamine, and terminal extensions of tetrasaccharide branches, bi- or triantennary, terminating with sialic acid (FSH) or sulfate (LH) residues. These carbohydrate structures can be more or less extended in length and are rich in sugar terminals, constituting the molecular basis of the gonadotropin heterogeneity evident after chromatographic separation.

Having a different terminal glycosylation, LH and FSH also have a different half-life. LH is rich in N-acetyl-glucosamine sulfate and is quickly removed from the circulation after interaction with specific liver receptors that recognize sulfate terminals. This rapid removal of sulfate LH from the blood results in rapid clearance of a relevant amount of the LH discharged in each secretory episode and "amplifies" the pulsatile features of LH in circulation. Conversely, FSH is predominantly sialylated and thereby protected from immediate capture and metabolism in the liver. As a result, LH and FSH half-lives are about 20 minutes and two hours, respectively (Jockenhövel et al. 1990). Therefore, although both gonadotropins are secreted simultaneously from the pituitary gland following a GnRH pulse, LH appears to be highly pulsatile and FSH much less so (Moyle and Campbell 1995).

The importance of **sugar residues** on gonadotropin activity has been investigated in vitro using glycosylation-deficient hormones. It was found that glycosylation is not critical for receptor binding but is important for receptor activation.

The use of recombinant variants of hCG and FSH defective in sialic acid or truncated at the mannose ramification revealed that glycosylation at position α 52 is necessary for the steroidogenic and cAMP response. Isoforms completely devoid of carbohydrates cannot be secreted by the producing cells and behave as competitive antagonists of the wild type. Overall, the current view is that glycosylation is fundamental for gonadotropin secretion and bioactivity, and strongly influences the half-life in circulation and in vivo biopotency.

It was found recently that two polymorphic variants of LH are present in the normal population. One of them has two amino acid exchanges in positions 8 and 15 of the β chain leading to a second glycosylation site in position 13. Approximately 12 % of Europeans produce this allelic variant. Under in vitro conditions, this variant displays increased bioactivity and shortened half-life. A difference in immunoactivity can be detected when certain monoclonal antibodies are used (Huhtaniemi et al. 1999).

3.2.3.2 Secretion of Gonadotropins

After the synthetic process is completed, LH and FSH are stored in different secretion granules, ready to be released upon stimulation with GnRH. A portion of molecules, however, is not stored in secretory granules, i.e. does not enter the regulated pathway of secretion and is, instead, constitutively secreted. FSH expecially follows the latter route. Storage in separate granules and the natural propensity to follow one of the two secretory pathways are the main reasons why the same GnRH stimulus can, under certain conditions, preferentially release one of the two gonadotropins. Low GnRH pulse frequency causes preferential release of FSH probably due to differential expression of the FSH receptor (Kaiser 1998).

LH and FSH are measurable in the pituitary gland as early as the 10th week of gestation and during the 12th week in peripheral blood. In fetal life and in infancy FSH is predominant over LH and the FSH/LH ratio is higher in females than in males. The relative abundance of the two gonadotropins changes during development.

It is noteworthy that before birth both male and female fetuses grow in an environment extraordinarily rich in potent, maternal estrogens.

It is testosterone that determines the initial phase of testicular migration and the development of male external genitalia. Testosterone is already produced by the fetal testicle during the 10th week of gestation, under the stimulation of fetal LH and maternal hCG. The role of maternal hCG in this crucial phase of gonadal development is suggested by the fact that a mutation of the LH β chain leading to a biologically inactive gonadotropin is associated with normal sexual differentiation (Huhtaniemi et al. 1999). Conversely, inactivating mutations of the LH receptor produce a clinical syndrome resembling complete androgen insensitivity, with a phenotype of female external genitalia (Themmen et al. 1998).

During infancy gonadotropins in serum are very low. The pulsatile secretion of gonadotropins becomes evident at the time of puberty, when LH and FSH pulses in serum are detected first during sleep, at night, and then progressively also during the day. Before puberty, gonadotropin levels are very low and GnRH secretion appears to be extremely limited, even in the presence of negligible steroid production by the gonads. High sensitivity of the hypothalamus to negative steroid feedback is believed to suppress GnRH production before puberty, but certainly other factors such as body mass, leptin and signals from the central nervous system are important to maintain the hypothalamo-pituitary-gonadal axis silent before the programmed time.

The steroid regulation of gonadotropin gene expression, synthesis and secretion is rather complex and shows many facets depending on the experimental model (Counis et al. 1991). In general, however, it is currently accepted that gonadal steroids exert their negative control on gonadotropins mainly at the hypothalamic level, depressing the release of GnRH. The steroid effect at the pituitary level is more complex, but there is considerable evidence that estrogens inhibit GnRH-stimulated gonadotropin synthesis and secretion at this level. In rodents, testosterone has a specific stimulatory effect on FSH gene expression, synthesis and secretion directly at the pituitary level. In primates, however, the effects of testosterone are always inhibitory.

Testosterone is the main testicular product suppressing FSH and LH secretion in men.

FSH secretion is, obviously, also under the control of some other factor(s) related to the efficiency of spermatogenesis, since oligoazoospermia is often accompanied by selective increase of serum FSH in the presence of normal testosterone levels. New assays for **inhibin B** permitted analysis of the relationship between **FSH and inhibin secretion** in man. A pronounced inverse correlation was established between serum concentrations of inhibin B and serum levels of FSH, testis size and sperm numbers. Clearly, inhibin B is the physiologically relevant form of inhibin in men (von Eckardstein et al. 1999). It appears at present that the serum levels of inhibin B directly reflect the integrity of the germinal epithelium and of the Sertoli cells. Whether the production and secretion of this inhibin is under the control of FSH remains to be clarified.

3.2.3.3 Mechanism of Action of Gonadotropins

LH and FSH exert their function via specific receptors (Simoni et al. 1997). The gonadotropin receptors also belong to the family of the G protein-coupled receptors and are characterized by a very large extracellular domain to which the hormone binds specifically, the usual membrane-spanning domain including 7 hydrophobic segments connected to each other through three extracellular and three intracellular tracts, and an intracellular carboxyterminal domain (Fig. 3.11).

The genes for LH and FSH receptors are localized on chromosome 2 and consist of 11 and 10 exons, respectively. The last exon encodes a small portion of the extracellular domain, the entire transmembrane domain and the intracellular C-terminus. The extracellular domain contains the high-affinity hormone binding site and is rich in leucine repeats, mainly located at the exon-intron boundaries, of unknown function. The 5'-flanking region of the two genes contains no conventional promoter and has multiple transcription start sites. Several alternatively spliced transcripts of LH and FSH receptors have been described, lacking one or more exons, but presently it is not known whether these RNA **isoforms** are translated into proteins of any physiological function. Furthermore, **allelic variants** with at least two amino acid exchanges have recently been described (Simoni et al. 1999).

The **mature receptor proteins** are glycosylated at several points, a process that does not seem to be involved in receptor activation and signal transduction but probably necessary for receptor folding and transport to the cell membrane. Upon **binding with the gonadotropin**, the receptor probably undergoes some conformational change resulting in activation of the G protein, cAMP production and activation of protein kinase A. Gonadotropins act mainly through stimulation of intracellular cAMP. More recently it has been shown that LH and FSH can also induce an increase of Ca^{++} influx in target cells, but the physiological importance of this mechanism is still unknown. cAMP remains, therefore, the main signal transducer and calcium could possibly act as a signal amplification or modulating mechanism. Following the hormone-receptor interaction there is an increase in cAMP concentrations and subsequent activation of protein kinaseses which, in turn, phosphorylate existing proteins such as enzymes, structural and transport proteins and transcriptional activators. Activating and inactivating mutations of the gonadotropin receptors have been identified. The biological consequences of these mutations are described below and in Chapt. 11.

3.2.4 Endocrine Regulation and Relative Importance of LH and FSH for Spermatogenesis

Both functions of the testis, androgen production and gamete development, are regulated by hypothalamus and hypophysis through a **negative feedback** mechanism (Fig. 3.8). **Testosterone** inhibits the secretion of **LH** and **FSH**. For FSH there is a further regulator, the protein hormone **inhibin B**.

> LH stimulates testosterone synthesis in the Leydig cells, whereas FSH controls spermatogenesis via the Sertoli cells. The intratesticular effect of testosterone is also important for spermatogenesis.

In certain animal species, e. g. Djungarian hamsters, FSH is the only hormone responsible for spermatogenesis, while LH and testosterone stimulate the development of androgen-dependent organs and sexual behavior. Conversely, in primates, both gonadotropins are necessary for spermatogenesis. The biological meaning of this **dual regulation system** is not clear yet (Nieschlag et al. 1999; Weinbauer and Nieschlag 1998).

For the interpretation of hormonal regulation and hormonal effects on spermatogenesis, the following **terminology** should be remembered:

- **Initiation:** first complete cycle of spermatogenesis during puberty,
- **maintenance:** hormonal requirements of intact spermatogenesis in the adult,
- **reinitiation:** hormonal requirements for the restimulation of gametogenesis after transitory interruption,
- **qualitatively normal spermatogenesis:** all germ cells are present although in subnormal numbers,
- **quantitatively normal spermatogenesis:** all germ cells are present in normal numbers.

The **initiation of spermatogenesis** normally occurs under the influence of **LH and FSH**. However, testosterone alone in extremely high doses is capable of inducing spermatogenesis. Complete spermatogenesis is seen in the vicinity of testosterone-producing Leydig cell tumors and in patients with activating mutations of the LH receptor (Fig. 3.12). The aim of treatment is to obtain sufficiently high intratesticular testosterone concentrations, which are crucial. This is normally pursued clinically by giving hCG, which contains high LH activity, together with FSH.

It is not known whether **FSH alone** can initiate all phases of germ cell maturation in man. It has been reported that spermatogenesis can be induced in patients with hypogonadotropic hypogonadism with human

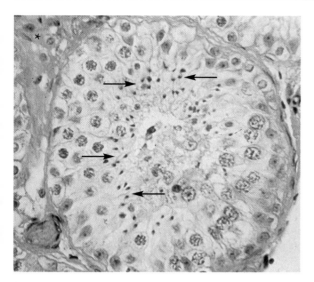

Fig. 3.12. Testicular histology of a 5.2-yrs old boy with an activating mutation of the LH receptor. Note complete spermatogenesis (*arrows*) and developed Leydig cells (*asterisk*). (Courtesy of Prof. Dr. W. Rabl, Pediatric Clinic of the Technical University Munich)

menopausal gonadotropins (hMG) (Jones and Darne 1993). Patients, however, had already also been treated with hCG so that in this case the effect cannot be considered to be solely dependent on FSH. Furthermore, the urinary FSH preparations used in human therapy until now also contained a certain LH-like activity, so that the final solution of this problem will be possible only using recombinant FSH. Two men bearing a defective FSH β subunit and suffering from azoospermia have been described (Lindstedt et al. 1998; Phillip et al. 1998). One of these patients was normally virilized. These observations suggest that FSH is necessary for the complete initiation of spermatogenesis in man.

> In summary, the results obtained to date indicate that both LH / testosterone and FSH are necessary for qualitatively and quantitatively normal development of spermatogenesis at puberty.

Experimental data obtained in volunteers help to clarify the hormonal contribution to the **maintenance and reinitiation of spermatogenesis**. High doses of testosterone suppress gonadotropin secretion through the negative feedback mechanism and lead to a drastic decrease of sperm numbers in the ejaculate. After administration of FSH the sperm production can reach only about 30 % of the original values. Similarly, hCG administration can also decrease sperm production through the negative

feedback of hCG-stimulated testosterone, although the hCG effect is not as powerful as that obtained by testosterone alone. However, sperm production can be completely restored by giving FSH. In this case too the different efficacy of testosterone and hCG results from the higher intratesticular testosterone concentration.

Spermatogenesis can be clearly reduced in non-human primates and in man by immunoneutralization of FSH (Moudgal and Sairam 1998). Patients with inactivating mutations of the FSH receptors were reported to produce sperm and can be fertile (Tapanainen et al. 1998). It is not entirely clear, however, whether the biological activity was totally abolished in those patients with sperm production and fertility. On the contrary, FSH alone can substantially maintain the spermatogenic process after inhibition of endogenous gonadotropin secretion. This is also suggested by the recent description of a hypophysectomized patient in which an activating mutation of the FSH receptor coexisted with normal spermatogenesis also in the absence of LH (Gromoll et al. 1996). Although the intratesticular testosterone concentrations were not known, the case of this patient suggests that the constitutive activation of the FSH receptor is sufficient for normal spermatogenesis. A possible function of testosterone could therefore be the preparation of the FSH receptor for FSH action.

> From a clinical viewpoint it is concluded that the synergic action of LH, testosterone and FSH is also necessary for the maintenance and possibly for reinitiation of normal spermatogenesis.

3.2.5 Local Regulation of Testicular Function

As described above, the regulation of testicular function is primarily controlled by central structures. The complexity of the testicular cell types and architecture also mandates a variety of local control and regulatory mechanisms. The categories of local interactions and communication can be classified as **paracrine**, referring to factors acting – mainly by diffusion – between neighboring cells; **autocrine**, referring to factors which are released from the cell and work back on the same cell and **intracrine**, referring to factors and substances which never leave the cell and whose site of production and action is the same cell. The term paracrinology has been generally used to describe local interaction and communication between remote cells. Interactions have also been described between the different testicular compartments (Fig. 3.13). Hence, the use of "paracrinology" to characterize all testicular interactions is not correct and the term "local interaction" appears more appropriate (Weinbauer and Wessels 1999).

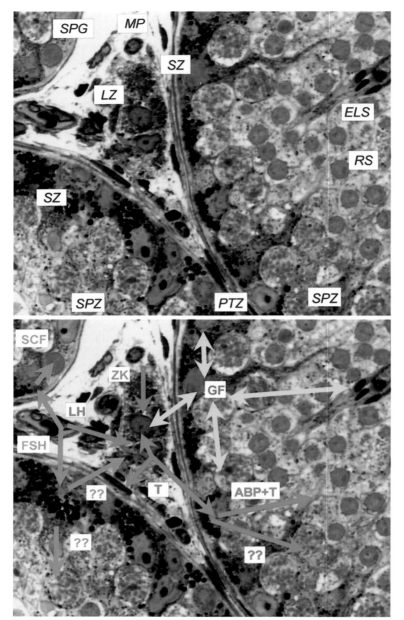

Fig. 3.13. Synopsis of classes of factors exerting local (paracrine and autocrine) effects within the testis. *ES* elongated spermatids, *ELS* elongating spermatids, *LZ* Leydig cells, *MP* macrophage, *RS* round spermatids, *SPZ* spermatocytes, *SPG* spermatogonia, *SZ* Sertoli cells, *PTZ* peritubular cells. *GF* growth facctors, *ABP* androgen binding protein, *T* testosterone, *LH* lutropin, *SCF* stem cell factor, *FSH* follitropin, *ZK* cytokine, *??* unknown factors (from Weinbauer and Wessels 1999)

For the majority of these factors the physiological relevance in vivo and their real meaning for testicular function is, however, not known. It has been demonstrated that the endocrine mechanisms play the central role in the regulation of testicular function. Probably **factors produced locally** are important for the **modulation of hormone activity** and local factors could thus be seen as **mediators of hormone action and intercellular communication**. From this point of view both gametogenesis and endocrine function of the testis are under local control. This view is supported by the fact that the androgen receptor is expressed in a stage-specific manner in the human testis (Fig. 3.14) (Suarez-Quian et al. 1999). While in the past years the Sertoli cell was seen as the coordinator and regulator of germ cell maturation, there are now indications that the germ cell also can influence the secretory activity of Sertoli cell through specific, not yet identified products. In other words, Sertoli cells are under the local control of germ cells, which need different metabolic substances depending on the spermatogenic phase (Franca et al. 1998).

A plethora of factors with potentially local testicular activity has accumulated: growth factors, immunological factors, opioids, oxytocin and vasopressin, peritubu-

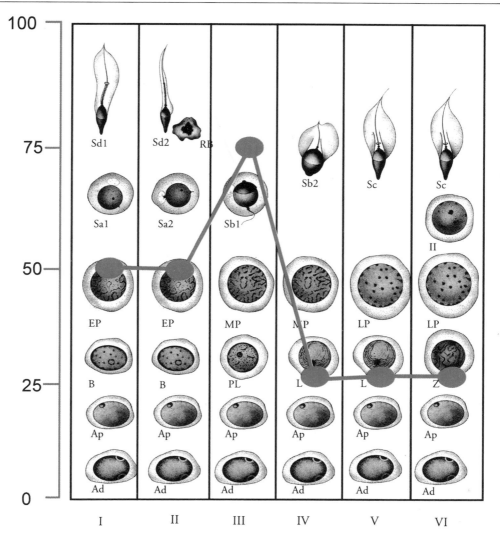

Fig. 3.14. Schematic representation of stage-specific expression of the androgen receptor (*red*) in Sertoli cell of the human testis. Germ cells do not express the androgen receptor. The ordinate indicates the proportion of Sertoli cells that express the androgen receptor. Highest expression is seen immediately after spermiation (stage III), coinciding with the initation of a new spermatogenic cycle. (Based upon Suarez-Quian et al. 1999)

lar cell modifying substance, renin and angiotensin, GHRH, CRH, ACTH, GnRH, calmodulin, ceruloplasmin, transport protein, glycoproteins, plasminogen activator, metalloproteases, dynorphin, PACAP, etc. Moreover, it is postulated that other, still unidentified protein factors could mediate the communication between interstitial and tubular compartments and between Sertoli cells and germ cells. Most of these interactions, either demonstrated or indirectly postulated, originate from results obtained in in-vitro studies. The physiological and biochemical evidence that intratesticular control mechanisms must participate in the regulation of testicular function is obvious and the physiological relevance for testicular function could be demonstrated for some factors. Gene-targeted animal models gain increasing importance in the efforts to unravel the hierarchy of testicular regulatory compounds and substances. These studies also revealed that some of these factors are redundant, i.e. their absence is compensated by backup mechanisms. A local factor with physiological meaning should fulfill the following criteria: production within the testis and action within the testis under in vivo conditions. The following paragraphs refer to the only three substances that meet these criteria and are currently relevant for men.

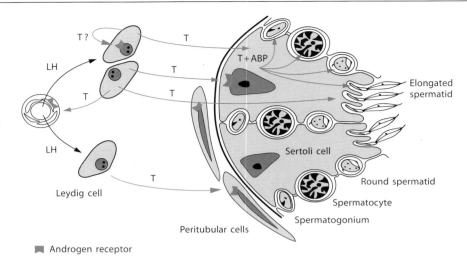

Androgen receptor

3.2.5.1 Testosterone

Testosterone, a classic endocrine factor, is also the **best documented local regulator of spermatogenesis** (Fig. 3.15). Testosterone is produced locally in the Leydig cells and acts locally in the seminiferous tubules. The elimination of testicular testosterone through application of ethane diemethane sulfonate (EDS), a toxin for Leydig cells, leads to profound alterations of germ cell maturation in the rat. Data obtained in mice suggest that the intratesticular transport of testosterone is pivotal for complete spermatogenesis (Takaimya et al. 1998). Thus, testosterone fulfills the requirements of a local regulator of gametogenesis. In boys with Leydig cell tumors, and high local androgen concentrations, seminiferous tubules adjacent to the tumor had complete spermatogenesis, while no sperm production could be seen in the tubules located in tumor-free areas. Similarly, activating mutations of the LH receptor prematurely induce qualitatively normal spermatogenesis (Fig. 3.12). These observations provide compelling evidence that testosterone can locally regulate spermatogenesis.

Testosterone has also other important physiological functions within the testis. In the non-human primate testosterone induces the formation of smooth muscle actin in the peritubular cells during prepubertal testicular maturation (Schlatt et al. 1993). Peritubular cells express the androgen receptor. The testosterone effect is significantly reinforced by FSH. Since FSH receptors are found only in Sertoli cells it follows that FSH influences androgen action indirectly through factors arising in the Sertoli cell. This indicates that as an endocrine factor FSH can also induce the formation of physiologically relevant, locally acting factors in the primate testis. Interestingly, recombinant FSH stimulates testosterone production (Levalle et al. 1998), lending further support to the importance of local interactions between Sertoli

Fig. 3.15. Local effects of testosterone in the human testis. Testosterone is synthesized and secreted in the Leydig cells under the control of LH. Testosterone is released into the blood circulation (endocrine component) and/or binds to testicular target cells (local component). Androgen receptors are found on Leydig cells, peritubular cells and Sertoli cells. Germ cells do not express androgen receptors. Testosterone induces smooth muscle actin production in the contractile peritubular cells and gametogenesis in the seminiferous tubules. Sertoli cells produce androgen binding protein (ABP). Testosterone influences cellular contacts between Sertoli cells and spermatids

cells, Leydig cells and peritubular cells in connection with the actions of androgens and gonadotropins. Testosterone stimulates the production of another factor in the peritubular cells, the **peritubular modifying substance** (PmodS), which influences the secretion of products from Sertoli cells (Skinner 1993). PmodS mediates stroma-epithelial interactions in general and also influences the prostate. The meaning of this observation for the physiology of Sertoli cells is unclear, since Sertoli cells possess receptors for androgens and are direct target cells for testosterone. Also, testosterone directly modulates Leydig cell function and androgen receptor expression in Leydig cells (Shan et al. 1997).

> Testosterone acts both as an endocrine and local (paracrine and autocrine) factor within the testis.

3.2.5.2 Growth factors

Growth factors bind to surface receptors and induce cell-specific differentiation events via specific signal transduction cascades. The main growth factors participating in the local regulation of spermatogenesis are **transforming growth factor** (TGF)-α and -β, **inhibin** and **activin, nerve growth factor** (NGF), **insulin-like growth factor** I (IGF-I) and **epidermal growth factor** (EGF).

Inhibin and activin have been detected not only in Sertoli cells, but also in Leydig cells of primates (Andersson et al. 1998; Toppari et al. 1998; Vliegen et al. 1993). Inhibins and activins are structurally related proteins. The heterodimer inhibin consists of an α subunit and a βA or βB subunit whereas activins are homodimers (βAβA or βBβB). It has been suggested that the inhibin βB subunit is expressed in human germ cells (Andersson et al. 1998). Generally, activins are considered to stimulate spermatogonial proliferation whereas inhibins exert inhibitory actions. Of considerable clinical interest are recent discoveries that serum concentrations of inhibin are correlated with spermatogenic activity, testis size and sperm production. This growth factor can actually be used as an endocrine indicator of local spermatogenic defects (von Eckardstein et al. 1999).

In vitro studies have suggested that the local function of inhibin and activin could be a modulation of steroidogenic activity in Leydig cells. Activins inhibit or stimulate Leydig cell steroidogenesis in a species-dependent manner. Generally, IGF-I and TGF-α exert a stimulatory activity in the testis, while TGF-β acts as an inhibitor. In the rat, the development of Leydig cells is sustained by an interplay between TGF-α and TGF-β. Several studies have demonstrated that the activity of LH on the Leydig cell is modulated by IGF-I. In the human Leydig cell the steroidogenic activity is also stimulated by EGF. This growth factor directly influences spermatogenesis: IGF-I concentrations are positively related to the number of pachytene spermatocytes (Weinbauer and Wessels 1999). In man, IGF-I shows the highest expression in these spermatocytes and stimulates DNA synthesis in mitotic germ cells. An important role of NGF for the structural organization of the human seminiferous tubules is postulated, since the culture of seminiferous tubules can be successful only in the presence of NGF. NGF has been localized in peritubular cells by immunocytochemistry. In the rat, NGF is an important regulator of meiotic division.

3.2.5.3 Cytokines

These are low molecular weight secretory proteins such as **interferon, tumor necrosis factor** (TNF), interleukins, leukemia inhibing factor (LIF), **stem cell factor** (SCF), **macrophage migration inhibiting factor** (MIF) that bind to cell surface receptors and provoke cell proliferation and differentiation. TNF and LIF are suspected to play a role in **Sertoli cell-germ cell interactions** and in the autocrine control of Sertoli cell proliferation (Be-

nahmed et al. 1997; Hara et al. 1998). MIF is produced specifically by Leydig cells (Meinhardt et al. 1999). Interestingly, MIF is found in Sertoli cells, basal germ cells and peritubular cells following elimination of Leydig cells, indicating that compensatory mechanisms maintain testicular MIF production. Whereas originally a testicular function had been proposed for interleukin-1, this concept is questioned by observations that interleukin-1 receptor type 1-deficient mice are fertile (Cohen and Pollard 1998). Unlike interleukins, SCF and its receptor (**c-kit**) are clearly essential local factors that govern germ cell migration during ontogenesis and spermatogonial differentiation in the adult testis (Orth et al. 1997; Schrans-Stassen et al. 1999). SCF is synthesized and secreted by Sertoli cells whereas the receptor is expressed on spermatogonial surfaces (Loveland and Schlatt 1997; Sandlow et al. 1997). Whether seminal SCF concentrations and spermatogenic disturbances are correlated (Fujisawa et al. 1998) requires further clarification. **C-kit** receptor is also found in seminoma and **carcinoma in-situ** cells (Rajper de Meyts and Skakkebaek 1994). In F344 rats, a strain with particularly high incidence of testicular tumors, 80% of tumor cells were found to express **c-kit** receptor (Kondoh et al. 1997). It is yet unclear, however, whether a direct relationship exists between SCF/**c-kit** expression and testicular tumor development.

The SCF/**c-kit** system provides an important in-vivo example for the need of local testicular interactions.

3.3 Testicular Descent

The testis is positioned caudally during the 10th–15th week of pregnancy until the entry of the **inguinal canal** (**transabdominal phase of descent**). The caudal ligament that derived from the caudal mesorchium and the renal anlage, converts into the **gubernaculum**. From week 25 of pregnancy onwards, the gubernaculum – following a transient period of extension and paralleled by the degeneration of the cranial ligament – is shortened. These events permit the transposition of the testis into the inguinal canal and along a peritoneal protrusion, the processus vaginalis, into the scrotum (**inguino-scrotal phase of descent**). By week 28 the testis and epididymis finally move through the inguinal canal. The gubernaculum degenerates. At birth, the testes reach at the bottom of the scrotum and in 97% of boys testicular descent is completed within another 12 weeks.

The incidence of positional anomalies of the testis is 2% and ranges among the most common congenital defects. These defects are associated with spermatogenic disturbances and increased risk of testicular tumor development (see Chapt. 8 for details). To date, the physiological and endocrine mechanisms that govern testicular descent are not known in detail. Animal studies sug-

gest that androgens induce the decay of the cranial ligament, a precondition for testicular descent (Emmen et
al. 1998). The formation of the gubernaculum seems to
depend on the production of an insulin-like factor by the
Leydig cells (Nef and Parada 1999; Zimmermann et al.
1999). Although patients with altered Muellerian-inhib-
iting hormone (MIS) or its receptor display positional
anomalies, it is not entirely clear whether MIS is involved in testicular descent. The inguino-scrotal phase
of testicular descent is thought to be independent of androgen actions (Hutson et al. 1997). Human gubernacu-
la were shown to contain binding sites for androgenic
hormones and the number of binding sites was reduced
in patients with maldescended testes (Hosie et al. 1999).
Some evidence exists for an involvement of the N. geni-
tofemoralis in testis desecent.

3.4. Vascularization, Temperature Regulation and Spermatogenesis

The **vascularization of the testis** has two main roles:
transport and mobilization of endocrine factors and
metabolites and **regulation of testicular temperature.**
The arterial supply of the testicular parenchyma follows
the lobular division of the seminiferous tubules. Each
lobulus is supplied by one artery from which segmental
arteries originate at a distance of about 300 μm from
each other, supplying blood to the lateral regions of the
lobuli (Ergün et al. 1994a and b). Segmental arteries and
capillaries become branched between the Leydig cells
and finally give rise to the venous system (Fig. 3.16). In
men, the testicular temperature is about 3–4 °C below
core body temperature and about 1.5–2.5 °C above the
temperature of scrotal skin (Mieusset and Bujan 1995).
For the maintenance of a physiologically lower temperature the testis relies on two thermoregulatory systems.
Heat can be transferred to the external environment
through the **scrotal skin**, as the scrotal skin is very thin,
possesses hardly any subcutaneous fat tissue and has a
very large surface. It is of interest that among mammals
a phylogenetic tendency towards the loss of the scrotum
has been suggested (Werdelin and Nilssone 1999). The
explanation has been put forward from the evolutionary
point of view that testicular descent is a costly event for
merely cooling the testis and is avoided or given up once
alternatives become available. The second regulatory
system is the **pampiniform plexus**. In this system, the
convoluted testicular artery is surrounded by several
veins coiling around the artery several times. Arterial
blood arriving at the testis is thereby cooled down by the
surrounding venous blood.

In case of a **varicocele**, a local disturbance of the
venous circulation, there is an **increase of the scrotal
temperature** (Lerchl et al. 1993). An increase of testicular
temperature results in damage of the spermatogenetic

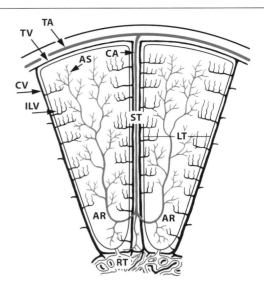

Fig. 3.16. Schematic representation of the testicular blood supply. Each lobulus is supplied by a recurrent artery. Segmental
arteries originate at a distance of about 300 μm from each other, become capillaries and then originate veins. *AR* recurrent
artery, *AS* segmental artery, *CA* centripetal artery, *CV* centrifugal vein, *ILV* intralobular vein, *LT* testicular lobulus, *RT* Rete
testis, *ST* testicular septum, *TA* testicular artery, *TV* testicular
vein. (Modified from Ergün et al. 1994a)

function of the testis. If the testicular temperature is increased in adults, the spermatogenic damage is reversible. Most importantly, however, substantial increase of
temperature must be achieved. Scrotal temperature elevations by 0.8–1° C over a period of 52 weeks in healthy
volunteers had no adverse effect on the number and
quality of spermatozoa (Wang et al. 1997). It is currently
unknown by which cellular and molecular mechanisms
spermatogenesis is destroyed in a heated testis (Setchell
1998). A possible explanation for the need of a cool testis is that a G protein essential for endocrine signal
transduction located in the testis is active only at 34 and
not at 37 °C (Iiri et al. 1994). Although testicular temperature is lower than body temperature in the majority of
mammals, this difference is not obligatory in every species. In elephants and whales the testes remain in the inguinal canal or in the abdominal cavity and yet functional, even at body temperature.

3.5 Immunology of the Testis

Gonocytes migrate to the testis even during prenatal development, but spermatogonia begin to differentiate into spermatozoa only at puberty. As the spermatogonia
proliferate and differentiate into spermatocytes, **novel
antigens** are expressed that are unique to these cells. At
the same time, adjacent Sertoli cells form complex net-
works of tight junctions that cause isolation of the tubu-

lar contents from the blood vascular compartment. The **blood-testis barrier** provides a **separation** between immune cells and products from most spermatogenic antigens. Because the spermatogenic cells are largely isolated from the immune system, they are not subjected to the usual mechanism that induces tolerance to self-antigens and thus remain autoimmunogenic. However, autoantigens are also expressed in cells located outside the inter-Sertoli cell tight junctions, e.g. in the basal compartment of the seminiferous epithelium and are recognized as foreign (Pöllänen and Cooper 1994). These antigens, however, do not stimulate the immune response and it is well known that allografts transplanted into the testis outside the barrier can survive much longer compared to other tissues. Thus, it would appear that the immune privilege of the testis is not only due to the blood-testis barrier, but also depends on a specific intratesticular regulation of the immune system function, possibly mediated by humoral factors (Hedger 1997). The physiological basis for this resides in the fact that only few or no T helper lymphocytes are present in the interstitium, and that immunocompetence will be activated to a rather low extent. Another mechanism that has been proposed is that Sertoli cells expressing the CD95 ligand and activated T lymphocytes bearing CD95 (FAS/Apo-1), will be eliminated by apoptosis (Bellgrau et al. 1995). The pattern of surface antigen expression changes dramatically during spermatogenesis. Differences in antigenic expression of more than 50% have been found between mature sperm and spermatogonia.

The normal cell population of the testis also includes **macrophages**. Testicular macrophages are found as early as week 7 of gestation and probably originate from hematopoietic precursor cells that migrate to the testis. Macrophages proliferate in the testis during postnatal life, probably under pituitary control, since hCG is able to increase the mitotic index of testicular macrophages in rats. In the adult, human testis macrophages represent about 25% of all interstitial cells. Morphologically and biochemically they are similar to macrophages resident in other tissues. Macrophages participate in normal immunological surveillance by presenting the antigens for cell-mediated immunity and are capable of phagocytosis. In man and in seasonally reproducing animals, macrophages are also found within the seminiferous epithelium. The physiological relevance of testicular macrophages for the immune response is not known.

Lymphocytes migrate through tissues as a part of the normal process of immune surveillance. **In the testis the activity of the immune system is thought to be inhibited by locally produced factors.** For example, Leydig cells are able to adhere to lymphocytes and suppress their proliferation. Normal testes of adult men have been shown to contain very few T lymphocytes and abundant macrophages, but no B lymphocytes are normally present.

An important role in the immune control of the testis is played by the endothelium. Testicular endothelial cells are less permeable to dyes than other organs, and the uptake of many substances from the circulation is cell-mediated. The maturation of testicular microvessels occurs at puberty and is hormone-dependent. Remarkably, in the rat endothelial cells express the hCG/LH receptor and hCG/LH influence the vascular permeability (Ghinea and Milgrom 1995). Most probably, the immune privilege of the testis is brought about by the interstitial cells rather than the blood testis barrier (Hedger 1997).

The number of mononuclear cells increases in case of testicular disease. In about 5% of testicular biopsies from infertile men lymphoid cells surround the tubules with markedly higher spermatogenic damage. Similarly, mononuclear infiltrates are often associated with carcinoma in situ. Seminomas generally show a very conspicuous infiltration of immunocompetent cells. Mumps can be complicated by a severe testicular inflammation in 35% of cases. As infertility ensues frequently, it is conceivable that an activation of the immune system triggers the immunological reaction of the germinal epithelium (Mahi-Brown 1994). Recently, it was postulated that the size and number of testicular mast cells correlates with spermatogenic defects (Jezek et al. 1999).

3.6 Testicular Androgens

Androgens are essential for the development and function of testes, maturation of secondary sexual characteristics, masculinization of the bone-muscle apparatus, libido, and stimulation of spermatogenesis. Physiologi-

Fig. 3.17. a Steroid biosynthesis in the Leydig cell. Steroid biosynthesis is induced by LH through activation of adenylyl cyclase. Starting material is cholesterol or acetate. The C atoms of cholesterol are numbered in order to follow better the different enzymatic modifications and their localization. StAR (Steroidogenic acute regulatory protein) plays a key role during steroidogenesis. StAR is localized to the inner mitochondrial membrane and governs cholesterol transport. **b** Peripheral transport of testosterone (T) in blood is achieved as a T-SHBG complex. Upon arrival at the target organ, T is released from SHBG and enters the cell probably via passive diffusion. **c** Cellular mechanism of action of T reaches the target cell through passive diffusion. In the target cell 5α-reduction to dehydrotestosterone (DHT) occurs only in certain organs. DHT or T binds to the androgen receptor and causes a change in the conformation, leading to cleavage from heatshock protein (HSP). The resulting T/DHT-androgen receptor complex can be activated through phosphorylation (not shown) and forms a dimer through combination of two complexes in diametrically opposed orientation. This dimer recognizes the androgen-sensitive region (ASR) of DNA, leading to stimulation of transcription and synthesis of androgen-dependent genes. Transactivation of the T/DHT androgen receptor complex can be modified by specific coactivators and corepressors. By means of this, cell-specific androgen effects are achieved

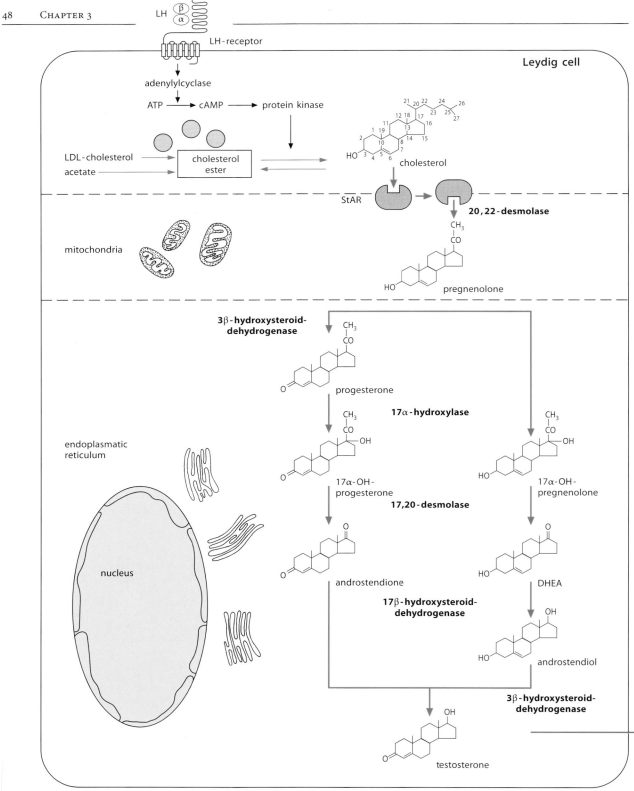

Δ^4-pathway Δ^5-pathway

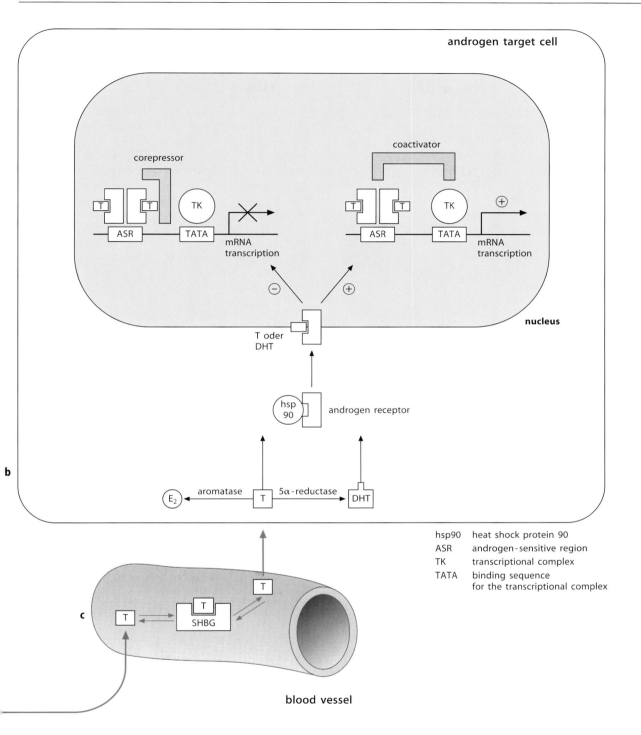

androgen target cell

coactivator

corepressor

TK

TK

ASR   TATA

ASR   TATA

mRNA
transcription

mRNA
transcription

⊖   ⊕

nucleus

T oder
DHT

hsp
90   androgen receptor

b

E₂   aromatase   T   5α-reductase   DHT

hsp90   heat shock protein 90
ASR   androgen-sensitive region
TK   transcriptional complex
TATA   binding sequence
         for the transcriptional complex

c   T   SHBG   T

blood vessel

cal effects of androgens depend on different factors such as number of androgen molecules and distribution of androgens and their metabolites inside the cell, interaction with the receptor and receptor activation. In turn, the androgen concentration in the organism depends on the synthesis rate, balanced by metabolic conversion and excretion (Mooradian et al. 1987; Rommerts 1998).

In men, **testosterone** is by far the most important and abundant androgen in blood. More than 95% of the existing androgens derive from the testis, which synthesizes about **6–7 mg testosterone per day**. The remaining contribution to androgen production derives mainly from the adrenals. The site of androgen production in the testis is the Leydig cell. Both synthesis and secretion are under regulation of pituitary LH and local paracrine factors (Saez 1994; Saez and Lejeune 1996).

Since Leydig cells cannot store androgens, **de novo biosynthesis** continuously takes place. The starting point for androgen synthesis is cholesterol, a fundamental substance of metabolism, with the typical steroid ring conformation energetically compatible with the transformation into androgens. Cholesterol can either be incorporated by the cell through receptor-mediated endocytosis from low-density lipoproteins (LDL), or can be synthesized de novo within the Leydig cell starting from acetyl-coenzyme A. Cholesterol is stored in cytoplasmic lipid droplets. The number of lipid droplets is inversely related to the rate of androgen synthesis in the Leydig cell, i. e. a high synthesis rate leads to a low content of lipid droplets and vice versa.

3.6.1 Synthesis of Androgens

Androgen synthesis requires the conversion of **cholesterol** to testosterone (Fig. 3.17). This transformation goes through 5 different enzymatic steps in which the side chain of cholesterol is shortened through oxidation from 27 C to 19 C. The steroidal A-ring assumes a keto configuration at position 3. The starting point for the transformation of cholesterol into testosterone is the shortening of the side chain through C 22 and C 20 hydroxylases, followed by cleavage of the bond between C 20 and C 22, leading to production of **pregnenolone**. The steps following pregnenolone formation occur in the endoplasmic reticulum either through the $\Delta 4$ or through the $\Delta 5$ **pathway**. The designation $\Delta 4$ or $\Delta 5$ refers to the localization of the double bond in the steroid. The $\Delta 5$ pathway is predominant over the $\Delta 4$ in human steroid synthesis. Along the $\Delta 4$ pathway, pregnenolone is dehydrated to **progesterone**, a key biological substance. The $\Delta 4$ pathway proceeds to the intermediate **17α-hydroxyprogesterone**. If the side chain is removed at this stage, the intermediate androstene-3,17-dione is produced, which, through further reduction at position C 17, is then transformed into testosterone. In the $\Delta 5$ synthesis path-

way, testosterone synthesis occurs through the intermediates **17-hydroxypregnenolone** and **dehydroepiandrosterone**.

For many years, the transformation of cholesterol into pregnenolone was considered the limiting step in testosterone synthesis. Meanwhile, however, it became clear that the key role is held by a regulatory mitochondrial protein. **The steroidogenic acute regulatory protein (StAR)** has a molecular weight of 30 kD and mediates the transport of sterols such as cholesterol from the outer towards the inner mitochondrial membrane (Stocco 1999). At this site cytochrome P450ssc (ssc = side chain cleavage) catalyzes the conversion into pregnenolone. The mechanism underlying the binding of StAR to cholesterol and the transmembrane transport must still be clarified. StAR mRNA expression is triggered by endocrine stimuli and rapid translation in steroidogenic cells. StAR is widely distributed in steroidogenic tissues including the adrenals and corpora lutea. The physiological importance of StAR is highlighted by the phenotype of patients with an inactivating mutation of the StAR gene. These patients suffer from life-threatening congenital adrenal hyperplasia as they are unable to produce the necessary amounts of steroids (Lin et al. 1995).

The enzyme **cytochrome P450ssc** is responsible for the different enzymatic reactions leading to the production of pregnenolone. Like other steroid synthetic enzymes, it belongs to the group of mono-oxygenases, containing the prosthetic hemogroup of hemoglobin and localized on the internal membrane of mitochondria. The intermediate compound pregnenolone is transformed into testosterone through the enzyme cytochrome P450 C17, also belonging to the group of mono-oxygeneses and located in the endoplasmic reticulum. The overall enzymatic system, however, is not capable of transforming every molecule of pregnenolone into testosterone so that several intermediates are produced.

Testosterone is the main secretory product of the testis, along with 5α-dihydrotestosterone (DHT), androsterone, androstenedione, 17-hydroxyprogesterone, progesterone and pregnenolone. The function of androsterone, progesterone and 17-hydroxyprogesterone in the testis is unknown. The transformation of testosterone into DHT takes place principally in the target organs, e. g. prostate. **Androstenedione** is important as a precursor for the production of extratesticular **estrogens** (Hall 1994). Only a very small portion of the testosterone produced is stored in the testis and the androgen is mainly secreted in blood. Testosterone concentration in the testicular lymphatic circulation and in the venous blood are very similar, but there are essential differences in the flow rate and velocity of both systems. Therefore, transport of testosterone in the general blood circulation occurs mainly through the spermatic vein (Sharpe 1994). The mechanism for testosterone transport from the Leydig cell into the blood or lymph is not completely known. Probably lipophilic steroids distributed within cells or small cell groups are released through passive diffusion.

3.6.2 Testosterone Transport in Blood

Testosterone is transported in plasma mainly bound to albumin or to **sex hormone binding globulin (SHBG)**. SHBG is a β globulin consisting of different protein subunits. It is produced in the testis and in the liver. SHBG is about 95 kDa in molecular weight, 30% of which is represented by carbohydrate, and possesses one androgen binding site per molecule.

In normal men, only 2% of total testosterone circulates freely in blood, while 44% is bound to SHBG and 54% to albumin. The binding affinity of testosterone to albumin is about 100 times lower compared to SHBG. However, since albumin concentration is much higher than that of SHBG, the binding capacity of both proteins for testosterone is about the same. The ratio of testosterone bound to SHBG over free SHBG is proportional to SHBG concentration. The dissociation of testosterone from binding proteins takes place in capillaries. The interaction of binding proteins with the endothelial glycocalyx leads to a structural modification of the hormonal binding site and thereby to a change in affinity. As a result testosterone is set free and can diffuse freely into the target cell. Hence, SHBG fulfills a central function in the **control of the availability of free testosterone**. Whether only free testosterone or also the fraction dissociating from SHBG constitutes the biologically active testosterone, is still a matter of debate (Griffin and Wilson 1994). Recent data suggest that the **testosterone-SHBG complex** itself is capable of binding to a specific membrane-bound receptor followed by the activation of adenylyl cyclase, synthesis of cAMP and modification of the transcriptional acitivity of the androgen receptor (Rosner et al. 1999).

SHBG is also capable of estradiol binding and is therefore also called testosterone-estradiol-binding globulin (TEBG). The type of binding is influenced by the different SHBG isoforms. For example, it could be demonstrated that post-translational changes in the carbohydrate structure of SHBG can lead to different binding affinity of the protein to testosterone and estradiol. SHBG concentration in serum is under hormonal regulation. In normal, healthy men with an intact hypothalamus-pituitary-testicular axis, an increase in plasma concentrations of SHBG leads to an acute decrease of free testosterone and simultaneous stimulation of testosterone synthesis, persisting until achievement of normal concentrations. Both increases and decreases of SHBG concentrations can be restored through this control system. SHBG concentration in man is about one third to one half of the concentration found in women. SHBG concentrations can be elevated in hypogonadal men.

3.6.3 Extratesticular Metabolism of Testosterone

Testosterone is a precursor of two important hormones: through 5α-reduction it gives rise to the highly biologically active hormone **5α-dihydrotestosterone (DHT)**, and through aromatization to estradiol. Estrogens influence testosterone effects by acting either synergistically or antagonistically. Moreover, estrogens have other specific effects which were originally described to be typical of testosterone. It has been found that inactivating mutations of the estrogen receptor or aromatase, preventing estrogen action on the bones, result in continuous linear growth and lack of epiphyseal closure. This important metabolic activity affecting bone had been previously seen as a typical androgen-dependent effect (Carani et al. 1997; Smith et al. 1994).

Reduction of testosterone to DHT occurs in the endoplasmic reticulum through the enzyme 5α-reductase. Two isoforms of this enzyme could be identified in humans. The gene for 5α-reductase type I is located on chromosome 5, while the gene for the 5α-reductase type II is on chromosome 2. The two isoforms are very similar to each other, but show different biochemical properties. Type I enzyme works optimally at alkaline pH, while the optimal pH for type II is acidic. Also, the tissue distribution of the two forms is different. Type I 5α-reductase has been localized in the skin, liver and brain, while type II is active in classical androgen-dependent tissues, such as the epididymis and prostate. At the cellular level, DHT sustains differentiation and growth and is particularly important for normal sexual development and virilization in men. Overall, testosterone effects result from influences of the hormone itself and of its metabolites estradiol and DHT. Changes in the property of type II 5α-reductase due to mutation can result in male pseudohermaphroditism (see Chap. 11). DHT is inactivated through reduction to 17-ketosteroids, and excreted in the urine.

Some androgen metabolites are excreted in free form, others are glucuronated by the liver before excretion. Owing to the high activity of enzymes metabolising steroids in the liver, the half-life of testosterone in plasma is only about 12 minutes, notwithstanding the protein binding.

3.6.4 Mechanism of Androgen Action

Testosterone dissociates from SHBG at the target organ and diffuses into the cells. The conversion of testosterone into DHT is organ-dependent. This occurs, for ex-

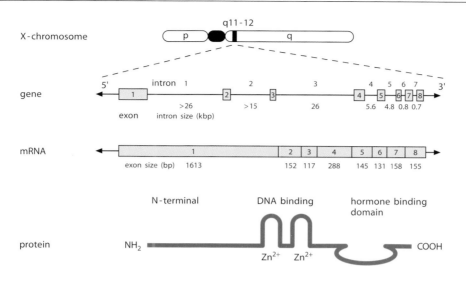

Fig. 3.18. Chromosomal localization of the androgen receptor and structure of the androgen receptor gene and protein. Upper figure: the gene for the androgen receptor is localized in the pericentromeric region of chromosome X, at the site Xq11–12. Middle figure: the entire gene encompasses a region of about 90 kilobase pairs (kbp) on genomic DNA. Different exons are represented by boxes 1–8, with corresponding intron sizes reported below. Exon 1 encodes the N-terminal region, exon 2–3 the DNA binding domain and exon 4–8 the steroid binding domain. Lower figure: schematic representation of the androgen receptor protein with the different functional domains

ample, in the prostate, where DHT is the main biologically active androgen (Mooradian et al. 1987). The first step in androgen action is binding to the androgen receptor which belongs to the family of steroid hormone receptors. These receptors have a typical mechanism of action: they bind to specific sequences of genomic DNA and induce stimulation of RNA synthesis. Mineralcorticoid, glucocorticoid, thyroid hormone, retinol, estrogen and progesterone receptors also belong to this family. These receptors share substantial similarities (Mangelsdorf et al. 1995). Members of this receptor family possess an N-terminal domain, a DNA-binding domain and a hormone-binding domain (Fig. 3.18).

While the DNA-binding domain and the hormone-binding domain show a high homology to the corresponding domains in the mineralocorticoid, glucocorticoid and progesterone receptors, the N-terminal domain has little similarity to the other steroid receptors. The precise function of this domain is not known yet, but it could participate in DNA binding, and transactivation and transrepression of the androgen receptor (Choong and Wilson 1998; Gast et al. 1998). An important characteristic of the N-terminal domain is the pres-

ence of CAG repeats, coding for glutamine. In normal men, about 17–29 of these repeats are present, while in patients with Kennedy disease, a disease affecting motoneurons, up to 72 such repeats are present (McLean et al. 1995, see also Chapt. 11). Data are available to suggest that glutamine repeats permit interaction with coactivators. Increased repeat length is associated with diminished coactivator interaction and transcriptional activity (Hsiao et al. 1999). These findings provide the first molecular basis for the understanding of the pathophysiology of Kennedy syndrome and the associated androgen insensitivity. The number of glutamine repeats of the androgen receptor has been associated with azoospermia or oligozoospermia. However, the results reported in these investigations are highly controversial and final conclusions are not yet warranted (Tut et al. 1997; Dowsing et al. 1999).

The **androgen receptor gene** is located on the **X-chromosome** and spans about 90 kb. The coding sequence, containing the sequence of nucleotides translated into amino acids, consists of 8 exons. The N-terminal domain is fully encoded by exon 1, while DNA-binding domain is encoded by exon 2 and 3 and steroid-binding domain by exons 4–8. Similar to all the other steroid receptors, the DNA-binding domain of the androgen receptor contains two zinc fingers. This domain is about 70 amino acids long and is localized between the N-terminal and the androgen-binding domain. In this part of the sequence, 8 cysteines are spatially arranged such that 4 sulphurs keep one zinc in place, giving rise to the typical structure of two overlapping helices. Exon 2 and 3 of the androgen receptor encode for the DNA-binding domain. While the first zinc finger, encoded by exon 2, is important for the specific binding of the androgen receptor to DNA, the second zinc finger, encoded by exon 3, stabilizes **DNA receptor interaction** due to its basic nature, interacting with the negatively charged phosphate groups of DNA, leading to dimerization of two receptor molecules. In immediate proximity to the DNA-binding domain, a short amino acid sequence is responsible for the transport of the receptor into the nucleus.

The androgen-binding domain of the androgen receptor encompasses about 30 % of the overall receptor (the DNA-binding domain about 10 %) and is responsible for the specific binding of androgens. This domain forms a hydrophobic pocket based upon 24 amino acids that enables the binding of testosterone (Wurtz et al. 1996). Experimental deletion of this domain results in increased gene transcription **in vitro**. Obviously, this part of the receptor is necessary for inducible and regulated gene transcription. This conclusion is also derived from the presence of particular sequences in this domain, which can bind the so-called heatshock proteins and thereby inactivate the receptor (Hippaku and Liao 1995). Most probably, the free receptor located in the cytosol (Paris et al. 1994) undergoes a conformational change owing to testosterone binding, giving rise to the hormone receptor complex. Heatshock proteins such as protein 90 (HSP 90) are responsible for the maintenance of the receptor in the inactive state and are released from the complex. The loss of this protein leads to uncovering of the functional domains of the receptor and is necessary for nuclear transport, dimerization and DNA binding. Moreover, androgen binding leads to receptor phosphorylation, a post-translational process, probably involved in receptor stabilization. DHT binds to the androgen receptor with higher affinity than testosterone, mainly because testosterone is more quickly dissociated from the receptor. Other steroids such as androstenedione, estradiol and progesterone bind to the androgen receptor with much lower affinity than testosterone.

The androgen receptor can interact with DNA in a homodimeric form consisting of two identical hormone receptor complexes. The time sequence of events is not known. Dimerization has been observed following androgen binding or only after interaction of the complex with DNA. The hormone receptor complex is now transferred from the cytosol into the nucleus of the cell where it recognizes specific sequences of genomic DNA. Interaction with DNA occurs through the two zinc fingers in the DNA-binding domain. Dimers bind to DNA sequences known as androgen responsive elements which contain typical palindromic sequences, i. e. DNA tracts with a nucleotide sequence independent of the reading direction. These DNA sequences are typical for androgen-dependent genes and function as binding sites for the androgen receptor. Palindromes partially explain the interaction of the androgen receptor with DNA in dimeric form. However, there are sequences capable of high affinity binding of the hormone receptor complex which show only minor resemblance to a palindromic sequence. Binding of testosterone to its receptor results

in the formation of a transcription complex consisting of androgen/androgen receptor, an RNA polymerase, several transcription factors and DNA. This transcription complex induces mRNA synthesis of androgen-dependent genes and, after mRNA translation, synthesis of new androgen-dependent proteins.

The activity of the transcriptional complex is regulated by co-activators and co-repressors. **Co-activators** increase and **co-repressors** decrease the transcriptional acitivity of the receptor. Functionally, the association between the transcriptional complex and DNA and hence receptor activity are modified. This family of proteins comprises CPB/3000, ARA 54 and testis-specific ARIP-3 (Moilanen et al. 1999). Since the androgen receptor is expressed ubiquitously in the body the question arises how tissue specificity of androgen action is achieved. It is currently assumed that this specificity is conveyed through tissue and organ-specific coactivators and corepressors. Current and future activities concentrate on selective androgen receptor modulators (SARMs), analogous to the SERMs for the estrogen receptor, in order to develop SARMs that, for example, only influence muscle growth but leave cardiovascular risk parameters unaltered (Vilar 1999).

Our understanding of the transactivation of the androgen receptor, i. e. the expression of androgen-dependent genes, has witnessed great advances during recent years. It was found that DHT activates other signal transduction pathways in prostate cell lines. DHT induced a transient stimulation of mitogen-activated protein (MAP) kinases which are known to be involved in the control of cell proliferation. These observation raise the exciting possibility that the androgen receptor can also act as a cytosolic activator.

Primary products of gene activation stimulated by the androgen receptor are not known yet. It is postulated that proteins are produced, which, in turn, can stimulate a cascade of other molecular events. Many secondary proteins, originating from primary androgen effects such as probasin and factor IX are known (Quigley 1998). One of them is the **prostate specific antigen** (PSA) (Quigley et al. 1995). The gene transcription of PSA is under androgen influence, since the PSA gene contains an androgen-binding element which can interact with the androgen receptor. Androgens, moreover, have other posttranscriptional effects on PSA. Androgens, however, not only have stimulating effects on gene transcription, but can also inhibit gene synthesis.

Androgen receptor defects such as deletions or inactivating mutations can profoundly alter **receptor function**. The resulting phenotype is highly variable ranging from undervirilization to testicular feminization.

Full elimination of the androgen receptor gene results in a female phenotype owing to the complete lack of all androgen activity (see Chapt. 11). Similar clinical consequences are also typical for mutations which severely damage the function of the androgen receptor, such as those in the DNA-binding or androgen-binding domain. Moreover, mutations in the N-terminal domain, which can decrease but not completely eliminate the function of the androgen receptor, might play a role in male idiopathic infertility. It would appear that the number of **CAG triplets** influences the transcriptional activity of the androgen receptor but its relationship to disturbances of spermatogenesis is unclear. Some oligozoospermic men bearing a mutation in the ligand-binding domain have been identified. It could be shown for the first time that the diminished ability for dimerization caused a reduction in transactivational activity. This affects the binding of coactivators and the formation of a functionally intact transcriptional complex (Ghadessy et al. 1999). Mutations in the androgen receptor could be also demonstrated in patients with prostate carcinoma, both in the primary tumor tissue and in metastases. However, it is not clear whether these mutations are the cause of the tumor development (McLean et al. 1995; Tilley et al. 1996).

No direct correlation has been found between the type of androgen receptor mutation and the phenotype. This suggests the involvement of additional factors besides the androgen receptor during androgen action.

3.6.5 Biological Actions of Androgens

In primates, the androgen receptor can be found not only in the classical androgen-dependent organs, such as muscles, prostate, seminal vesicles, epididymis and testes, but also in almost every tissue, e.g. hypothalamus, pituitary, kidney, spleen, heart, salivary glands (Dankbar et al. 1995). In the testis, the androgen receptor is expressed in peritubular cells, Leydig cells and Sertoli cells, while the germ cells to do not seem to express it. The regulation of androgen receptor expression at the transcriptional and translational level is complex and depends on factors such as age, cell type and tissue. Generally, androgens have a positive effect on stabilization of the receptor protein, so that androgen administration leads to inhibition of receptor degradation and thereby to an increase in androgen receptor protein levels. The effects of androgens on the androgen receptor mRNA are opposite. In this case, androgen administration leads to down-regulation of the androgen receptor mRNA by shortening of the mRNA half-life.

Androgens are important in every phase of human life. During the **embryonal stage**, testosterone determines the **differentiation of the sexual organs**, during puberty, the further development toward the **adult male**

phenotype which is then maintained along with important anabolic **functions**. DHT is the main androgen acting on **epididymis**, **vas deferens**, **seminal vesicles** and **prostate**, originating from testosterone through 5α-reductase. These tissues are particularly dependent on continuous androgen action. In addition, testosterone aromatization to estrogens plays an important role in prostate growth. Estrogen concentrations in prostate stromal tissue are clearly increased in case of benign prostate hyperplasia (BPH). In the epididymis, seminal vesicles and vas deferens the lack of testosterone can result in regression of the secretory epithelia, eventually leading to aspermia (ejaculation failure). The testosterone effects in the epididymis, seminal vesicle and vas deferens are mediated through testosterone, DHT and estradiol.

Both testosterone and DHT are necessary for normal **penis** growth, which is positively correlated with the increasing testosterone concentrations during puberty. However, androgen receptors are no longer expressed in the penis of adult men and any androgen deficiency after puberty results in only minor decrease of penis size. Similarly, testosterone administration to adults is not capable of increasing penis size.

Testosterone is the main androgen present in **muscles**, which have very low 5α-reductase activity. Testosterone has direct anabolic effects both in smooth and in striated muscles with an increase of muscular mass and hypertrophy of the fibres. The number of muscular fibres, however, does not change. Loss of testosterone leads to muscular atrophy. As consequence of testosterone action, mRNA synthesis and glycogen synthesis increase in the striated muscles. Testosterone also has an anabolic effect in the heart, increasing mRNA synthesis.

Both androgens and estrogens induce an increase of the **bone density** by stimulating mineralization, while the lack of these steroids results in osteoporosis. At the beginning of puberty, the increase in linear growth of bones is directly correlated with increasing testosterone concentrations. At the end of puberty, depending on the presence of testosterone, epiphyseal closure occurs, an event that can be consistently delayed in the presence of low testosterone concentrations. It is clear now that the androgen action on bone metabolism is mediated through estradiol (Carani et al. 1997). Conversely, the administration of high testosterone doses can induce precocious epiphyseal closure. This effect can be used therapeutically in cases of excessively tall stature (see Chapt. 15).

The effect of androgens on **skin and dependent organs** vary in the different cutaneous districts and are mediated by testosterone and, probably, DHT. Depending on testosterone, the growth of sebaceous glands can be stimulated and **sebum production** in the face, upper part of the back and in the skin of the chest can be induced. Testosterone contributes to the development of acne vulgaris, while estrogens can diminish sebum concentration. The effects of DHT and testosterone on the **hair** are influenced by the androgen sensitivity of the hair follicle. While axillary hair and the lower part of pubic hair start growing even in the presence of low androgen concentrations, much higher androgen levels are necessary for the growth of beard, upper part of the pubic hair and chest hair. The **hairline** is determined both by genetic factors and individual distribution of the androgen receptor and depends on the androgen milieu. High 5α-reductase activity has been observed in bald men, while in patients with 5α-reductase deficiency or hypogonadism there is no regression of the hair line. Since the growth of the scalp hair is related to increased 5α-reductase activity, increased activity of this enzyme with consequences for hair loss could be an expression of the precocious aging of the hair follicles.

During puberty, there is a testosterone-dependent growth of the length of the **larynx** of about 1 cm. This size increase, together with the length and mass of the vocal cords, leads to a lowering of vocal register. To maintain a high soprano voice, young males in the 16th–19th century were castrated before puberty. A deep voice is directly related to androgens so that a lower register can also be induced in women by testosterone. The depth of voice in a man is correlated with the duration of the pubertal phase after which the androgen receptors are lost. Once reached, register remains unchanged and no modification of the voice can be obtained after puberty in hypogonadal patients.

In the **central nervous system (CNS)** testosterone can be either aromatized or reduced to DHT. The individual activities of the different enzymes and distribution of receptors are not homogeneous in the CNS, but rather vary according to the brain region. The influence of androgens on development and on neural organization of the brain before birth is under discussion. Testosterone has important psychotropic effects (Christiansen 1998). There is a close relationship between androgen milieu and normal corporeal and spiritual performance and activity as well as good general mood and self-confidence. The frequency and presence of sexual phantasies, morning erections, frequency of masturbation or copulation and sexual activity are strictly related to blood testosterone concentrations in the normal-to-subnormal range. On the other hand, androgen deficiency is often accompanied by loss of interest, lethargy, depressive mood, loss of libido and sexual inactivity (Nieschlag et al. 1992). Androgens are also important for other male characteristics such as aggressive behaviour, initiative and concentration capacities. A connection with spatial orientation and mathematical and composition skills is also postulated.

The function of the **liver** is also influenced by steroid hormones. A sexual dimorphism is known both for protein synthesis in the liver and for many liver enzyme systems. This is reflected by the existence of different reference ranges for hepatic enzymes depending on the sex. As far as protein production is concerned, estrogens and testosterone/DHT have often antagonist effects, e. g. on SHBG synthesis. Testosterone and estrogens, however, can also have synergistic effects, for example on α-1-antitrypsin.

The influence of androgens on the **hematopoietic system** is twofold. Through the androgen-dependent, receptor-mediated erythropoietin synthesis there is a stimulation of blood red cell production. On the other hand, androgens also directly affect the hematopoietic stem cells and lead to increased synthesis of hemoglobin. These effects can also be demonstrated in vitro on the granulopoietic and thrombopoietic stem cells, although the role of androgens in this field is still unclear. Effects of testosterone on **blood circulation** are presently an important matter of investigation. It is well known that sclerosis of the coronary arteries is one of the most frequent causes of death in Western industrialized countries and that the risk of contracting this disease is twice as high in men compared to women. For this sex-dependent disease, differences in hormone secretion between sexes are supposed. This view derives from the observation that suppression of testosterone concentrations in serum leads to a subsequent increase in high density lipoprotein (HDL) concentrations. Influences of testosterone and estradiol on coagulation and fibrinolysis are also discussed. Androgen deficiency is associated with an elevation of the levels of plasminogen activator type 1 which, in turn, can lead to decreased fibrinolysis. On the other hand, testosterone is capable of stimulating the expression of thromboxane A2-receptors on thrombocytes causing increased aggregability in the primary phase of blood clotting. This is an example of the consequences of anabolic steroid abuse.

3.6.6 Androgen Secretion at Different Ages

Fetal sex determination can be separated into two phases:

- Sex determination,
- Sexual differentiation.

Sex determination is primarily under genetic control and is mediated by the "sex determining gene on the Y chromosome" (Sry) and other transcription factors. These factors govern testicle formation and male germ cell development (Parker et al. 1999) (Fig. 3.19). Sexual differentiation refers to the hormonal induction and regulation of the maturation of the secondary reproductive organs. During the first weeks of gestation, the external genitalia are indistinguishable between the sexes and have the potential of developing in the female or in

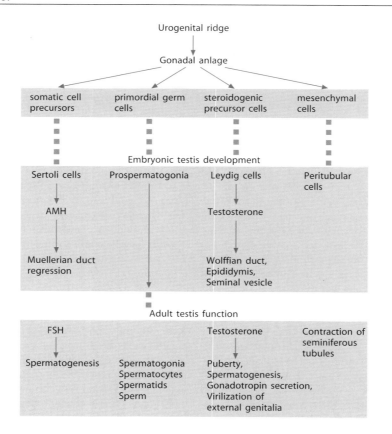

Fig. 3.19. Schematic representation of the cellular and molecular interactions during determination and differentiation of male development from embryonic to the adult phase. Differentiation and function of the various cells are depicted following vertical lines. Steps of differentiation are denoted by dotted lines, endocrine steps by red arrows. *AMH* Anti-Muellerian hormone

the male direction. Under the influence of DHT the differentiation of the bipotent structures starts at the 8th week of gestation towards the male phenotype. DHT induces the growth of the gonadal ridge and the fusion of the genital folds and streaks. At the same time, DHT stimulates prostate differentiation from the sinus genitalis. After the end of the differentiation process, at about week 14 of gestation, DHT influences the continuous growth of the external sexual organs, in particular the penis. At the moment of differentiation of the external sexual organs, fetal testosterone production is maximal. This occurs between weeks 9 and 14 of gestation, after which testosterone production decreases. During this period, enough testosterone is produced for the enzymatic transformation into DHT. hCG plays the main role in stimulating fetal testosterone production. In the second half of pregnancy, fetal LH becomes the main stimulator of Leydig cells (Huhtaniemi 1996).

In the male **newborn**, serum testosterone concentrations are comparable to those found in normal adults, decrease then at the end of the first week of life, increase again in the second month of life to a new height and fall by the 6th month of life to very low levels such as those found in female babies. Up to the 7th year of life, androgen concentrations in serum are very low, although there is a remarkable increase of free testosterone levels. During this phase, Leydig cells can be stimulated to produce testosterone through the exogenous administration of hCG.

At the age of about 7 years androgen production starts increasing, first due to increased secretion of dehydroepiandrosterone by the adrenal gland (**adrenarche**). At the age of about 10 years gonadotropin secretion starts, first with pulsatile discharge of LH by the pituitary only during sleeping hours. This nocturnal LH pulsatility becomes progressively evident, also during the day, in the course of **pubertal maturation** until the pattern typical for the adult man is reached. FSH also starts increasing, along with basal LH and testosterone serum concentrations. The clinical modifications during puberty follow the hormonal modifications in a characteristic sequence.

Normal testosterone concentrations in peripheral serum range between 12 and 30 nmol/l. Testosterone concentrations in blood follow a circadian rhythm with higher levels in the morning hours and about 25% lower levels in the evening. The situation in **elderly men** is described in Chapter 21.

3.7 References

Alastalo TP, Lonnstrom M, Leppa S, Kaarniranta K, Pelto-Huikko M, Sistonen L, Parvinen M (1998) Stage-specific expression and cellular localization of the heat shock factor 2 isoforms in the rat seminiferous epithelium. Exp Cell Res 240:16–27

Andersson AM, Müller J, Skakkebaek NE (1998) Different roles of prepubertal and postpubertal germ cells and Sertoli cells in the regulation of serum inhibin B levels. J Clin Endocrinol Metab 83:4451–4458

Aslam H, Rosiepen G, Krishnamurthy H, Arslan M, Clemen G, Nieschlag E, Weinbauer GF (1999) The cycle duration of the seminiferous epithelium remains unaltered during GnRH antagonist-induced testicular involution in rats and monkeys. J Endocrinol 161:281–288

Baskin DG, Hahn TM, Schwartz MW (1999) Leptin sensitive neurons in the hypothalamus. Horm Metab Res 31:345–350

Bellgrau D, Gold D, Selawry H, Moore J, Franzusoff A, Duke RC (1995) A role for CD95 ligand in preventing graft rejection. Nature 377:630–632

Benahmed M (1997) Role of tumor necrosis factor in the male gonad. Contracept Fertil Sex 25:569–571

Boime I, Ben-Mehamed D (1999) Gycoprotein hormone structure-function and analog design. Rec Prog Horm Res 54:271–288

Brinkworth MH, Weinbauer GF, Bergmann M, Nieschlag E (1997) Apoptosis as a mechanism of germ cell loss in elderly men. Int J Androl 20:222–228

Cavicchia JC, Sacerdote FL, Ortiz L (1996) The human blood-testis barrier in impaired spermatogenesis. Ultrastruct Pathol 20:211–218

Carani C, Qin K, Simoni M, Faustini-Fustini M, Serpente S, Boyd J, Korach KS, Simpson ER (1997) Effect of testosterone and estradiol in a man with aromatase deficiency. N Engl J Med 10:91–95

Chemes HE (1996) Leydig cell development in humans. In: Payne AH, Hardy MP, Russell LD (eds) The Leydig cell. Cache River Press, Vienna, pp 175–202

Choong CS, Wilson EM (1998) Trinucleotide repeats in the human androgen receptor: a molecular basis for disease. J Mol Endocrinol 21:235–257

Christiansen K (1998) Behavioural correlates of testosterone. In: Nieschlag E, Behre HM (eds) Testosterone: action, deficiency, substitution. Springer, Berlin Heidelberg New York, pp 107–142

Clouthier DE, Avarbock MR, Maika SD, Hammer RE, Brinster RL (1996) Rat spermatogenesis in mouse testis. Nature 381:418–421

Cohen PE, Hardy MP, Pollard JW (1997) Colony-stimulating factor-1 plays a major role in the development of reproductive function in male mice. Mol Endocrinol 11:1636–1650

Cohen PE, Pollard JW (1998) Normal sexual function in male mice lacking a functional type I interleukin-1 (IL-1) receptor. Endocrinology 139:815–818

Cooper TG, Raczek S, Yeung CH, Schwab E, Schulze H, Hertle L (1992) Composition of fluids obtained from human epididymidal spermatocoeles. Urol Res 20:275–280

Counis R, Justiz M (1991) Regulation of pituitary gonadotropin gene expression. Outline of intracellular signaling pathways. Trends Endocrinol Metab 2:181–187

Dankbar B, Brinkworth MH, Schlatt S, Weinbauer GF, Nieschlag E, Gromoll J (1995) Ubiquitous expression of the androgen receptor and testis-specific expression of the FSH receptor in the cynomolgus monkey (*Macaca fascicularis*) revealed by a ribonuclease protection assay. J Steroid Biochem Mol Biol 55:35–41

de Rooij DG (1998) Stem cells in the testis. Int J Exp Pathol 79:67–80

Dowsing AT, Yong EL, Clark M, Mc Lachlan RI, de Kretser DM, Trounson AO (1999) Linkage between male infertility and trinucleotide repeat expansion in the androgen-receptor gene. Lancet 354:640–643

Emmen JM, McLuskey A, Grootegoed JA, Brinkmann AO (1998) Androgen action during male sex differentiation includes suppression of cranial suspensory ligament development. Hum Reprod 13:1272–80

Ergün S, Luttmer W, Fiedler W, Holstein AF (1998) Functional expression and localization of vascular endothelial growth factor and its receptors in the human epididymis. Biol Reprod 58:160–168

Ergün S, Stingl J, Holstein AF (1994a) Segmental angioarchitecture of the testicular lobes in man. Andrologia 26:143–150

Ergün S, Stingl J, Holstein AF (1994b) Microvasculature of the human testis in correlation to Leydig cells and seminiferous tubules. Andrologia 26:255–262

Evans JJ (1999) Modulation of gonadotropin levels by peptides acting at the anterior pituitary gland. Endocr Rev 20:46–67

Fan NC, Peng C, Krisinger J, Leung PCK (1995) The human gonadotropin-releasing hormone receptor gene: complete structure including multiple promoters, transcription initiation sites and polyadenylation signals. Mol Cell Endocrinol 107:R1–R8

Fernald RD, White RB (1999) Gonadotropin-releasing hormone genes: phylogeny, structure and functions. Front Neuroendocrinol 20:224–240

Franca LR, Ogawa T, Avarbock MR, Brinster RL, Russell LD (1998) Germ cell genotype controls cell cycle during spermatogenesis in the rat. Biol Reprod 59:1371–1377

Fujisawa M, Kanzaki M, Okuda Y, Okada H, Arakawa S, Kamidono S (1998) Stem cell factor in human seminal plasma as a marker for spermatogenesis. Urology 51:460–463

Gast A, Schneikert J, Cato AC (1998) N-terminal sequences of the human androgen receptor in DNA binding and trans-repressing functions. J Steroid Biochem Mol Biol 65:117–123

Ghadessy FJ, Lim J, Abdullah AAR, Panet-Raymond V, Choo CK, Lumbroso R, Tut TG, Gottlieb B, Pinsky L, Trifiro MA, Yong EL (1999) Oligospermic infertility associated with an androgen receptor mutation that disrupts interdomain and coactivator (TIF2) interactions. J Clin Invest 103:1517–1525

Gharib SD, Wierman ME, Shupnik MA, Chin WW (1990) Molecular biology of the pituitary gonadotropins. Endocr Rev 11:177–199

Ghinea N, Milgrom E (1995) Transport of protein hormones through the vascular endothelium. J Endocrinol 145:1–9

Griffin HG, Wilson JD (1994) Disorders of the testes and male reproductive tract. In: Wilson JD, Foster DW (eds) Testbook of endocrinology. Saunders Company, Philadelphia, pp 799–852

Griswold MD, Russell LD (1999) Sertoli cells, function. In: Knobil E, Neill JD (eds) Encyclopedia of reproduction. Academic, San Diego, pp 371–380

Gromoll J, Simoni M, Nieschlag E (1996) An activating mutation of the follicle-stimulating hormone receptor autonomously sustains spermatogenesis in a hypophysectomized man. J Clin Endocrinol Metab 81:1367–1370

Hall PF (1994) Testicular steroid synthesis: organization and regulation. In Knobil E, Neill JD (eds) The physiology of reproduction. Raven, New York, pp 1334–1362

Hara T, Tamura K, de Miguel MP, Mukouyama Y, Kim H, Kogo H, Donovan PJ, Miyajima A (1998) Distinct roles of oncostatin M and leukemia inhibitory factor in the development of primordial germ cells and Sertoli cells in mice. Dev Biol 201:144–153

Harderlin JP, Julliard AK, Moniot B, Soussi-Yanicostas N, Verney C, Schwanzel-Fukuda M, Ayer-Le Lievre C, Petit C (1999) Anosmin-1 is a regionally restricted component of basement membranes and interstitial matrices during organogenesis: implications for the developmental anomalies of X chromosome-linked Kallmann syndrome. Dev Dyn 215:26–44

Harris GC, Nicholson HD (1998) Characterisation of the biological effects of neurohypophysial peptides on seminiferous tubules. J Endocrinol 156:35–42

Hayes FJ, Crowley WF Jr (1998) Gonadotropin pulsations across development. Horm Res 49:163–168.

Hedger MP (1997) Testicular leukocytes: what are they doing? Rev Reprod 2:38–47

Hippaku RA, Liao S (1995) Androgen receptors and action. In: De Groot LJ (ed) Endocrinology. Saunders, Philadelphia, pp 2336–2351

Hoffman WH, Kovacs KT, Gala RR, Keel BA, Jarrell TS, Ellegood JO, Burek CL (1991) Macroorchidism and testicular fibrosis associated with autoimmune thyroiditis. J Clin Invest 14:609–616

Holstein AF (1999) Spermatogenese beim Menschen: Grundlagen und Klinik. Ann Anat 181:427–436

Holstein AF, Maekawa M, Nagano T, Davidoff MS (1996) Myofibroblasts in the lamina propria of human seminiferous tubules are dynamic structures of heterogenous phenotype. Arch Histol Cytol 59:109–125

Holstein AF, Roosen-Runge EC (1981) Atlas of human spermatogenesis. Grosse, Berlin

Hosie S, Wessel L, Waag KL (1999) Could testicular descent in humans be promoted by direct androgen stimulation of the gubernaculum testis? Eur J Pediatr Surg 9:37–41

Hsiao PW, Lin DL, Nakao R, Chang C (1999) The linkage of Kennedy's neuron disease to ARA24, the first identified androgen receptor polyglutamine region-associated coactivator. J Biol Chem 29:20229–20234

Huhtaniemi I (1996) Ontogeny of the luteinizing hormone action in the male. In: Payne ADH, Hardy MP, Russell LD (eds) The Leydig cell. Cache River Press, Vienna, pp 365–382

Huhtaniemi I, Jiang M, Nilsson C, Petterson K (1999) Mutations and polymorphisms in gonadotropin genes. Mol Cell Endocrinol 151:89–94

Hutson JM, Hasthorpe S, Heyns CF (1997) Anatomical and functional aspects of testicular descent and cryptorchidism. Endocr Rev 18:259–80

Hutson JC (1998) Interactions between testicular macrophages and Leydig cells. J Androl 19:394–398

Iiri T, Herzmark P, Nakamoto JM, van Dop C, Bourne HR (1994) Rapid GDP release from Gs alpha in patients with gain and loss of endocrine function. Nature 371:164–168

Jezek D, Banek L, Hittmair A, Pezerovic-Panijan R, Goluza T, Schulze W (1999) Mast cells in testicular biopsies of infertile men with 'mixed atrophy' of seminiferous tubules. Andrologia 31:203–10

Jockenhövel F, Fingscheidt U, Khan SA, Behre HM, Nieschlag E (1990) Bio- and immunoactivity of FSH in serum after intramuscular injection of highly purified urinary human FSH in normal men. Clin Endocrinol 33:503–521

Johnson L (1994) A new approach to study the architectural arrangement of spermatogenic stages revealed little evidence of a partial wave along the length of the human seminiferous tubules. J Androl 15:435–441

Johnson L (1995) Efficiency of spermatogenesis. Microsc Res Tech 32:385–422

Johnson L, McKenzie KS, Snell JR (1996) Partial wave in human seminiferous tubules appears to be a random occurrence. Tissue Cell 28:127–36

Jones TH, Darne JF (1993) Self-administered subcutaneous human menopausal gonadotropin for the stimulation of testicular growth and the initiation of spermatogenesis in hypogonadotropic hypogonadism. Clin Endocrinol 38:203–208

Kaiser UB (1998) Molecular mechanisms of the regulation of gonadotropin gene expression by gonadotropin-releasing hormone. Mol Cells 8:647–656

Karten MJ, Rivier J (1986) Gonadotrophin-releasing hormone analog design. Structure-function relationships towards the development of agonists and antagonists: rationale and perspective. Endocr Rev 7:44–66

Kerr JB (1992) Functional cytology of the human testis. Bailliere's Clin Endocrinol Metab 6:235–250

Kondoh G, Yomogida K, Dohmae K, Nozawa M, Koga M, Nonomura N, Miki T, Okuyama A, Nishimune Y (1997) Coexpression of multiple Sertoli cell and Leydig cell marker genes in the spontaneous testicular tumor of F344 rat: evidence for phenotypical bifurcation of the interstitial cell tumor. Jpn J Cancer Res 88:839–845

Krishnamurthy H, Weinbauer GF, Aslam H, Yeung CH, Nieschlag E (1998) Quantification of apoptotic testicular germ cells in normal and methoxyacetic acid-treated mice as determined by flow cytometry. J Androl 19:710–717

Lapthorn AJ, Harris DC, Littlejohn A, Lustbader JW, Canfield RE, Machin KJ, Morgan FJ, Isaacs, NW (1994) Crystal structure of human chorionic gonadotropins. Nature 369:455–461

Lerchl A, Keck C, Spiteri-Grech J, Nieschlag E (1993) Diurnal variations in scrotal temperature of normal men and patients with varicocele before and after treatment. Int J Androl 16:195–200

Levalle O, Zylbersztein C, Aszpis S, Aquilano D, Terradas C, Colombani M, Aranda C, Scaglia H (1998) Recombinant human follicle-stimulating hormone administration increases testosterone production in men, possibly by a Sertoli cell-secreted nonsteroid factor. J Clin Endocrinol Metab 83:3973–3976

Li C, Chen P, Smith MS (1999) Morphological evidence for direct interaction between arcuate nucleus neuropeptide Y (NPY) neurons and gonadotropin-releasing hormone neurons and the possible involvement of NPY Y1 receptors. Endocrinology 140:5382–5390

Lin D, Sugawara T, Strauss JF, Clark BJ, Stocco DM, Saenger P, Rogol A, Miller WL (1995) Role of steroidogenic acute regulatory protein in adrenal and gonadal steroidogenesis. Science 267:1828–1831

Lindstedt G, Nystrom E, Matthews C, Ernest I, Janson PO, Chatterjee K (1998) Follitropin (FSH) deficiency in an infertile male due to FSHbeta gene mutation. A syndrome of normal puberty and virilization but underdeveloped testicles with azoospermia, low FSH but high lutropin and normal serum testosterone concentrations. Clin Chem Lab Med 36:663–665

Lopez FJ, Merchenthaler IJ, Moretto M, Negro-Vilar A (1998) Modulating mechanisms of neuroendocrine cell activity: the LHRH pulse generator. Cell Mol Neurobiol 18:125–146

Loveland KL, Schlatt S (1997) Stem cell factor and c-kit in the mammalian testis: lessons originating from Mother Nature's gene knockouts. J Endocrinol 153:337–44

MacLean HE, Warne GL, Zajac JD (1995) Defects of androgen receptor function: from sex reversal to motor neurone disease. Mol Cell Endocrinol 112:133–141

Mahi-Brown CA (1994) Autoimmune orchitis. Immunol Allergy Clin North America 14:787–801.

Mangelsdorf DJ, Thummel C, Beato, M, Herrlich P, Schutz G, Umesono K, Blumberg B, Kastner P, Mark M, Chambon P (1995) The nuclear receptor superfamily: the second decade. Cell 83:835–839

McEwen BS, Alves SE (1999) Estrogen actions in the central nervous system. Endocr Rev 20:279–307

Meinhardt A, Bacher M, O'Bryan MK, McFarlane JR, Mallidis C, Lehmann C, Metz CN, de Kretser DM, Bucala R, Hedger MP (1999) A switch in the cellular localization of macrophage migration inhibitory factor in the rat testis after ethane dimethane sulfonate treatment. J Cell Sci 112:1337–44

Meistrich ML, van Beek MEAB (1993) Spermatogonial stem cells. In: Desjardins C, Ewing LL (eds) Cell and molecular biology of the testis. Oxford University Press, New York, pp 266–295

Mieusset R, Bujan L (1995) Testicular heating and its possible contributions to male infertility: a review. Int J Androl 18:169–184

Millar R, Conklin D, Lofton-Day C, Hutchinson E, Troskie B, Illing N, Sealfon SC, Hapgood J (1999) A novel human GnRH receptor homolog gene: abundant and wide tissue distribution of the antisense transcript. J Endocrinol 162:117–126

Moilanen AM, Karvonen U, Poukka H, Yan W, Toppari J, Jänne O, Palvimo JJ (1999) A testis-specific androgen receptor coregulator that belongs to a novel family of nuclear proteins. J Biol Chem 274:3700–3704

Mooradian, AD, Morley, JE, Korenman, SG (1987) Biological actions of androgens. Endocr Rev 8:1–27

Moudgal NR, Sairam MR (1998) Is there a true requirement for follicle stimulating hormone in promoting spermatogenesis and fertility in primates? Hum Reprod 13:916–919

Moyle WR, Campbell, RK (1995) Gonadotropins. In: DeGroot JL, Besser M, Burger HG, Jameson LJ, Loriaux DL, Marshall JC, Odell WD, Potts JT Jr, Rubenstein AH (eds) Endocrinology. Saunders, Philadelphia, pp 230–241

Nef S, Parada LF (1999) Cryptorchidism in mice mutant for Insl3. Nat Genet 22:295–299

Ngan ES, Cheng PK, Leung PC, Chow BK (1999) Steroidogenic factor-1 interacts with a gonadotrope-specific element within the first exon of the human gonadotropin-releasing hormone receptor gene to mediate gonadotrope-specific expression. Endocrinology 140:2452–2462

Nieschlag E (1992) Testosteron, Anabolika und aggressives Verhalten bei Männern. Dtsch Ärtzebl 89:2967–2972

Nieschlag E, Simoni M, Gromoll J, Weinbauer GF (1999) Role of FSH in the regulation of spermatogenesis: clinical aspects. Clin Endocrinol (Oxf) 51:139–146

Nieschlag E, Weinbauer GF, Cooper TG, Wittkowski W (1999) Reproduktion. In: Deetjen P, Speckmann ET (eds). Physiologie. Urban & Fischer, München pp 521–540

Orth JM, Qiu J, Jester WF Jr, Pilder S (1997) Expression of the c-kit gene is critical for migration of neonatal rat gonocytes in vitro. Biol Reprod 57:676–683

Paris F, Weinbauer GF, Blüm V, Nieschlag E (1994) The effect of androgens and antiandrogens on the immunohistochemical localization of the androgen receptor in accessory reproductive organs of male rats. J Steroid Biochem Mol Biol 48:129–137

Parker KL, Schimmer BP, Schedl A (1999) Genes essential for early events in gonadal development. Cell Mol Life Sci 55:831–838

Petersen PM, Pakkenberg B, Giwercman A (1996) The human testis studied using stereological methods. Acta Stereologica 15:181–185

Phillip M, Arbelle JE, Segev Y, Parvari R (1998) Male hypogonadism due to a mutation in the gene for the beta-subunit of follicle-stimulating hormone. N Engl J Med 338:1729–1732

Pineau C, McCool S, Glucksman MJ, B Jg, Pierotti AR (1999) Distribution of thimet oligopeptidase (E.C. 3.4.24.15) in human and rat testes. J Cell Sci 112:3455–3462

Pöllänen P, Cooper TG (1994) Immunology of the testicular excurrent ducts. J Reproduct Immunol 26:167–216

Quigley CA (1998) The androgen receptor: Physiology and pathophysiology. In: Nieschlag E, Behre HM (eds) Testosterone: Action, deficiency, substitution, 2nd edn. Springer, Berlin Heidelberg New York, pp 33–107

Quigley HA, De Bellis A, Marschke KB, El-Awady MK, Wilson EM, French FS (1995) Androgen receptor defects: Historical, clinical and molecular perspectives. Endocr Rev 16:271–321

Rajpert-de-Meyts E, Skakkebaek NE (1994) Expression of the c-kit protein product in carcinoma-in-situ and invasive testicular germ cell tumours. Int J Androl 17:85–92

Rommerts FFG (1998) Testosterone: an overview of biosynthesis, transport, metabolism and nongenomic actions. In: Nieschlag E, Behre HM (eds) Testosterone: action, deficiency, substitution, 2nd edn. Springer, Berlin Heidelberg New York, pp 1–33

Rosiepen G, Chapin RE, Weinbauer GF (1995) The duration of the cycle of the seminiferous epithelium is altered by administration of 2,5-hexanedione in the adult Sprague-Dawley rat. J Androl 16:127–135

Rosner W, Hryb DJ, Khan MS, Nakhla A, Romas NA (1999) Sex hormone-binding globulin mediates steroid hormone signal transduction at the plasma membrane. J Steroid Biochem Mol Biol 69:481–485

Saez JM (1994) Leydig cells: Endocrine, paracrine, and autocrine regulation. Endocr Rev 5:574–611

Saez JM, Lejeune H (1996) Regulation of Leydig cell functions by hormones and growth factors. In: Payne ADH, Hardy MP, Russell LD (eds) The Leydig cell. Cache River Press, Vienna, pp 383–406

Sandlow JI, Feng HL, Sandra A (1997) Localization and expression of the c-kit receptor protein in human and rodent testis and sperm. Urology 49:494–500

Saunders PT, Gaughan J, Saxty BA, Kerr LE, Millar MR (1996) Expression of protamine P2 in the testis of the common marmoset and man visualized using non-radioactive insitu hybridization. Int J Androl 19:212–219

Schlatt S, Weinbauer GF (1994) Immunohistochemical localization of proliferating cell nuclear antigen as a tool to study cell proliferation in rodent and primate testes. Int J Androl 17:214–22

Schlatt S, Weinbauer GF, Nieschlag E (1991) Inhibin-like and gonadotropin-like immunoreactivity in pituitary cells of male monkeys (*Macaca fascicularis* and *Macaca mulatta*). Cell Tissue Res 265:203–209

Schlatt S, Weinbauer GF, Arslan M, Nieschlag E (1993) Appearance of alpha-smooth muscle actin in peritubular cells of monkey testes is induced by androgens, modulated by follicle-stimulating hormone, and maintained after hormonal withdrawal. J Androl 14:340–350

Schlatt S, Arslan M, Weinbauer GF, Behre HM, Nieschlag E (1995) Endocrine control of testicular somatic and premeiotic germ cell development in the immature testis of the primate *Macaca mulatta*. Eur J Endocrinol 133:235–47

Schlatt S, Rosiepen G, Weinbauer GF, Rolf C, Brook PF, Nieschlag E (1999) Germ cell transfer into rat, bovine, monkey and human testis. Hum Reprod 14:144–150

Schrans-Stassen BHGJ, van de Kant HJ, de Rooij DG, van Pelt AM (1999) Differential expression of c-kit in mouse undifferentiated and differentiating type A spermatogonia. Endocrinology 140:5894–5900

Schulze W, Rehder U (1984) Organization and morphogenesis of the human seminiferous epithelium. Cell Tissue Res 237:395–407

Schwanzel-Fukuda M (1999) Origin and migration of luteinizing hormone-releasing hormone neurons in mammals. Microsc Res Tech 44:2–10

Seeburg PH, Mason AJ, Young III WS, Steart TA, Nikolics K (1989) The gene encoding GnRH and its associated peptide GAP: some insights into hypogonadism. J Steroid Biochem 33:687–691

Setchell BP (1998) Heat and the testis. The Parkes Lecture. J Reprod Fertil 114:179–194

Setchell BP (1999) Blood-Testis Barrier. In: Knobil E, Neill JD (eds) Encyclopedia of reproduction. Academic, San Diego, pp 375–381

Shan LX, Bardin CW, Hardy MP (1997) Immunohistochemical analysis of androgen effects on androgen receptor expression in developing Leydig and Sertoli cells. Endocrinology 138:1259–1266

Sharpe R (1994) Regulation of spermatogenesis. In: Knobil E, Neill JD (eds) The physiology of reproduction. Raven, New York, pp 1363–1434

Sherwood NM, Lovejoy DA, Coe IR (1993) Origin of mammalian gonadotropin-releasing hormones. Endocr Rev 14:241–254

Simoni M, Gromoll J, Höppner W, Kamischke A, Krafft T, Stähle D, Nieschlag E (1999) Mutational analysis of the folliclestimulating hormone receptor in normal and infertile men: identification and characterization of two discrete FSH receptor isoforms. J Clin Endocrinol Metab 84:751–755

Simoni M, Gromoll J, Nieschlag E (1997) The follicle-stimulating hormone receptor: biochemistry, molecular biology, physiology and pathophysiology. Endocr Rev 18:739–773

Sinha Hikim AP, Swerdloff RS (1999) Hormonal and genetic control of germ cell apoptosis in the testis. Rev Reprod 4:38–47

Skinner MK (1993) Secretion of growth factors and other regulatory products. In Russel LD, Griswold MD (eds) The Sertoli cell. Cache River Press, Clearwater, pp 237–248

Smith EP, Boyd J, Frank GR, Takashi H, Cohen RM, Specker B et al (1994) Estrogen resistance caused by a mutation in the estrogen receptor gene in a man. N Engl J Med 331:1056–1061

Steger K (1999) Transcriptional and translational regulation of gene expression in haploid spermatids. Anat Embryol (Berl) 199:471–487

Steger K, Rey R, Louis F, Kliesch S, Behre HM, Nieschlag E, Hoepffner W, Bailey D, Marks A, Bergmann M (1999a) Reversion of the differentiated phenotype and maturation block in Sertoli cells in pathological human testis. Hum Reprod 14:136–143

Steger K, Tetens F, Bergmann M (1999b) Expression of connexin 43 in human testis. Histochem Cell Biol 112:215–220

Stephan JP, Syed V, Jegou B (1997) Regulation of Sertoli cell IL-1 and IL-6 production in vitro. Mol Cell Endocrinol 134:109–118

Stocco DM (1999) An update on the mechanism of action of the Steroidogenic Acute Regulatory (StAR) protein. Exp Clin Endocrinol Diabetes 107:229–235

Suarez-Quian CA, Martinez-Garcia F, Nistal M, Regadera J (1999) Androgen receptor distribution in adult human testis. J Clin Endocrinol Metab 84:350–358

Takaimya K, Yamamoto A, Furukawa K, Zhao J, Fukumoto S, Amashiro S, Okada M, Haraguchi M, Shin M, Kishikawa M, Shiku H, Auzawa S, Furukawa K (1998) Complex gangliosides are essential in spermatogenesis of mice: possible roles in the transport of testosterone. Proc Natl Acad Sci USA 95:12147–12152

Tapanainen JS, Vaskivuo T, Aittomaki K, Huhtaniemi IT (1998) Inactivating FSH receptor mutations and gonadal dysfunction. Mol Cell Endocrinol 145:129–135

Teerds KJ (1996) Regeneration of Leydig cells after depletion by EDS: A model for postnatal Leydig cell renewal. In: Payne AH, Hardy MP, Russell LD (eds) The Leydig cell. Cache River Press, Vienna, pp 203–220

Themmen AP, Martens JW, Brunner HG (1998) Activating and inactivating mutations in LH receptor. Mol Cell Endocrinol 145:137–142

Tilley WD, Buchanan G, Hickey TE, Bentel JM (1996) Mutations in the androgen receptor gene are associated with progression of human prostate cancer to androgen independence. Clin Cancer Res 2:277–285

Toppari J, Kaipia A, Kaleva M, Laato M, de Kretser DM, Krummen LA, Mather JP, Salmi TT (1998) Inhibin gene expression in a large cell calcifying Sertoli cell tumour and serum inhibin and activin levels. APMIS 106:101–112; discussion 112–113

Tripiciano A, Filippini A, Ballarini F, Palombi F (1998) Contractile response of peritubular myoid cells to prostaglandin F2alpha. Mol Cell Endocrinol 138:143–150

Tut TG, Ghadessy FJ, Trifiro MA, Pinsky L, Yong EL (1997) Long polyglutamine tracts in the androgen receptor are associated with reduced trans-activation, impaired sperm production and male infertility. J Clin Endocrinol Metab 82:3777–3782

Venables J, Eperon I (1999) The roles of RNA-binding proteins in spermatogenesis and male infertility. Curr Opin Genet Dev 9:346–354

Vilar AN (1999) Selective androgen receptor modulators (SARMs): a novel approach to androgen therapy for the new millenium. J Clin Endocrinol Metab 84:3459–3462

Vliegen MK, Schlatt S, Weinbauer GF, Bergmann M, Groome NP, Nieschlag E (1993) Localization of inhibin/activin subunits in the testis of adult nonhuman primates and men. Cell Tissue Res 273:261–268

von Eckardstein S, Simoni M, Bergmann M, Weinbauer GF, Gassner P, Schepers AG, Nieschlag E (1999) Serum inhibin B in combination with serum follicle-stimulating hormone (FSH) is a more sensitive marker than serum FSH alone for impaired spermatogenesis in men, but cannot predict the presence of sperm in testicular tissue samples. J Clin Endocrinol Metab 84:2496–2501

Wang C, McDonald V, Leung A, Superlano L, Berman N, Hull L, Swerdloff RS (1997) Effect of increased scrotal temperature on sperm production in normal men. Fertil Steril 68:334–339

Weinbauer GF, Nieschlag E (1992) LH-RH antagonists: state of the art and future perspectives. In: Höffken K (ed) Peptides in oncology. Springer, Berlin Heidelberg New York, pp 113–136

Weinbauer GF, Nieschlag E (1998) The role of testosterone in spermatogenesis. In: Nieschlag E, Behre HM (eds) Testosterone: action, deficiency, substitution, 2nd edn. Springer, Berlin Heidelberg New York, pp 143–168

Weinbauer GF, Nieschlag E (1999) Testicular physiology of primates. In: Weinbauer GF, Korte R (eds) Reproduction in nonhuman primates. Waxmann, Muenster, pp 13–26

Weinbauer GF, Wessels J (1999) Paracrine control of spermatogenesis. Andrologia 31:249–262

Weinbauer GF, Respondek M, Themann H, Nieschlag E (1987) Reversibility of long-term effects of GnRH agonist administration on testicular histology and sperm production in the non-human primate. J Androl 8:319–329

Werdelin L, Nilsonne A (1999) The evolution of the scrotum and testicular descent in mammals: a phylogenetic view. J Theor Biol 196:61–72

Wurtz J, Bourguet W, Renaud J, Vivat V, Chambon P, Moras D, Gronemeyer H (1996) A canonical structure for the ligand binding domain of nuclear receptors. Nature Struct Biol 3:87–94

Zhengwei Y, McLachlan RI, Bremner WJ, Wreford NG (1997) Quantitative (stereological) study of the normal spermatogenesis in the adult monkey (*Macaca fascicularis*). J Androl 18:681–687

Zhengwei Y, Wreford NG, Royce P, de Kretser DM, McLachlan RI (1998a) Stereological evaluation of human spermatogenesis after suppression by testosterone treatment: heterogeneous pattern of spermatogenic impairment. J Clin Endocrinol Metab 83:1284–1291

Zhengwei Y, Wreford NG, Schlatt S, Weinbauer GF, Nieschlag E, McLachlan RI (1998b) Acute and specific impairment of spermatogonial development by GnRH antagonist-induced gonadotrophin withdrawal in the adult macaque (*Macaca fascicularis*). J Reprod Fertil 112:139–147

Zimmermann S, Steding G, Emmen JM, Brinkmann AO, Nayernia K, Holstein AF, Engel W, Adham IM (1999) Targeted disruption of the Insl3 gene causes bilateral cryptorchidism. Mol Endocrinol 13:681–691

CHAPTER 4

Physiology of Sperm Maturation and Fertilization 4

T.G. COOPER · C.-H. YEUNG

4.1 Secondary Male Accessory Sex Organs and Formation of the Ejaculate

The primary sex organ, the testis, concerned with the manufacture of androgens and spermatozoa, is in continuity with its extra-testicular pathways (the **ductuli efferentia**, **epididymis** and **ductus deferens**), that transmit sperm to the urethra. Also discharging their secretions into the urethra are the more distal secondary sexual organs, the **prostate** and **seminal vesicles**, and the **periurethral glands** (of Littré) and **bulbourethral** glands (of Cowper) (Fig. 4.1).

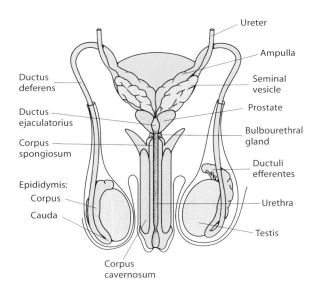

Fig. 4.1. Scheme showing the morphological relationship between the accessory glands of reproduction. From Nieschlag et al. (1999)

4.2 Anatomy of the Human Epididymis and Sperm Transport through it

Spermatozoa shed from the seminiferous epithelium together with fluid secreted by the Sertoli cells are wafted through the tubuli recti into the cavities of the rete testis as the fluid is drawn along by its absorption in the testicular efferent ducts. The sperm then pass into 12–18 **efferent ducts** (each 0.2–0.5 m long) forming the globus major of the epididymis (**caput epididymidis**) that eventually unite to form the single tubule of the epididymis. The efferent ducts comprise ciliated and non-ciliated cells whose arrangement, appearance and height form at least five different tubule types (Yeung et al. 1991). They provide a resorptive epithelium that concentrates spermatozoa entering the ducts from the testis by mediating the transfer of ions and water from the tubule lumen to the interstitium and they may also have a secretory role.

The single duct of the epididymis is coiled into lobules forming the grossly discernible isthmus (**corpus epididymidis**) and a somewhat smaller globus minor (**cauda epididymidis**) and the total length of the tubule is 5–6 m in man (von Lanz and Neuhäuser 1964). The epididymis proper has a pseudostratified epithelium, containing a population of **principal cells** of various heights (generally shorter distally) and **basal cells** that do not extend to the lumen and also a population of wandering **lymphocytes**. The fixed cells are both resorptive and secretory in nature and they maintain a unique microenvironment in which sperm can remain viable for over two weeks. **Basal cells** share some characteristics with macrophages (Yeung et al. 1994).

> The time for sperm to pass through the epididymis lies between 2 and 11 days (Johnson and Varner 1988) and in this organ the sperm mature and are stored prior to ejaculation.

4.3 Epididymal Secretion and Absorption

Epididymal epithelial functions include the estrogen-dependent water resorption in the efferent ducts, which is driven by the **absorption** of Na+ ions, and the androgen-dependent **secretion** of components that modify the epididymal spermatozoa in preparation for fertilization and keep the mature sperm quiescent before ejaculation. The absorption of fluid further concentrates the spermatozoa and epididymal secretions in the lumen. Epididymal secretions are important for some changes undergone by the maturing spermatozoa, whereas others are time-dependent phenomena (see Cooper 1995b, 1998). However, little is known in detail about these secretions and what they do in man, although some ideas are emerging. Changes in ion concentrations and viscous proteins within the epididymal canal prevent the motility of sperm within this organ (see 4.6.3).

Three low molecular weight secretions are present in high concentrations in the epididymis: **glycerophosphocholine** (**GPC**), synthesized from circulating lipoproteins (and possibly from sperm cells themselves), **L-carnitine**, which is not synthesized in the epididymis but concentrated from the circulation, and **myo-inositol**, which is both transported and synthesized by the epididymal epithelium. Of many hydrolytic enzymes the neutral form of α-glucosidase is the predominant secretion of the human epididymis, and its absence from seminal plasma is used clinically as an indication of distal ductal occlusion in cases of azoospermia (Cooper 1996; see Chapter 6). The amounts of the epididymal secretions α-**glucosidase**, GPC and **carnitine** in semen vary greatly between fertile men (Cooper et al. 1991) and seminal GPC provides a low prognostic value for IVF success and carnitine none (Jeyendran et al. 1989). The role of **glucosidase** is unknown and its inhibition in rats only temporarily and partially decreases their fertility (Cooper and Yeung 1999). Some specific human **epididymal secretions** are involved in gamete recognition (see Cooper 1998; Kirchhoff 1999).

4.4 Erection and Ejaculation

The **ejaculatory** process consists of two sequential processes under control of the **autonomic nervous system**. Under psychological, visual, auditory and tactile stimuli, **parasympathetic** impulses travelling over the nervi erigentes liberate acetylcholine that vasodilates the pudendal arteries. This increases blood flow into the corpora cavernosum and spongiosum and compresses venous outflow, thus increasing turgidity of the penis and causing an **erection**. Parasympathetic impulses also lead to secretion by the urethral and bulbourethral gland.

The next phase, **emission** (the passage of spermatozoa into the urethra) is under **sympathetic** control with nerve impulses travelling over the rami communicantes and hypogastric nerves to liberate adrenaline that initiates contraction of the smooth muscles surrounding the ampulla, ductuli deferentia and terminal cauda epididymidis.

At **ejaculation** proper, **parasympathetic** fibres from the lower lumbar and upper sacral centres initiate contraction of the bulbocavernous muscles, leading to forcible ejection of sperm from the urethra at the same time as ascending impulses give rise to the sensation of **orgasm**.

Finally, **detumescence** of the penis is caused by **sympathetic** release of noradrenaline causing dilation of the penile vasculature and penile flaccidity.

4.5 Seminal Plasma

In fertile men the sequence in which the accessory glands contribute their secretions to the ejaculate is fixed: the **bulbourethral glands** secrete an alkaline solution with glycoproteins to neutralise the urinary tract and lubricate the tract before ejaculation; the **prostate**, **epididymis** and **ductuli deferentia** contract together, discharging spermatozoa and prostatic secretions; finally the **seminal vesicles** contract and expel the pellet of spermatozoa to the outside with their secretions. Coagulation of semen occurs as a result of interaction of components of the prostate and a protein from the seminal vesicles (**seminogelin**). Liquefaction that occurs within 20–30 min in vitro is a result of dissolution of the coagulum by the action of **prostate-specific antigen** (PSA).

Of all the accessory glands that contribute to the ejaculate, the **seminal vesicles** provide the bulk volume but proper functioning of all the organs is necessary to provide sufficient fluid of the optimum composition for a normal ejaculate. The major secretions of the sex organs that appear in seminal plasma (**fructose** for seminal vesicles; **zinc**, **acid phosphatase**, **citric acid**, **prostate-specific antigen** for the prostate, **carnitine**, **glycerophosphocholine**, **neutral α-glucosidase** for the epididymis) are analysed clinically to diagnose possible causes of infertility – the amount of secretion providing information about the presence and functioning of the glands (see Chap. 6 for more details).

4.6 The Process of Natural Fertilization

> **Fertilization** is the event that brings together the haploid chromatin content of both gametes in the formation of a new individual.

As seen above, after natural intercourse only sperm from the distal cauda epididymidis enter the ejaculate and can fertilize the freshly ovulated egg. These sperm have to **survive** in the female tract, **move** to the oviduct, **penetrate** the egg investments and **fuse** with the oocyte before they can deliver their **chromatin** into the egg's cytoplasm to have it decondense eventually to form a **male pronucleus**, **zygote** and viable **embryo**. The sperm also has to **activate the egg** to permit resumption of the second meiotic division (expelling the **second polar body** and forming the **female pronucleus**) as well as deliver-

ing centrioles that organise the formation of the first **mitotic spindle** (Figs. 4.2 and 4.3).

A parallel event that the sperm have to undergo while they move through the female tract is **capacitation** in which they are prepared for eventual interaction with the egg (see Fig. 4.2).

Upon completion of sperm transport and capacitation the **acrosome reaction** is stimulated by contact with the zona pellucida. The acrosome reaction is important for aiding the passage of the sperm through the zona pellucida, by releasing a soluble acrosomal protease (**acrosin**) from the acrosome and exposing bound acrosin on the inner acrosomal membrane. The acrosome reaction is also important, via modification of the equatorial segment of the acrosome, for the eventual **fusion** of the sperm cell with the **egg membrane** (see below).

Fertilization in vivo involves a sequence of complex processes which require participation of various specific sperm proteins or surface components. Advances in transgenic animal studies have revealed that single factors are often dispensable, suggesting the likelihood of back-up systems for each process. The role of the epididymis in the development of the ability of sperm to perform each process is discussed in a later section of this chapter (Sect. 4.8). Although the fertilization process described above is the normal sequence of events in vivo for sperm from fertile men, other routes of insemination are often employed in assisted reproduction techniques to help infertile men (see Sect 4.11; Fig. 4.2; see Chap. 17). Physiologically young spermatozoa from the proximal epididymis may be able to perform some steps of fertilization, depending on their state of maturity when introduced into the female tract or when incubated with oocytes in vitro. Whereas most information about the acquisition of sperm fertilizing ability has come from animal studies, assisted reproduction techniques have permitted the collection of information about some of these processes in man (see below).

4.6.1 Movement of Sperm through the Female Tract

Ejaculated spermatozoa have to reach the oviductal **ampulla** to fertilize eggs at this location. During intercourse spermatozoa are deposited in the **vagina** within the coagulum and migrate out of this during its liquefaction in the vagina and **cervix**. Around ovulation the cervical crypts secrete a mucus in which the alignment of its glycoprotein constituents favours the passage of sperm cells (Mortimer 1995). However, mucus can represent a barrier to sperm passage when anti-sperm antibodies are present in it. Antibody-coated spermatozoa are anchored by their tails, leading to a "shaking" phenomenon. This observation has diagnostic significance in the in vitro **cervical mucus contact test** (see Chap. 6). In addition to sperm suffering from sub-normal tail flagella-

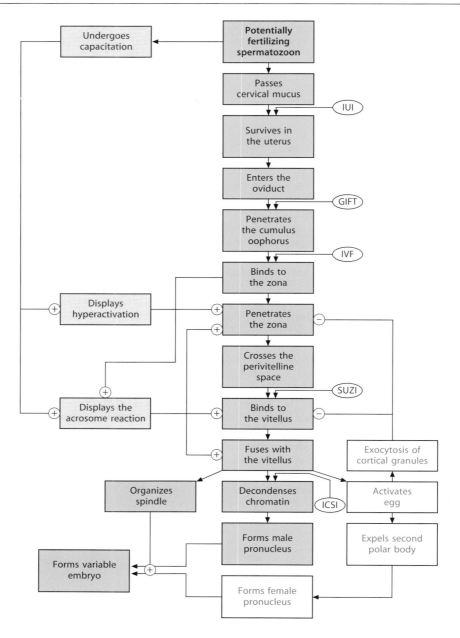

Fig. 4.2. Scheme of events taken by the fertilizing spermatozoon after natural mating. *Pink rectangular boxes*, sequential events; *grey rectangular boxes*, concomitant events of capacitation. *IUI, GIFT, IVF, SUZI, ICSI*, entry points of sperm provided by intra-uterine insemination, gamete intra-fallopian transfer, in vitro fertilization, sub-zonal insemination, intracytoplasmic sperm injection, respectively. *White boxes*, events undergone by the egg. (+), positive influence (feed-forward activation), (−) negative influence (feed-back inhibition)

tions, morphologically abnormal spermatozoa also suffer a hindrance when penetrating cervical mucus, as a result of hydrodynamic considerations (resistance to passage of the head) (Katz et al. 1990).

Whereas it is clear that sperm cells themselves have to migrate out of cervical mucus, the extent to which they are slowly released from a pool sequestered in cervical crypts is debated (Mortimer 1995). In addition to their own movements, bulk movement of spermatozoa is assisted by movements of the female tract, stimulated by seminal **prostaglandins** originating from the seminal vesicles and by peristalsis on the side of the dominant

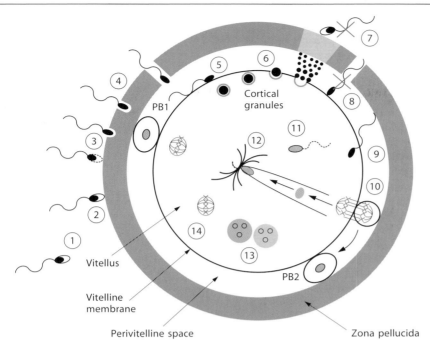

Fig. 4.3. The sequence of events leading to fertilization. After the intact, capacitated spermatozoon penetrates the cumulus oophorus (*1*) it makes contact with the zona pellucida (*2*) which induces the acrosome reaction on the surface of the zona (*3*). The acrosome-reacted sperm drives its way through the zona substance (*4*) into and across the perivitelline space (PVS). Fusion of the acrosome-reacted sperm with the vitellus (*5*) initiates membrane-mediated calcium-dependent electrical spikes and introduces sperm-associated egg activating factors that promote migration of the cortical granules to the egg surface where their contents are liberated into the PVS (*6*) and diffuse across it to alter the zona substance such that subsequent spermatozoa cannot bind to the zona, the "zona block to polyspermy" (*7*). The granules' membranes are now the egg membrane and block fusion of acrosome-reacted sperm that may be in the PVS, the "vitelline block to polyspermy" (*8*). Penetration of the fertilizing spermatozoon (*9*) further activates the egg, overcoming the metaphase promoting factors, so that the second meiotic division ensues, leading to second polar body (PB2) and the female pronucleus (*10*). Meanwhile the sperm chromatin decondenses in the cytoplasm (*11*), its protamine is replaced by histone and the male pronucleus forms. The sperm's centriole organizes microtubule spindles that spread throughout the ooplasm (*12*) and eventually contact the female pronucleus and draw it to that of the male (*13*). Eventual alignment of sister chromatids leads to syngamy (*14*)

follicle (Kunz et al. 1996). Whether the human uterotubal junction is a serious obstacle to spermatozoa is not known (Mortimer 1995), but it permits greater entry of sperm in the late follicular phase (Kunz et al. 1996). The composition of tubal fluid is such that proximal migration of spermatozoa is arrested until ovulation, when movement of the sperm cells is stimulated by factors in

follicular fluid released upon ovulation (Hunter 1987). The factors in this fluid that stimulate motility have yet to be identified. Progesterone is one component of the fluid that has recently been considered to stimulate motility, possibly by way of non-genomic membrane receptors, but there is current debate over whether chemokinesis (involving increased motile vigour) or chemotaxis (involving changes in direction) are relevant to these changes in sperm behaviour (Eisenbach 1999).

4.6.2 Penetration of Spermatozoa through the Egg Investments

After reaching the site of fertilization in the **ampulla** of the oviduct, individual sperm cells still have to pass through two layers of egg-coatings before they can contact the oocyte directly. The outer coat is the **cumulus oophorus** which consists of **granulosa cells** embedded in a viscoelastic matrix composed mainly of hyaluronic acid (Dandekar et al. 1991) and the inner coat is the **acellular zona pellucida** of the oocyte which consists of a meshwork of the glycoproteins ZP1, ZP2 and ZP3 (Green 1997). ZP1 is the zona's protein backbone held together by inter-molecular disulphide bonds and extending from it are attached ZP2 and ZP3 subunits that are rich in terminal carbohydrate residues. Although lytic enzymes on the sperm surface, such as the **hyaluronidase** PH-20 (Lin et al. 1994), may be involved in facilitating the passage of sperm through the **cumulus**, and acrosomal **acrosin** may aid sperm passage through the **zona pellucida**, the necessity for mechanical force from the sperm itself is demonstrated by the **physical distortion** of the cumulus matrix (Dandekar et al. 1992) and by **stress lines** in the zona pellucida created by the penetrating spermatozoon (Phillips 1991).

This force is generated by a type of sperm movement known as **hyperactivation**, which has been well described **in vitro** for laboratory animals and occurs in the **oviduct**. This motility is recognised as vigorous thrashing of the sperm tail, flagellating with **large bend amplitudes** and resulting in a darting, non-progressive motion of the sperm head. Such movement provides the sperm with an increased thrust compared to the forward progressive, high beat-frequency and low amplitude flagellation of uncapacitated freshly ejaculated or mature epididymal sperm. It also increases the chances of collision with the cumulus because it enlarges the area swept out by the sperm track. For humans, hyperactivation is not as well defined as for laboratory animals (Mortimer and Swan 1995) and only a small portion of sperm may be hyperactivated at any time. Although it is a result of an altered pattern of tail flagellation, hyperactivated motility of human sperm is largely performed by computer image analysis of patterns of the track of the head, ranging from thrashing, star-spin, erratic, circular or helical, depending on the conditions of measurement and settings of the equipment. The classification of hyperactivated motility still has to be standardised, but it is positively correlated with **zona binding, acrosome reaction, zona-free oocyte penetration** and **fertilizing capacity**. Human sperm require glucose for this form of motility (Hoshi 1992).

> Infertility can be caused by reduced sperm motility as a consequence of mitochondrial dysfunction, so that insufficient energy is produced (Folgero et al. 1993) or by **axonemes** that cannot respond to exogenous ATP with flagellation (Yeung et al. 1988).

4.6.3 Sperm Motility

> **Motility** is essential for sperm migration out of cervical mucus, partly responsible for their reaching the site of fertilization, and obligatory for **penetrating** the egg's cellular and acellular investments (cumulus or zona pellucida).

The structural basis of sperm **flagellation** is the sperm tail with its central axoneme and the associated **outer dense fibres**. The proximal part is circumscribed by the **mitochondria** and is known as the **mid-piece** (Fig. 4.4).

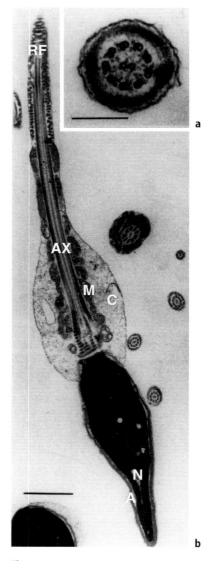

Fig. 4.4. a Transverse section through the principal piece reveals that the axoneme is composed of a central pair of microtubules surrounded by 9 tubule doublets that are connected to each other and to the central pair. Bar, 0.2 μm. (From Neugebauer et al. 1990, with permission) **b** Longitudinal section of a normal spermatozoon: sperm head with nucleus (*N*) and acrosome (*A*). The mid-piece comprises the axoneme (*AX*) and associated outer dense fibres, mitochondria (*M*) and cytoplasm (*C*). The principal piece contains the axoneme and fibrous sheath (*RF*). Bar, 1 μm

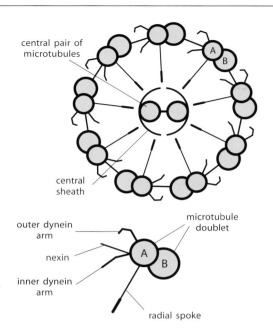

central pair of microtubules

central sheath

outer dynein arm

nexin

inner dynein arm

microtubule doublet

radial spoke

Fig. 4.5. Components of the axoneme are represented schematically. The axonemal complex comprises 9 microtubule doublets interlinked by nexin and connected to the central sheath of the central pair by radial spokes

This provides energy from respiratory substrates, although in man glycolysis can provide additional energy for motility (Yeung et al. 1996).

The axonemal complex (Fig. 4.5) is comprised of nine **microtubule doublets, circularly arranged,** interlinked by **nexin** and connected to the **central sheath** of the central pair of microtubules by **radial spokes**. The motor of flagellation is the row of outer and inner **dynein arms** protruding from each doublet. When the dynein **ATPase** is activated in one longitudinal half of the axoneme, the arms pull on the adjacent doublets with repetitious formation and breakage of dynein bridges, and the sliding movement of the doublets so produced is translated into flagellar bending. When active sliding is switched to the doublets on the other half of the flagellum, bend-formation occurs in the opposite direction. The mechanisms for the co-ordination of microtubule sliding into flagellar oscillation are still not fully elucidated but working hypotheses (see Yeung 1995) include the "**switch-point**" **model** and the more recent "**geometric clutch**" **model** (Lindemann and Kannous 1997).

Not all axonemal anomalies lead to total immotility of the sperm cell, in particular the lack of outer dynein arms which is in agreement with the interpretation of different functions for different types of dynein arms. Bend initiation and the maintenance of the angle of the

propagating bend are each attributed to the inner arms, whereas the outer arms are not essential for flagellation but generate force to overcome the viscous bending resistance in the regulation of bend growth and beat frequency.

> Various types of **axonemal defects** in ejaculated human spermatozoa have been identified clinically as the cause of sperm immotility in **infertile** men. These include absence of dynein arms, central pairs, linking components or outer dense fibres, and disorganisation of axonemal components (Zamboni 1992; Chemes et al. 1998) (see Sect. 6.5.6 and 8.8).

4.6.4 The Importance of Capacitation in Fertilization

During the time that sperm cells pervade the female tract they also undergo a process ("**capacitation**"), that enables them to fertilize eggs (see Fig. 4.2). This process is demonstrated by the inability of even ejaculated sperm cells to fertilize eggs immediately on contact with eggs *in vitro,* but which do so after a capacitation period has elapsed. In man this period is extremely variable in duration (Yanagimachi 1994). This is a necessary consequence of sperm being prevented from undergoing precocious fertilization events in the male and lower female tract by inhibitors or "**decapacitation factors**". During the process of capacitation these factors are removed from the sperm cells, permitting fertilization at the appropriate place. Thus capacitation can be considered a reversal in the female tract of a mechanism in the male tract to keep sperm quiescent before the right moment in fertilization (Visconti et al. 1998).

Some of the decapacitation factors are acquired in the **epididymis**, others only at ejaculation from **seminal vesicle** secretions, and these factors are removed somewhere within the female tract (uterus and oviduct). A loss of cholesterol from sperm membranes is important in mediating this process in man since sterols and their sulphates are present in spermatozoa and sterol binding proteins are present in follicular fluid (Zarintosh and Cross 1996). Consequences of **capacitation** are the ability of the sperm to undergo **hyperactivation** (see below), to interact with eggs and to undergo the **acrosome reaction** (see Fig. 4.2), both of which are associated with the phosphorylation of proteins by activated protein kinases.

Another consequence of capacitation may be for the sperm that are bound to cells of the oviductal epithelium to free themselves and move towards the freshly ovulated oocyte (Smith 1998).

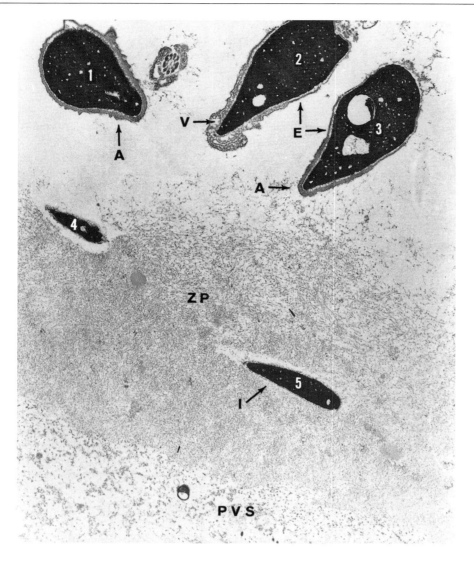

4.6.5 Binding of Sperm to the Zona Pellucida

Despite vigorous movement of the spermatozoon, an initial loose contact between the gametes gives way to a firmer binding between carbohydrate groups O-linked to the **zona pellucida protein** ZP3 and a "**zona receptor**" on the sperm. A variety of proteins associated with the sperm surface have been considered capable of mediating this sperm-zona binding and different sperm membrane sugar residues are involved in different species (Töpfer-Peterson 1999). In particular fucose or fucoidan and mannose are reported to inhibit sperm-zona binding and N-acetylglucosamine (Brandelli et al. 1996) and mannose-ligands (Benoff et al. 1997) can induce the acrosome reaction.

Interaction with both carbohydrate and protein moieties of ZP3 triggers acrosomal exocytosis which is

Fig. 4.6. Human spermatozoa outside and within the zona pellucida 8 h after in vitro fertilization with salt-stored human zonae. Sperm 1 and 3 have unreacted acrosomes and the plasma membranes over the anterior acrosome (A) and equatorial segment (E) are intact. Sperm 2 shows changes in the acrosomal membranes that may represent fusion and vesiculation (V). Sperm within the zona have lost their plasma membrane and outer acrosomal membranes. The inner acrosomal membrane (I) is in contact with the zona substance (ZP). (From Overstreet and Hembree 1976, with permission)

mediated by intracellular events, such as raised intracellular Ca^{2+}, pH and cyclic AMP concentrations and transmembrane phosphoproteins phosphorylated by tyrosine kinases (Visconti et al. 1998). Receptors for ZP3 on human sperm have not been unequivocally identified but candidates are integral membrane proteins present on testicular spermatozoa, others are epididymal secre-

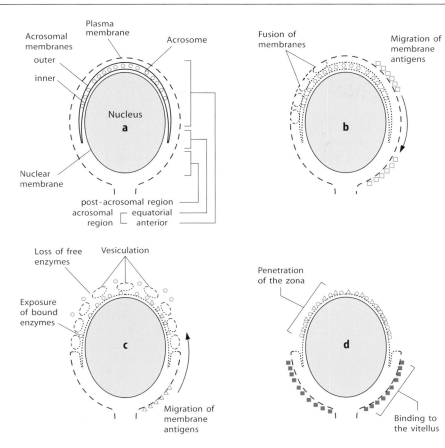

Fig. 4.7a–d. Scheme of events occurring during the acrosome reaction. **a** The membranes of the sperm head; **b** the fusion of outer acrosomal and overlying plasma membrane and migration of components to the posterior head; **c** formation and loss of acrosomal vesicles with attendant exposure of bound, and loss of soluble, lytic enzymes and migration of components to the anterior head; **d** the final state with membrane domains exposed for further sperm-egg interactions

tions. There is current debate as to whether progesterone acts on the surface of the sperm head directly or by priming the sperm to respond to other acrosomal exocytotic stimuli, including ZP3 (Revelli et al. 1998).

> A cause of **infertility** may be the dysfunction of such non-genomic progesterone receptors (Tesarik and Mendoza 1992).

4.6.6 The Acrosome Reaction and Penetration of the Zona Pellucida

It is generally agreed that the **acrosome reaction** of importance to sperm penetration occurs on the surface of the **zona pellucida** (Cross et al. 1988; Morales et al. 1994; see Fig. 4.6). If the **acrosome reaction** occurs outside the **cumulus** the sperm cannot migrate through this investment, as acrosome-reacted sperm are short-lived.

The **acrosome reaction** involves changes in the various membranes of the sperm head. First the plasma membrane over the **acrosome** fuses with the underlying **outer acrosomal membrane** and this leads to the forma-

tion of hybrid vesicles that are eventually shed as the sperm moves through the **zona pellucida** (Figs. 4.6 and 4.7). One consequence of this is the release of soluble, and exposure of a bound, sperm protease (**acrosin**) that can digest the substance of the zona. Together with increased flagellar propulsion (**hyperactivation**) the sperm is driven through the zona and each sperm penetrating the egg generates a **penetration slit** through which the sperm gains entry to the perivitelline space. The slit formed by each spermatozoon entering the perivitelline space is suggestive of local dissolution of the zona by the penetrating sperm and the sperm-bound trypsin-like enzyme acrosin exposed after the acrosome reaction is considered responsible for this. The vigour of sperm cells alone, in the absence of enzymes, has been debated to be sufficient for zona penetration (Bedford 1998). However, as high molecular weight α-acrosin (**proacrosin**) can also function as a zona binding protein, another postulated role for it is **secondary binding** to the zona by acrosome reacted spermatozoa, involving the zona protein ZP2 (Green 1997).

The nature of the "zona lysin" is still debated since lectin-treated, trypsin and acrosin-resistant zona are still penetrated by spermatozoa and transgenic mice with a mutant proacrosin gene, lacking acrosin activity, are capable for fertilization both in vivo and in vitro (Baba et al. 1994; Adham et al. 1997). That fertilization occurs in the absence of proacrosin in these transgenic mice suggests that neither proacrosin nor acrosin are essential for fertilization in these animals. Other factors, possibly PH-20 (a sperm **surface hyaluronidase**) or an **acrosomal hyaluronidase**, which can digest the zona, may function as enzyme and zona-receptor in these transgenic animals or purely physical activity is necessary (Bedford 1998).

> **Infertility** can be associated with failure of several aspects of attachment of the sperm to the egg: failure of bound cells to undergo a normal acrosome reaction (Liu and Baker 1994) and an inability of sperm to intrude into the zona or incomplete penetration of the zona (Bedford and Kim 1994).

4.6.7 Fusion of Sperm with the Vitellus

Once a sperm cell is **capacitated**, changes in the sperm tail (a vigorous flagellation termed **hyperactivation**) and the sperm head are noticeable. The most obvious changes occurring in the proximal sperm head are those associated with the **acrosome reaction**. However, subtle changes in the **equatorial region** of the acrosome and **post-acrosomal region** also occur (see Figs. 4.7 and 4.3). Unlike the proximal acrosomal region there is no vesiculation of the equatorial region of the acrosome which is now considered to be the site of initial **sperm-egg contact** (Yanagimachi 1994). Components that may be responsible for interaction with the zona pellucida that are present on the sperm plasma membrane overlying the acrosome are not lost with the membranes at the time of vesiculation and may be involved in the next step of sperm-egg fusion.

Once inside the **perivitelline space** the normally penetrating sperm is already **acrosome-reacted** so that the changes in the post-acrosomal and equatorial regions that permit fusion with the egg have already taken place

(Fig. 4.3). (In the case of SUZI, unselected cells may be introduced into this space and the acrosome reaction would have to occur within the perivitelline space.)

For ejaculated sperm cells there is considerable evidence that integrin-ligands (**disintegrins**) are present on the sperm surface and interact with **integrins** (cell adhesion molecule receptors) associated with the vitelline membrane. Competitive inhibition of sperm-egg contact have indicated that peptides containing the **RGD (arg-gly-asp) sequence** of amino acids are involved in contact of an acrosome-reacted sperm cell with the vitellus. Capacitated sperm cells express the RGD-containing **adhesion protein** on the equatorial segment of the acrosome (Bronson and Fusi 1996), a region that comes in contact with the oolemma during fertilization.

> **Infertility** can result when acrosome-reacted spermatozoa are defective in their fusing ability (Tesarik and Thebault 1993).

4.6.8 Egg Activation

Sperm enter the egg after fusion of the egg membrane with the sperm membrane at the equatorial region, forming a mosaic membrane. This action at the membrane stimulates **calcium release** from intracellular egg reserves (Fig. 4.3, Tesarik et al. 1995). Some sperm components (sperm-associated oocyte-activation factors, SAOAF) are required to set in train the **calcium oscillations** in the egg that accompany sperm penetration (Dozortsev et al. 1995b) and these calcium fluxes promote the exocytosis of **cortical granules** that are superficially situated in the unfertilized egg (Fig. 4.3). (During ICSI membrane-intact sperm are injected (Nagy et al. 1994; Sathananthan et al. 1996) and other methods of egg activation are required.)

The granules act to inhibit **polyploidy** by preventing a second sperm entering the egg by action at two levels, the vitellus and the zona. Firstly, fusion of the cortical granules with the vitelline membrane immediately alters the composition of the egg membrane to that of the interior membrane of the granules, for which sperm have no affinity; this constitutes the "**vitelline block to polyspermy**". Secondly, the contents of the granules are released into the perivitelline space. Of these, glycosidases alter the zona glycoprotein ZP3 to ZP3f that lacks the carbohydrates that the sperm primary receptor recognizes, and proteases degrade ZP2 to ZP2f that is unable to bind to acrosome-reacted spermatozoa (Wassarman 1992). This constitutes the "**zona block to polyspermy**" (see Fig. 4.3).

Sperm cytosolic oocyte activation factors develop during spermatogenesis and are present in round spermatids but are absent from primary and secondary spermatocytes (Sousa et al. 1996).

> Infertility stemming from failure of egg activation may be due to insufficient SAOAF and be overcome by injection of SAOAF from other sperm (Palermo et al. 1997).

4.6.9 Male Pronucleus Formation

Within the testis sperm **chromatin** is highly condensed and arginine-rich histones are replaced by even more basic highly charged **protamines** during spermiogenesis (see Chap. 3) which fit into the spiral grooves of nucleic acid (Barone et al. 1994). Within a few hours of sperm-egg fusion the sperm head swells as the disulphide bonds of the nucleoprotein protamine are reduced by **glutathione** in the egg cytoplasm and **nucleoplasmin** displaces the protamines, exchanging them for histones (Montag et al. 1992). After nucleoprotein degeneration, restrictions on the DNA template are removed, and the **male pronucleus** is generated, around which a membrane forms (Fig. 4.3). Eventually the tail and paternal mitochondrial DNA is lost.

Fusion of sperm with egg also inactivates the metaphase-promoting factor, leading to extrusion of the **second polar body** from the egg, the **female pronucleus** is then formed from its haploid chromosome complement (Fig. 4.3). At the same time, the centromere from the fertilizing spermatozoon is activated, which is responsible for organising the microtubule spindles that pervade the fertilized egg, make contact with the female pronucleus and draw both pronuclei together for the first mitotic division (Navara et al. 1995; Sathananthan et al. 1996). Both male and female pronuclei move together and the chromosomes condense during the prophase of **syngamy** before breakdown of the nuclear membrane at which time paternal and maternal sets of chromosomes become visible. These interact on the spindle during the first cleavage division.

> Some **infertile** men have sperm that cannot be "activated" in the ooplasm (Brown et al. 1995) and infertility may result when penetrating sperm cannot organize the cytoskeletal structures necessary for the mitotic spindle (Asch et al. 1995).

4.7 Early Embryonic Development

After formation of the **zygote**, cleavage divisions occur in the oviduct and after 2.5–3 days the fertilized egg enters the uterus where division continues to the **morula** stage (consisting of 16 totipotent cells) and **blastocyst** (32–64 cells). During transport both the uterus and embryo undergo morphological and biochemical changes: the uterus becomes receptive for blastocysts to survive (dependent on ovarian progesterone and estrogens) and the embryo develops to a form that is eventually dependent on the maternal circulation. Within the uterine cavity the blastocyst expands and becomes asymmetrical; the outer layer defining the future **trophectoderm** and the inner cells the **inner cell mass**. At a late cleavage stage **compaction** of the blastocyst occurs, when it acquires gap and tight junctions and epithelial differentiation begins. The formation of an enveloping epithelium (**trophectoderm**) isolates the developing embryo from the external environment and directional ion transport by the trophectoderm leads to fluid secretion into the blastocyst cavity (**blastocoele**) and the creation of different ion concentrations inside the conceptus.

Implantation is a unique association of the embryo with the endometrium that is necessary for **placentation** (a haemochorial placenta forms). After 3 days free in the uterus (6–7 days after fertilization), the blastocyst comes in close apposition to the uterine epithelial cells and awaits a signal from it to initiate changes for implantation. In a pre-implantation phase the fertilized egg **hatches** from the zona pellucida. This is a necessary event for implantation that requires steroid-dependent lytic factors. The free blastocyst enters the endometrium on day 20–21 after fertilization and during implantation the unattached 'free' blastocyst becomes fixed in the uterus in an intimate relationship with the endometrium. During attachment/adhesion of the embryo to the endometrial wall fibroblast-like cells of the uterine stroma are transformed into giant cells dependent on progesterone. Invasion of the uterine luminal epithelial cells, penetration of the basal lamina and eventual tapping of maternal blood vessels are synchronized by progesterone and estrogens.

4.8 Sperm Maturation in the Epididymis

The process occurring in the proximal epididymis (caput and corpus epididymidis) whereby sperm gain their ability to fertilize eggs is termed **sperm maturation** and it is associated with many physiological, biochemical and morphological changes in the spermatozoa (Cooper 1998). Most studies have been made in animals and show that although ejaculated sperm from healthy males can fertilize eggs, spermatozoa leaving the testis are incapable of doing so when inseminated into the female tract or in vitro. Such studies on fertility cannot be done for ethical reasons in man, and there are few morphological signs of **sperm maturation** in humans (Bedford 1994), but there are data on the ability of sperm from various regions of the epididymis to interact with eggs.

4.8.1 Evidence from Surgical Anastomoses

The **fertilizing capacity** of sperm from various regions of the human epididymis can be inferred by pregnancies following operations in which occluded parts of the duct are bypassed by connection of the existing patent ductus deferens to the epididymis above the site of blockage (Fig. 4.8). Pregnancies established after coitus occur from 6 months to 2 years later whether connection is made at the levels of cauda, corpus or caput, with more success when sperm have passed through more of the duct (see Cooper 1995a).

While this may be interpreted as indicating that the human epididymis has some beneficial influence on the spermatozoa, proximal connections to the efferent ducts and even testicular tubules have also resulted in **pregnancies**. In all these cases sperm have been trapped for unknown periods of time in the caput epididymidis or testis before their release into the newly created outlet and long periods of time elapse before paternity results. There is current debate as to whether an effect of the epididymis can be ruled out or whether accumulated **epididymal secretions** above this site of blockage have influenced the sperm cells (see Cooper 1993; Temple-Smith et al. 1998). It is not known if, after this operation, the **efferent ducts** or the **ductus deferens** secrete factors that interact with the sperm, but it is known that some glycoprotein secretions of the human epididymis are also expressed in the latter organ (Kirchhoff 1995).

4.8.2 Evidence from Assisted Reproduction

Another avenue of approach to determining the "**fertility profile**" of the epididymis is the application of **assisted reproduction techniques** (see Chap. 17). Under these experimental conditions, though, where the challenges to spermatozoa are completely different from those encountered *in vivo*, various stages of fertilization may be manifested *in vitro* by what were hitherto considered "immature" spermatozoa. Thus, in contrast to epididymovasostomies, in which sperm are deposited through natural copulatory activity into, and have to survive in, the female tract, assisted reproductive technologies bypass most of the natural barriers overcome by sperm after a normal ejaculation (Cooper 1995a).

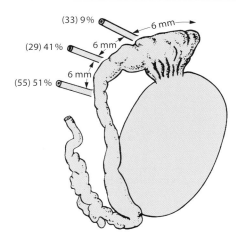

Fig. 4.8. Scheme indicating how epididymal occlusion can be overcome by anastomosing the remaining patent vas deferens to an unobstructed region. The length of the epididymis through which sperm pass naturally varies with the site of attachment. The pregnancy rates (%) increase the more distal the connection (number of patients in parenthesis). From Bedford (1988)

Data are available from **in vitro fertilization (IVF)** where sperm are taken from various regions of occluded ducts, especially from men with **congenital bilateral aplasia of the vas deferens** and **cystic fibrosis**, where no vasal structures are present and surgical correction is not possible. Pregnancies can result from fertilization of eggs by sperm obtained from cauda, corpus, caput (**micro-epididymal sperm aspiration, MESA**), the efferent ducts and testicular sperm from epididymal cysts (Hirsch et al. 1996) and testicular biopsies (**testicular sperm extraction, TESE**). Where comparisons have been made, sperm from more proximal regions of the tract are, however, less competent to initiate pregnancies as judged by high embryonic losses (Fig. 4.9 h).

With more invasive reproductive technologies (see Chap. 17) human testicular spermatozoa produce pregnancies by **subzonal insemination (SUZI)** and **intracytoplasmic sperm injection (ICSI)**. Even immature germ cells, obtained from the ejaculate or testicular biopsies can initiate pregnancies *via* intracytoplasmic injection methods termed **ELSI** (elongated spermatid injection), **ROSI** (round spermatid injection) or **ROSNI** (round spermatid nucleus injection) (see Lacham-Kaplan and Trounson 1997). Where comparisons have been made on the application of **ICSI** with testicular spermatozoa, the rate of 2 pronuclear embryos is lower and the transfer rate and pregnancy rates are lower with testicular sperm compared to epididymal sperm cells (Van Steirteghem et al. 1995). This demonstrates that even for humans the germ cell acquires some functional capabilities beyond the testis related to embryo formation.

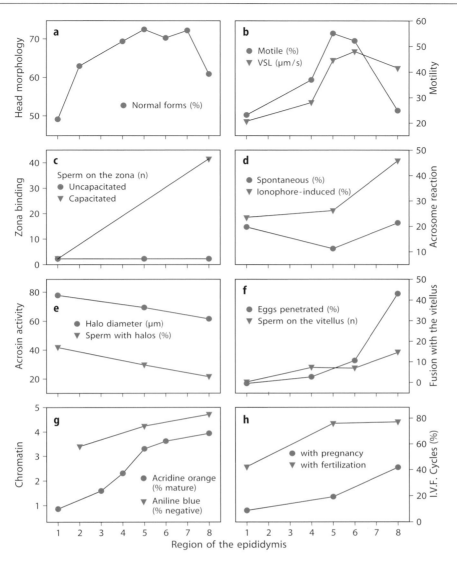

Fig. 4.9 a–h. Summary of changes to human spermatozoa removed from different regions of the epididymis. **a** normal sperm head morphology (uniform head shape, from Soler et al. 2000); **b** motility (percentage and straight-line velocity) (from Yeung et al. 1993); **c** binding ability of uncapacitated cells is low (Delpech et al. 1982) but only mature capacitated cells bind to the zona (from Moore et al. 1992); **d** spontaneous acrosomal loss is constant in all epididymal regions but ionophore-induced acrosome reactions occur only to corpus and cauda sperm (Yeung et al. 1997); **e** acrosin activity as detected on substrates declines or is less accessible upon maturation (Haidl et al. 1994); **f** penetration of zona-free hamster eggs by capacitated, acrosome-reacted sperm increases as sperm mature (Moore et al. 1983); **g** chromatin assumes the mature compacted form of packaging as assessed by aniline blue binding to nucleoproteins (Haidl et al. 1994) and acridine orange binding to nuclei acids (Golan et al. 1996); **h** fertilization and pregnancy rates are higher when distal epididymal sperm are used in IVF (Patrizio et al. 1994). Regions of epididymis: *1* efferent ducts; *2–3* proximal corpus; *4* midcorpus; *5–6* distal corpus; *7–8* cauda epididymidi

4.8.3 Development of Sperm Motility

Spermatozoa released from the testis are equipped with the structural complex for flagellation although they are immotile. Some sluggishly motile spermatozoa can be obtained from the testis of patients with **congenital absence of the ductus deferens** or **obstructive azoospermia**, although the incidence of spontaneous testicular sperm motility seems to occur only in association with epididymal or ductus deferens blockage (Jow et al. 1993). Induction of motility is a time-dependent phenomenon and it is now common practice to incubate testicular sperm *in vitro* to induce motility before using them for ICSI (Edisiringhe et al. 1996). The axonemal complex of testicular spermatozoa is already functional in some but not all cells, since flagellation can be induced by ATP in a low percentage of testicular sperm permeated with Triton X–100.

In passing through the epididymis, sperm from the testis not only acquire the potential for motility, but also develop the pattern of movement from an immature into a mature form. The mature status of the sperm axoneme is attained before that of the intact sperm (Yeung 1995), indicating that developments in second messenger signalling occur later. Although the profiles of change found in consecutive segments of the epididymis differ in various mammalian species, there is a general trend of increase in parameters including motility percentage, **velocity** of forward progression (VSL) and **straightness** of swim-path (Fig. 4.9b). The increase in VSL is largely a consequence of development in the coordination of flagellation, reflected by the parallel increase in the linearity of progression, in addition to an increase in the vigour of flagellation as reflected by the curvilinear velocity. These maturational changes in sperm kinematics occur along the proximal half of the epididymis and are accomplished in the mid-corpus epididymidis. There is little change in the amplitude of head displacement along the axis of progression.

The **heterogeneity** of the sperm population in any one region of the epididymis attests to differing rates of maturation in motility among individual sperm cells. Young mature spermatozoa from the mid-corpus epididymidis, where kinematic values are maximal, are most homogenous. In several animals studied, especially in man, there is a decline to various extents in either percentage motility or VSL, or both, within the cauda epididymidis, often accompanied by a decrease in homogeneity of the sperm population. This probably reflects ageing of the mature spermatozoa, and the extent of such decline is related to the periods of **sexual inactivity** (Yeung et al. 1993; Bedford 1994).

The nature of the stimulus to sperm motility development within the epididymis is not clear, but changes in intracellular pH, Ca^{2+}, cAMP levels (see Yeung 1995) and protein phosphatase (Vijayaraghavan et al. 1996), have been postulated for animal spermatozoa. Epididymal sperm possess a novel **adenylyl cyclase** and they can be stimulated by **bicarbonate** that is produced by epithelial cells containing carbonic anhydrase. Equally important are the phosphodiesterase activities that regulate cAMP production and A kinase anchoring protein (AKAP) which is derived from the pro-AKAP acquired in the testis (Turner et al. 1998) and partially processed to the mature form in the epididymis.

The increased vigour of the more mature sperm cells, as indicated by VCL, provides them with an efficiency which is lacking from more proximal cells with respect to their escaping from cervical mucus, migrating within the female tract and penetrating the egg investments. They have less of an advantage in vitro when contact with eggs is provided technically, as in IVF, although

penetration of the zona here is still required. For **subzonal insemination** (SUZI), where the zona is breached mechanically to bring the sperm cell into the perivitelline space, motility is not required for fertilization since even immotile sperm (e.g. from men with the ciliary disturbance Kartagener's syndrome) may fuse with the egg. After penetrating the egg the sperm normally stops beating (Yanagimachi 1994) so that motility is not required once the sperm nucleus has entered the egg, and stopping movement by damaging the sperm membrane is a normal and necessary practice in ICSI techniques (Dozortsev et al. 1995a; see Chap. 17).

4.8.4 Development of Sperm-Zona Binding Capacity

Capacitated spermatozoa from the caput epididymidis bind to the zona pellucida to a lower extent than those from the ejaculate, which provides evidence for an epididymal maturation of the zona binding process (Fig. 4.9c). Many sperm "zona receptors" have been identified in different species; some are present on testicular sperm and are modified during epididymal transit by changes in size or location on the sperm head, others are secretion products of the epididymis (Cooper 1996). Recently, a human **epididymal secreted glycoprotein** (P34H) has been shown to be involved in zona binding (Boué et al. 1996; Legare et al. 1999).

> Some cases of **infertility** are associated with failure of attachment of the sperm to the zona (Bedford and Kim 1994) and reduced epididymal P34H in sperm (Boué et al. 1996).

4.8.5 Development of the Ability to Undergo the Acrosome Reaction

When epididymal sperm are incubated under conditions considered capacitating for mature cells, "**spontaneous**" **acrosome reactions** are constant in all epididymal regions (Fig. 4.9d). Attempts to induce the acrosome reaction in human epididymal sperm by incubation with calcium ionophore (Fig. 4.9d) or prolonged incubation at 4°C (Haidl et al. 1994) lead to a higher rate of acrosome reactions by mature than immature spermatozoa, demonstrating a maturation in the ability of sperm cells to respond to external stimuli with an acrosome reaction. This may reflect changes in sperm sterols (Haidl and Opper 1997). Provided that they undergo the acrosome reaction, immature sperm should have sufficient acrosin for zona penetration, since spermatozoa are packaged with their full complement of acrosin in the testis and caput epididymidal spermatozoa contain as much, if not more, **acrosin** as sperm from the cauda (Fig. 4.9 e).

> **Infertility** may be caused by acrosome reaction insufficiency (Tesarik and Mendoza 1993).

4.8.6 Development of the Potential to Fuse with the Vitellus

The ability of epididymal sperm to bind to and fuse with the hamster vitelline membrane occurs beyond the caput and is maximal in the cauda epididymidis (Fig. 4.9 f). As sperm have to be both capacitated and acrosome-reacted in order to fuse with the egg, and immature sperm are less competent to undergo the acrosome reaction (Fig. 4.9 d), it is unclear whether the reduced ability of immature sperm to fuse reflects their failure to be **capacitated** or to be **acrosome-reacted** or whether the **equatorial region** of the sperm has been modified inappropriately if the acrosome reaction occurs.

RGD (arg-gly-asp) tripeptide sequences are involved in **sperm-vitellus recognition** (Bronson and Fusi 1996) and the human **epididymis** secretes a soluble form of fibronectin, an RGD-containing cell adhesion protein, possibly responsible for sperm-egg interaction (Miranda and Tezón 1992). Other secreted proteins include the FLB1 and SOB2 antigens (Boué et al. 1995; Lefevre et al. 1997) and testicular sperm proteins containing the metalloproteinase-like domains (Frayne et al. 1998) that may be involved in sperm-oolemma contact.

4.8.7 Condensation of Sperm Chromatin and Ability to Form Pronuclei

In all species studied, there is an accumulation of disulphide bonds in the chromatin material of maturing sperm in the epididymis due to oxidation of sulphydryl (SH) groups of DNA-binding proteins (**protamines**). Chromatin condensation occurs to sperm in the epididymis (Bedford 1994) as indicated by decreased staining by aniline blue, a dye that interacts with **histones**, and by acridine orange, that binds to the nucleic acid, as sperm mature (Fig. 4.9 g), reflecting the oxidation of sulphydryl bonds on nucleoproteins. Providing that the egg contains sufficient reducing power in the ooplasm, no problems will be encountered with decondensing mature sperm cell nuclei; consequently there is no problem during ICSI treatment in decondensing immature sperm heads which contain fewer S-S bonds.

4.8.8 Development of the Ability to Contribute to a Healthy Embryo

In many species epididymal spermatozoa that have developed the competence to fertilize eggs may not produce viable embryos. **Delayed fertilization**, delayed cleavage, and **pre-** and **post-implantation** losses have been documented in many species (Mieusset 1995). The cause of this has hardly been investigated, but observations on the **methylation of genes** within spermatozoa in the epididymis (Ariel et al. 1994) may throw light on this. Methylation of some genes prevents their transcription so that without methylation, unscheduled DNA synthesis may occur that could result in asynchronous cell division if it applied to genes expressed in the early embryo. This suggests that the epididymis has control over genes expressed in the next generation and differences in methylation states of sperm at the time of syngamy may be responsible for asynchronous development of the embryos.

Despite fertilization by human epididymal sperm occurring in vitro, transfer of embryos does not always result in pregnancies. Comparison of the number of cycles that produce pregnancies with those in which fertilization occurs (see Cooper 1995) clearly reveals that human sperm from the proximal occluded epididymides are not able to generate embryos of such good quality as sperm obtained more distally (Fig. 4.9h). This view is confirmed by recent findings on the application of ICSI to testicular spermatozoa which have shown that the formation rate of 2 pronuclear embryos is lower (Lacham-Kaplan and Trounson 1999) and the transfer rate and **pregnancy rates** are lower with testicular sperm compared to epididymal sperm cells. The stage of sperm development when parental imprinting occurs (the parent-of-origin-specific expression of only one allele of a gene) is unknown for man but in mice it is already established in round spermatids.

Thus **nuclear chromatin** is not developed into its final form at the time of spermatozoon formation in the testis and a period in the epididymis is required for the mature state to be achieved (see 4.8.7). As this fully condensed chromatin requires some time to be decondensed in the egg, it may constitute a timing device before pronuclei are formed that permits synchrony with female pronucleus formation.

4.9 Sperm Storage in the Epididymis

Spermatozoa within the epididymal canal are quiescent. This is partially enforced by lower concentrations of sodium and higher concentrations of potassium in **epididymal fluid** than are found in serum as a result of the transporting activities of the epithelium. Low **sodium**

ion concentrations prevent the sodium-dependent increase in intracellular pH that normally promotes motility once the cells are released from the tract at ejaculation or in vitro. Low intracellular pH, brought about by the penetrating acids (e. g. lactate), may also inhibit the initiation of motility within the epididymis.

The **storage capacity** of the human epididymis is small (Bedford 1994) and **transport** of sperm through it rapid (see 4.2). Ejaculated sperm are unlikely to have been held for long periods in the epididymis and after about 2 weeks of abstinence sperm appear in the urine (Barratt and Cooke 1988). When aged spermatozoa are cleared from the epididymis by multiple ejaculations within a short period of time after a two-week period of **sexual abstinence**, they are still viable. By this method of accumulating sperm in the epididymis, an increase in the number of morphologically normal and motile spermatozoa can be achieved by multiple ejaculation at the end of the abstinence period (Cooper et al. 1993). Although the fertilizing potential of sperm stored so long has to be proven, this strategy may be beneficial for increasing the sperm output of oligozoospermic patients.

During their time in the epididymis sperm are likely to be protected from lipid peroxidation by certain secre-

tory products of the epididymis such as **superoxide dismutase** and **glutathione peroxidase** (Williamson et al. 1998) and from damage by leaking acrosomal enzymes by a secreted **acrosin inhibitor** (Kirchhoff 1999). Experimenal retention of the epididymis (but not testis) in the abdomen reduces the size and **storage capacity** of the epididymis and our clothed lifestyle which limits **scrotal cooling** may influence spermatozoa contained in the epididymis with undesirable consequences for fertility (Bedford 1994).

> It is possible that dysfunction of epididymal sperm storage can be a cause of **infertility** (De-Kretser et al. 1998).

4.10 Immune Protection of Autoantigenic Spermatozoa in the Epididymis

As spermatozoa are formed many years after the **immune system** develops its ability to distinguish "self" from "non-self", they will be considered "foreign"

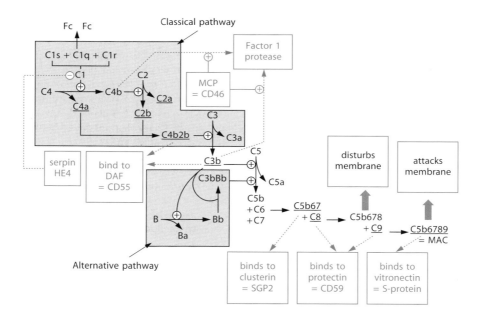

Fig. 4.10. A scheme outlining putative complement regulators in the male reproductive tract. *Black text*, sequential events; *grey boxes*, classical and alternative pathways; *red text*, immunoprotective pathways. In the *classical pathway*, the C1 component interacting with appropriately situated Fc fragments of immunoglobulins stimulates production of a cascade of proteases (C4b, C2b) that combine to yield C4b2b which cleaves C3 to C3b. In the *alternative pathway*, C3b is produced spontaneously or by conversion of Factor B to Bb and production of the protease C3bBb. *Both pathways* generate C3b which converts C5 to C5b, and which in turn sequentially combines with other complement components C6, C7, C8 and C9 to yield a mem-

brane attack protein (MAC). Protection from attack (*red text*) is at the level of (i) inhibition of initial C1 protease by serine protease inhibitors (*e. g.* serpins), (ii) destruction of the proteases C4b and C3b by Factor I protease, involving a sperm membrane cofactor protein (MCP, CD46), (iii) binding of the proteases C4b2b and C3b by decay accelerating factor (DAF, CD55), (iv) binding of components of the membrane attack complex by clusterin (SGP-2), protectin (CD59) and vitronectin (S-protein) on sperm cells. CD46, CD55 and CD59 are present on testicular spermatozoa and the epididymis secretes SGP-2 and serpin, HE4

should they be recognised by the immune system. Various strategies have been adopted to hide them from immunological surveillance. Firstly, sperm are **segregated** within the epididymal tubule. Unless this is ruptured, as may occur after vasectomy, injury or disease, or in cases of agenesis of the ductus deferens by continuous accumulation of sperm cells, they are to a large extent separated from circulating **immune effector cells**. However, the **tight junctional complexes** in the epididymis that prevent paracellular transport are not as effective as those in the testis and antigenic material can gain access to the interstitium either through these tight junctions or by circumventing the barrier altogether by transcytosis.

A second line of defence operating under normal conditions, indicated by the lack of anti-sperm immune response despite the leakage of antigens, comprises **immunosuppression** by factors in the epididymis that reduce lymphocyte activation (Pöllänen and Cooper 1994). **Macrophages** that are able to present sperm autoantigens to the immune system are only occasionally found in the normal epididymal epithelium but they are abundant in the interstitial tissues. Cell-mediated antigenic responses against sperm are effectively paralysed as spermatozoa lack both the MHC-I- and MHC-II-antigens that are required for the responses of CD4+- or CD8+-lymphocytes and co-stimulatory molecules are normally absent. Should circulating antibodies be produced, their escape from capillaries is limited (Pöllänen et al. 1995). **Complement**-assisted destruction of sperm in the lumen is minimal because of low levels of complement and the high levels of **complement regulatory proteins** on spermatozoa. The latter are present on developing germ cells in the testis (e.g. CD46, CD55 and CD59) and are secreted by the epididymal epithelium into epididymal fluid (e.g. SGP-2: Ibrahim et al. 1999) (see Fig. 4.10).

DeKretser et al. (1998) have shown that **antisperm antibodies** are present in the serum of men with epididymal occlusion, whether of obstructive or congenital origin. The incidence is higher when occlusion is more distal which suggests that there are regional abilities of the duct to suppress antigen responses. The macrophage-like expression of basal cells of the human epididymis (Yeung et al. 1994) may indicate their involvement in removal of sperm auto-antigens.

4.11 Assisted Reproduction

Providing that an infertile man has some sperm production in the testis, several treatment modalities are available to him. Such assisted reproduction strategies are explained in Chapter 17 and involve obtaining spermatozoa from the ejaculate, the epididymis and, in an increasing number of cases, spermatids from the testis

itself (Van Steirteghem et al. 1995). When the ductus deferens is present, bypassing the blocked epididymis by anastomosing the vas deferens to the proximal patent duct (**epididymovasostomy**) can return sperm to the ejaculate so that by normal intercourse these spermatozoa follow the pathways outlined above. Sperm employed for **intra-uterine insemination** (IUI) still have to survive in and ascend the female tract but bypass the vagina. Where sperm numbers are so low as to preclude these interventions various other assisted reproductive strategies are used and what is demanded of sperm here depends on where the sperm are obtained and in what situation they are used. Technologies have been introduced that demand less, or at least something different, from the fertilizing sperm cells. For example, in **gamete intra-fallopian transfer** (GIFT) sperm are placed directly in the oviduct and avoid cervical and uterine passage; with **fertilization in vitro** (IVF) sperm avoid all contact with the female body and usually do not have to penetrate the cumulus oophorus since it is shed in the presence of high sperm numbers; with **sub-zonal insemination** (SUZI) spermatozoa are introduced directly into the perivitelline space and do not have to penetrate the zona pellucida; and **intra-cytoplasmic sperm injection** (ICSI), as its name implies, bypasses even the egg membrane (see Fig. 4.2).

Clearly, what is required for a testicular spermatid to fertilize an egg after microinjection into the egg cytoplasm is only the latter part of what is required of a normally ejaculated spermatozoon and whether "fertilization" is the correct term to describe what is achieved in these cases of assisted reproduction is questionable. The evidence compiled above indicates that for nearly every step in the normal fertilization process, the ability of sperm cells to perform that step is modified in the epididymis. Clearly, when these steps are bypassed by assisted reproduction techniques, the dependence of fertilization on the maturational status of the spermatozoa is less apparent. Furthermore, infertility similarly can stem from the inability of sperm cell to undergo any one of these sequential steps.

4.12 References

Adham IM, Nayerna K, Engel W (1997) Spermatozoa lacking acrosin protein show delayed fertilization. Mol Reprod Dev 46:370–376

Ariel M, Cedar H, McCarry J (1994) Developmental changes in methylation of spermatogenesis-specific genes include reprogramming in the epididymis. Nature Genetics 7:59–63

Asch A, Simerly C, Ord T, Ord VA, Schatten G (1995) The stage at which human fertilization arrests: microtubule and chromosome configurations in inseminated oocytes which failed to complete fertilization and development in humans. Hum Reprod 10:1897–1906

Baba T, Azuma S, Kashiwabara S-I, Toyada Y (1994) Sperm from mice carrying a targeted mutation of the acrosin gene can penetrate the oocyte zona pellucida and effect fertilization. J Biol Chem 269:31845–31849

Barone JG, De Lara J, Cummings KB, Ward WS (1994) DNA organization in human spermatozoa. J Androl 15:139–144

Barratt CLR, Cooke ID (1988) Sperm loss in the urine of sexually rested men. Int J Androl 11:201–207

Bedford M (1988) The bearing of epididymal function in strategies for in vitro fertilization and gamete intrafollicular transfer. Proc NY Acad Sci USA 541:284–291

Bedford JM (1994) Status and state of the human epididymis. Hum Reprod 9:2187–2199 1994

Bedford JM (1998) Mammalian fertilization misread? Sperm penetration of the Eutherian zona pellucida is unlikely to be a lytic event. Biol Reprod 59:1275–1287

Bedford JM, Kim HH (1993) Sperm/egg binding patterns and oocyte cytology in retrospective analysis of fertilization in vitro. Hum Reprod 8:453–463

Benoff S, Hurley IR, Mandel FS, Cooper GW, Hershlag A (1997) Induction of the human sperm acrosome reaction with mannose-containing neoglycoprotein ligands. Mol Hum Reprod 3:827–837

Boué F, Blais J, Sullivan R (1996) Surface localization of P34H, an epididymal protein, during maturation, capacitation, and acrosome reaction of human spermatozoa. Biol Reprod 54:1009–1017

Boué F, Duquenne C, Lassalle B, Lefevre A, Finaz C (1995) FLB1, a human protein of epididymal origin that is involved in the sperm-oocyte recognition process. Biol Reprod 52:267–278

Brandelli A, Miranda PV, Tezón JG (1996) Voltage-dependent calcium channels and Gi regulatory protein mediate the human sperm acrosomal exocytosis induced by N-acetylglucosaminyl/mannosyl neoglycoprotein. J Androl 17:522–529

Bronson RA, Fusi FM (1994) Integrins and human reproduction. Mol Hum Reprod 2:153–168

Brown DB, Hayes EJ, Uchida T, Nagamani M (1995) Some cases of human male infertility are explained by abnormal in vitro human sperm activation. Fertil Steril 64:612–622

Chemes HE, Olmeda SB, Carrere C, Oses R, Carizza C, Leisner M, Blaquier J (1998) Ultrastructural pathology of the sperm flagellum: association between flagellar pathology and fertility prognosis in severely asthenozoospermic men. Hum Reprod 13:2521–2526

Cooper TG (1993) The human epididymis – is it necessary? Int J Androl 16:245–250

Cooper TG (1995a) Functions of the human epididymis. In: Hamamah S, Mieusset R, Dacheux JL (eds) Frontiers in Endocrinology. Epididymis: role and importance in male infertility treatment. Ares Serono Symposia, Rome, pp 1–12

Cooper TG (1995b) The epididymal influence on sperm maturation. Reprod Med Rev 4:141–161

Cooper TG (1996) Physiology and evaluation of epididymal function. In: Comhaire FH (ed) Male infertility. Clinical investigation, cause, evaluation and treatment. Chapman and Hall Medical, London, pp 97–119

Cooper TG (1998) Epididymis: In: Neill JD, Knobil E (eds) Encyclopedia of reproduction, vol 2. Academic, San Diego, pp 1–17

Cooper TG, Yeung CH (1999) Recent biochemical approaches to post-testicular, epididymal contraception. Hum Reprod Update 5:141–152

Cooper TG, Yeung CH, Nashan D, Jockenhövel F, Nieschlag E (1990) Improvement in the assessment of human epididymal function by the use of inhibitors on the assay of α-glucosidase in seminal plasma. Int J Androl 13:297–305

Cooper TG, Jockenhövel F, Nieschlag E (1991) Variations in semen parameters from fathers. Hum Reprod 6:859–866

Cooper TG, Keck C, Oberdieck U, Nieschlag E (1993) Effects of multiple ejaculations after extended periods of sexual abstinence on total, motile and normal sperm numbers, as well as accessory gland secretions, from healthy normal and oligozoospermic men. Hum Reprod 8:1251–1258

Cross NL, Morales P, Overstreet JW, Hanson FW (1988) Induction of acrosome reactions by the human zona pellucida. Biol Reprod 38:235–244

Dandekar P, Aggeler J, Talbot P (1992) Structure, distribution and composition of the extracellular matrix of human oocytes and cumulus masses. Hum Reprod 7:391–398

De Kretser DM, Huidobro C, Southwick GJ, Temple-Smith PD (1998) The role of the epididymis in human infertility. J Reprod Fertil Suppl 53:271–275

Delpech S, Lecomte P, Lecomte C (1988) Etude in vitro chez l'homme de la liaison des spermatozoids epididymaires a la zone pellucida. J Gynecol Obstet Biol Reprod 17:339–342

Dozortsev D, Rybouchkim A, DeSutter P, Qian C (1995a) Human oocyte activation following intracytoplasmic injection: the role of the sperm cell. Hum Reprod 10:403–407

Dozortsev D, Rybouchkin A, DeSutter P, Dhont M (1995b) Sperm plasma membrane damage prior to intracytoplasmic sperm injection: a necessary condition for sperm nucleus decondensation. Hum Reprod 10:2960–2964

Edirisingher WR, Junk SM, Matson PL, Yovich JL (1996) Changes in motility patterns by in-vitro culture of fresh and frozen/thawed testicular and epididymal spermatozoa: implication for planning treatment by intracytoplasmic sperm injection. Hum Reprod 11:2474–2476

Eisenbach M (1999) Sperm chemotaxis. Rev Reprod 4:56–88

Fogdestam I, Fall M, Nilsson S (1986) Microsurgical epididymovasostomy in the treatment of occlusive azoospermia. Fertil Steril 46:925–929

Folgerø T, Bertheussen K, Lindal S, Torbergsen T, Øian P (1993) Mitochondrial disease and reduced sperm motility. Hum Reprod 8:1863–1868

Frayne J, Jury JA, Barker HL, Hall L (1998) The MDC family of proteins and their processing duing epididymal transit. J Reprod Fertil Suppl 53:149–155

Green DP (1997) Three-dimensional structure of the zona pellucida. Rev Reprod 2:147–156

Golan R, Cooper TG, Oschry Y, Oberpenning F, Schulze H, Shochat L, Lewin LM (1996) Changes in chromatin condensation of human spermatozoa during epididymal transit as determined by flow cytometry. Hum Reprod 11:1457–1462

Haidl G, Opper C (1997) Changes in lipids and membrane anisotropy in human spermatozoa during epididymal maturation. Hum Reprod 12:2720–2723

Haidl G, Badura B, Schill W-B (1994) Function of human epididymal spermatozoa. J Androl 15:23S–27S

Hirsch AV, Dean NL, Mohan PJ, Shaker AG, Bekir JS (1996) Natural spermatocoeles in irreversible obstructive azoospermia-reservoirs of viable spermatozoa for assisted conception. Hum Reprod 11:1919–1922

Hunter RHF (1987) Human fertilization in vivo, with special reference to progression, storage and release of competent spermatozoa. Hum Reprod 2:329–323

Ibrahim NM, Troedsson MHT, Foster DN, Loseth KJ, Farris JA, Blaschuk O, Crabo BG (1999) Reproductive tract secretions and bull spermatozoa contain different clusterin isoforms that cluster cells and inhibit complement-induced cytolysis. J Androl 20:230–240

Jeyendran RS, van der Ven HH, Rosecrans R, Perez-Pelaez M, Al-Hasani S, Zaneveld LJD (1989) Chemical constituents of human seminal plasma: relationship to fertility. Andrologia 21:423–428

Johnson L, Varner DD (1988) Effect of daily sperm production but not age on transit time of spermatozoa through the human epididymis. Biol Reprod 39:812–817

Jow WW, Steckel J, Schlegel PN, Magid MS, Goldstein M (1993) Motile sperm in human testis biopsy specimens. J Androl 14:194–198

Katz DF, Morales P, Samuels SJ, Overstreet JW (1990) Mechanisms of filtration of morphologically abnormal human sperm by cervical mucus. Fertil Steril 54:513–503

Kirchhoff C (1995) Molecular biology of sperm maturation in the human epididymis. Reprod Med Rev 4:121–139

Kirchhoff C (1999) Gene expression in the epididymis. Int Rev Cytol 188:133–202

Kunz G, Beil D, Deininger H, Wildt L, Leyendecker G (1996) The dynamics of rapid sperm transport through the female genital tract: evidence from vaginal sonography of uterine peristalsis and hysterosalpingoscintigraphy. Hum Reprod 11:627–632

Lacham-Kaplan O, Trounson A (1997) Fertilization and embryonic development capacity of epididymal and testicular sperm and immature spermatids and spermatocytes. Reprod Med Rev 6:55–68

Lefevre A, Ruis CM, Chokomian S, Duquenne C, Finaz C (1997) Characterization and isolation of SOB2, a human sperm protein with a potential role in oocyte membrane binding. Mol Hum Reprod 3:507–516

Legare C, Gaudreault C, St-Jacques S, Sullivan R (1999) P34H sperm protein is prefentially expressed by the human corpus epididymidis. Endocrinology 140:3318–3327

Lin Y, Mahan K, Lathrop WF, Myles DG, Primakoff P (1994) A hyaluronidase activity of the sperm plasma membrane protein PH-20 enables sperm to penetrate the cumulus cell layer surrounding the egg. J Cell Biol 125:1157–1163

Lindemann CB, Kanous KS (1997) Model for flagellar motility. Int Rev Cytol 173:1–72

Liu DY, Baker HWG (1994) Disordered acrosome reaction of spermatozoa bound to the zona pellucida: a newly discovered sperm defect causing infertility with reduced sperm-zona pellucida penetration and reduced fertilization in vitro. Hum Reprod 9:1694–1700

Mieusset R (1995) Spermatozoa and embryo development. In: Hamamah S, Mieusset R, Dacheux JL (eds) Frontiers in Endocrinology. Epididymis: role and importance in male infertility treatment. Ares Serono Symposia, Rome, pp 105–128

Miranda PV, Tezón JG (1992) Characterization of fibronectin as a marker for human epididymal sperm maturation. Mol Reprod Dev 33:443–450

Montag M, Tor V, Liow S-L, Ng S-C (1992) In vitro decondensation of mammalian sperm and subsequent formation of pronuclei-like structures for micromanipulation. Mol Reprod Dev 33:338–346

Moore HDM, Hartmann TD, Pryor JP (1983) Development of the oocyte-penetrating capacity of spermatozoa in the human epididymis. Int J Androl 6:310–318

Moore HDM, Curry MR, Penfold LM, Pryor JP (1992) The culture of human epididymal epithelium and in vitro maturation of epididymal spermatozoa. Fertil Steril 58:776–783

Morales P, Vigil P, Franken DR, Kaskar K, Coetzee K, Kruger TF (1994) Sperm-oocyte interactions: studies on the kinetics of zona pellucida binding and acrosome reaction of human spermatozoa. Andrologia 26:131–137

Mortimer D (1995) Sperm transport in the female genital tract. In: Grudzinskas JG, Yovich JL (eds) Gametes. The Spermatozoon. CUP, Cambridge, pp 157–174

Mortimer ST, Swan MA (1995) Variable kinematics of capacitating human spermatozoa. Hum Reprod 10:3178–3182

Navara CS, Simerly C, Zoran S, Schatten G (1995) The sperm centrosome during fertilization in mammals: implications for fertility and reproduction. Reprod Fertil Devel 7:747–754

Neugebauer DC, Neuwinger J, Jockenhovel F, Nieschlag E (1990) 9+0 Axoneme in spermatozoa and some nasal cilia of a patient with totally immotile spermatozoa associated with thickened sheath and short midpiece. Hum Reprod 5:981–986

Nieschlag E, Weinbauer GF, Cooper TG, Wittkowski W. (1999) Reproduktion. In: Deetjen P, Speckmann E-J (eds) Physiologie, 3rd edn. Urban and Schwarzenberg, Munich, pp 521–539

Overstreet JW, Hembree WC (1976) Penetration of the zona pellucida of non-living human oocytes by human spermatozoa. Fertil Steril 27:815–831

Palermo GD, Avrech OM, Colombero LT, Wum H, Wolny YM, Fissore RA, Rosenwaks Z (1997) Human sperm cytosolic factor triggers Ca2+ oscillations and overcomes activation failure of mammalian oocytes. Mol Human Reprod 3:367–374

Patrizio P, Ord T, Silber SJ, Asch RH (1994) Correlation between epididymal length and fertilization rate in men with congenital absence of the vas deferens. Fertil Steril 61:265–268

Phillips DM (1991) Structure and function of the zona pellucida. In: Familiari G, Makabem S, Motta PM (eds) Ultrastructure of the ovary. Kluwer Academic, The Hague, pp 63–72

Pöllänen P, Cooper TG (1994) Immunology of the testicular excurrent ducts. J Reprod Immunol 26:167–216

Pöllänen P, Saari T, Cooper TG (1995) Regulation of the transport of immunoglobulin into the male rat reproductive tract. J Reprod Immunol 28:111–136

Revelli A, Massobrio M, Tesarik J (1998) Nongenomic actions of steroid hormones in reproductive tissues. Endocrine Rev 19:3–17

Sathananthan AH, Ratnam SS, Ng SC, Tarin JJ, Gianaroli L, Trounson A (1996) The sperm centriole: its inheritance, replication and perpetutation in early human embryos. Hum Reprod 11:345–356

Smith TT (1998) The modulation of sperm function by the oviductal epithelium. Biol Reprod 58:1102–1104

Soler C, Pérez-Sánchez F, Schulze H, Bergmann M, Oberpenning F, Yeung C-H, Cooper TG (2000) Objective evaluation of the morphology of human epididymal sperm heads. Int J Androl 23:77–84

Sousa M, Mendoza C, Barros A, Tesarik J (1996) Calcium responses of human oocytes after intracytoplasmic injection of leukocytes, spermatocytes and round spermatids. Mol Hum Reprod 2:853–857

Temple-Smith PD, Zheng SS, Kadioglu T, Southwick GJ (1998) Development and use of surgical procedures to bypass selected regions of the mammalian epididymis: effects on sperm maturation. J Reprod Fertil Suppl 53:183–195.

Tesarik J, Mendoza C (1992) Defective function of a nongenomic progesterone receptor as a sole sperm anomaly in infertile patients. Fertil Steril 58:793–797

Tesarik J, Mendoza, C (1993) Sperm treatment with pentoxifylline improves the fertilizing ability in patients with acrosome reaction insufficiency. Fertil Steril 60:141–148

Tesarik J, Thebault A (1993) Fertilization failure after subzonal sperm insertion associated with defective functional capacity of acrosome-reacted spermatozoa. Fertil Steril 60:369–371

Tesarik J, Sousa M, Mendoza C (1995) Sperm-induced calcium oscillation of human oocytes show distinct features in oocyte center and periphery. Mol Reprod Devel 41:257–263

Töpfer-Peterson, E (1999) Carbohydrate-based interactions on the route of a spermatozoon to fertilization. Human Reprod Update 5:314–329

Turner RMO, Johnson LR, HaigLadewig L, Gerton GL, Moss SB (1998) An X-linked gene encodes a major human sperm fibrous sheath protein, hAKAP82. J Biol Chem 273:32135–141

Van Steirteghem AC, Nagy Z, Liu J, Joris, C; Janssenswillen C, Silber S, Devroey P (1995) Embryo development after ICSI using testicular, epididymal and ejaculated spermatozoa. In: Hamamah S, Mieusset R, Dacheux JL (eds) Frontiers in Endocrinology. Epididymis: role and importance in male infertility treatment. Ares Serono Symposia, Rome, pp 141–147

Vijayaghavan S, Stephens DT, Trautman K, Smith GD, Khatra B, da Cruz e Silva EF, Greengard P (1996) Sperm motility development in the epididymis is associated with decreased glycogen synthase kinase-3 and protein phosphatase 1 activity. Biol Reprod 54:709–718

Visconti PE, Galantino-Homer H, Moore GD, Bailey JL, Ning X, Fornes M, Kopf GS (1998) The molecular basis of sperm capacitation. J Androl 19:242–248

von Lanz T, Neuhäuser G (1964) Morphometrische Analyse des menschlichen Nebenhodens. Z Anat Entwickl 124:126–152

Wassarman PM (1992) Regulation of mammalian fertilization by gamete adhesion molecules. In: Nieschlag E, Habenicht U-F (eds) Spermatogenesis, fertilization, contraception. Molecular, cellular and endocrine events in male reproduction. Springer, Berlin Heidelberg New York, pp 345–366

Williamson K, Frayne J, McLaughlin EA, Hall L (1998) Expression of extracellular superoxide dismutase in the human male reproductive tract, detected using antisera raised against a recombinant protein. Mol Hum Reprod 4:235–242

Yanagimachi, R (1994) Mammalian fertilization. In: Knobil E, Neill JD (eds) The physiology of reproduction, 2nd edn. Raven, New York, pp 189–317

Yeung CH (1995) Development of sperm motility. In: Hamamah S, Mieusset R, Dacheux JL (eds) Frontiers in endocrinology. Epididymis: role and importance in male infertility treatment. Ares Serono Symposia, Rome, pp 73–86

Yeung CH, Bals-Pratsch M, Knuth UA, Nieschlag E (1988) Investigation of the cause of low sperm motility in asthenozoospermic patients by multiple quantitative tests. Int J Androl 11:289–299

Yeung CH, Cooper TG, Bergmann M, Schulze H (1991) Organization of tubules in the human caput epididymidis and the ultrastructure of their epithelia. Am J Anat 191:261–279

Yeung CH, Cooper TG, Oberpenning F, Schulze H, Nieschlag E (1993) Changes in movement characteristics of human spermatozoa along the length of the epididymis. Biol Reprod 49:274–280

Yeung CH, Nashan D, Cooper TG, Sorg C, Oberpenning F, Schulze H, Nieschlag E (1994) Basal cells of the human epididymis – antigenic and ultrastructural similarities to tissue-fixed macrophages. Biol Reprod 50:917–926

Yeung CH, Cooper TG, Majumder GC, Rolf C, Behre HM (1996) The role of phosphocreatine kinase in the motility of human spermatozoa supported by different metabolic substrates. Mol Hum Reprod 2:591–596

Yeung CH, Perez-Sanchez F, Soler C, Poser D, Kliesch S, Cooper TG (1997) Maturation of human spermatozoa (from epididymides selected from prostatic carcinoma patients) with respect to their morphology and ability to undergo the acrosome reaction. Hum Reprod Update 3:205–213

Zamboni L (1992) Sperm structure and its relevance to infertility. Arch Pathol Lab Med 116:325–344

Zarintosh RJ, Cross NL (1996) Unesterified cholesterol content of human sperm regulates the response of the acrosome to the agonist, progesterone. Biol Reprod 55:19–24

CHAPTER 5

Classification of Andrological Disorders

5

E. NIESCHLAG

5.1 Classification Based on Localization of Origin and Cause

Infertility and hypogonadism are the symptoms of a wide range of disorders to be dealt with in the following chapters. It is the physician's task to recognize the subtle nuances of these symptoms and to use appropriate ancillary techniques in order to come to the appropriate diagnosis. In andrology, as in all areas of medicine, a diagnosis as exact as possible is a prerequisite for optimal therapeutic direction. The best therapy cannot be given without knowledge of the pathological basis of the underlying disorder.

The **causes of male infertility and hypogonadism** are located at various levels of the organism. The **testes** themselves may be affected; the causes for infertility may lie in the **excurrent seminal ducts** or in the **accessory sex glands**; there may be a disturbance of **semen deposition**, but also central structures such as the **hypothalamus** and the **pituitary** or the **androgen target organs** may be afflicted.

> The **first principle** in classifying disorders of male infertility and hypogonadism is therefore the topographic **localization** of the cause. The **nature** of the cause may serve as a **second principle** of classification, e.g. endocrine, genetic, inflammatory etc.

Such a classification is used in this volume. An overview is shown in Table 5.1, which also indicates the diagnostic criterion to determine whether an individual disorder is connected with signs of androgen deficiency, infertility or both symptoms.

In addition to this vertical classification of disorders, factors must be considered targeted at several specific levels or being of general importance. Thus, **general and systemic diseases** may affect all or several of the above-mentioned levels at the same time and may thus exert their impact on testicular function and fertility; therefore general and systemic diseases will be dealt with in a separate chapter (Chap. 12). The impact of **toxins and environmental factors** on fertility is not yet fully understood and requires further intensive research; these issues are summarized in a special chapter (Chap. 13). In all disorders **psychological factors** play an important role, in some they may even be their cause; therefore, psychology of male infertility is reviewed in an individual chapter (Chap. 19). In addition, there is a large group of patients in whom no clear cause of infertility can be identified. These patients most likely represent a heterogeneous group whose so-called **idiopathic infertility** may have very different causes. It is a compelling task of andrology to investigate these causes by intensive research. In these patients, seminal parameters may be normal or subnormal and may then be described by the terminology of oligo-, astheno- and teratozoospermia. Such symptomatic description fails to provide any clue to pathophysiology. Idiopathic infertility will be dealt with in the context of therapeutic measures (Chap. 16).

There may be special aspects of fertility, infertility and genetic risks for the offspring of **older men**; endocrine alterations and the possibility of hormone replacement therapy in senescence are of increasing interest. A special chapter is devoted to male senescence (Chap. 21).

For some time disturbances of sexual differentiation were summarized under the term **intersexuality**. Since the transition from a completely normal to an intersexual phenotype may be indistinct and since the causes of disturbed sexual differentiation can be identified according to the levels of classification used here, we have dispensed with the term **intersexuality** as a nosological entity. For psychological reasons it is also advisable to eliminate this discriminating term when dealing with patients and to use terminology based on the pathophysiology. The different **disorders of sexual differentiation** (as far as the male sex is concerned) are classified according to the above-mentioned principles and can be found either under "Disorders at the Testicular Level" (Chap. 8) (e.g. male pseudohermaphroditism based on disorders of testosterone biosynthesis or Leydig cell

Table 5.1. Classification of disorders of testicular function based on localization of cause

Localization of disorder	Disorder	Cause	Androgen deficiency	Infertility
Hypothalamus/ pituitary	Kallmann syndrome	Congenital disturbance of GnRH secretion, defect of the Kal-X gene	+	+
	Idiopathic hypogonadotropic hypogonadism	Congenital disturbance of GnRH secretion	+	+
	Prader-Labhart-Willi syndrome	Congenital disturbance of GnRH secretion	+	+
	Constitutionally delayed puberty	Delayed biological clock	+	+
	Secondary disturbance of GnRH secretion	Tumors, infiltrations, trauma, irradiation, disturbed circulation, malnutrition, systemic diseases	+	+
	Hypopituitarism	Tumors, infiltrations, trauma, irradiation, ischemia, surgery GnRH receptor mutation	+	+
	Pasqualini syndrome	Isolated LH-deficiency	+	(+)
	Hyperprolactinemia	Adenomas, medications, drugs	+	+
Testes	Congenital anorchia	Fetal loss of testes	+	+
	Acquired anorchia	Trauma, torsion, tumor, infection, surgery	+	+
	Testicular maldescent	Testosterone-, MIH-deficiency, congenital anatomical hindrance	(+)	+
	Varicocele	Venous insufficiency?	(–)	+
	Orchitis	Infection and destruction of germinal epithelium	(–)	+
	Sertoli-cell-only syndrome	Congenital/acquired	–	+
	Spermatogenic arrest	Congenital/acquired	–	+
	Globozoospermia	Absence of acrosome formation	–	+
	Immotile cilia syndrome	Absence of dynein arms	–	+
	Klinefelter syndrome	Meiotic non-dysjunction	+	+
	46XX-male	Translocalization of part of Y-chromosome	+	+
	47XYY-Male	Meiotic non-dysjunction	(+)	(+)
	Noonan syndrome	Congenital	+	+
	Structural chromosomal anomalies	Deletions, translocations	–	+
	Persistent oviduct	MIH receptor mutation	–	(–)
	Gonadal dysgenesis	Genetic disturbances of gonadal differentiation	+	+

Table 5.1. (continued)

Localization of disorder	Disorder	Cause	Androgen deficiency	Infertility
	Leydig cell hypoplasia	LH-receptor mutation	+	(+)
	Male pseudohermaphroditism	Enzymatic defects in testosterone synthesis	+	+
	True hermaphroditism	Genetic disturbance in gonadal differentiation	+	+
	Testicular tumors	Congenital/acquired?	+	+
	Disorder caused by exogenous factors or systemic diseases	Medication, irradiation, heat, environmental and recreational toxins, liver cirrhosis, renal failure	+	+
	Idiopathic infertility	?	–	+
Excurrent seminal ducts and accessory sex glands	Infections	Bacteria, viruses, chlamydia	–	+
	Obstructions	Congenital anomalies, infections, vasectomy, appendectomy, herniotomy, kidney transplantation	–	+
	Cystic fibrosis	Mutation of the CFTR-gene	–	+
	CBAVD (congenital bilateral aplasia of the vas deferens)	Mutation of the CFTR-gene	–	+
	Young syndrome	Mercury poisoning?	–	+
	Disturbance of liquefaction	?	–	+
	Immunologic infertility	Autoimmunity	–	+
Disturbed semen deposition	Ectopic urethra	Congenital	–	(+)
	Penis deformations	Congenital/acquired	–	(+)
	Erectile dysfunction	Multifactorial origin	(+)	(+)
	Disturbed ejaculation	Congenital/acquired	–	+
	Phimosis	Congenital	–	(+)
Androgen target organs	Testicular feminization	Complete androgen receptor defect	+	+
	Reifenstein syndrome	Incomplete androgen receptor defect	+	+
	Prepenile bifid scrotum + hypospadias	Incomplete androgen receptor defect	+	+
	Bulbospinal muscular atrophy	Androgen receptor defect	(+)	–
	Perineoscrotal hypospadias with pseudovagina	5α-reductase deficiency	+	+
	Estrogen resistence	Estrogen receptor defect	(–)	(–)
	Estrogen deficiency	Aromatase deficiency	(–)	(–)
	Gynecomastia	?	(+)	(–)
	Androgenic alopecia	?	–	–

Table 5.2. Percentage distribution of diagnoses of 10,469 consecutive patients attending the Institute of Reproductive Medicine of the University of Münster. In case of several disorders the leading diagnosis was counted. Because of the nature of the specialization of the Institute, hypogonadism appears overrepresented, including mainly Klinefelter syndrome, IHH, Kallmann syndrome and pituitary insufficiency

Diagnosis	%
Idiopathic infertility	31.1
Varicocele	15.6
(Endocrine) hypogonadism	8.9
Infections (subclinical)	8.0
Maldescended testes	7.8
Disturbances of semen deposition (including erectile dysfunction, hypospadias etc.)	5.9
Immunological factors	4.5
General and systemic diseases	3.1
Obstructions	1.7
Gynecomastia	1.1
Testicular tumors (incidental diagnosis in infertility workup)	0.3
Semen cryopreservation in malignant disease	6.5
Remainder	5.5

hypoplasia) or under "Disorders of Androgen Target Organs" (Chap. 11) (e. g. testicular feminization and Reifenstein syndrome).

Prevalence and incidence of the various disorders – to whatever extent known – will be reported in the appropriate paragraphs. Table 5.2 provides an overview of the frequency of individual disorders as they may occur in a larger center of andrology/reproductive medicine.

5.2 Classification According to Therapeutic Possibilities

Unlike the previously described classification of andrological disorders based on localization of origin and cause, a purely pragmatic classification based on treatment modalities is also possible. Such a classification would largely ignore pathophysiological considerations, with the primary question of whether and how to treat the patient receiving priority. When talking to patients it is useful to have therapeutic possibilities at one's fingertips. For this reason, such an overview is presented and briefly explained in Table 5.3.

As described in the following chapters, there is a series of fertility disturbances whose pathophysiological origins are known and which can be **treated rationally**. For some diseases for which the cause is known there are **no rational therapies** available. For others, e. g. anomalies of testicular descent and infections, **preventive treatment** can avoid infertility. Techniques of assisted reproduction (intrauterine insemination, in vitro fertilization and intracytoplasmic sperm injection) offer effective treatment of male infertility which can, however, only be considered **symptomatic therapy** as they do not eliminate the cause of disturbed fertility (see Chap. 17). Thus they are applied independently of the diagnosis and exclusively on the basis of ejaculate parameters or extractability of sperm from the epididymis or testis.

Prior to the introduction of assisted reproduction (especially before ICSI) many **empirical therapies** were used for male infertility. These were and continue to be used indiscriminately in various diagnoses. This applied most frequently to **varicocele**, **immunological infertility** and especially **idiopathic infertility**. Together these cases comprise almost half the patients with disturbed fertility (see Table 5.2). Because of the dimensions of the problem empirical treatment of idiopathic infertility is dealt with in a separate chapter, whereas varicocele (see Sec. 8.4) and immunological infertility (see Sec. 9.7) are discussed in the context of the volume's classification.

Table 5.3. Classification of male infertility according to therapeutic possibilities

Disorder	Therapy	Disscussed in section of this volume
Rational Therapy		
IHH and Kallmann syndrome	GnRH oder gonadotropins	7.1
Pituitary insufficiency	Gonadotropins	7.1
Prolactinoma	Dopamin agonists	7.7
Infections	Antibiotics	9
Chronic general diseases (Renal insufficiency, diabetes mellitus)	Treatment of underlying disease	12
Medications, drugs, toxins	Elimination	12/13
Obstructive azoospermia	Epididymovasostomy, vasovasostomy	9.2
Retrograde ejaculation	Imipramine	10.3
Preventive Therapy		
Maldescended testes	GnRH/hCG/orchidopexy	8.3
Delayed puberty	Testosterone/GnRH/hCG	7
Infections	Timely use of antibiotics	9.1
Exogenous factors (X-rays, drugs, poisons)	Elimination	12/13
Malignant disease	Gonadal protection/ cryopreservation of sperm	18
No Therapy		
Bilateral anorchia	[Testosterone substitution]	8.1
Complete SCO syndrome	–	8.6
Gonadal dysgenesis	[Testosterone substitution]	8.15
Empirical Therapy		
Idiopathic infertility	Various medications	16
Immunological infertility	Immunosuppression	9.8
Varicocele	Intervention/counselling	8.4
Symptomatic Treatment		
Severe fertility disturbance	Assisted reproduction (IUI, IVF, ICSI, TESE)	17

CHAPTER 6

Diagnosis of Male Infertility and Hypogonadism   **6**

H. M. BEHRE · C. H. YEUNG · A. F. HOLSTEIN · G. F. WEINBAUER
P. GASSNER · E. NIESCHLAG

In this chapter the diagnostic methods of andrology are presented with particular emphasis on the two main topics, male **infertility** and male **hypogonadism**. Regarding special diagnostic procedures, reference is made to separate chapters of this book, e.g. erectile dysfunction (Chap. 10) or special gynecological diagnostics (Chap. 14).

The diagnostic procedures of hypogonadism and infertility mainly consist of a comprehensive anamnesis, a clinical examination, endocrinological laboratory diagnostics and – in case of infertility – semen analysis. On suspicion of certain clinical findings, additional examinations are needed.

6.1 Anamnesis

The anamnesis provides important information for the assessment of testicular function. Impairment of general performance, a diminution of beard growth and a decrease in shaving frequency, a decrease in erection frequency, particularly spontaneous nocturnal and morning erections, and a lessening of sexual desire and phantasies provide important information on possible androgen deficiency. Because of a concomitant decrease in libido, patients' complaints may be muted in contrast to those generated by erectile dysfunction not caused by testosterone deficiency. Important aspects emerge from suspicions aroused by particular clinical pictures. In the case of a suspected pituitary tumor, for example, the field of vision should be checked for impairment; in the case of a suspected Kallmann syndrome, disturbances of the olfactory sense have to be considered.

As regards **medical history**, onset of puberty, voice mutation and the beginning of beard growth have to be recorded. Any testicular maldescent and the age at which medical therapy (hCG or GnRH) or surgery (orchidopexy) were carried out are of importance. Herniotomy, possibly with subsequent testicular damage, is recorded. Since general diseases (diabetes mellitus, liver or kidney diseases) can lead to hypogonadism and/or infertility, the relevant symptoms have to be recorded (see Chap. 12). Recurrent bronchitis or sinusitis in childhood or adulthood indicate diseases of the respiratory system which may, e.g. in the case of Kartagener syndrome, Young syndrome or cystic fibrosis, be associated with infertility. Infectious diseases with or without clinically manifest orchitis or epididymitis can lead to androgen deficiency and/or infertility. Sexually transmitted diseases (syphilis, gonorrhoea, AIDS) and their respective treatments must be recorded. The **family medical history**, including data on the fertility status of parents, siblings and other relatives, provides essential information for a possible genetic cause of hypogonadism and infertility.

An exact **drug history** is important, since a multitude of substances can lead to side-effects of androgen deficiency and infertility (e.g. sulfasalazine, anti-hypertensive drugs, antibiotics, cytostatic agents, anabolic hormones) (see Chap. 12). Occupational exposure to heat and chemicals can lead to infertility (see Chap. 13). In addition, exposure to **exogenous toxins**, which may impair spermatogenesis and testicular testosterone production, should be carefully recorded (see Chap. 13). Athletic activities, particular habits and nicotine and alcohol abuse are to be registered.

Since involuntary childlessness is a problem common to the **couple**, the medical history should be taken in the presence of both partners. In case of infertility, the duration of barrenness, unprotected intercourse and intercourse frequency are documented. Periodic separations, e.g. because of shiftwork or frequent travel, are recorded. Indications for dyspareunia should also be pursued. Professional or private stress factors which may lead to conflicts between the partners are explored. Earlier pregnancies with the present partner or in another partnership are also recorded. Both previously performed and anticipated infertility examinations of the female partner should be noted.

6.2 Physical Examination

A thorough physical examination provides an overview of all organ systems and of diseases which may be associated with hypogonadism and/or infertility. In the following sections, special examinations are mentioned when hypogonadism or infertility are suspected. It should be kept in mind that the clinical presentation of hypogonadism is dependent on the time of manifestation (Table 6.1). If androgen deficiency becomes manifest after puberty, clinical symptoms can be discrete.

6.2.1 Body Proportions, Skeletal Structure, Fat Distribution

If androgen deficiency exists at the time of normal onset of puberty, **eunuchoid tall stature** will result because of delayed or absent pubertal development with delayed epiphyseal closure. Consequently, arm span will exceed body length and the legs become longer than the trunk. Because of these characteristic body proportions these patients are short when sitting ("**sitting dwarfs**") and tall while standing ("**standing giants**"). Patients may remain short if other central disorders are present, especially those affecting thyroid function or growth factors. However, bodily proportions will develop similarly to those seen in eunuchoid tall stature. Onset of androgen deficiency after puberty will not result in a change of bodily proportions, although the **musculature can be**

Table 6.1. Symptoms of hypogonadism relative to age of manifestation

Affected organ/function	Before completed puberty	After completed puberty
Larynx	No voice mutation	No voice mutation
Hair	Horizontal pubic hairline, straight frontal hairline, diminished beard growth	Diminishing secondary body hair
Skin	Absent sebum production, lack of acne, pallor, skin wrinkling	Decreased sebum production, lack of acne, pallor, skin wrinkling
Bones	Eunuchoid tall stature, osteoporosis	Osteoporosis
Bone marrow	Low degree anemia	Low degree anemia
Muscles	Underdeveloped	Atrophy
Prostate	Underdeveloped	Atrophy
Penis	Infantile	No change of size
Testes	Possibly maldescended testes, small volume	Decrease of testicular volume
Spermatogenesis	Not initiated	Involuted
Libido and potency	Not developed	Loss

atrophic depending on the duration and degree of androgen deficiency.

Long-standing androgen deficiency leads to **osteoporosis** which can result in severe **lumbago** and pathological spine and hip **fractures** (Jackson et al. 1992). The androgen deficiency does not directly cause an increase in subcutaneous fatty tissue; however, **fat distribution** will have female characteristics (hips, buttocks, lower abdomen) (Marin et al. 1995) and the **lean body mass** will decrease.

6.2.2 Voice, Hair, Skin

If hypogonadism is present before normal puberty, **no voice mutation** will occur because of a lack of laryngeal growth. Often patients are addressed as females despite advanced age, especially on the telephone, with negative effects on the patient's self-esteem. When hypogonadism develops after puberty, the voice, already mutated, remains unchanged.

The **frontal hairline** remains straight, **beard growth** is lacking or sparse, shaving is seldom or never necessary, and the **upper pubic hairline** remains horizontal. **Temporal hair recession** or **balding** will not occur but secondary sexual hair and body hair become sparser (Randall 1998). When evaluating hair distribution as a a possible indication of androgen deficiency, **ethnic differences** must be considered (Santner et al. 1998).

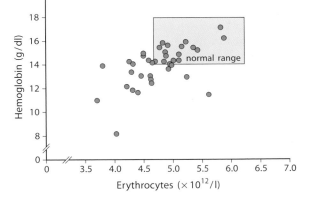

Fig. 6.1. Concentration of hemoglobin and erythrocytes in blood in 39 consecutively examined patients with hypogonadism before testosterone substitution therapy

Another typical feature is early, **fine wrinkling of the perioral and periorbital skin**. Additionally, because sebaceous gland stimulation is absent, the skin remains dry (Imperato-McGinley et al. 1993). Anemia (Fig. 6.1), along with decreased blood circulation of the skin, causes **pallor**.

6.2.3 Olfactory Sense

The existence of **hyposmia** or **anosmia**, which are important diagnostic indicators of Kallmann syndrome, are recorded following specific questioning and systematic examination. Patients with Kallmann syndrome are unable to smell aromatic substances (e. g. vanilla, lavender). Substances irritating to the trigeminal nerve (e. g. ammonia) are, however, recognizable.

6.2.4 Mammary Gland

Gynecomastia is defined as enlargement of the mammary gland in the male. It must be distinguished by palpation or sonography from pure **lipomastia**. In most cases gynecomastia is bilateral, more rarely unilateral without side preference. In cases of marked, especially unilateral enlargement, and suspicious findings at palpation, a **mammography** should be performed for diagnosis of a possible mammary cancer. Gynecomastia can cause breast tension and the mammillae may be sensitive to touch. In most cases, however, gynecomastias are asymptomatic.

Gynecomastia develops frequently in pubescent boys at the age of about 14 years and disappears within 2–3 years. Concomitant obesity augments and prolongs the clinical picture. Gynecomastia can occasionally persist into adulthood without clinical significance. It may appear in the aging male. Small, firm testes in combination with gynecomastia are typical for Klinefelter syndrome. Gynecomastia can also be present in other forms of primary hypogonadism or diseases of androgen target organs. Hyperprolactinemia can lead to gynecomastia which is caused more often by concomitant hypogonadism than by the increased prolactin itself.

> Rapidly developing gynecomastia may indicate an **endocrinologically active testicular tumor** (Braunstein 1993). The symptom triad gynecomastia, loss of libido and testicular tumor is characteristic. **Careful palpation and sonography of the testes is obligatory in all cases of gynecomastia.**

Testicular tumors (Leydig cell tumor; embryonic carcinoma, teratocarcinoma, chorioncarcinoma, combination tumor) lead either directly or via elevated hCG secretion to increased estradiol production by the Leydig cells. Chronic, general illnesses (e. g. liver cirrhosis, terminal renal failure under hemodialysis, hyperthyroidism) can also cause gynecomastia. A large number of **drugs**, with quite different mechanisms of action, may exacerbate gynecomastia (see Sect. 11.4).

6.2.5 Testis

The normal testis has a firm **consistency**. When LH and FSH stimulation are absent the testes are usually soft; small, very firm testes are typical for Klinefelter syndrome. Fluctuating to tightly elastic consistency indicates a hydrocele which is confirmed through diaphanoscopy or, preferably, through ultrasonography. Differences in testicular consistency between the two sides, a very hard testis or an uneven surface raise suspicion of a testicular tumor. Testicular size is determined by palpation and comparison to testis-shaped models of defined sizes (Prader orchidometer). A healthy European man has, on average, a **testicular volume** of 18 ml per testis; the normal range lies between 12 and 30 ml. A higher testicular volume is known as megalotestis (Meschede et al. 1995). Accurate testicular volume measurement, especially in the case of undescended testes or intrascrotal pathological processes, is possible with the use of ultrasonography. Normal testicular volume in combination with azoospermia indicates an obstruction of the seminal duct, as testicular volume correlates with sperm production, although within wide margins (Fig. 6.2).

The presence of **maldescended testes** or **anorchia** should be recorded. In the case of **cryptorchidism**, the testis lies intra-abdominally or retroperitoneally above the inguinal canal and cannot be palpated. The **inguinal testis** is a testis fixed in the inguinal canal. The **retractile testis** is located at the orifice of the inguinal canal and can be temporarily moved to the scrotum, or migrates spontaneously between the scrotum and the inguinal canal, e. g. in response to cold or coitus. In the case of an **ectopic testis**, the testis lies outside the normal path of descent (see Sect. 8.3).

Palpation is performed with the patient standing. A supine position is chosen if a testis in not palpable or difficult to palpate. Cold and excitement of the patient

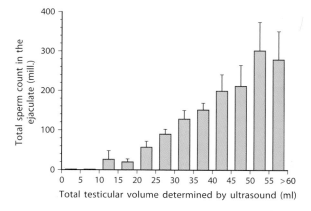

Fig. 6.2. Correlation between sonographically measured testicular volume and total sperm count in the ejaculate of 246 patients of the Institute of Reproductive Medicine, Münster

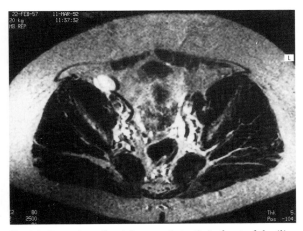

Fig. 6.3. Detection of a right ectopic testis in front of the iliac muscle by nuclear magnetic resonance tomography in a 35 year-old man. Sonography of the scrotal content and the inguinal region failed to detect testicular tissue on either side. A normal increase of testosterone had been shown by hCG test. After surgical removal, histology revealed a seminoma (pT1N0M0). The patient was asymptomatic and remained free of metastases. No testicular tissue is detectable on the left side

are to be avoided since they can induce a cremasteric reflex and thus cause retraction of the testis. Ultrasonography is especially indicated for maldescended testes. In cases of bilateral cryptorchidism or ectopic testes, measuring anti-Muellerian hormone (AMH) or performing an hCG-test distinguishes the condition from anorchia (see Sect. 6.4.5 and 6.4.6). When testes are unpalpable, they can be localized by **magnetic resonance tomography**, as the imaging method of choice (Fig. 6.3).

6.2.6 Epididymis

The normal epididymis can be palpated as a soft organ in a cranio-dorsal position relative to the testis. Smooth cystic distensions indicate a distal **obstruction**; indurations indicate an obstruction caused by diseases such as gonorrhoea or epididymitis. **Spermatoceles** appear as tense-elastic spherical formations, mainly in the area of the head of the epididymis. Painful swelling of the epididymis indicates acute or chronic **inflammation**, soft tumorous swelling of the epididymis can be found in rare cases of a tuberculoma.

6.2.7 Pampiniform plexus

A **varicocele**, a distension of the venous pampiniform plexus, usually appearing on the left side, will be diagnosed by careful palpation of the standing patient. During the Valsalva maneuver, with increasing abdominal pressure, the veins distend. Depending on the results of palpation, the varicocele is assigned to one of the following grades. I° **varicocele** can be palpated only during the Valsalva maneuver. II° **varicocele** can be palpated without a Valsalva maneuver. III° **varicocele** is a visible distension of the pampiniform plexus.

While III° varicoceles can be easily diagnosed, diagnosis of smaller varicoceles depends largely on the experience of the investigator. In addition, palpation can be complicated by previous surgery, hydroceles or maldescended testes. Here, Doppler sonography or ultrasonography offer the best methods for diagnosis.

6.2.8 Deferent Duct

The deferent duct can be palpated between the vessels of the spermatic chord in the upright, standing patient. Absence of the deferent duct leads to obstructive azoospermia. Obstructive azoospermia caused by congential malformation of the epididymis and/or deferent duct (unilateral or bilateral **congenital aplasia of the vas deferens = CBAVD**) is found in approximately 2 % of infertile patients attending infertility clinics (see Chap. 9). Partial obliterations or aplasias of the deferent duct can escape palpation. In such cases, surgical exploration of the scrotal content is indicated.

6.2.9 Penis

The penis remains infantile if hypogonadism becomes manifest before onset of normal puberty. If hypogonadism appears after puberty, changes of penile size will not occur. Among Europeans the erect penis is between 11 and 15 cm long (Baker and Bellis 1995). During examination of the penis, the urethral orifice has to be localized, as even minor forms of **hypospadias** can lead to infertility. **Phimosis** is diagnosed by retraction of the prepuce. **Deviations** of the penis during erection and resulting problems of cohabitation should be described by the patient and be documented by autophotography (see Chap. 10).

6.2.10 Prostate and Seminal Vesicles

Rectal examination reveals the normal prostate gland to have a smooth surface and the size of a horse chestnut. In cases of hypogonadism prostate volume remains small and the normal age-dependent increase in volume is not seen. A doughy, soft consistency points to prostatitis, general enlargement to benign prostatic hyperplasia (BPH), knobby surface and hard consistency to a carcinoma. Significantly more information can be obtained from simultaneous transrectal sonography of the prostate and seminal vesicles (see Sect. 6.3).

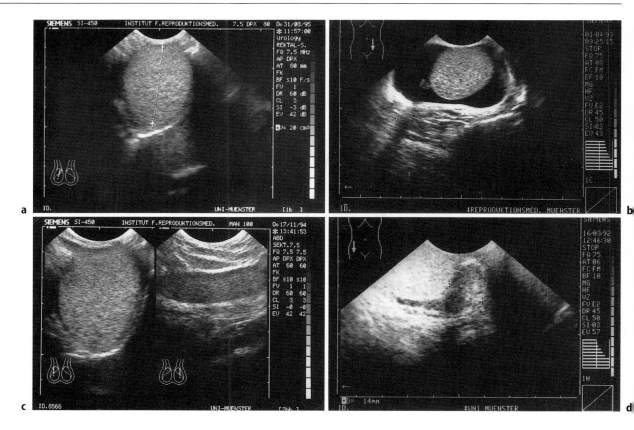

Fig. 6.4 a–d. Scrotal sonography with a 7.5 MHz sector scanner (Siemens SI 450, Erlangen). **a** Determination of testicular volume applying the area-length-diameter-calculation: testicular volume 20 ml. Homogeneous testis with normal echogenicity. **b** Hydrocele. The echo-free edge surrounds the testis with homogeneous parenchyma. **c** The right testis shows normal homogeneity and echogenicity. The left testis shows decreased echogenicity following maldescent and orchidopexy in childhood. **d** Enlarged and hypoechogenic epididymis (cauda epididymis: 14 mm in diameter) in acute epididymitis (infection with Chlamydia trachomatis)

6.3 Ancillary Methods of Investigation

6.3.1 Scrotal Ultrasonography

Ultrasonography allows imaging diagnostics of the scrotal content without side-effects. Normal testis and epididymis display homogenous parenchymal echogenicity. **Determination of testicular volume** by palpation can be difficult in the case of hydroceles, thickened scrotal skin, epididymal fibrosis and particularly, in the case of cryptorchidism. Here, ultrasonography allows objective determination of testicular volume. Using a rotation ellipsoid formula, precise and reproducible determination of testicular volume is possible, which is of importance for longitudinal therapeutic studies (e.g. treatment with gonadotropins in hypogonadotropic hypogonadal patients) (Fig. 6.4 a) (Behre et al. 1989). A **hydrocele** appears as an echo-free area around the testis (Fig. 6.4 b). It can occur following surgery or result from testicular tumors, or from chronic and recurrent inflammations of the testis or epididymis.

In **varicocele**, enlargement of the venous diameter of the pampiniform plexus can be registered and the increase in the diameter of individual veins can be measured during the Valsalva maneuver (Fig. 6.5 a). For the diagnosis of **testicular tumors**, today sonography is the

method of choice since even unpalpable, intratesticular tumors can be recognized. These tumors appear as hyperechogenic or, mostly, as hypoechogenic or mixed areas (Fig. 6.6 a–c). Regarding differential diagnosis, hypoechogenic areas may be caused by abscesses, hematomas or intratesticular cysts (Fig. 6.7 a). In the case of cryptorchidism, the testis frequently shows diminished echogenic appearance (Fig. 6.4 c). Differential diagnosis of hyperechogenic areas are fibrotic changes (e.g. after mumps orchitis or testicular biopsy) and, rarely microlithiasis testis (Fig. 6.7). Focal hyperechogenic or, more rarely, hypoechogenic areas may occur after testicular sperm extraction (TESE) (Ron-El et al. 1998).

Since infertile patients have an increased prevalence of **testicular tumors**, ultrasonography has become in-

Fig. 6.5 a–c. Diagnosis of a varicocele. **a** Sonography shows an increase of the vein diameter of the pampiniform plexus in a patient with varicocele (VC) during the Valsalva maneuver. In this example of a I° VC the vein diameter dilates from 2.3 to 4.2 mm. In a III° VC, ultrasonography shows multiple, severely dilated scrotal veins of the pampiniform plexus even without the Valsalva maneuver. **b** Venous backflow in the pampiniform plexus during Valsalva maneuver documented by Doppler sonography (10 MHz probe). **c** In case of varicocele the retrograde venous flux can be directly visualized by color-coded duplex sonography during Valsalva maneuver. Left: prior, and right during Valsalva maneuver

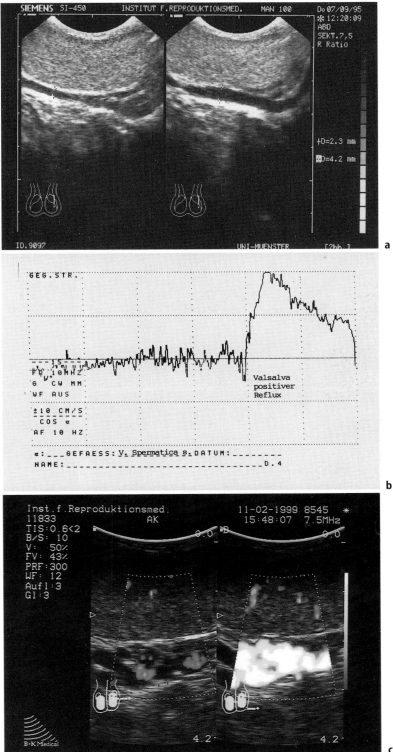

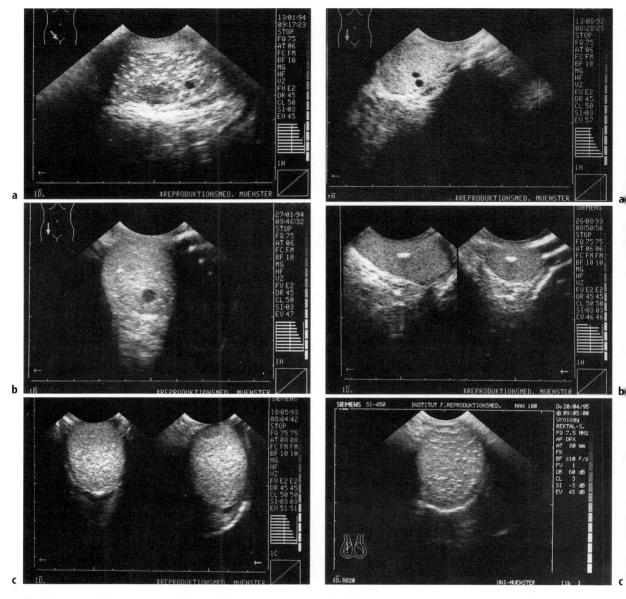

Fig. 6.6 a–c. Scrotal sonography with a 7.5 MHz sector scanner (Siemens SI 450, Erlangen, Germany). **a** Inhomogeneous parenchyma with hyperechoic and hypoechoic areas. After surgical removal, histology showed a seminoma of the testis (pT1 No Mo). **b** Hypoechoic area at the lower testicular pole; small hyperechoic areas and otherwise echonormal parenchyma of the testis. Histology revealed a seminoma (pT1 No Mo). **c** Hypoechoic area at the upper testicular pole. Histology showed a Leydig cell tumor

Fig. 6.7 a–c. Scrotal sonography with a 7.5 MHz sector scanner (Siemens SI 450, Erlangen, Germany). **a** Intratesticular multiple cysts: echo-free, smoothly limited round areas with dorsal echo enhancement in an otherwise homogenous testis. **b** Intratesticular calcifications with dorsal echo extinction. **c** Inhomogeneous parenchyma with numerous small, hyperechoic areas and otherwise inconspicuous echogenicity of the testis ("snowsquall"). Histology revealed a Sertoli-cell-only syndrome

creasingly important for the screening of infertile patients (Behre et al. 1995). Among 8000 patients who attended the Institute of Reproductive Medicine because of infertility, we diagnosed four patients with a **carcinoma in situ** (testicular intraepithelial neoplasia, always precancerous) and 19 patients with **testicular tumor**, of which three were benign Leydig cell tumors. A remarkable finding is the different distribution of testicular tumors observed, if the 3800 patients seen before and the 4200 seen after the introduction of sonography for routine andrological diagnosis are considered separately. In the first group of 3800, only one carcinoma in situ and one testicular tumor were found as incidental observations (after biopsy for evaluation of spermatogenesis and after a pathological finding at palpation). In the latter group we discovered a carcinoma in situ in three and a testicular tumor in 18 of the 4200 patients because of conspicuous results from sonography, subsequently confirmed by histology. In only five of the 18 patients with testicular tumors could a suspicious resistance be palpated; all patients with carcinoma in situ were inconspicuous at palpation.

Acute **epididymitis** results in a hypoechogenic and enlarged sonographical picture of the epididymis (Fig. 6.4d). An accompanying hydrocele is frequently found. Chronic epididymitis causes hyperechogenicity because of fibrotic changes of the epididymis. A spermatocele appears as an echo-free, even, round area within the epididymis.

Using sonography we obtained pathological findings in 53% of 3518 consecutively examined patients attending our clinic primarily because of infertility (Table 6.2). 0.4% of these patients had testicular tumors. This high rate of testicular tumors among patients attending infertility clinics was recently confirmed (0.5% in 1375 patients; Pierik et al. 1999). The incidence of testicular tumors is thus markedly higher than in the general male population; in Europe the overall incidence ranges from 0.8 to 7.6 per 100,000 man years (Ekbom and Akre 1998).

> Because of the high incidence of pathology detected by sonography and because of the high sensitivity and specificity of the method, we perform ultrasonography of the scrotal contents in every patient attending our infertility clinic.

6.3.2 Doppler Sonography

Doppler sonography enables blood flux through the pampiniform plexus to be measured. By this method any reflux of blood can be detected acoustically during a Valsalva maneuver and bidirectional flow can be registered (Fig. 6.5b). Color-coded duplex sonography can make venous reflux visible (Fig. 6.5c) (Chiou et al. 1997; Corund et al. 1999). Doppler or duplex sonography is well suited to determine the therapeutic results of surgical or radiological treatment of varicocele and can be used for objective evaluation of relapsing varicoceles.

6.3.3 Thermography

Since a varicocele with venous stasis can cause increased temperature of the affected testis and scrotal content, the temperature difference between both sides can provide information about the pathophysiological consequences of a varicocele. Thermography can be performed with thermosensitive films (WHO 1993) or continuously over 24 hours by means of a portable gauge

Table 6.2. Diagnoses by scrotal sonography in 3518 consecutive male patients attending the Institute of Reproductive Medicine, Münster, because of infertility

Sonographic Findings	Cases (n)	Proportion (%)
Without pathological findings	1604	45.6
Inhomogeneities of testicular parenchyma	424	12.2
Testicular cysts	24	0.7
Testicular tumors	15	0.4
Hydroceles	268	7.6
Epididymal enlargements/ inhomogeneities	365	10.4
Spermatoceles	146	4.2
Varicoceles	672	19.1

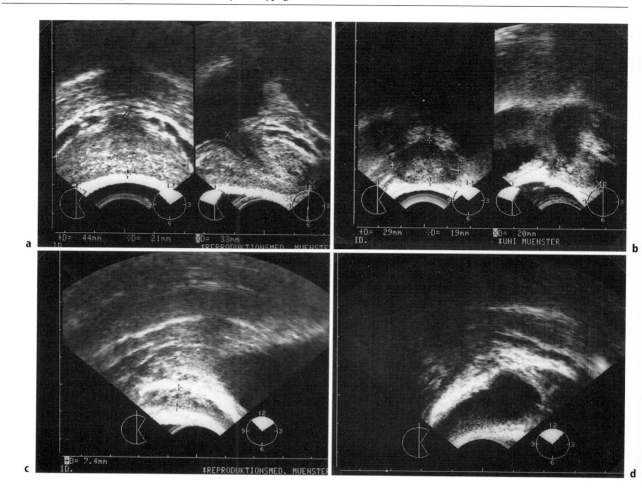

with thermal measuring devices (thermoport) (Jocken-hövel et al. 1990; Lerchl et al. 1993). Thermographic techniques have failed to become established in routine diagnosis.

6.3.4 Transrectal Ultrasonography of the Prostate Gland and the Seminal Vesicles

Transrectal sonography of the prostate (Fig. 6.8a, b) and the seminal vesicles (Fig. 6.8c, d) has a firm place in the diagnosis of hypogonadism and infertility (Behre et al. 1995). **Transrectal sonography of the prostate** can be applied for diagnosis of prostatitis, benign prostatic hyperplasia and prostate carcinoma. It allows intraprostatic cysts and dilatations of the ejaculatory duct to be ascertained as the cause or result of obstructions (see Chap. 9). Transverse and longitudinal scans, planimetry or, even better, three-dimensional imaging enable prostate volume to be determined exactly (Behre et al. 1994; Tong et al. 1998). Reduced **prostate volume,** characteristic of hypogonadal patients increases during a few

Fig. 6.8a–d. Transrectal sonography (7.5 MHz Endo-P-probe, Siemens Sonoline SI 450, Erlangen, Germany). **a** Normal prostate in transverse (left figure) and longitudinal scans (right figure). Exact determination of prostate volume by the planimetric method or – as shown here – by the formula for an ellipsoid. Prostate volume: 21 ml. Normal, healthy man. **b** Hypoechoic and small prostate gland (volume 6 ml) in an hypogonadal patient without substitution therapy. **c** Display of a normal seminal vesicle. **d** Dysfunction of the seminal vesicle. No depletion of an enlarged seminal vesicle is seen after ejaculation (as shown here). Diameter of the seminal vesicle: 22 mm

months of testosterone therapy to the age-appropriate normal range without, however, exceeding it, as shown by transrectal volume measurements (Behre et al. 1994). **Prostate specific antigen** (PSA) and **uroflow** are important parameters for monitoring prostate function. Especially in patients over 45 years, regular monitoring of the prostate is of particular importance to prevent any prostate carcinoma, whose growth might be stimulated by testosterone therapy, from being overlooked.

Transrectal ultrasonography of the seminal vesicles can be performed before and after ejaculation and may thus reveal agenesis or aplasia, as well as dysfunction of the seminal vesicles. The extent of such conditions, often associated with infertility, is largely unknown (Mesche- de et al. 1997). Patients with congenital aplasia of the vas deferens (CBAVD) are characterized by low ejaculate volume, azoospermia and low fructose in serum, often associated with aplasia, hypoplasia or cystic dilatations of the seminal ducts (Eckardstein et al. 2000). Transrec- tal sonography can also be applied to the diagnosis of prostatovesiculitis (Purvis and Christiansen 1993).

6.3.5 Further Imaging Techniques

On suspicion of pathological processes in the pituitary or hypothalamus, **magnetic resonance tomography (MRT)** is the method of choice and is superior to con- ventional X ray of the sella region or computer tomogra- phy. Magnetic resonance tomography (or computer to- mography) is applied when cryptorchidism or anorchia (unilateral or bilateral) is suspected and when testicular tissue cannot be visualized by sonography of the scro- tum or the inguinal canal (Fig. 6.3).

In younger hypogonadal patients and in boys with delayed puberty, **bone age** is determined by X ray of the left hand according to the appearance of the bones and extent of epiphyseal maturation (e.g. by comparison to the anatomical atlas by Greulich and Pyle 1959). Spinal alterations caused by osteoporosis due to androgen de- ficiency can be diagnosed by traditional X rays only in advanced stages. Osteoporosis can be diagnosed early with high accuracy and reproducibility by planimetric methods, such as **DPA (dual photon absorptiometry)** and **DXA (dual energy X ray absorptiometry)** or volu- metric methods such as **quantitative computer tomog- raphy of the lumbar spine (QCT)** or **peripheral QCT** of the tibia or radial bone (**pQCT**) (Fischer et al. 1993). Recently **quantitative ultrasonography (QUS)**, free of radioactivity and its incumbent risks, has become an es- tablished method for screening patients and for moni- toring therapy (Wüster et al. 1998). These methods can be applied for long-term objective monitoring of bone density of patients under androgen substitution therapy as an adjunct to hormone measurement (Behre et al. 1997).

6.4 Endocrine Laboratory Diagnosis

The main constituent of endocrine laboratory diagnosis of testicular disorders is the determination of the gona- dotropins LH and FSH as secretions of the anterior pitu- itary, of testosterone as the most important secretion of the Leydig cells and of inhibin B as the product of the Sertoli cells. When hypothalamic or pituitary disease are suspected, a GnRH stimulation test or, for patients with elevated prolactin, a TRH stimulation test should be per- formed. The hCG test evaluates the endocrine reserve capacity of the testes. For special diagnostic questions, additional hormone determinations are performed, e.g. determinations of prolactin and estradiol in the case of gynecomastia or hCG and estradiol upon suspicion of testicular tumor. For disturbances of sexual differentia- tion, different steroids are measured in order to localize enzyme defects. Determining androgen receptor levels or dihydrotestosterone and androgen metabolizing en- zymes (e.g. 5α-reductase) in the target organs may be necessary (see detailed descriptions in Chap. 3 and 11).

6.4.1 Gonadotropins

The evaluation of serum levels of LH and FSH in combi- nation with testosterone provides important informa- tion to pinpoint the localization of hypogonadism, which is decisive for adequate therapy.

> High gonadotropin levels in serum in combina- tion with low testosterone levels indicate testicular origin of hypogonadism (**primary hypogona- dism**); low gonadotropin levels point to a central cause (**secondary hypogonadism**).

For differentiation between low normal and pathologi- cally low LH and FSH levels, highly sensitive fluoro- immunoassays are recommended.

When interpreting basal **LH** values, the physiological **pulsatility of pituitary secretion** with ensuing oscilla- tions of serum levels has to be considered. A normal man shows approximately 8 to 20 LH pulses per day. Pa- tients with primary hypogonadism have increased aver- age serum concentrations, as well as elevated LH pulse frequency. When hypothalamic GnRH fails to be secret- ed, only sporadic LH pulses or none at all can be mea- sured. High LH levels occurring in combination with high testosterone serum concentrations indicate an androgen receptor defect (**androgen resistance**) (see Chap. 11).

FSH displays only minor serum level oscillations, and therefore a single point measurement is representative. **To a certain extent, FSH serum concentrations mirror spermatogenesis.** High FSH levels in the presence of a small, firm testis (<6 ml) and azoospermia are diag- nostic indicators for Klinefelter syndrome; low FSH levels indicate a hypothalamic or pituitary deficiency (Fig. 6.9). If testicular volume exceeds 6 ml and azoospermia or severe oligozoospermia is simulta- neously present, then elevated FSH indicates primary

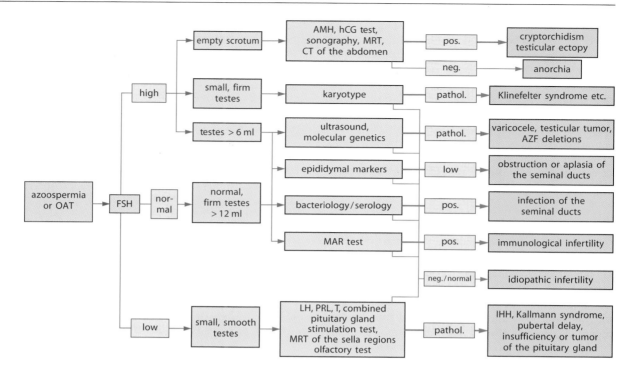

Fig. 6.9. Flow scheme for differential diagnosis of male fertility disorders indicating the importance of FSH, along with semen analysis

impairment of spermatogenesis. Within wide margins, the extent of FSH elevation is correlated with the number of seminiferous tubules lacking germ cells (Sertoli cell-only tubules) (Fig. 6.10) (Bergmann et al. 1994; Eckardstein et al. 1999).

Normal FSH values in combination with azoospermia, normal testicular volume and low levels of glucosidase in the ejaculate, raise suspicion of an obstruction or aplasia of the deferent duct (Fig. 6.9). This constellation, possibly accompanied by ambiguous findings, justifies bilateral testicular biopsy; in case of normal testicular biopsy, reconstructive surgery of the epididymis or deferent duct or techniques of assisted reproduction are indicated (Weidner et al. 1995).

For the determination of gonadotropin levels in serum, competitive assays, e.g. radioimmunoassays (RIA), or sensitive non-competitive immunoassays such as immunoradiometric assays (IRMA), immunofluorometric assays (IFMA) or enzyme-linked immunosorbant assays (ELISA), are available (Nieschlag 1998). In addition, sensitive **in vitro bioassays** for LH and FSH have been developed recently. In most cases, bioactivity and immunoactivity of gonadotropins are well correlated, so that in vitro bioassays are unnecessary for routine clinical diagnosis (Simoni and Nieschlag 1991).

Mutations of gonadotropin genes are rare. Inactivating mutations of the LH-ß subunit lead to infertility and failure of spontaneous puberty to occur. Inactivating mutations of the FSH-ß subunit cause azoospermia and, hence, infertility (Huhtaniemi et al. 1999). Similarly, rare mutations of the **gonadotropin receptor gene** are divided into activating and inactivating mutations. Activating LH receptor mutations cause precocious puberty, whereas inactivating mutations cause Leydig cell hypoplasia and hypogonadism. Inactivating FSH receptor mutations lead to variable disturbances of spermatogenesis. The only activating FSH receptor mutation described so far maintained spermatogenesis in a hypophysectomized male (overview in Simoni et al. 1997 and in Sect. 8.17).

6.4.2 GnRH, GnRH Test, GnRH Receptor

Because of extremely low serum concentrations, **GnRH** cannot be measured in peripheral blood by immunoassay.

The **GnRH test** is performed to determine the gonadotropin reserve capacity of the pituitary and is particularly indicated for low-normal LH and FSH values, which cannot always be differentiated from pathologically low basal values.

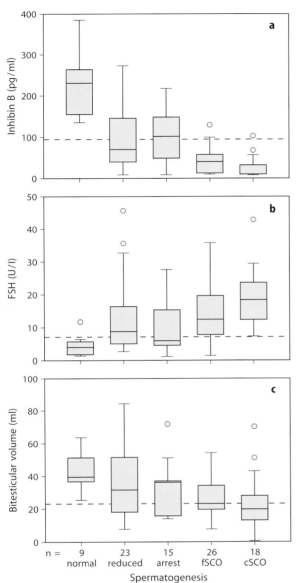

Fig. 6.10 a–c. Box plot showing serum concentrations of inhibin B (**a**) and FSH (**b**) as well as total testicular volume (**c**) in 91 infertile men divided into 5 groups according to testicular histology (*normal*: normal spermatogenesis; *reduced*: qualitatively reduced spermatogenesis; arrest: spermatogenic arrest; *fSCO*: focal Sertoli-cell-only syndrome; *cSCO*: complete Sertoli-cell-only syndrome). Broken line shows lower normal levels for inhibin B and total testicular volume as well as upper normal levels of FSH (Eckardstein et al. 1999)

The rise of LH should be at least threefold 30 to 45 minutes after injection of 100 µg GnRH; the increase in FSH should be 1.5 times over basal. However, the results should be judged by an experienced clinician.

If a hypothalamic disorder is suspected during the first GnRH test and no rise of gonadotropins is observed, a **GnRH pump test** should be performed. After pulsatile GnRH treatment (5 µg GnRH every 120 minutes) for 36 hours to 7 days, the GnRH test is repeated. A significant rise in gonadotropin levels after 7 days points to hypothalamic disease; no rise is typical for pituitary insufficiency (see Sect. 7.1). An additional GnRH test after 36 hours serves to differentiate constitutionally delayed puberty from idiopathic hypogonadotropic hypogonadism (see Sect. 7.5). For further differentiation, medical imaging procedures (e. g. MRT) are necessary. When basal gonadotropin levels are high, which points to a primary testicular disorder, no additional information can be gained from a GnRH test.

Recently **GnRH receptor mutations** were also identified as the cause of hypogonadotropic hypogonadism (Pralong et al. 1999; see Chap. 7).

6.4.3 Prolactin, TRH Stimulation Test

The determination of **prolactin** in male patients of an infertility clinic does not play such a pivotal role as it does in the female. Unclear fertility disorders, erectile dysfunction and loss of libido, gynecomastia, galactorrhea or other symptoms that indicate a pituitary disorder and suspicion of pituitary tumor should prompt prolactin serum measurements, which are performed by competitive or non-competitive immunoassay. When interpreting results, it should be remembered that numerous drugs, particularly psychiatric medication, and stress increase prolactin secretion.

In most cases pituitary adenomas with endocrine activity produce prolactin (see Chap. 7). Endocrine stimulation tests can be applied to differentiate a prolactinoma from hyperprolactinemia with other causes. For the male the thyreotropin releasing hormone (TRH) stimulation test is best suited. Typically patients with a prolactinoma show a diminished increase of prolactin after TRH administration because of autonomous prolactin production by the tumor, whereas patients with hyperprolactinemia of non-tumor origin respond normally. A prolactin rise of less than 30 % over basal after 200 µg TRH i.v. provides a diagnostic hint for a macroprolactinoma (Gsponer er al. 1999) Because of the wide scatter of test results from normal men, no borderline values for microprolactinomas can be given (Le Moli et al. 1999).

6.4.4 Testosterone, Free Testosterone, Salivary Testosterone, SHBG

Testosterone in serum is the laboratory value most important for confirming a clinical suspicion of hypogonadism and for monitoring testosterone substitution therapy. When interpreting testosterone values, **diurnal variations** should be considered as they cause morning serum concentrations to be approximately 20–40 % higher than evening values (Fig. 6.11).

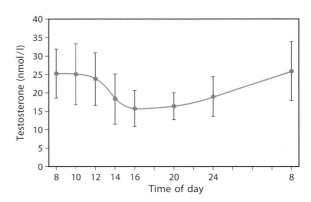

Fig. 6.11. Circadian rhythm of testosterone concentrations in young men (median ± SD, data from Behre et al. 1992)

Short, intensive physical exercise can increase serum testosterone concentrations, whereas extended exhausting physical exercise and high-performance sports can bring about a decrease. Nearly all chronic diseases, particularly those of the liver, kidneys and the cardiovascular system, as well as stress, anesthesia, drugs and certain medication (e.g. ketoconazole) can prompt a decrease in testosterone levels. Low levels of testosterone are found more often in elderly males. This decrease is in part physiological, but may be partially caused by disease or, in particular, by a combination of different diseases (multimorbidity) (see Chap. 21) (Gray et al. 1999).

Considering these factors, normal serum testosterone concentration in the adult male lies between 12 and 40 nmol/l during the first half of the day; concentrations below 10 nmol/l are certainly pathological; values between 10 and 12 require additional testing. Prepubertal boys and castrates have serum levels below 4 nmol/l.

Serum concentrations are determined by radioimmunoassay, enzyme immunoassay, fluoroimmunoassay or chemiluminence assay (Nieschlag 1998). Testosterone remains stable even after repeated freezing and thawing. Normally, a single morning blood sample is sufficient for the assessment of testosterone serum levels; serum pooling is not necessary (Vermeulen and Verdonck 1992).

In blood, testosterone is bound to protein, specifically to **sex hormone binding globulin (SHBG)**. Only approximately 2 % of testosterone is unbound and available as free testosterone for biological activity. The concentration of free testosterone, as a measure of biologically available testosterone, is determined by equilibrium dialysis or as the serum fraction of total testosterone which is not precipitated by ammonium sulfate. These methods, however, are too complicated for clinical routine. Calculating free testosterone from the serum concentration of total testosterone and SHBG using a standardized formula has proved to be a simple and reliable method for estimating testosterone bioactivity (Vermeulen et al. 1999).

Since generally total testosterone is well correlated with free testosterone, separate determination of free testosterone is only necessary in certain cases. As an example, hyperthyroidism and antiepileptic drugs cause an increase in SHBG levels and thereby increased testosterone concentration in serum, without a parallel increase of the biologically active free testosterone fraction. In extreme obesity low testosterone levels are measured, however, in combination with low SHBG values; accordingly, the free testosterone fraction remains normal.

Testosterone can also be measured in **saliva** (normal range 200–500 pmol/l). Salivary concentrations are correlated with free testosterone in serum. This determination is especially suited for monitoring testosterone substitution therapy since the patient can produce samples without the help of medical personnel (Tschöp et al. 1998).

6.4.5 hCG Test

The **endocrine reserve capacity of the testis** can be tested by stimulation with human chorionic gonadotropin (hCG). hCG has predominantly LH activity and stimulates testosterone production of the Leydig cells. Today, the test is predominantly used for differentiation between cryptorchidism or ectopy of the testis (rise in testosterone levels present, but diminished) and anorchia (absent testosterone rise) (Fig. 6.9). On the first day of the examination, basal blood samples are obtained between 8.00 and 10.00 h; immediately thereafter a single injection of 5000 I.E. hCG is given i.m. Further blood samples are obtained after 48 and/or 72 hours. The rise of testosterone should be 1.5–2.5-fold. Lesser values indicate primary hypogonadism; higher values signal secondary hypogonadism. Failure of values in the castrate range to increase indicates anorchia or complete testicular atrophy. Decreasing reserve capacity of the Leydig cells is a characteristic of the elderly man (see Chap. 21).

6.4.6 Anti-Muellerian Hormone

Anti-Muellerian hormone (AMH), also known as **Muellerian inhibiting substance** (MIS), is a testicular hormone secreted by the immature Sertoli cell and is responsible for the regression of the Muellerian ducts in the male fetus.

Determining serum levels of AMH is a sensitive and specific test providing evidence for the existence of a testis in the prepubertal male (Lee et al. 1997). Normal values for boys show the presence of testicular tissue; undetectable serum concentrations indicate **anorchidism**. Compared to the hCG test, the AMH test is equally specific, but more sensitive and hence its predictive value is higher in prepubertal boys (Lee et al. 1997).

AMH serum concentrations are significantly higher in prepubertal boys with normal testicular function than in boys with disturbed testicular function (Lee et al. 1997). Extremely high values are seen in men with idiopathic hypogonadotropic hypogonadism, where they are caused by deficient pubertal maturation of the Sertoli cell and where they are comparable to values seen in prepubertal boys (Young et al. 1999). hCG or testosterone therapy reduces these levels significantly (Young et al. 1999).

6.4.7 Inhibin B

Inhibin is produced by the Sertoli cells in the testes and plays a role in the regulation of FSH secretion in the pituitary (see Chap. 3). The original inhibin radioimmunoassays could not differentiate between various inhibin isoforms and were unable to provide any information about the physiological importance of the substance. Once specific immunoassays became available, it was possible to identify inhibin B as the serum isoform most important for the male (Hayes et al. 1998).

Inhibin B shows a marked **circadian rhythm**, with high values in the morning, descending to lowest levels in the late afternoon (Carlssen et al. 1999). In healthy and infertile men morning serum concentrations of inhibin B are correlated with FSH serum levels, sperm concentration and testicular volume (Fig. 6.10) (Jensen et al. 1997; Pierik et al. 1998; Eckardstein et al. 1999). As a direct secretory product of the Sertoli cell, inhibin B is slightly more sensitive than FSH as a parameter for evaluating spermatogenesis (Jensen et al. 1997; Eckardstein et al. 1999). However, neither inhibin B nor FSH nor a

combination of the two can accurately predict the presence of sperm in testicular biopsies, information which is of great relevance for azoospermic patients who are to undergo testicular sperm extraction (TESE) prior to ICSI therapy (Tournaye et al. 1997; Eckardstein et al. 1999).

6.4.8 Further Diagnosis including Techniques of Molecular Biology

Determining serum concentrations of 17β **estradiol, hCG, androstenedione** or **5α-dihydrotestosterone (DHT)** and **5α-reductase** activity in skin fibroblasts may be necessitated by particular findings, e. g. gynecomastia, suspected testicular tumor, enzyme defects in testosterone biosynthesis or resistance of androgen target organs (see detailed descriptions in Chap. 8 and 11).

Molecular analysis of the **androgen receptor gene** and **androgen binding studies** are indicated when androgen resistance in the target organs is suspected (Quigley 1998; see detailed description in Chap. 11). Recent studies imply that even if mutations of the androgen receptor gene do not cause decreased androgen binding, they may still cause marked oligozoospermia and thus infertility via disturbed signal transduction (Ghadessy et al. 1999).

The importance of **estrogen receptor mutations** and **aromatase deficiency** are described in Chap. 11.

6.5 Semen Analysis

Semen analysis is performed for evaluation of fertility disorders with or without symptoms of androgen deficiency.

> For standardization and to make results from different laboratories comparable, the examination of the ejaculate should always be performed according to the *Guidelines of the World Health Organization*, which are explained in detail in the *WHO Laboratory Manual for the Examination of the Human Ejaculate and Sperm-Cervical Mucus Interaction* (WHO 1999). This laboratory handbook belongs in every andrology laboratory and is to be considered as a supplement to this book.

Therefore only the essential aspects of ejaculate analysis and selected sperm function tests are described in this chapter.

For comparability of results patients should observe a period of **abstinence** of between 48 hours and 7 days.

Because of the normal variability of the various parameters an estimation of fertility potential should be based on at least two semen analyses performed at an interval of 4–12 weeks. The ejaculate should be obtained at the clinic by masturbation into a wide-mouthed, clean glass container with a graduated cylinder, which makes transfer into other vials unnecessary (Fig. 6.12). A private room should be available with adjoining sanitary facilities; appropriate illustrated literature, background music and/or video tapes should provide a suitable atmosphere.

6.5.1 Physical Examination

The **ejaculate volume** is measured in the graduated glass container (Fig. 6.12) and should total at least 2 ml. A normal ejaculate has a homogenous grey-opalescent **appearance** and liquefies at room temperature within 60 min; thereafter the microscopic examination can begin. A **yellowish** appearance and purulent smell indicate infections, a **reddish-brown** color indicates the presence of red blood cells (**hematospermia**). For all following examinations the ejaculate has to be mixed well. If the **pH** exceeds 8, infection should be suspected; pH-values lower than 7.2 together with azoospermia indicate malformation or obstruction of the epididymis, the deferent ducts, the seminal vesicles or the ejaculatory ducts (Eckardstein et al. 2000).

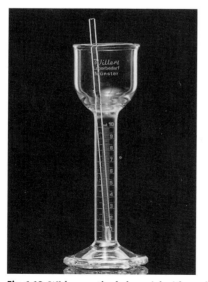

Fig. 6.12. Wide-mouthed glass vial with graduated cylinder and stirring rod

6.5.2 Microscopic Examination

Microscopic examination can be accomplished with a normal light microscope, however, a **phase contrast microscope** delivers better results. **Sperm agglutination** in the fresh semen sample is suggestive of immunological infertility. However, adherence of sperm to debris or other elements of the ejaculate, which is observed occasionally, has to be distinguished but is not considered pathological.

Sperm motility is examined in the fresh sample at a magnification of 400–600x. The examination should be performed preferably at 37°C or at room temperature (between 20 and 24°C) within 60 minutes after ejaculation. The quality of motility is expressed according to the classes "a" to "d", which are defined as follows:

a) rapid progressive motility (>25 μm/s),
b) slow or sluggish progressive motility,
c) non-progressive motility (<5 μm/s),
d) immotility.

Cut-off velocity values have been introduced in the WHO Handbook (WHO 1999) to standardize the grading of sperm.

Sperm concentration is determined in a counting chamber (e.g. Neubauer improved chamber) after dilution in a bicarbonate-formalin solution containing gentian violet or trypan blue solution. Azoospermia must be confirmed by the absence of sperm in the sediment after high-speed centrifugation of the ejaculate.

Besides sperm cells the ejaculate contains **epithelial cells** of the urogenital tract and so-called **round cells** (spermatogenic cells and leukocytes). A distinction between white blood cells and spermatogenic cells is achieved by peroxidase staining, which specifically stains active **leukocytes**, or by CD45 staining which is a pan-leukocyte marker.

Sperm morphology is examined in a fixed microscopic preparation of an aliquot of a well-mixed semen sample, best stained according to Papanicolaou (Fig. 6.13). Normal sperm have a regular oval-shaped head (length 4–5.5 μm, width 2.5–3.5 μm) with an intact midpiece and an intact tail. The acrosome should be clearly visible and cover 40–70% of the sperm head area. Abnormal forms of spermatozoa are manifold: large or small oval heads outside the above-mentioned dimensions and tapering, pyriform and vacuolated heads ($>20\%$ of the head area occupied by unstained vacuolar areas). Sperm without acrosomes have globular heads (**globozoospermia**). Some spermatozoa have double heads; heads with irregular forms are classified as amorphous. The midpiece and the tail can show defects, tails can be coiled, broken, or doubled. Heads can be separated from tails (decapitation forms) (Fig. 6.13).

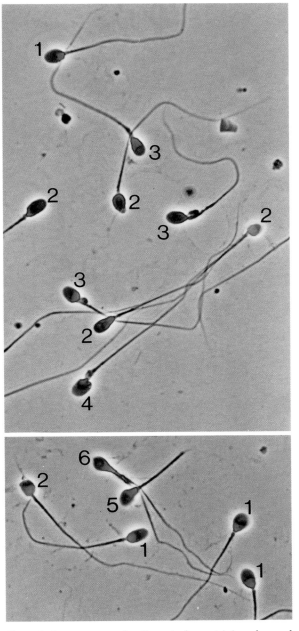

Fig. 6.13. Sperm smear after Papanicolaou staining observed with phase contrast optics (×1000) showing normal morphology (*1*), heads of abnormal size or shape (*2*), midpiece defects (*3*), both head and midpiece defects on the same cell (*4*), both head and tail defects (*5*) and all head, midpiece and tail defects on the same sperm (*6*)

6.5.3 Biochemical Analysis

Different chemical substances can be measured in the ejaculate which are secreted by specific organs or compartments of the reproductive system and can thus serve as a marker for their function. As a general principle, a decrease in the concentration of the markers indicates a dysfunction of the secreting organs or a distal obstruction of the efferent system.

The determination of specific substances for each level of the efferent system allows a rough localization of the disorder. However, it should be considered that in the case of bilateral organs, only bilateral dysfunction will cause significant changes of the biochemical markers.

Prostate function can be gauged by the measurement of **zinc, citric acid** and **prostatic acid phosphatase. Prostaglandins** and **fructose** are secreted mainly by the **seminal vesicles.** Low fructose concentrations in the seminal plasma may indicate bilateral agenesis or severe dysfunction of the seminal vesicles or obstruction of the ejaculatory ducts. As an indicator of endocrine activity, fructose does not have the significance formerly attributed to it. In cases of low fructose levels, transrectal ultrasonography of the seminal vesicles before and after ejaculation should be performed for further diagnosis (Fig. 6.8c, d).

Neutral α-glucosidase, L-carnitine and **glycerophosphocholine** can be considered as markers for **epididymal function.** Neutral α-glucosidase has a higher specificity and sensitivity for judgement of epididymal function. As the assay is simpler, cheaper and faster than others, measurement of this parameter should be the first choice (Cooper 1990). A severely diminished or undetectable amount of neutral α-glucosidase in the presence of normal FSH and normal testicular volume is an indication that azoospermia might be caused by bilateral epididymal obstruction or obstruction of the efferent ducts (Fig. 6.9).

6.5.4 Immunological Tests

Sperm agglutinations in the fresh semen sample point to the presence of specific sperm antibodies. Not all antibodies directed against sperm cause agglutination; some, for example, are cytotoxic and can cause motility disorders. For the determination of antibodies of the IgA or IgG class directed against sperm antigens, the **mixed antiglobulin reaction test (MAR test)** has proven to be useful. For this test, a fresh semen sample and IgG- or IgA-coated latex particles or sheep erythrocytes are mixed together with antiserum directed against IgA or IgG antibodies. If the respective antibodies are present on the sperm surface, the particles or cells will be bound to the spermatozoa by the antiserum. The proportion of these bound sperm can then be quantified. If more than 50 % of the spermatozoa are IgG or IgA antibody-coated immunological infertility is likely (Abshagen et al. 1998) (Fig. 6.9). Because of variability of the test results, diagnosis should be based on two or three MAR tests and should be complemented by sperm mucus interaction tests (postcoital test, Kremer test) (Paschke et al. 1994).

The significance of sperm antibodies measurable in serum, e. g. by the TAT test, is controversial and their determination in the routine workup of the infertile couple has no clinical relevance.

6.5.5 Microbiology

Nowadays in Europe the classic venereal diseases such as gonorrhea or syphilis are of minor importance in infertile men (see Sect. 9.1). The predominent microorganisms found are Chlamydia trachomatis or Ureaplasma urealyticum, as well as gram-negative bacteria typical of urogenital infections (Purvis and Christansen 1993). These microorganisms can be identified directly in the urine, ejaculate, prostate exprimate or urethral swab. Leukocyte concentrations higher than 1 million/ml ejaculate and/or a significant growth of microorganisms in the ejaculate culture indicate an infection of the efferent seminal system (see Sect. 9.1.2) (WHO 1993) (Fig. 6.9). Whereas the determination of different microorganisms in an aerobic ejaculate culture is unproblematic, the proof of chlamydia requires special examination techniques. Today, the direct determination of chlamydia in the ejaculate by means of PCR (polymerase chain reaction) can be considered as the "gold standard" (see Sect. 9.1.2).

6.5.6 Electron Microscopy

In fertile as well as infertile men spermatozoa display considerable morphological variability when judged by light microscopy, so that a clear definition of a normal sperm cell is problematic. In a minority of infertile patients specific anomalies of sperm cells can often be found only by electron microscopy. In this case head defects with and without defects of the nucleus and tail defects have to be differentiated from each other.

The head defect in **globozoospermia** is a hereditary disturbance of spermiogenesis, where the Golgi apparatus of the spermatid forms an acrosome, which remains without contact with the spermatid nucleus. Upon release of the spermatid from the seminiferous epithelium (spermiation), the acrosome remains within the Sertoli

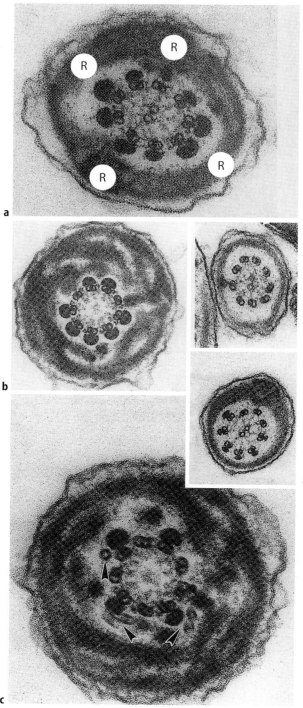

Fig 6.14.a Cross-section of normal sperm tail through the principal piece as indicated by the fibrous sheath (R), showing the 9+2 axonemal structure (see Fig. 6.4. for nomenclature) and the corresponding outer dense fibers. Abnormal tail structures are indicated by deletion of central tubules (**b, c**), absence of the inner (**b**) or both outer and inner (**d, e**) dynein arms, ectopic location of microtubules (arrow in c) and fibrous sheath dysplasia (**b, c**). (From Zamboni 1992 with permission)

Sample record form for ejaculate and hormone analysis						Pat. No.:	
Name, Surname:				Date of birth:			
Date of sample							
Duration of abstinence (days)							
Therapy							
Time of sample collection							
Start of analysis							
Volume (ml)							
Consistency							
pH							
Motility (%)	(a) rapid progression						
	(b) slow progression						
	(c) non-progressive motility						
	(d) immotile						
Count	(million/ml)						
	(million per ejaculate)						
Morphology	normal (%)						
	head defects (%)						
	neck or midpiece defects (%)						
	tail defects (%)						
	cytoplasmic droplets (%)						
	specific defects						
Eosin test (% stained cells)							
HOS test (% swollen sperm)							
Round cells (million/ml)							
Leukocytes (million/ml)							
Agglutinationen (%)							
MAR test	IgG (%)						
	IgA (%)						
α-Glucosidase (≥ 11 mU/ejaculate)							
Fructose (≥ 13 µmol/ejaculate)							
Zinc (≥ 2,4 µmol/ejaculate)							
Other tests							
Technician							
LH	(2-10 U/l)						
FSH	(1-7 U/l)						
Prolactin	(≤ 500 mU/l)						
Testosterone	(≥ 12 nmol/l)						
Estradiol	(≤ 250 pmol/l)						
SHBG	(11-71 nmol/l)						
PSA	(≤ 4 µg/l)						

neg. = negative test   < std. (value) = undetectable   n.e. = not evaluable   n.p. = not possible

Fig. 6.15. Form for continuous documentation of ejaculate and hormone investigations

Table 6.3. Normal values of semen variables according to WHO Guidelines (1999)

Ejaculate volume	≥2.0 ml
pH	7.2
Sperm concentration	≥20 million spermatozoa/ml
Total sperm count	≥40 million spermatozoa/ejaculate
Motility	≥50% spermatozoa with forward progression (categories a + b) or ≥25% spermatozoa with rapid progression (category a)
Morphology	≥30% spermatozoa with normal forms[a]
Vitality	≥50% vital spermatozoa, e.g. sperm excluding the eosin dye
MAR test	<50% of spermatozoa with adherent particles or erythrocytes
Leukocytes	<1 million/ml
α-Glucosidase (neutral)	≥11 mU/ejaculate
Citric acid	≥52 μmol/ejaculate
Acid phosphatase	≥200 U/ejaculate
Fructose	≥13 μmol/ejaculate
Zinc	≥2.4 μmol/ejaculate

[a] The 4th edition of the WHO Guidelines (1999) provides no reference values for normal sperm morphology, so that the percentage value of the 3rd edition (1992) is maintained here. Currently, multicenter studies are underway to determine new reference values. Data from assisted reproduction indicate that fertilization rates in vitro decrease if normal sperm morphology falls below 15%.

cell, so that the spermatozoon lacks the acrosome necessary for fertilization. The heads of the normally motile spermatozoa appear globular under light microscopic examination of the ejaculate. So-called **pinhead sperm** are actually sperm tails without heads and can be very motile.

A normal **sperm tail** has 9 microtubule doublets, which are arranged concentrically around two central microtubuli (9 + 2). The doublets are equipped with dynein arms joined by nexin and are connected with the central tubuli by radial spokes (Fig. 4.5 and 6.14a). The best-known defect associated with sperm immotility is the absence of the dynein arms, in particular, the inner arms (Fig. 6.14), which generate sliding of the microtubules to induce flagellation (see Chap. 4). Other flagellar defects are manifested as disorganization of the microtubules and outer dense fibers, dysplasia of the fibrous sheath, and deviations from the normal central pair (9+2 microtubule structure) (Zamboni 1992; Chemes et al. 1998), including the deletion of the central pair (9 + 0) (Neugebauer et al. 1990). The **immotile cilia syndrome** is characterized by a general absence or reduction of ciliar movements in all respective organs and, when accompanied by a situs inversus and bronchiectasis, is known as **Kartagener syndrome**.

6.5.7 Documentation, Normal Values, Nomenclature and Classification of Semen Parameters

The documentation of semen and hormone parameters is best managed using an evaluation sheet containing several columns in which the values of ejaculate examinations at different timepoints can be entered (Fig. 6.15). This enables straightforward evaluation and comparison of the results of several examinations.

Normal values of ejaculate parameters are listed in Table 6.3. For standardized description of different combinations of possible defects the recommended nomenclature is given in Table 6.4.

The investigation of ejaculate parameters plays a central role in the evaluation of male fertility. Since the occurrence of a pregnancy depends on many factors, particularly on the reproductive functions of the female (see Chap. 14), examination of merely the ejaculate parameters is of limited value for prognosis of the couple's fertility. Sharp discrimination between a fertile and infertile male is not possible based solely on the parameters and diagnoses mentioned above. This is only possible in the case of azoospermia. Otherwise, semen parameters have value only in relation to female reproductive functions since subnormal semen parameters can

Table 6.4. Describing terminology for the semen variables according to WHO Guidelines (1999)

Normozoospermia	Normal ejaculate as defined in Table 6.3
Oligozoospermia	<20 million spermatozoa/ml
Asthenozoospermia	<50% spermatozoa with forward progression (categories "a" and "b") and <25% spermatozoa with category "a" movement
Teratozoospermia	[<30% spermatozoa with normal morphology] (see Table 6.3)
Oligoasthenoteratozoo-spermia (OAT)	Signifies disturbance of all 3 variables (combinations of only 2 prefixes may also be used)
Azoospermia	No spermatozoa in the ejaculate
Parvisemia	Ejaculate volume <2 ml
Aspermia	No ejaculate

be compensated by optimal reproductive functions of the female partner and may be compatible with fertility.

6.5.8 Objective Semen Analysis (CASA)

Systematic investigations have shown that the estimation of concentration, motility and morphology of sperm is influenced by significant subjective factors (Neuwinger et al. 1990). In addition to standardization of ejaculate analysis by uniform laboratory methods, achieved by use of the Laboratory Manual of the World Health Organization (WHO 1999), intensive efforts are being made to establish objective laboratory methods. In clinical practice, however, the classic investigation of the ejaculate maintains its central role in the assessment of fertility.

DNA flow cytometry allows objective and precise determination of sperm concentration (Hacker-Klom et al. 1999). The haploid spermatozoa differ with regard to their DNA staining pattern from all other cells of the ejaculate and are therefore unequivocally measurable. Since this method allows several thousand cells to be counted in very short time, high precision is possible because statistical counting errors are minimized.

Sperm concentration can also be automatically analyzed by computer-aided sperm analysis (CASA). Counting the number of sperm cells identified by the size and contrast of the digitized video image of the sperm heads has been hampered by the presence of non-sperm particles (including round cells in the semen recognized by the programme as spermatozoa). Attempts to overcome the problem posed by this contamination include (a) additional criteria of the oval-shaped head based on measurements of the major and minor axis and their ratio (e. g. Hamilton-Thorne Systems), (b) tail-detection algorithm which scans for projections along the axis of the sperm head and excludes particles of sim-

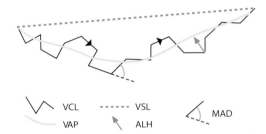

Fig. 6.16. Sperm movement parameters (in selection) recorded by computer-assisted sperm analysis (CASA). *VCL* curvelinear velocity (μm/s); *VAP* average path velocity (μm/s); *VSL* straight-line velocity (μm/s); *ALH* amplitude of lateral head displacement (μm); *MAD* mean angular displacement (degree); *from these calculated parameters:* *LIN* linearity = VSL/VCL; *STR* straightness = VSL/VAP; *WOB* wobble = VAP/VCL

ilar size but without a tail projection (Cell Motion Analyzer) and (c) recognition by additional fluorescent staining of DNA (Hamilton-Thorne Systems). However, the reliability of these methods to determine sperm concentrations accurately, especially for low sperm numbers, has yet to be established.

The evaluation of sperm motility is especially influenced by subjective factors. Among the various methods for objective measurements, the tracking of video images of individual sperm cells by CASA is the best developed. Besides determining the proportion of motile sperm, these systems allow measurements of additional parameters, such as sperm velocity, linearity, amplitude of lateral head displacement and beat cross frequency of the head (Fig. 6.16) (WHO 1999). Correlation with pregnancy rates in vivo or after in-vitro fertilization (IVF) showed that evaluation of sperm motility by CASA indeed has predictive value for fertility (De Geyter et al. 1992, 1998; Barratt et al. 1993; Irvine et al. 1994).

Standardization of **sperm morphology** is the least developed of all parameters. Computer-aided video techniques will probably also be applied in the future (Kruger et al. 1995).

The achievement of objectivity in the assessment of ejaculate parameters has thus been only partially successful. Therefore, in clinical practice well-controlled conventional semen analysis (see next section) remains fundamental in the evaluation of fertility. CASA investigations are to be considered optional and supplementary for the routine examination of an infertile couple.

6.5.9 Quality Control

The need for effective quality control of ejaculate analysis was demonstrated by a significant discrepancy between different evaluations of sperm concentration and morphology of identical samples analyzed by different laboratories (Neuwinger et al. 1990). Since then initial steps have been taken to establish a strict quality control programme in the andrology laboratory (Cooper et al. 1992; Clements et al. 1995). **Internal quality control** is of importance for maintaining standards throughout the year and for coping with changes in personnel. This includes regular determinations of the inter- and intra-technician coefficients of variations for the evaluation of sperm concentration, motility and morphology (Cooper et al. 1992). In this case the use of video-recording or cryopreserved samples has been shown to be advantageous (Clements et al. 1995). In large andrology laboratories the periodic calculation of monthly means of all the various determinations can be used for early recognition of a systematic bias in the methods used (WHO 1999) or to monitor the introduction of new assessment criteria (e.g. the change of velocity cut-off for grade "a" sperm at $25\mu m/s$). Determinations of biochemical marker substances in seminal plasma are subjected to the usual internal quality controls of the clinical laboratory.

All andrology laboratories should enroll in **external quality control** schemes. These provide information on the overall agreement between laboratories and are thus essential if multicenter clinical studies are to be performed at separate centers. There are schemes for monitoring sperm concentration, motility, morphology and anti-sperm antibodies. Providing that all technicians in the same laboratory are in good agreement (determined from internal QC), any technician may analyze the external QC sample. Regular feedback of the results to the technicians is mandatory in enforcing consistent application of selection criteria so that eventual agreement with designated values can be reached (Cooper et al. 1999).

6.6 Sperm Function Tests

Sperm function tests were developed to detect abnormalities of sperm survival, transport in the female genital tract and for the different steps of fertilization. Sperm function tests can be divided into vitality tests, sperm mucus interaction tests (in vivo and in vitro) and tests that examine capacitation, acrosome reaction, zona binding and ovum penetration (a detailed description of these physiological steps can be found in Chap. 4). As the different tests examine different aspects of sperm function, a combination of different tests is required to assess the fertility potential of sperm. Although some function tests show good correlation with pregnancy rates of in vitro fertilization programmes, there is no universally accepted fixed set of standard function tests.

Recently much advancement has been made in the characterization of sperm defects, including DNA damage, chromatin condensation status and decondensation efficiency, sperm enzymes and surface antigens related to sperm function, signal transduction mechanisms and exposure of surface binding sites on capacitation, and oxidative damage. With the progress of research and development, introduction of more sperm function tests in the future would be a matter of course. Meanwhile, only well-established sperm function tests, including those recommended in the WHO Handbook (1999), are described in this chapter.

6.6.1 Vitality Tests

When the percentage motility of a sample is low, these tests are used in order to determine whether sperm have lost their flagellation because of metabolic dysfunction or axonemal defects, or are simply dead (necrozoospermia).

The **HOS test** is a simple test of the integrity and compliance of the semipermeable plasma membrane of the sperm tail (Jeyendran et al. 1984). Sperm in the ejaculate are diluted with a hypoosmotic solution so that water enters the cell osmotically. Intact sperm are indicated by the swelling of the tail into various sizes and shapes to accommodate the increase in cell volume, whereas dead cells retain their normal tail shape because of leaky membranes.

The **eosin test** is based on the fact that eosin is excluded by live cells. The damaged cell membrane of dead sperm can be penetrated and therefore such cells are stained specifically.

> With the availability of intracytoplasmic sperm injection (ICSI) vitality tests have regained interest, as dead cells can be distinguished from vital cells which can be used for ICSI.

6.6.2 Sperm-Mucus Interaction Tests

Cervical mucus is the first barrier that sperm encounter in their migration up the female tract. During almost the entire menstrual cycle the mucus is highly viscous and becomes hydrated and penetrable by sperm only for a few preovulatory days. Mucus penetration serves the natural process of selection for spermatozoa with normal morphology and motility (see Chap. 4). Penetration failure may be due to hostile mucus, such as acidity caused by bacterial infection. Therefore mucus quality is very important for the assessment of sperm mucus interaction. Sperm function tests are divided into **in vivo postcoital tests** and the different **in vitro tests**.

The **in vivo postcoital test** is performed within a few days prior to ovulation on the day after nocturnal coitus with the aim to examine penetration into, as well as the survival of sperm in cervical mucus. In addition to the collection and scoring of mucus described below, a vaginal pool sample is collected and examined to confirm the disposition of sperm in the vagina. The number of sperm in the mucus is counted in a calibrated, high-magnification microscopic field, and sperm motility is assessed by grades. The presence of motile sperm independent of the number indicates a normal test result (Oei et al. 1995). A test with negative results should be repeated at different times of the mid-cycle to ensure that the result is not due to incorrect timing.

For the **in vitro sperm-mucus interaction test**, sexual abstinence should be observed by the couple for three days to ensure the absence of sperm in the mucus from previous intercourse. The optimal time for the collection of mucus receptive to sperm may vary considerably among women. If the secreted volume or quality is insufficient, secretion can be increased by administration of ethinyl estradiol. It should be noted, however, that in this case the mucus no longer reflects the physiological situation, where no hormones are given.

After aspiration from the endocervical canal, the mucus is evaluated using a scoring system provided by the WHO (1999).

- Volume,
- consistency (viscosity),
- ferning (crystallization of drying mucus on slide into fern-like patterns),
- spinnbarkeit (elasticity),
- cellularity (the number of leukocytes or other cells present),
- pH

From the combined score, the mucus is assessed as favorable or unfavorable for sperm interaction.

The purpose of the **in vitro sperm cervical mucus contact test (SCMC test)** is to indicate antibodies on sperm or in mucus and other detrimental factors in the mucus. The test should be performed immediately after semen liquefaction to mimic the physiological situation. One drop each of semen and mucus is placed on a slide and mixed. On contact with the mucus, motile sperm should continue swimming with normal flagellation. The presence of "shaking sperm" ($>25\%$) noted on examination immediately and again after 30 minutes is considered positive. The semen alone serves as a control for sperm activity. Cross-over testing using donor semen sample and donor mucus should then be performed to identify whether the antibodies are on sperm or in mucus.

In the **in vitro slide test** for mucus penetration, a drop of mucus is placed on the slide under the center of the cover slip. Semen is allowed to seep in from the edge of the cover slip to form an interface with the mucus. After 30 minutes' incubation, sperm from normal semen should have penetrated into the mucus along finger-like projections of seminal fluid with greater than 90% motility.

In the **in vitro capillary test (Kremer test)**, mucus is loaded into a flat capillary tube which is then sealed at one end, and the open end put horizontally into a reservoir of semen. After incubation for two hours at $37°C$, both the distance travelled by the vanguard sperm and the densities of sperm at 1 and 4.5 cm along the tube are scored. The result is classified as "good", "fair", "poor" or "negative penetration" according to a scoring system. If the test shows impaired penetration of sperm, a cross-over test should be performed where the ejaculate and cervical mucus of the infertile couple as well as that of a fertile donor couple are tested. This can determine whether the reason for the impaired test result is primarily on the male or the female side.

In view of the marked variability of human cervical mucus quality, one useful substitute is high molecular weight **hyaluronic acid polymer** which provides test results highly correlated to Kremer tests and gives the best reproducibility (Neuwinger et al. 1991). However, this test has not yet entered clinical routine.

6.6.3 Sperm Capacitation

Before fertilization can occur, sperm undergo the capacitation process in the female tract by which they acquire cell-surface changes and exhibit **hyperactivation**, characterized by vigorous non-progressive motion with forceful, large amplitude bending (see Chap. 4). The physiological endpoint of such **capacitation** changes is the acrosomal reaction (see next section). The capacitation status can be tested in vitro in ejaculated sperm washed and incubated in albumin-containing culture medium as used in IVF.

The characteristic **hyperactivated motility patterns** can be observed in capacitated sperm contained in 50–200 µm deep chambers. By the use of computerized motion analysis (CASA) with pre-set cinematic criteria to sort out different subpopulations of motile sperm, hyperactivated sperm can be distinguished from non-hyperactivated ones, mainly by having high VCL, low LIN (calculated as VSL/VCL) and by the large ALH values of the former (see Fig. 6.16) (Grunert et al. 1990). The clinical significance of such CASA data is reflected by their correlation to IVF outcomes or artificial insemination pregnancy rates (De Geyter et al. 1998; Wang et al. 1993; Johnston et al. 1994).

Changes of the sperm head during capacitation are reflected by characteristic alterations in chlortetracycline (**CTC**)-staining patterns, which can be detected by fluorescence microscopy (Lee et al. 1987). In addition to the capacitation status, the acrosome reaction can be simultaneously evaluated since acrosome-reacted sperm show a staining pattern different from that of capacitated sperm with acrosomes still intact.

6.6.4 Acrosome Reaction

As fluorescence microscopes become more common, the once widely used dyes for **acrosome reaction** such as triple stain and trypan blue are gradually being replaced by fluorescent lectins and antibodies which give more intense and less ambiguous staining (Aitken and Brindle 1993) and enable the application of flow cytometry (see Cooper and Yeung 1998). The most common probes used include peanut lectins which label the outer acrosomal membrane, pea lectin, which labels the acrosomal content and the commercially available antibody CD46, which targets the inner acrosomal membrane (Fénichel et al. 1989). Washed or swum-up sperm are tested after incubation under capacitation conditions, often with the addition of the calcium ionophore A23187 or progesterone to replace the physiological stimulation by zona pellucida (see Chap. 4). The use of a supravital stain is normally included to differentiate dead sperm which are labelled non-specifically. Since different markers target different acrosomal compartments, they give different results and reaction-dynamics. Nevertheless, test results have been shown to correlate well with fertilizing capacity either with lectins or antibodies (Wang et al. 1983; Fénichel et al. 1991). Since the acrosome reaction occurs in vivo on the zona and the zona pellucida is the physiological trigger, testing the zona-bound sperm is most relevant (Liu and Baker 1996).

6.6.5 Zona-Binding Assays

Since **sperm-zona binding** in human is species-specific, human zonae are used exclusively. They are obtained from surplus oocytes or oocytes that failed to fertilize in IVF programmes. Oocytes are used either fresh, or, more practically, after storage in high salt concentration which does not alter zona properties including those of sperm-binding and penetration. Owing to the high intra- and interindividual variability of oocyte quality, it is essential to have an internal control for each oocyte and to use several oocytes in order to interpret test results accurately. Besides biological variability, the limited source of oocytes is another hindrance to the widespread use of the zona-binding test, although it is the best single predictor for IVF success so far. With recent success in recombinant ZP3 and ZP2 (van Duin et al. 1994; Lacy et al. 1995), which are the zona pellucida glycoproteins responsible for primary and secondary sperm binding respectively, standardized binding tests independent of human material may soon be developed.

In the **hemizona test** the zona pellucida is cut into exactly two halves using a micromanipulator. One half is incubated with the patient's capacitated sperm, the other half with the fertile donor's sperm as control. Binding ability is expressed as the hemizona index (HZI = no. of bound sperm/bound donor sperm × 100).

For the **competitive binding assay**, patient and donor sperm for control are labelled with different fluorochromes (green with FITC and red with TRITC) and co-incubated with zonae. The binding rate ratio of patient/donor sperm reflects the binding capacity of the test sample relative to the control.

6.6.6 Hamster-Ovum-Penetration Test

The final steps of sperm/egg interaction involve the binding of sperm to the oolemma and eventual fusion of the two membranes to allow the penetration of the sperm nucleus into the ooplasm. This sperm function is tested by the use of eggs from hamsters (**hamster ovum penetration test, HOP test**) induced to superovulate by the injection of hormones. These hamster oocytes are denuded by removing the cumulus and zona with hyarulonidase and trypsin respectively. Since only acrosome-reacted sperm can bind to the oolemma, either overnight preincubation or a short preincubation plus induction of acrosome reaction by ionophore A23187 is required before coincubation with hamster oocytes (WHO 1999). Although the test has been used clinically for a number of decades, its diagnostic value is still controversial, probably owing to the difficulty in optimizing the test protocol, which can lead to false negative results (Aitken 1994).

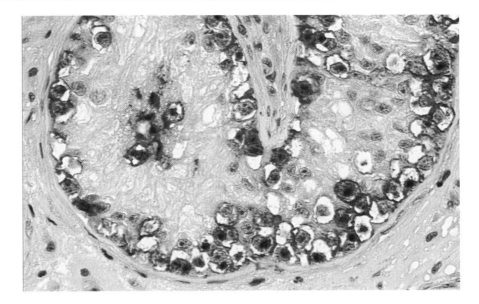

6.6.7 Reactive Oxygen Species and Sperm Function

In the past decade, there has been significant albeit incomplete understanding of the influence of **reactive oxygen species (ROS)** on male reproduction (Aitken 1995; Ochsendorf 1998; deLamarinde and Gagnon 1999). Ejaculated sperm are normally protected from oxidative stress by antioxidative enzymes present in the seminal plasma, mostly originating from the prostate (Yeung et al. 1998), and in sperm themselves. High production of ROS by large numbers of active leukocytes in semen, as in the case of infections, or by abnormal sperm with excessive cytoplasm, leads to peroxidation damage and impairment of sperm functions including motility, longevity and fertilizing ability. This may be the underlying cause of some male infertility. However, the low levels of ROS generation by normal sperm are essential for capacitation, including hyperactivation and acrosome reaction. ROS known to affect various sperm functions include superoxide, hydrogen peroxide, lipid peroxide and their radicals, and nitric oxide.

Various assays have been been developed to monitor ROS generation in semen or sperm, their ROS scavenging capacities or activities of different protective enzyzmes, or the resultant lipid peroxidation in sperm. The usefulness of these measurements in clinical semen analysis is under study. The question whether administering **antioxidants** to men with subnormal semen quality has any beneficial effects is controversial (Rolf et al. 1999).

Fig. 6.17. Identification of carcinoma in situ (CIS; testicular intraepithelial neoplasia, TIN) of the testis by immunocytochemical detection of placental alkaline phosphatase (PLAP) in a paraffin section. PLAP-positive CIS cells are stained red. Stains: Alkaline phosphatase-antialkaline phosphatase, new fuchsin and hematoxyline counterstain

6.7 Testicular Biopsy

The measurement of FSH and glucosidase have replaced invasive testicular biopsy as routine diagnostics for evaluation of male fertility in recent years. However, when findings are ambiguous, a bilateral testicular biopsy allows **differentiation** between an **obstruction of the efferent seminal ducts** and **damage of the seminiferous tubules**. In cases of azoospermia, only testicular biopsy can clarify whether haploid germ cells are still present and whether they can be used for ICSI (see Sect. 17.5.2). For this reason **cryopreservation of testicular tissue** (Schulze et al. 1999) is to be carried out following the biopsy. Prior to intended reconstructive surgery of the efferent ducts bilateral biopsy should clarify whether spermatogenesis is intact or whether damaged epithelium is the cause of infertility.

The second main indication for testicular biopsy is the identification of a **carcinoma in situ of the testis** (Fig. 6.17), for which biopsy is well suited because of its high sensitivity and specificity. Any inhomogeneity of the testicular parenchym seen in sonography should make testicular biopsy mandatory (see Sect. 6.3.1). If orchidectomy is performed because of a clinically manifest testicular tumor, a testicular biopsy of the contralateral side should be evaluated since in such patients the incidence of a contralateral tumor or carcinoma in situ is clearly increased (up to 5%) (Von der Maase et al. 1986; Dieckmann 1993). Similarly, bilateral testicular biopsy should be performed in the event of **orchidopexy for cryptorchidism** in an adult to exclude a possible carcinoma in situ.

6.7.1 Testicular Tissue Sampling

Testicular biopsy can be performed under local anesthesia. The spermatic chord is infiltrated distally from the external abdominal ring using 10 ml Mepivacain (1%) or Ropivacain (7.5 mg/ml) (Schulze and Knuth 2000). Additionally, the scrotal skin can be anesthetised in the incision area. The testis is then exposed by scrotal incision. Tissue of the size of a rice kernel is removed through a 10 mm incision in the tunica albuginea. After preparation for histology the biopsy should show approximately 30 cross-sections of testicular tubules. Subsequently the individual layers are closed. Deepseated sutures from the scrotal skin to the tunica albuginea are to be avoided since they often cause postoperative complaints. Moreover, the lymph drainage passages for the scrotal skin and the testes, which are normally separated, should not be joined to allow uncontrolled communication.

6.7.2 Fixation and Further Tissue Processing

To enable correct evaluation of testicular tissue it should be fixed in 5.5% **glutaraldehyde** for light microscopy in semithin sections or in **Bouin's solution** for additional immunohistochemical determinations e. g. placental alkaline phosphatase for carcinoma in situ. If tissue from a testicular biopsy is to be analyzed by **semithin histology** as well as by **paraffin section histology**, a fixation method should be used which is compatible with both techniques (Benson and Busch 1996). **Fixation of testicular tissue in the usual formalin solution is not suitable** because the poor preservation of parenchyma structures does not allow correct evaluation of spermatogenesis or identification of a carcinoma in situ (Fig. 6.17).

For **semithin histology** the biopsy is fixed in solution I (5.5% glutaraldehyde in 0.05 M phosphate buffer) and solution II (1% OsO4 in a phosphate buffer-saccarose mixture) and subsequently embedded in epoxy resin (glycid ether) (for method see Holstein and Wulfhekel 1971). 1 µm sections, so-called semithin sections, are achieved using a semithin microtom (glass or diamond cutter "histo Diotome", Diatome Ltd, Biel, Switzerland) and the sections are stained with toluidine blue /pyronine or according to Laczkó and Levai (1975).

Semithin section histology is the optimal method for routine diagnosis of testicular biopsies because of excellent tissue preservation, making evaluation of cytological details of germ cells possible. **Developmental stages of spermatids**, for example, can be judged in semithin sections (see Fig. 6.19 c–e) to determine which are suitable for **testicular sperm extraction** (TESE) and used in assisted reproduction (see Sect. 17.6.1; Schulze and Knuth 2000). Tissue embedded in glycid ether can, if necessary, be used to make ultrathin sections for further investigation in the **transmission electron microscope** (Holstein and Roosen-Runge 1981; Holstein et al. 1988).

Alternatively, **paraffin section histology** can be used, especially when additional **immunocytochemical investigations** are planned. This requires samples to be fixed in Bouin's solution (Böck 1989), which must always be freshly mixed. It consists of 15 ml saturated hydrous picric solution, 5 ml formaldehyde (96%) and 1 ml glacial acetic acid (100%).

After dehydration and intermedium the fixated tissue is transferred to paraffin. Usually 5µm thick sections are made using a sliding microtom. Staining with periodic acid and Schiff's reagent makes changes in the tubule walls and the acrosome visible. Staining of the acrosome permits evaluation of the maturational stages of the spermatids, but not with the same precision and sharpness which is achieved with the semithin section method.

Immunocytochemical methods of detection can be performed with paraffin sections. Immunocytochemical demonstration of placental alkaline phosphatase (PLAP) is of particular clinical importance for the detection of **carcinoma in situ cells** (Fig. 6.17). Approximately 90% of tumor cells can be found with this method (Heidenreich et al. 1998)

6.7.3 Histological Examination of the Testicular Biopsy

When evaluating a testicular biopsy the primary goal is **exclusion of a tumor or a carcinoma in situ**. In addition, histological diagnosis of focal or total Sertoli-cell-only syndrome or of spermatogenetic arrest can be made. In the case of **complete Sertoli-cell-only syndrome (SCO) (germinal cell aplasia)**, the seminiferous tubules are reduced in diameter and show no spermatogenic cells aside from Sertoli cells. A variable proportion of tubules will have still some germinal cells in the case of a **focal SCO** syndrome. FSH values are elevated in patients with SCO syndrome in most cases; the FSH serum levels are correlated positively with the degree of germinal cell aplasia (Fig. 6.10). **Spermatogenic arrest** is defined as an interruption in the development of spermatogonia to mature sperm at the level of spermatogonia, primary or secondary spermatocytes or round spermatids.

In semithin sections 100 cross-sections of testicular tubules are evaluated per biopsy. The status of spermatogenesis is evaluated at every cross-section; the me-

Table 6.5. Assessment of the spermatogenic status. (Score count based upon De Kretser and Holstein 1976)

Score	Histological criteria	Diagnosis
10	>20 mature spermatids/tubule, Germinal epithelium height 80 μm, Spermiation common	Intact spermatogenesis
9	>20 mature spermatids/tubule, Germinal epithelium height <80 μm, Spermiation rare	Reduced spermatogenesis (hypospermatogenesis)
8	<20 mature spermatids/tubule, Germinal epithelium height <80 μm, Spermiation absent	Reduced spermatogenesis (hypospermatogenesis)
7	No mature spermatids, Numerous round immature spermatids	Disturbed differentiation of spermatids
6	No mature spermatids, Few round immature spermatids	Disturbed differentiation of spermatids
5	No spermatids, Numerous primary spermatocytes	Primary spermatocyte maturation arrest
4	No spermatids, Few primary spermatocytes	Primary spermatocyte maturation arrest
3	No spermatids, No primary spermatocytes, Only spermatogonia	Spermatogonial arrest
2	No germ cells, Only Sertoli cells	Sertoli-cell-only
1	Degenerating Sertoli cells, No germinal epithelium	Tubular atrophy

Table 6.6. Reference values for determining the score count from a testicular biopsy.

Tubular diameter	Intact spermatogenesis	> 180 μm
	Reduced spermatogenesis	180 μm
	Arrested spermatogenesis	< 180 μm
	Sertoli-cell-only	~ 150 μm
Thickness of the lamina propria	Intact spermatogenesis	~ 8 μm
	Reduced spermatogenesis	> 8 μm
	Arrested spermatogenesis	> 8 μm
	Sertoli-cell-only	> 10 μm
	Tubular sclerosis	> 12 μm
Height of the germinal epithelium	Intact spermatogenesis	~ 80 μm
	Reduced spermatogenesis	< 80 μm
	Arrested spermatogenesis	~ 60 μm
	Sertoli-cell-only	< 20 μm

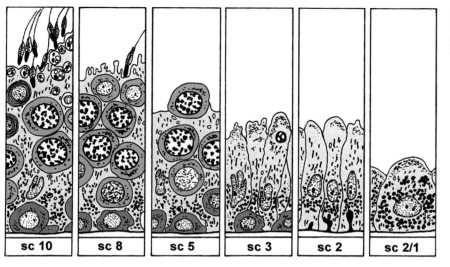

Fig. 6.18. Schematic diagram for use in establishing "score count" (*sc*) of germinal epithelium in testicular tubules

Table 6.7. Defects associated with a poor score count.

Germinal epithelium	Loss of germ cells, vacuolization, Sertoli cell lipid accumulation
Germ cells	Malformation of spermatids: spermiogenesis arrest (Holstein and Roosen-Runge 1981), acrosome defects, acrosome loss, aberrant nuclear condensation, tail defects, giant cells, malformation of spermatocytes: megalospermatocytes, etc. malformations of spermatogonia: multinuclear or polyploid, etc.
Tumor cells	Intra- or intertubular (CIS = carcinoma in situ, TIN = testicular intraepithelial neoplasia)
Tubular lumen	Released immature germ cells, sequestration of Sertoli cells, macrophages, lymphocytes
Lamina propria	Thickened, concretions, diverticula
Leydig cells	Number, distribution and morphology (hyperplasia, hypoplasia, hypertrophy, tumor)
Lymphocytes	Diffuse, periarterial, peritubular (orchitis?)
Extracellular matrix	Increased, interstitial fibrosis
Arterioles	Thickened intima, sclerosis

dian represents the **biopsy score count** (Table 6.5, Fig. 6.18).

When determining the score count, the values listed in Table 6.6 should be used. When the score count is poor, information on the quality of the germ cell epithelium, germ cells, testicular tubules and intertubular space is necessary. This information allows conclusions about the nature and possibly about the cause of disturbed fertility to be drawn (Table 6.7 and Fig. 6.19–6.21).

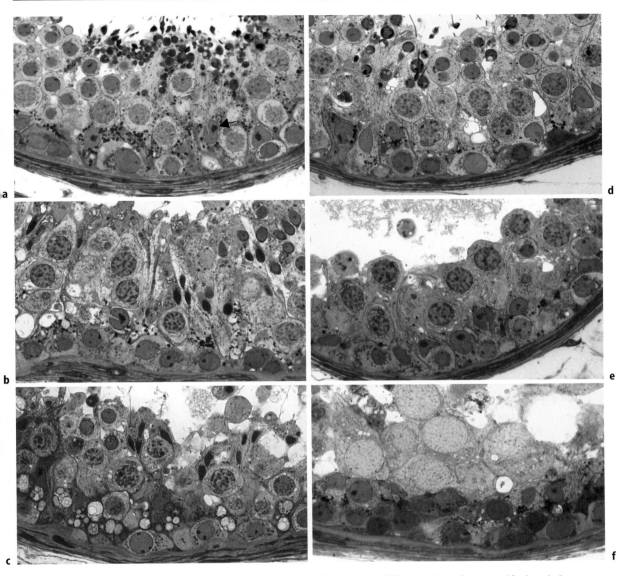

Fig. 6.19. a Intact spermatogenesis (sc 10). The germinal epithelium consists of spermatogonia, primary and some secondary spermatocytes and spermatids which move into the lumen of the testicular tubule (spermiation). Cytoplasm derived from the spermatids remaining in the germinal epithelium (residual bodies) are heavily stained. Nuclei of Sertoli cells show a heavily stained nucleolus (*arrow*). Section of testicular tubule of a 34 year-old man with obstructive azoospermia. Stain: toluidine blue – pyronine, ×1100. **b** Reduced spermatogenesis (sc 9). Germinal epithelium on the lamina propria (stained red) showing spermatogonia, spermatocytes I, spermatids (spermiogenesis stage 7 and stage 4; Holstein and Roosen-Runge 1981) and Sertoli cells with numerous lipid droplets. Testicular tubule of a 42 year-old man with prostate cancer. Stained according to Laczkó and Levai (1975), ×1100. **c** Reduced spermatogenesis (sc 8). Mature spermatids are still produced, but the germinal epithelium is low, Sertoli cells contain numerous lipid droplets, appropriate to patient's age. 52 year-old infertile patient. Stained according to Laczkó and Levai (1975), ×1100.

d Disturbed differentiation of spermatids (sc 7). Immature spermatids are still produced (spermiogenesis stage I), however, development to mature spermatids is lacking. 36 year-old infertile patient. Stain according to Laczkó and Levai (1975), ×1100. **e** Spermatogenic arrest at the level of spermatocyte stage I (sc 5). Spermatocytes I are still being produced, no spermatids are detectable. Severe disturbance of spermatogenesis seen in contralateral testis of a 26 year-old patient with seminoma. Stain according to Laczkó and Levai (1975), ×1100. **f** Disturbed meiosis in primary spermatocytes. A group of primary spermatocytes (megalospermatocytes) with very large, weakly stained nuclei stemming from absent pairing of homologous chromosomes (disturbed meiosis) (Holstein et al. 1988). Megalospermatocytes, which fail to develop into spermatids, can occur in small groups in the germinal epithelium at all ages, but can account for almost 100 % of spermatocytes in some patients. 43 year-old infertility patient. Stain according to Laczkó and Levai (1975), ×1100

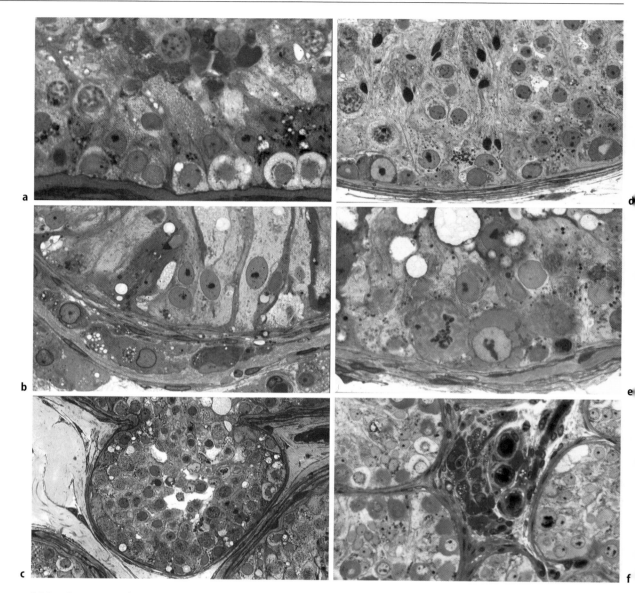

6.20. a Spermatogenic arrest at the level of spermatogonial stage (sc 3). Lamina propria (stained red) thickened by increased accumulation of extracellular matrix. Type A pale spermatogonia are present; spermatogenesis, however, does not occur. Large vacuoles in adluminal compartment of germinal epithelium contain large amounts of glycogen (stained red). 32 year-old infertile patient. Stained according to Laczko and Levai (1975), × 1100. **b** Sertoli-cell-only (SCO) syndrome (sc 2). Germinal epithelium consists only of Sertoli cells with smoothly contoured nuclei. Several Sertoli cells (dark stain) show degenerate processes. Leydig cells are present in the markedly thickened lamina propria. This position of Leydig cells is often found in cryptorchidism. 41 year-old infertile patient. Stain according to Laczkó and Levai (1975), × 1100. **c** Diverticulum of a testicular tubule. Germinal epithelium is expressed through an opening in the myofibroblast layer of the lamina propria and is covered by only a thin layer of fibroblasts. Residual spermato-

genic activity can be noted. Diverticula, a sign of advanced age, are rare in men below 40 years. 68 year-old man, × 570. **d** Early form of testicular tumor (CIS = carcinoma in situ). A tumor cell with large nucleus, prominent nucleolus and dark stained cytoplasm is located in the basal compartment of the germinal epithelium. Cytoplasm is heavily stained because of high glucogen content. Spermatogenesis up to mature spermatids is present in the adluminal compartment of the epithelium. 27 year-old infertile patient. × 1100. **e** Intratubular tumor cells can be differentiated well from spermatogonia by staining glycogen mass in cytosplam red. Leftmost of the three tumor cells is in process of mitosis. Sertoli cells contain very large lipid droplets. Spermatogenesis is extinguished. × 1800. **f** Hypoplastic testicular tubules from testis of a 34 year–old man with seminoma. These tubules contain immature Sertoli cells, pale spermatogonia type A pale and tumor cells stained red. Stained according to Laczkó and Levai (1975), × 750

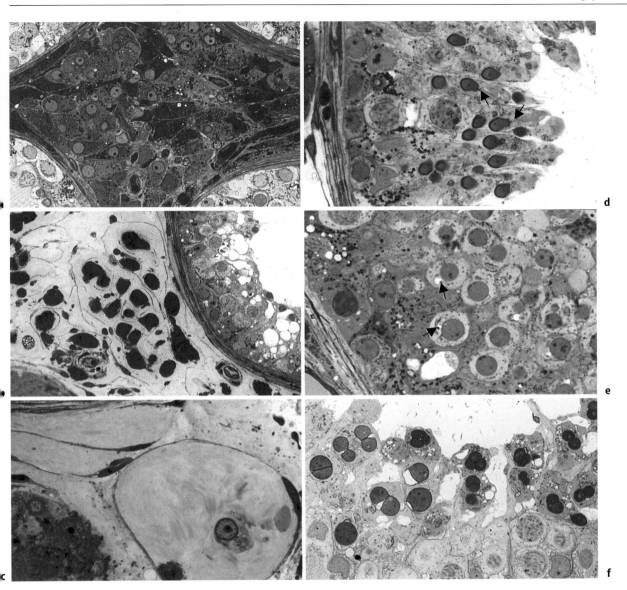

Figure 6.21. a Leydig cell hyperplasia. The number of Leydig cells in the interstitium is markedly reduced and the cells contain cytoplasm to a varying degree. Some cells exhibit degenerative changes. 31 year-old patient. Toluidine blue, ×750. **b** Hypoplasia of Leydig cells. Note extracellular matrix between Leydig cells. Cell size is markedly reduced. The germinal epithelium is highly vacuolized. Lack of spermatid formation. 39 year-old patient. Toluidine blue-pyronin, ×750. **c** Leydig cell atrophy. Dramatic accumulation of extracellular matrix. Leydig cells are atrophic. Thin co-cells (Holstein and Davidoff 1997) compartmentalize the interstitium. Stained according to Laczkó and Levai (1975), ×1100. **d** Cytological characteristics of spermatids. Immature spermatids (step 3 of spermiogenesis, Holstein and Roosen-Runge 1981) containing acrosome cap and nuclear insertion of flagellum (*arrow*). This insertion is evident from a dark granulum on the nuclear membrane opposite the acrosome in semithin sections. The granulum corresponds to the centriols which are necessary for pronuclear fusion following sperm impregnation of the egg. This is the

reason why only spermatids from maturational step 3 onwards can be used for ICSI. 31 year-old patient with complete spermatogenesis and obstructive azoospermia. Toluidine blue-pyronin, ×1400. **e** Morphogenesis of round-headed and acrosome-less spermatids. The proacrosomic granule (*arrow*) does not attach to the nucleus. The acrosome is a small granulum stained dark blue and without orientation to the nucleus. In this case, acrosomal development is uncoupled from that of the nucleus and the nucleus remains without an acrosome during further development. Sperm devoid of acrosome cannot penetrate the zona pellucida of the oocyte, resulting in infertility. 33 year-old infertile patient. Toluidine blue-pyronin, ×1400. **f** Multinuclear immature spermatids. Two or four immature spermatids (step 1 or 2 of spermiogenesis) share an acrosomic vesicle. Multinucleated spermatids are infertile even after maturation. Generally these cells already disintegrate in the tubular lumen and highlight a disturbance of spermatid differentiation. 41 year-old infertile patient, ×1200

6.8 Molecular and Cytogenetics

The genetic investigation of patients with fertility disorders plays an important role. Besides Klinefelter syndrome, in which hypogonadism and infertility are known to be of genetic origin, today, mainly because of improved cyto- and molecular genetic methods, chromosomal defects can be found in up to 10% of infertile patients (patients with severe oligozoospermia, azoospermia, Sertoli-cell-only syndrome, spermatogenetic arrest or patients with a positive family anamnesis for infertility, e.g. infertility of the brother). However, the connection between the fertility disorder and the genetic abnormality remains speculative in many cases (de Braekelaar and Dao 1991).

The most common autosomal aberrations are **reciprocal translocations, Robertsonian translocations** and **pericentric inversions**. The prevalence of chromosomal abnormalities increases with decreasing semen quality and is highest in azoospermia (Meschede and Horst 1997). Chromosome anomalies were found in couples investigated consecutively and treated with ICSI in 9 out of 432 men (2%) and in 24 out of 432 women (5.5%) (Meschede et al. 1998).

The evaluation of buccal mucosa cell smears for detection of **Barr bodies (sex chromatin)** is a simple and quick diagnostic screening method. A negative finding does not exclude a chromosome anomaly of any other kind, e.g. of the autosomes or the Y chromosome. **Chromosome analysis (karyotyping)** is performed in a human genetics laboratory on peripheral lymphocytes. Chromosome analysis allows the detection of numerical or structural chromosome aberrations.

Because of extreme DNA condensation, conventional band differentiation in mature spermaozoa is only possible after a prior hamster-ovum-penetration test (see Sect. 6.6.6). The technique is very time-consuming for routine diagnosis.

As an alternative, chromosome analysis by means of **fluorescence in situ hybridization (FISH)** is becoming increasingly important. This method is based on marking single chromosomes with specific DNA sequences to which fluorescent stains are bound covalently. The DNA probes attach to the complementary sequences of the chromosome DNA sequence and, upon exposure to UV light, show a characteristic emission pattern. The light signals within a cell show the number of copies of the chromosome in question. Because of the small size of a sperm, the number of chromosomes analyzed simultaneously is generally limited to three. Many studies initially concentrated on identifying numeric chromosome aberrations in fertile volunteers (Downie et al. 1997; Guttenbach et al. 1997; Martin et al. 1998) and agreed upon a rate of 0.1 to 0.4% per chromosome; chromosome 21, X and Y seem to be more severely afflicted.

Since introduction of ICSI, studies on patients with disturbed spermatogenesis have become increasingly important. Although it is not yet possible to examine sperm intended for microinjection for chromosome aberrations, FISH analyses have provided an important basis for estimating risks of abortion and aneuploidy. According to most recent findings, the rate of aneuploidy in sperm of oligoasthenozoospermic men is higher by a factor of 1.5 to 3 than in sperm of normal fertile volunteers (McInnes et al. 1998; Columbero et al. 1999; Pang et al. 1999; Pfeffer et al. 1999). It follows that there will be a concomitant relative increase in the rate of abortions or in the risk of aneuploid offspring, which, however, because of the low absolute frequency, is negligible.

Chromosome analysis of sperm prior to ICSI benefits men with constitutional chromosome aberrations and patients seeking paternity after chemotherapy. FISH analysis of sperm from Klinefelter patients (47, XXY) showed a high proportion of gonosomal aneuploid sperm (Foresta et al. 1998), whereas additional Y chromosomes in 47,XYY men seem to be largely eliminated by mechanisms of meiotic selection (Mennicke et al. 1997). Comparative studies in men before, during and after chemotherapy have rarely been performed to date, as often spermatogenesis is permanently eliminated as a result of treatment. In a few cases, however, a significant rise in gonosomal disomies during and shortly after treatment was observed which could not be found two years after termination of therapy (Martin et al. 1997, 1999).

Advances in the diagnosis of hypogonadism and infertility can be expected in the future through development of new molecular diagnostic tests. Single gene defects of the Y chromosome are increasingly found as a cause of impaired sexual development or spermatogenesis. The importance of **Y chromosome microdeletions** (Azoospermia Factor[AZF]) for diagnosing infertility is discussed in detail in Sect. 8.13.2. The European Academy of Andrology has recently issued guidelines and initiated an external quality control program for molecular diagnosis of Y chromosome deletions (Simoni et al. 1999).

Deletions or mutations of the **testis determining gene** on the short arm of the Y chromosome (**SRY**) lead to a female phenotype in chromosomally male patients (**XY females**). Transfer of the SRY to an X chromosome during paternal meiosis can produce a male phenotype in genetic females (**XX males**) (see Sect. 8.10). There is a strong association between bilateral congenital deferent duct aplasia and mutations in the **cystic fibrosis transmembrane conductance regulator gene** (**CFTR gene**; see detailed description in Chap. 9). Intensive research is focused on the evaluation of mutations in the **FSH receptor gene** as possible causes for male infertility (see details in Chap. 3).

Regarding **indications necessitating karyotyping and/or molecular genetic diagnostics**, only general guidelines can be presented here. More detail is given in the description of certain diseases in other chapters. In normally androgenized infertile patients chromosome analysis should be performed if **azoospermia** or severe **oligozoospermia** (< 5 million sperm/ml) are present and if another cause (e. g. obstruction, previous chemotherapy etc.) cannot be identified. Karyotyping is also indicated in the case of a positive **family anamnesis** for infertility, especially if brothers of the patients are affected. In patients with endocrine hypogonadism the clinical picture will indicate whether chromosome analysis would be useful. If Klinefelter syndrome is suspected, chromosome analysis is essential. Previous pathological pregnancies (two or more **miscarriages, stillborn infant** with abnormalities) should be reasons for chromosomal analysis in both partners. The Guidelines for Assisted Reproduction issued by the German Medical Board in December 1998 recommend chromosome analysis in both partners in cases of non-obstructive azoospermia or severe oligozoospermia (< 5 million sperm/ml), as well as prior to ICSI (Bundesärztekammer 1998) (see Chap. 17). For couples wishing to apply methods of **microassisted reproduction**, a karyotype is generally recommended. This aspect is presented in greater detail in Chapter 17.

The clinical role of molecular genetic analysis in the AZF gene locus has not yet been fully clarified. While it is not yet part of **routine** diagnostics for patients with idiopathic infertility, it is potentially a promising adjunct to the diagnostic spectrum. The present Guidelines for Assisted Reproduction only point out that molecular analysis of the AZF gene locus can be offered in cases of non-obstructive azoospermia and severe oligozoospermia (Bundesärztekammer 1998). In congenital bilateral aplasia of the vas deferens (CBAVD) (see Chap. 9), however, genetic counselling is mandatory, including detailed mutation analysis of the cystic fibrosis receptor gene (CFTR gene) and, if positive, a sweat test (see Chap. 9) with ultrasonographic examination of the urogenital tract. The results will indicate whether the female partner requires molecular genetic exploration.

6.9 References

Abshagen K, Behre HM, Cooper TG, Nieschlag E (1998) Influence of sperm surface antibodies on spontaneous pregnancy rates. Fertil Steril 70:355–356

Aitken RJ, Brindle JP (1993) Analysis of the ability of three probes targetting the outer acrosomal membrane or acrosomal contents to detect the acrosome reaction in humareaction in human spermatozoa. Hum Reprod 8:1663–1669

Aitken J (1994) On the future of the hamster oocyte penetration assay. Fertil Steril 62:17–19

Aitken RJ (1995) Free radicals, lipid peroxidation and sperm function. Reprod Fertil Dev 7:659–668

Baker RR, Bellis MA (1995) Human sperm competition. Copulation, masturbation and infidelity. Chapman and Hall, London

Barratt CLR, Tomlinson MJ, Cooke ID (1993) Prognostic significance of computerized motility analysis for in vivo fertility. Fertil Steril 60:520–525

Behre HM, Nashan D, Nieschlag E (1989) Objective measurement of testicular volume by ultrasonography: evaluation of the technique and comparison with orchidometer estimates. Int J Androl 12:395–403

Behre HM, Klein B, Steinmeyer E, McGregor GP, Voigt K, Nieschlag E (1992) Effective suppression of luteinizing hormone and testosterone by single doses of the new gonadotropin-releasing hormone antagonist cetrorelix (SB-75) in normal men. J Clin Endocrinol Metab 75:393–398

Behre HM, Bohmeyer J, Nieschlag E (1994) Prostate volume in testosterone-treated and untreated hypogonadal men in comparison to age-matched controls. Clin Endocrinol 40:341–349

Behre HM, Kliesch S, Schädel F, Nieschlag E (1995) Clinical relevance of scrotal and transrectal ultrasonography in andrological patients. Int J Androl 18 [Suppl]:2 27–31

Behre HM, Kliesch S, Leifke E, Link TM, Nieschlag E (1997) Long-term effect of testosterone therapy on bone mineral density in hypogonadal men. J Clin Endocrinol Metab 82:2386–2390

Benson DM, Busch R (1996) Fixation of testicular tissue for immunohistochemical and ultrastructural examination. Andrologia 28:27–33

Bergmann M, Behre HM, Nieschlag E (1994) Serum FSH and testicular morphology in male infertility. Clin Endocrinol 40:133–136

Böck P (1989) Romeis Mikroskopische Technik. Urban and Schwarzenberg, Munich

Braunstein GD (1993) Current concept: gynecomastia. N Engl J Med 328:490–495

Büchter D, Behre HM, Kliesch S, Nieschlag E (1998) Pulsatile GnRH or human chorionic gonadotropin/human menopausal gonadotropin as effective treatment for men with hypogonadotropic hypogonadism: a review of 42 cases. Eur J Endocrinol 139:298–303

Bundesärztekammer (1998) Richtlinien zur Durchführung der Assistierten Reproduktion. Dtsch Ärztebl 95:A3166–A3171

Carlsen E, Olsson C, Petersen JH, Andersson AM, Skakkebaek NE (1999) Diurnal rhythm in serum levels of inhibin B in normal men: relation to testicular steroids and gonadotropins. J Clin Endocrinol Metab 84:1664–1669

Chemes HE, Olmedo SB, Carrere C, Oses R, Carizza C, Leisner M, Blaquier J (1998) Ultrastructural pathology of the sperm flagellum: association between flagellar pathology and fertility prognosis in severely asthenozoospermic men. Hum Reprod 13:2521–2526

Chiou RK, Anderson JC, Wobig RK, Rosinsky DE, Matamoros A Jr, Chen WS, Taylor RJ (1997) Color Doppler ultrasound criteria to diagnose varicoceles: correlation of a new scoring system with physical examination. Urology 50:953–956

Clements S, Cooke ID, Barratt CLR (1995) Implementing comprehensive quality control in the andrology laboratory. Hum Reprod 10:2096–2106

Colombero LT, Hariprashad JJ, Tsai MC, Rosenwaks Z, Palermo GD (1999) Incidence of sperm aneuploidy in relation to semen characteristics and assisted reproductive outcome. Fertil Steril 72:90–96

Cooper TG (1990) Secretory proteins from the epididymis and their clinical relevance. Andrologia 22 [Suppl 1]:155–165

Cooper TG, Yeung CH (1998) A flow cytometric technique using peanut agglutinin for evaluating acrosomal loss from human spermatozoa. J Androl 19:542–550

Cooper TG, Neuwinger J, Bahrs S, Nieschlag E (1992) Internal quality control of semen analysis. Fertil Steril 58:172–178

Cooper TG, Atkinson AD, Nieschlag E (1999) Experience with external quality control in spermatology. Hum Reprod 14:765–769

Corund F, Belin X, Amar E, Delafontaine D, Helenon O, Moreau JF (1999) Varicocele: strategies in diagnosis and treatment. Eur Radiol 9:536–545

De Braekeleer M, Dao TN (1991) Cytogenetic studies in male infertility: a review. Hum Reprod 6:245–250

De Geyter Ch, De Geyter M, Schneider HPG, Nieschlag E (1992) Interdependent influence of follicular fluid oestradiol concentration and motility characteristics of spermatozoa on in-vitro fertilization results. Hum Reprod 7:664–670

De Geyter C, De Geyter M, Koppers B, Nieschlag E (1998) Diagnostic accuracy of computer-assisted sperm motion analysis. Hum Reprod 13:2512–2520

De Kretser DM, Holstein AF (1976) Testicular biopsy and abnormal germ cells. In: Hafez ESE (ed) Human semen and fertility regulation in men, Mosby, St. Louis, pp 332–343

deLarmirande E, Gagnon C (1999) The dark and bright sides of reactive oxygen species on sperm function. In: Gagnon C (ed) The male gamete: from basic science to clinical application. Cache River Press, Vienna, pp 455–467

Dieckmann KP (1993) Carcinoma in situ (testikuläre intraepitheliale Neoplasie) des Hodens. In: Hertle L, Pohl J (eds) Urologische Therapie. Urban and Schwarzenberg, Munich, pp 456–458

Downie SE, Flaherty SP, Matthews C (1997) Detection of chromosomes and estimation of aneuploidy in human spermatozoa using fluorescence in-situ hybridization. Mol Hum Reprod 3:585–598

Eckardstein S v, Simoni M, Bergmann M, Weinbauer GF, Gassner P, Schepers AG, Nieschlag E (1999) Serum inhibin B in combination with serum follicle-stimulating hormone (FSH) is a more sensitive marker than serum FSH alone for impaired spermatogenesis in men, but cannot predict the presence of sperm in testicular tissue samples. J Clin Endocrinol Metab 84:2496–2501

Eckardstein S v, Cooper TG, Rutsch K, Meschede D, Horst J, Nieschlag E (2000) Seminal plasma characteristics as indicators of cystic fibrosis transmembrane conductance regulator (CFTR) gene mutations in men with obstructive azoospermia. Fertil Steril 73:1226–1231

Ekbom A, Akre O (1998) Increasing incidence of testicular cancer – birth cohort effect. Acta Pathol Microbiol Immunol Scand 106:225–229

Fénichel P, Hsi BL, Farahifar D, Donzeau M, Barrier-Delpech D, Yeh CJG (1989) Evaluation of the human sperm acrosome reaction using a monclonal antibody, GB24, and fluorescence-activated cell sorter. J Reprod Fertil 87:699–706

Fénichel P, Donzeau M, Farahifar D, Basteris B, Ayraud N, Hsi L (1991) Dynamics of human acrosome reaction: relation with in vitro fertilization. Fertil Steril 55:699–706

Fischer M, Felsenberg D, Kempers B (1993) Methoden der Knochendichtemessung – heutiger Stand. Klinikarzt 22:15–21

Foresta C, Galeazzi C, Bettella A, Stella M, Scandellari C (1998) High incidence of sperm sex chromosome aneuploidies in two patients with Klinefelter's syndrome. J Clin Endocrinol Metab 83:203–205

Ghadessy FJ, Lim J, Abdullah AA, Panet-Raymond V, Choo CK, Lumbroso R, Tut TG, Gottlieb B, Pinsky L, Trifiro MA, Yong EL (1999) Oligospermic infertility associated with an androgen receptor mutation that disrupts interdomain and coactivator (TIF2) interactions. J Clin Invest 103:1517–1525

Gray A, Feldman HA, McKinlay JB, Longcope C (1991) Age, disease, and changing sex hormone levels in middle-aged men: results of the Massachusetts Male Aging Study. J Clin Endocrinol Metab 73:1016–1025

Greulich WW, Pyle SI (1959) Radiographic atlas of skeletal development of the hand and wrist, 2nd edn. Stanford University Press, Stanford

Grunert JH, De Geyter Ch, Nieschlag E (1990) Objective identification of hyperactivated human spermatozoa by computerized sperm motion analysis with the Hamilton-Thorn sperm motility analyser. Hum Reprod 5:593–599

Gsponer J, De Tribolet N, Deruaz JP, Janzer R, Uske A, Mirimanoff RO, Reymond MJ, Rey F, Temler E, Gaillard RC, Gomez F (1999) Diagnosis, treatment, and outcome of pituitary tumors and other abnormal intrasellar masses. Retrospective analysis of 353 patients. Medicine 78:236–269

Guttenbach M, Engel W, Schmid M (1997) Analysis of structural and numerical chromosome abnormalities in sperm of normal men and carriers of constitutional chromosome aberrations. A review. Hum Genet 100:1–21

Hacker-Klom UB, Göhde W, Nieschlag E, Behre HM (1999) DNA flow cytometry of human semen. Hum Reprod 14:2506–2512

Hayes FJ, Hall JE, Boepple PA, Crowley WF (1998) Differential control of gonadotropin secretion in the human: endocrine role of inhibin. J Clin Endocrinol Metab 83:1835–1841

Heidenreich A, Sesterhenn IA, Mostofi FK, Moul JW (1998) Immunohistochemical expression of monoclonal antibody 43–9F in testicular germ cell tumours. Int J Androl 21:283–288

Holstein AF, Roosen-Runge EC (1981) Atlas of human spermatogenesis. Grosse, Berlin

Holstein AF, Wulfhekel U (1971) Die Semidünnschnitt-Technik als Grundlage für eine cytologische Beurteilung der Spermatogenese des Menschen. Andrologie 3:65–69

Holstein AF, Davidoff M (1997) Compartmentalization of the intertubular space in the human testis. Adv Exp Med Biol 424:161–162

Holstein AF, Roosen-Runge EC, Schirren C (1988) Illustrated pathology of human spermatogenesis. Grosse, Berlin

Huhtaniemi I, Jiang M, Nilsson C, Pettersson K (1999) Mutations and polymorphisms in gonadotropin genes. Mol Cell Endocrinol 151:89–94

Irvine DS, Macleod IC, Templeton AA, Masterton A, Taylor A (1994) A prospective clinical study of the relationship between the computer-assisted assessment of human semen quality and the achievement of pregnancy in vivo. Hum Reprod 9:2324–2334

Imperato-McGinley J, Gautier T, Cai LQ, Yee B, Epstein J, Pochi P (1993) The androgen control of sebum production. Studies of subjects with dihydrotestosterone deficiency and complete androgen insensitivity. J Clin Endocrinol Metab 76:524–528

Jackson JA, Riggs MW, Spiekerman AM (1992) Testosterone deficiency as a risk factor for hip fractures in men: a case-control study. Am J Med Sci 304:4–8

Jensen TK, Andersson AM, Hjollund NH, Scheike T, Kolstad H, Giwercman A, Henriksen TB, Ernst E, Bonde JP, Olsen J, McNeilly A, Groome NP, Skakkebaek NE (1997) Inhibin B as a serum marker of spermatogenesis: correlation to differences in sperm concentration and follicle-stimulating hormone levels. A study of 349 Danish men. J Clin Endocrinol Metab 82:4059–4063

Jeyendran RS, Van der Ven HK, Perez-Palaez M, Crabo BG, Zaneveld LJD (1984) Development of an assay to assess the functional integrity of the human sperm membrane and its relationship to other semen characteristics. J Reprod Fertil 70:219–228

Jockenhövel F, Gräwe A, Nieschlag E (1990) A portable digital data recorder for long-term monitoring of scrotal temperatures. Fertil Steril 54:694–700

Johnston RC, Mbizvo MT, Summerbell D, Kovacs GT, Baker HWG (1994) Relationship between stimulated hyperactivated motility of human spermatozoa and pregnancy rate in donor insemination: A preliminary report. Hum Reprod 9:1684–1687

Kruger TF, Dutoit TC, Franken DR, Menkveld R, Lombard CJ (1995) Sperm morphology: assessing the agreement between the manual method (strict criteria) and the sperm morphology analyzer IVOS. Fertil Steril 63:134–141

Lacey HA, Pinarbasi E, Hornby DPH (1995) Subcloning of human ZP2 cDNA for in vitro prokaryotic and eukaryotic expression. Annual Conference of the Society for the Study of Fertility, Dublin

Laczkó J, Lévai G (1975) A simple differential staining method for semi-thin sections of ossifying cartilage and bone tissues embedded in Epoxy resin. Mikroskopie 31:1–4

Lee MA, Trucco GS, Bechtol KB, Wummer N, Kopf GS, Blasco L, Storey BT (1987) Capacitation and acrosome reactions in human spermatozoa monitored by a chlortetracycline fluorescence assay. Fertil Steril 48:649–658

Lee MM, Donahoe PK, Silverman B, Hasegawa T, Hasegawa Y, Gustafson ML, Chan Y, MacLaughlin DT (1997) Measurements of serum müllerian inhibiting substance in the evaluation of children with nonpalpable gonads. N Engl J Med 336:1480–1486

Le Moli R, Endert E, Fliers E, Mulder T, Prummel MF, Romijn JA, Wiersinga WM (1999) Establishment of reference values for endocrine tests. II: Hyperprolactinemia. Nether J Med 55:71–75

Lerchl A, Keck C, Spiteri-Grech J, Nieschlag E (1993) Diurnal variations of scrotal temperature in normal men and patients with varicocele before and after treatment. Int J Androl 16:195–200

Liu DY, Baker HWG. (1996) A simple method for assessment of the human acrosome reaction of spermatozoa bound to the zona pellucida: a lack of relationship with ionophore A23187 induced acrosome reaction. Hum Reprod 11:551–557

Marin P, Oden B, Björntorp P (1995) Assimilation and mobilization of triglycerides in subcutaneous abdominal and femoral adipose tissue in vivo in men: effects of androgens. J Clin Endocrinol Metab 80:239–243

Martin RH (1998) Genetics of human sperm. J Ass Reprod Genet 15:240–245

Martin RH, Ernst S, Rademaker A, Barclay L, Ko E, Summers N (1997) Analysis of human sperm karyotypes in testicular cancer patients before and after chemotherapy. Cytogenet Cell Genet 78:120–123

Martin RH, Ernst S, Rademaker A, Barclay L, Ko E, Summers N (1999) Analysis of sperm chromosome complements before, during and after chemotherapy. Cancer Genet Cytogenet 108:133–136

McInness B, Rademaker A, Greene CA, Ko E, Barclay L, Martin R (1998) Abnormalities for chromosomes 13 and 21 detected in spermatozoa from infertile men. Hum Reprod 13:2787–2790

Mennicke K, Diercks P, Schlieker H, Bals-Pratsch M, al Hasani S, Diedrich K, Schwinger E (1997) Molecular cytogenetic diagnostics in sperm. Int J Androl 20 [Suppl 3]:11–19

Meschede D, Horst J (1997) Genetic counselling for infertile male patients. Int J Androl 20 [Suppl 3]:20–30

Meschede D, Behre HM, Nieschlag E (1995) Endocrine and spermatological characteristics of 135 patients with bilateral megalotestis. Andrologia 27:207–212

Meschede D, Dworniczak B, Behre HM, Kliesch S, Claustres M, Nieschlag E, Horst J (1997) CFTR gene mutations in men with bilateral ejaculatory-duct obstruction and anomalies of the seminal vesicles. Am J Hum Genet 61:1200–1202

Meschede D, Lemcke B, Exeler JR, De Geyter C, Behre HM, Nieschlag E, Horst J (1998) Chromosome abnormalities in 447 couples undergoing intracytoplasmic sperm injection – prevalence, types, sex distribution and reproductive relevance. Hum Reprod 13:576–582

Moeller H (1993) Clues to the aetiology of testicular germ cell tumours from descriptive epidemiology. Eur Urol 23:8–15

Nashan D, Behre HM, Grunert JH, Nieschlag E (1990) Diagnostic value of scrotal sonography in infertile men: report on 658 cases. Andrologia 22:387–385

Neugebauer DC, Neuwinger J, Jockenhövel F, Nieschlag E (1990) 9+0 axoneme in spermatozoa and some nasal cilia of a patient with totally immotile spermatozoa associated with thickened sheath and short midpiece. Hum Reprod 5:981–986

Neuwinger J, Behre HM, Nieschlag E (1990) External quality control in the andrology laboratory: an experimental multicenter trial. Fertil Steril 54:308–314

Neuwinger J, Cooper TG, Knuth UA, Nieschlag E (1991) Hyaluronic acid as a medium for human sperm migration tests. Hum Reprod 6:396–400

Nieschlag E (1998) Hodenfunktionen. In: Thomas L (ed) Labor und Diagnose, 5th edn. TH-Books Verlagsgesellschaft, Frankfurt, pp 1124–1133

Nieschlag E, von zur Mühlen A, Sippell W (1993) Männliche Gonaden. In: Deutsche Gesellschaft für Endokrinologie (ed) Rationelle Diagnostik in der Endokrinologie einschließlich Diabetologie und Stoffwechsel. Thieme, Stuttgart, pp 186–212

Ochsendorf FR (1998) Infection and reactive oxygen species. Andrologia 30 [Suppl 1]:81–86

Oei SG, Helmerhorst FM, Keirse MJNC (1995) When is the postcoital test normal? A critical appraisal. Hum Reprod 10:1711–1714

Pang MG, Hoegerman SF, Cuticchia AJ, Moon SY, Doncel GF, Acosta AA, Kearns WG (1999) Detection of aneuploidy for chromosomes 4, 6, 7, 8, 9, 10, 11, 12, 13, 17, 18, 21, X and Y by fluorescence in-situ hybridization in spermatozoa from nine patients with oligoasthenoteratozoospermia undergoing intracytoplasmic sperm injection. Hum Reprod 14:1266–1273

Paschke R, Schulze Bertelsbeck D, Bahrs S, Heinecke A, Behre HM (1994) Seminal sperm antibodies exhibit an unstable spontaneous course and an increased incidence of leucocytospermia. Int J Androl 17:135–139

Pfeffer J, Pang M-G, Hoegerman SF, Osgood Ch J, Stacey MW, Mayer J, Oehninger S, Kearns WG (1999) Aneuploidy frequencies in semen fractions from ten oligoasthenoteratozoospermic patients donating sperm for intracytoplasmic sperm injection. Fertil Steril 72:472–478

Pierik FH, Vreeburg JT, Stijnen T, De Jong FH, Weber RF (1998) Serum inhibin B as a marker of spermatogenesis. J Clin Endocrinol Metab 83:3110–3114

Pierik FH, Dohle GR, van Muiswinkel JM, Vreeburg JT, Weber RF (1999) Is routine scrotal ultrasound advantageous in infertile men? J Urol 162:1618–1620

Pralong FP, Gomez F, Castillo E, Cotecchia S, Abuin L, Aubert ML, Portmann L, Gaillard RC (1999) Complete hypogonadotropic hypogonadism associated with a novel inactivating mutation of the gonadotropin-releasing hormone receptor. J Clin Endocrinol Metab 84:3811–3816

Purvis K, Christiansen E (1993) Infection in the male reproductive tract. Impact, diagnosis and treatment in relation to male infertility. Int J Androl 16:1–13

Quigley CA (1998) The androgen receptor: physiology and pathophysiology. In: Nieschlag E, Behre HM (eds) Testosterone – action, deficiency, substitution, 2nd edn. Springer, Berlin Heidelberg New York, pp 33–106

Randall VA (1998) Androgens and hair. In: Nieschlag E, Behre HM (eds) Testosterone – action, deficiency, substitution, 2nd edn. Springer, Berlin Heidelberg New York, pp 169–186

Rolf C, Cooper TG, Yeung CH, Nieschlag E (1999) Antioxidant treatment of patients with asthenozoospermia or moderate oligoasthenozoospermia with high-dose vitamin C and vitamin E: a randomized, placebo-controlled, double-blind study. Hum Reprod 14:1028–1033

Ron-El R, Strauss S, Friedler S, Strassburger D, Komarovsky D, Raziel A (1998) Serial sonography and colour flow Doppler imaging following testicular and epididymal sperm extraction. Hum Reprod 13:3390–3393

Santner SJ, Albertson B, Zhang GY, Zhang GH, Santulli M, Wang C, Demers LM, Shackleton C, Santen RJ (1998) Comparative rates of androgen production and metabolism in Caucasian and Chinese subjects. J Clin Endocrinol Metab 83:2104–2109

Schulze W, Knuth UA (2000) Diagnostics of testicular dysfunction: Testicular biopsy. In: Shalet SM, Wass JAH (eds) Oxford textbook of endocrinology. Oxford University Press, Oxford (in press)

Schulze W, Thoms F, Knuth UA (1999) Testicular sperm extraction: comprehensive analysis with simultaneously performed histology in 1418 biopsies from 766 subfertile men. Hum Reprod 14 [Suppl 1]:82–96

Simoni M, Nieschlag E (1991) In vitro bioassays of follicle-stimulating hormone: methods and clinical applications (review). J Endocrinol Invest 14:983–997

Simoni M, Gromoll J, Nieschlag E (1997) The follicle-stimulating hormone receptor: biochemistry, molecular biology, physiology, and pathophysiology. Endocr Rev 18:739–773

Simoni M, Bakker E, Eurlings MC, Matthijs G, Moro E, Muller CR, Vogt PH (1999) Laboratory guidelines for molecular diagnosis of Y-chromosomal microdeletions. Int J Androl 22:292–299

Tschöp M, Behre HM, Nieschlag E, Dressendorfer RA, Strasburger CJ (1998) A time-resolved fluorescence immunoassay for the measurement of testosterone in saliva: monitoring of testosterone replacement therapy with testosterone buciclate. J Clin Chem Lab Med 36:223–230

Tong S, Cardinal HN, McLoughlin RF, Downey DB, Fenster A (1998) Intra- and inter-observer variability and reliability of prostate volume measurement via two-dimensional and three-dimensional ultrasound imaging. Ultrasound Med Biol 24:673–681

Tournaye H, Verheyen G, Nagy P, Ubaldi F, Goossens A, Silber S, Van Steirteghem AC, Devroey P (1997) Are there any predictive factors for successful testicular sperm recovery in azoospermic patients? Hum Reprod 12:80–86

van Duin M, Polman JEM, de Breet ITM, van Ginneken K, Bunschoten H, Grootenhuis A, Brindle J, Aitken RJ (1994) Recombinant human zona pellucida protein ZP3 produced by Chinese hamster ovary cells induces the human sperm acrosome reaction and promotes sperm-egg fusion. Biol Reprod 51:607–617

Vermeulen A, Verdonck G (1992) Representativeness of a single point plasma testosterone level for the long term hormonal milieu. J Clin Endocrinol Metab 74:939–942

Vermeulen A, Verdonck L, Kaufman JM (1999) A critical evaluation of simple methods for the estimation of free testosterone in serum. J Clin Endocrinol Metab 84:3666–3672

Wang C, Lee GS, Leung A, Surrey ES, Chan SYW (1993) Human sperm hyperactivation and acrosome reaction and their relationships to human in vitro fertilization. Fertil Steril 59:1221–1227

Weidner W, Schroeder-Printzen I, Weiske WH, Haidl G (1995) Microsurgical aspects of the treatment of azoospermia. The BMFT Study Group for Microsurgery. Int J Androl 18 [Suppl 2]:63–66

WHO Laborhandbuch zur Untersuchung des menschlichen Ejakulats und der Spermien-Zervikalschleim-Interaktion (1999) Übersetzung von: Nieschlag E, Nieschlag S, Bals-Pratsch M, Behre HM, Knuth UA, Meschede D, Niemeier M, Schick A, 4th edn. Springer, Berlin Heidelberg New York

WHO Manual for the standardized investigation and diagnosis of the infertile couple (1993) Rowe PJ, Comhaire FH, Hargreave TB, Mellows HJ (eds). Cambridge University Press, Cambridge

Wüster C, Heilmann P, Pereira-Lima J, Schlegel J, Anstatt K, Soballa T (1998) Quantitative ultrasonometry (QUS) for the evaluation of osteoporosis risk: reference data for various measurement sites, limitations and application possibilities. Exp Clin Endocrinol Diabetes 106:277–288

Yeung CH, Cooper TG, DeGeyter M, DeGeyter C, Rolf C, Kamischke A, Nieschlag E (1998) Studies on the origin of redox enzymes in seminal plasma and their relationship with results of in-vitro fertilization. Mol Human Reprod 4:835–839

Young J, Rey R, Couzinet B, Chanson P, Josso N, Schaison G (1999) Antimüllerian hormone in patients with hypogonadotropic hypogonadism. J Clin Endocrinol Metab 84:2696–2699

Zamboni L (1992) Sperm structure and its relevance to infertility. An electron microscopic study. Arch Pathol Lab Med 116:325–344

CHAPTER 7

Diseases of the Hypothalamus and the Pituitary Gland   7

H. M. Behre · E. Nieschlag · D. Meschede · C. J. Partsch

7.1 Idiopathic Hypogonadotropic Hypogonadism (IHH) and Kallmann Syndrome

7.1.1 Definition and Prevalence

> **Idiopathic hypogonadotropic hypogonadism (IHH)** and **Kallmann syndrome** (Kallmann et al. 1944) are closely related diseases sharing **disturbed hypothalamic secretion of GnRH** as their core pathophysiological feature. Hypogonadism resulting from the GnRH deficiency is the only clinical manifestation of idiopathic hypogonadotropic hypogonadism. In addition, patients with Kallmann syndrome feature **anosmia** and occasionally some other physical anomalies.

Among males Kallmann syndrome in its fully developed form has a prevalence of about 1 in 10000. The prevalence in males is four times higher than in females (Seminara et al. 1998).

7.1.2 Etiology and Pathogenesis

Deficiency of hypothalamic GnRH constitutes the basic **endocrine abnormality** in both idiopathic hypogonadotropic hypogonadism and Kallmann syndrome. Secondary to this, the secretion of gonadotropins from the pituitary is impaired (see Sect. 3.1.2). Owing to LH and FSH deficiency, the gonads can neither produce sperm nor sufficient quantities of testosterone. For the X chromosomal recessive variant of Kallmann syndrome the mechanism underlying the defective GnRH secretion is well characterized. **During normal embryonic development** precursors of the **GnRH neurones migrate from the nasal olfactory epithelium to their ultimate anatomical destination in the basal hypothalamus** (Fig. 7.1). This migratory movement is disturbed in embryos with X-linked Kallmann syndrome. Here, the precursors of GnRH neurons do not leave the olfactory epi-

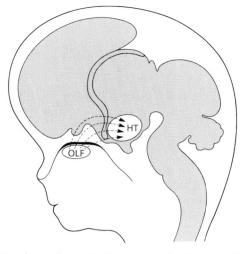

Fig. 7.1. Scheme illustrating the embryonal migration of GnRH neurones (OLF: nasal olfactory epithelium; HT: hypothalamus)

thelium and are thus unable to stimulate the pituitary gonadotrophs (Schwanzel-Fukuda et al. 1989).

As indicated by a positive family history or results of mutation analysis, a primary genetic basis of Kallmann syndrome or IHH is certain in a minority of patients (Meschede and Horst 1999). However, 65 % of the patients represent sporadic cases. The pedigree of patients with a positive family history suggests an autosomal dominant, autosomal recessive or X chromosomal recessive inheritance of the disease (Waldstreicher et al. 1996). The gene responsible for the X chromosomal recessive form is known (Franco et al. 1991). It has been mapped to the short arm of the X chromosome (Meitinger et al. 1990) and is termed **KAL-1** (previously KAL, KALIG-1 or ADMLX). Its protein product is called anosmin-1. It seems to be an extracellular regulator of the directed outgrowth of axons.

KAL-1 is a large gene spanning approximately 200,000 base pairs. Numerous different types of deletions of the entire gene or single exons and point mutations have been characterized (for review see Meschede and Horst 1999). Mutations in the KAL-1 gene are rare in sporadic cases of Kallmann syndrome or IHH (Georgopoulos et al. 1997).

Several well documented familial cases show that Kallmann syndrome, IHH and isolated anosmia without concomitant GnRH deficiency should be regarded as a disease spectrum. These disorders, previously considered as distinct, can be found in close relatives. This can be explained as variable phenotypic expression of a uniform gene defect.

7.1.3 Clinical Picture

Absent or incomplete pubertal development with severe hypogonadism is the **clinical hallmark** of both idiopathic hypogonadotropic hypogonadism and Kallmann syndrome. The testis has a mean volume of about 3 ml (normal for adult men: ≥12 ml). The patients frequently present with uni- or bi-lateral cryptorchidism, or orchidopexy has previously been performed. The scrotum may be hypoplastic and hypopigmented. Other signs of hypogonadism include underdevelopment of the penis and prostate, absent or sparse pubic, axillary and body hair, lack of beard growth, enuchoid body proportions and a female distribution pattern of adipose tissue (Fig. 7.2). Gynecomastia is a rare finding. Untreated men with idiopathic hypogonadotropic hypogonadism and Kallmann syndrome are infertile because of aspermia or azoospermia. Without endocrine substitution these patients have no or reduced sexual activities. Osteoporosis may occur as a secondary complication of longstanding hypogonadism.

The variability of the clinical picture with regard to clinical severity and age of onset should be noted. Besides the fully expressed disease, minor forms with partial pubertal development or onset of GnRH deficiency in adulthood have been described (Seminara et al. 1998).

Anosmia, notably absent in idiopathic hypogonadotropic hypogonadism, represents the second cardinal symptom of Kallmann syndrome. This clinical symptom differentiates it from IHH. The inability to perceive olfactory stimuli results from **aplasia or hypoplasia of the olfactory bulbs and tracts**. The insensitivity only relates to aromatic olfactants; mucosal irritants such as ammonia evoke a normal reaction.

In addition to hypogonadism and anosmia, **other anomalies may be associated with Kallmann syndrome** (Schwankhaus et al. 1989; Waldstreicher et al. 1996). 5–10 % of patients show impaired hearing or oral anomalies such as cleft lip or high arched palate. Synkinesis of the extremities or unilateral renal aplasia may occur especially in patients with the X-linked disease. Numerous other malformations and functional problems have been described in single case reports, but these probably represent coincidental findings.

7.1.4 Diagnosis

If idiopathic hypogonadotropic hypogonadism or Kallmann syndrome is suspected, the most important endocrine parameters to be checked are the **basal serum levels of LH, FSH, testosterone, and estradiol**. Measurement of prolactin, TSH, ACTH, IGF-1, growth and thyroid hormones, and cortisol allows for evaluation of the other hypothalamic-pituitary axes. In addition, **GnRH**

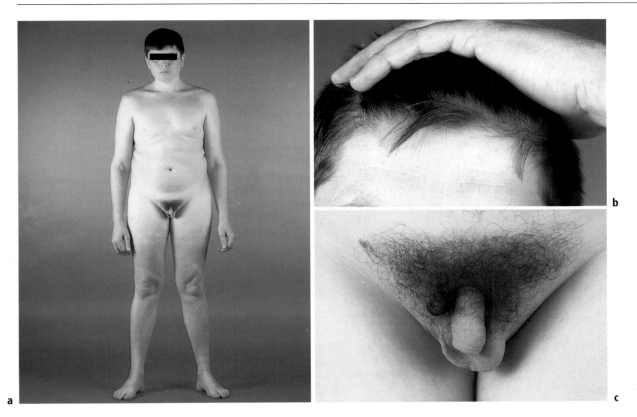

Fig. 7.2 a–c. 33-year-old patient with Kallmann syndrome before (remarkably late) initiation of treatment with testosterone and subsequent treatment with hCG/hMG. Infertility was the primary complaint. Typical presentation with signs of hypogonadism already present before puberty: **a** arm span larger than height (eunuchoid body proportions), female distribution pattern of adipose tissue, no beard growth; **b** straight frontal hair line and **c** straight pubic hair line, infantile penis and scrotum, and markedly subnormal volume of the testes. Voice mutation had not occurred yet in this patient. Gonadotropin and testosterone levels were subnormal, but LH and FSH concentrations increased appropriately in response to a GnRH bolus. Hematocrit was severely reduced, the prostate was small, ejaculate analysis revealed azoospermia. Bone density as measured by quantitative computed tomography was reduced to 24% of the age-adjusted normal value

tests (see Sect. 6.4.2), performed both before and after a period of pulsatile GnRH stimulation, are mandatory.

Typically patients with Kallmann syndrome and idiopathic hypogonadotropic hypogonadism have markedly subnormal basal levels of LH, FSH and testosterone (hypogonadotropic hypogonadism). Responsiveness of the gonadotropins to GnRH stimulation is poor or altogether absent. This should not be misinterpreted as a sign of a primary abnormality at the pituitary level. Obviously the gonadotrophs only respond to a GnRH stim-

ulus in a physiological fashion after a certain period of "priming".

To differentiate between real pituitary pathology and the reversible unresponsiveness due to the lack of preceding exposure to GnRH, the **GnRH pump test** is performed. For a period of seven days 5 μg GnRH are applied subcutaneously every 90 to 120 minutes using a portable minipump. If the gonadotropin response to a GnRH bolus has normalized after such pretreatment, a hypothalamic source of the hypogonadism is indicated. In contrast, a primary pituitary problem must be suspected if the gonadotrophs remain functionally resistant to a GnRH bolus. Another important differential diagnosis is that between idiopathic hypogonadotropic hypogonadism / Kallmann syndrome and constitutional pubertal delay. GnRH bolus testing after 36 hours of pulsatile GnRH pretreatment with a minipump may be helpful in this situation (see Sect. 7.5.4).

Typically, patients with congenital hypogonadotropic hypogonadism have significantly increased serum levels of anti-Muellerian hormone, which can be lowered by hCG or testosterone therapy (Young et al. 1999a).

It should be noted that in a small minority of patients with idiopathic hypogonadotropic hypogonadism or Kallmann syndrome, basal levels of FSH in the low-normal range may be found, while basal LH is clearly subnormal (see Sect. 7.8) (Spratt et al. 1987).

Table 7.1. Therapeutic options for stimulation of spermatogenesis in patients with idiopathic hypogonadotropic hypogonadism or Kallmann syndrome

Drug	Trade name	Administration	Dose
Pulsatile GnRH	Lutrelef	Subcutaneous, external minipump (Zyklomat pulse)	5–20 µg per pulse every 120 min
Alternatively to pulsatile GnRH Human chorionic gonadotropin (hCG)	Choragon, Predalon Pregnesin, Primogonyl	Intramuscular or subcutaneous	1000–2500 IU 2 times per week (Monday and Friday)
in combination with Human menopausal gonadotropin (hMG)	Humegon, Menogon, Pergonal	Intramuscular or subcutaneous	150 IU 3 times per week (Monday, Wednesday, Friday)
or with highly purified or recombinant FSH	Fertinorm, Gonal F, Puregon	Subcutaneous	150 IU 3 times per week

Proving **anosmia** in Kallmann syndrome is usually a straightforward procedure. The patient can be asked to close his eyes and identify an aromatic substance such as perfumed soap or coffee. More sophisticated testing with a standardized set of olfactants may sometimes be necessary. Mucosal irritants (e.g. ammonia) and gustatory stimuli are perceived normally in patients with Kallmann syndrome.

Imaging procedures should include testicular and renal **ultrasound** (the latter to detect renal agenesis) and **nuclear magnetic resonance imaging** of the hypothalamic-pituitary region. It is of utmost importance not to overlook any intracranial mass which may present with clinical symptoms indistinguishable from idiopathic hypogonadotropic hypogonadism or Kallmann syndrome. Measurement of **bone density** should be included in the routine diagnostic workup (see Sect. 6.3.5).

As Kallmann syndrome is a genetic disorder, it is important to take a meticulous **family history**. The patient should be specifically questioned about relatives with hypogonadism, infertility, or anosmia. If the X chromosomal recessive form of the Kallmann syndrome is suspected, mutation analysis of the KAL-1 gene should be performed. In patients desiring children, genetic counselling should be offered before initiation of therapy. The recurrence risk can be up to 50% in autosomal dominant Kallmann syndrome or IHH.

7.1.5 Therapy

Treatment in newly diagnosed patients with idiopathic hypogonadotropic hypogonadism or Kallmann syndrome is initiated by applying **testosterone** for several months (see Chap. 15). This leads to rapid virilization, a higher level of general physical well-being and activity, and increased sexual drive. Most patients welcome these dramatic physical and psychological changes. Once the initial goal of rapid virilization has been achieved, treatment is redirected at stimulating gametogenesis up to the point that mature spermatozoa are produced. Medication is changed from testosterone to either GnRH or gonadotropins. This therapeutic approach is beneficial both for patients who desire fertility soon, as well as for those who want to have children later on. In the latter group spermatogenesis, once driven to full maturation, can probably be restimulated more effectively when fertility is actually desired (Büchter et al. 1998).

The **pulsatile application of GnRH** by means of a portable minipump most closely simulates normal physiology (Table 7.1). The pump delivers a small bolus of GnRH (usually 5–20 µg/pulse) every 120 minutes. Application is via a subcutaneous needle that has to be changed on a regular basis. The GnRH pulses induce the secretion of gonadotropins from the pituitary. In turn, the gonadotropins stimulate gonadal steroid production and gamete maturation. **Alternatively**, treatment with

Fig. 7.4 a, b. Kallmann syndrome: testicular histology **a** before and **b** during hCG/hMG therapy with elongated spermatids present. (Provided by Prof. C.A. Paulsen, MD, University of Washington, Seattle)

Fig. 7.3. Sperm concentrations in infertile patients with hypogonadotropic hypogonadism (*IHH/KalS* idiopathic hypogonadotropic hypogonadism and Kallmann syndrome; *HYP* hypogonadism due to pituitary dysfunction). The diagram shows sperm concentrations over the course of hCG/hMG or pulsatile GnRH treatment up to the point when the female partner conceived. Stimulation of spermatogenesis was achieved sooner in "HYP" patients with a larger baseline testicular volume. Taken that the reproductive functions in the female partner are optimal, pregnancies occur with sperm concentrations of less than 3 million/ml. It may be necessary to continue treatment over prolonged periods of time. Therapy should not be terminated prematurely

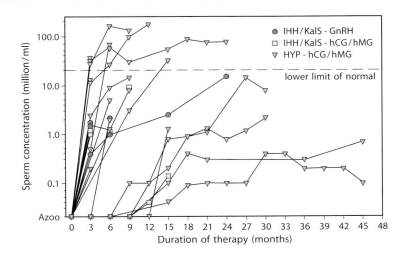

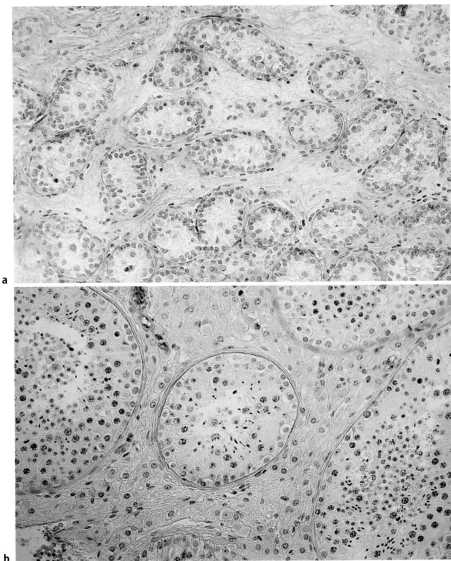

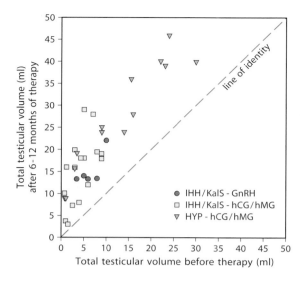

Fig. 7.5. Testicular volume measured by ultrasonography in patients with hypogonadotropic hypogonadism (*IHH/KalS* idiopathic hypogonadotropic hypogonadism and Kallmann syndrome; *HYP* hypogonadism due to pituitary dysfunction) before treatment and during a 6–12 month course of hCG/hMG or pulsatile GnRH. Note the significantly larger baseline testicular volume in "HYP" patients, who, for example, in a case of pituitary tumor, develop hypogonadism after puberty. However, among "idiopathic hypogonadotropic hypogonadism/KalS" patients a marked increase in testicular size can also be achieved

human chorionic gonadotropin (**hCG**, corresponding to LH) and human menopausal gonadotropin (**hMG**, corresponding to FSH) can be considered. In the male hCG and hMG must be injected intramuscularly or subcutaneously two and three times per week, respectively (Table 7.1). As an alternative to hMG, highly purified FSH (Burgues and Calderon 1997; European Metrodin HP Group 1998) or recombinant FSH (Kliesch et al. 1995; Liu et al. 1999) can be used for therapy. In the future recombinant hCG or LH will probably be available.

Treatment is continued either until sperm appear in the ejaculate or a pregnancy has been induced (Fig. 7.3). There is a good chance of achieving fertility in men with Kallmann syndrome, and sperm production can be induced in nearly all patients (Fig. 7.4) (Liu et al. 1988; Schopohl et al. 1991; Büchter et al. 1998; European Metrodin HP Group 1998; Barrio et al. 1999; Liu et al. 1999). This may necessitate treatment courses with GnRH or gonadotropins that extend over two and more years (Fig. 7.3). Cryptorchidism or markedly subnormal testicular volume is not a contraindication to therapy. Nearly all such patients respond to treatment with a substantial increase in testicular volume (Fig. 7.5).

Gonadotropins and GnRH appear to be similarly efficient in stimulating spermatogenesis (Büchter et al. 1998). Both GnRH and hCG/hMG therapy are costly and

can only be justified when fertility is actually desired or, in the initial phase of treatment, when spermatogenesis is to be stimulated up to the point of sperm production. Once either goal has been achieved, therapy is switched back to testosterone, which is cheaper and fully sufficient to compensate the androgen deficiency. Testosterone substitution (possibly interrupted when fertility is desired) has to be lifelong to preserve secondary sexual characteristics and androgen-dependent functions and to prevent osteoporosis.

7.2 Prader-Labhart-Willi Syndrome

7.2.1 Etiology and Pathogenesis

Roughly one in 10,000 individuals has Prader-Labhart-Willi syndrome (PLWS) (1956). Because of the complex disturbance of their physical and mental development (Cassidy 1997), patients with PLWS are most often seen by pediatricians. As **the disease must be considered in the differential diagnosis of delayed and incomplete puberty**, it should be familiar to the andrologist. Although Prader, Labhart and Willi were the first to describe the syndrome, it is often referred to as Prader-Willi-syndrome.

The **genetic basis** of the mostly sporadic, but occasionally familial Prader-Labhart-Willi syndrome is complex and cannot be described in detail in this chapter. Probably the phenotype is not caused by the loss or functional disturbance of a single gene but of a gene cluster in the region 15q11–q13 located on the proximal long arm of chromosome 15. This chromosomal region carries a **genomic imprint**. Genomic imprinting can modify the expression of genes according to their parental origin (Morison and Reeve 1998). Among various candidate genes the role of the SNRPN (small nuclear ribonucleoprotein polypeptide N) is the most established in the pathophysiology of the Prader-Labhart-Willi syndrome. This gene is essential for parental imprinting of the proximal long arm of chromosome 15 (Dittrich et al. 1996).

In 75 % of Prader-Labhart-Willi syndrome patients, a **deletion in the chromosomal region 15q11–13** is detectable. It is always the paternally inherited chromosome 15 which carries the deletion. Some of these deletions may be detected by conventional chromosome analysis, others are sub-microscopic microdeletions. In addition, other structural chromosomal anomalies such as translocations or marker chromosomes may be observed in patients with PLWS. In another 25 % of the patients, **maternal uniparental disomy** of 15q11–13 is the mechanism underlying Prader-Labhart-Willi syndrome. Here **both** copies of the critical chromosomal region are contributed by the mother. Under normal circumstances, they should be inherited in a biparental fashion. As in deletion cases, the active paternal allele of the Prader-Labhart-Willi syndrome gene cluster is lacking. A few patients with Prader-Labhart-Willi syndrome have "**imprinting mutations**" which interfere with the process of parental imprinting of critical chromosomal regions during gametogenesis (Ohta et al. 1999).

7.2.2 Clinical Picture and Diagnosis

Newborns and infants with Prader-Labhart-Willi syndrome often come to clinical attention because of **generalized and profound muscular hypotonia**. Motor development is delayed, and feeding frequently poses a major problem in the first year of life. While the **children fail to thrive in infancy, as toddlers they tend to become obese**, often to a remarkable extent. Hyperphagia persisting into adulthood may be difficult to control. In about 10 % of the patients diabetes mellitus develops as a sequel of obesity. Men with Prader-Labhart-Willi syndrome have an average **final adult height of 155 centimeters**. Even in relation to the short stature, hands and feet appear small, and the hands tend to be narrow. General **hypopigmentation** can be observed in every third patient. Aberrant craniofacial features in Prader-Labhart-Willi syndrome include almond-shaped palpebral fissures and a narrow forehead, but usually the face does not appear very dysmorphic. **Mental retardation** is present in most, but not all patients with Prader-Labhart-Willi syndrome. Typically, retardation is mild with an IQ ranging at around 60 to 70. The mental handicap may be more pronounced in some cases. Various behavior disorders are seen in childhood as well as adulthood (Cassidy 1997).

The **genitalia are hypoplastic** in the vast majority of males with Prader-Labhart-Willi syndrome. Children typically have a micropenis, uni- or bi-lateral maldescended testes, and a hypoplastic scrotum. **Pubertal development is delayed and incomplete**. While the penis and testes are small and the general state of virilization poor, pubic hair may be normally developed. **Testosterone, LH and FSH serum levels are subnormal**. It takes several days of pretreatment until GnRH evokes a sufficient gonadotropin response, indicating that the hypogonadism in Prader-Labhart-Willi syndrome is primarily **hypothalamic** (Jeffcoate et al. 1980). In addition, Leydig cell function may be impaired, as indicated by a subnormal response of testosterone to injected hCG. Testicular biopsies show atrophy of the seminiferous tubules. It is presumed that all men with Prader-Labhart-Willi syndrome are **infertile**, but this issue has not been systematically studied.

The clinical diagnosis of Prader-Labhart-Willi syndrome should always be confirmed by **DNA analysis**. A reliable and highly sensitive molecular test is based on analyzing the methylation pattern in the "critical" gene region (Gillesen-Kaesbach et al. 1995). However, this test does not differentiate between deletion, uniparental disomy and an imprint mutation. For further analysis, additional special tests and blood samples of the parents are needed.

7.2.3 Therapy

No causal treatment of Prader-Labhart-Willi syndrome is available. **Testosterone** can be given to compensate the endocrine hypogonadism (see Chap. 15). Whether or not such hormonal treatment is initiated has to be decided on an individual basis, taking into account the psychosocial situation of the patient. Some pilot studies demonstrated positive effects of growth hormone therapy on longitudinal growth (Hauffa 1997).

7.2.4 Bardet-Biedl and Laurence-Moon Syndromes

Along with the Prader-Labhart-Willi syndrome, the Bardet-Biedl and Laurence-Moon syndromes were previously incorrectly considered as disorders with primary hypothalamic hypogonadism. The **Bardet-Biedl** and **Laurence-Moon** syndromes are very rare familial disorders with autosomal recessive inheritance. Genes responsible for the Bardet-Biedl syndrome are mapped to chromosomes 2, 3, 11, 15 and 16 (Young et al. 1999b). The Bardet-Biedl and Laurence-Moon syndromes have in common obesity, progressive retinal dystrophy and mental retardation. Beyond these features, patients with Bardet-Biedl syndrome may have hexadactyly, while individuals with Laurence-Moon syndrome display progressive neurological problems, including spastic paraplegia and ataxia (Green et al. 1989; Beales et al. 1999).

Hypogonadism and hypogenitalism occur as facultative features in both conditions. It appears that, in contrast to previous thinking, the hypogonadism does **not** have a **hypothalamic or pituitary** basis. With few exceptions adult male patients have normal LH and FSH serum levels, and FSH may actually be increased. GnRH testing shows a regular gonadotropin response. Furthermore, the serum testosterone concentration is usually within the normal range. Neither ejaculate parameters nor testicular histology have been systematically studied in the Bardet-Biedl and Laurence-Moon syndromes. Some case reports suggest that spermatogenesis may be compromised to a variable degree. However, paternity of males with Bardet-Biedl syndrome has been described (Beales et al. 1999).

7.3 Cerebellar Ataxia and Hypogonadism

Cerebellar ataxias constitute a highly **heterogenous group** of disorders. So far, no generally accepted classification scheme exists (Baraitser 1997; Koeppen 1998). **Most cerebellar ataxias are genetically determined.** Several dozen hereditary conditions featuring cerebellar ataxia are known. The so-called pure forms become symptomatic only through cerebellar dysfunction. Another group of disorders combines this feature with extracerebellar signs and symptoms. One of these associations is that between cerebellar ataxia and hypogonadism (Baraitser 1997).

Within this category ataxias with hypo- and hypergonadotropic hypogonadism are to be distinguished. The term cerebellar ataxia with hypergonadotropic hypogonadism has been applied to several different conditions such as the Marinesco-Sjögren syndrome, ataxia teleangiactasia (the Louis-Bar syndrome) and even untypical cases of Klinefelter syndrome. It is beyond the scope of this book to discuss this poorly characterized group of patients.

Similarly, **cerebellar ataxia with hypogonadotropic hypogonadism** does not represent a single entity. The autosomal recessive Boucher-Neuhäuser syndrome is best defined: it is characterized by absent or incomplete pubertal development with low levels of LH, FSH, testosterone and estradiol, signs of spinocerebellar ataxia and an atypical chorioretinal dystrophy (Rump et al. 1997). The increase of gonadotropins following GnRH administration is subnormal, even after GnRH pretreatment. This makes pituitary involvement probable. There are similarities between the Boucher-Neuhäuser syndrome and Holmes cerebellar ataxia (hypogonadotropic hypogonadism, (spino)-cerebellar ataxia, nystagmus, possibly mental retardation; De Michele et al. 1993) and the Oliver-McFarlane syndrome (hypogonadotropic hypogonadism, growth retardation, retinal degeneration, trichomegaly of eyelashes and sparse hair; Sampson et al. 1989).

7.4 Congenital Adrenal Hypoplasia with Hypogonadotropic Hypogonadism

The cytomegalic form of congenital adrenal hypoplasia is a rare, X-chromosomal recessive disease with a **prevalence** of approximately 1:12,500 (Kelch et al. 1984). It is usually associated with **hypogonadotropic hypogonadism** and can also occur in combination with Duchenne-type muscular dystrophy and/or glycerol kinase deficiency as a "microdeletion syndrome" (Budarf and Emanuel 1997). The LH and FSH deficiency is not present during the first years of life, but develops later (Bassett et al. 1999; Kaiserman et al. 1998; Peter et al. 1998; Ta-

kahashi et al. 1997). Whether the hypogonadism is caused by a pituitary or hypothalamic dysfunction is not known. In some patients a hypothalamic dysfunction was detected (Kletter et al. 1991; Partsch and Sippell 1989); treatment with pulsatile GnRH was without success in others (Caron et al. 1999a; Habiby et al. 1996; Kletter et al. 1991). In addition, a gonadal defect has been suggested (Caron et al. 1999a). Therefore, it is recommended that first the level of dysfunction should be determined in each patient, and the therapeutic strategy should only be chosen subsequently (see Sect. 7.1, 7.8 and Chap. 15). The patients need lifelong substitution with gluco- and mineralo-corticoids. Their dose must be increased in stressful situations and particularly prior to surgical procedures. **Withdrawal trials** are absolutely **contraindicated.**

In the majority of the patients the disease is caused by **mutations of the DAX-1 gene** (Peter et al. 1998) which is located on the short arm of the X chromosome in the region Xp21.3–21.2. However, mutations of the DAX-1 gene are not found in all patients, so genetic heterogeneity has to be assumed (Muscatelli et al. 1994; Zanaria et al. 1994; Yanase et al. 1996). The clinical presentation can be quite variable within one family (Merke et al. 1999). It should be noted that adrenal insufficiency may have its onset after the neonatal period.

7.5 Constitutional Delay of Development

7.5.1 Normal Onset of Puberty and Definition of Delayed Puberty

Normal male puberty starts with the growth of the scrotum and a change in color and texture of the scrotal skin (stage G2 at 11.2 ± 3 years; mean ± twice the standard deviation; Fig. 7.6). A unilateral increase of testicular volume to ≥ 3 ml (11.8 ± 1.8 years) is the most reliable sign for the onset of puberty (Largo and Prader 1983). Thereafter pubertal hair growth, penis growth, growth spurt, beard growth and voice mutation follow. Because of the wide variability in the age of onset of puberty, a **healthy boy** aged between 13 and 14 years could equally well show all, as well as no signs of puberty (Fig. 7.6) (Largo and Prader 1983). Recently, the data by Largo and Prader have been confirmed in a large-scale cross-sectional German study (Willers et al. 1996).

> Delayed puberty (pubertas tarda) is present in a boy by definition if **pubertal** development (**genital development, testicular growth**) has **not started by the age of 14 years** (see Fig. 7.6).

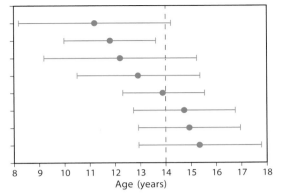

Start of genital development   G2
Unilateral testicular volume ≥ 3 ml
Start of pubic hair development   P2
Start of penile growth   G3
Peak height velocity
Adult penis   G5
Adult pubic hair   P5
End of pubertal testicular growth

Age (years)

Fig. 7.6. Schematic diagram of normal pubertal development. Means ± twice the standard deviation are presented. The broken line represents the upper age limit for normal onset of puberty. Pubertal development commencing thereafter is defined as pubertas tarda

7.5.2 Etiology and Pathogenesis of Constitutional Delay of Puberty

> **Constitutional delay of puberty (CDP)** is by far the **most common cause** of **delayed puberty (pubertas tarda)**. In males the **prevalence** may be as high as 1:40.

Activation of the GnRH pulse generator with the subsequent increase of hormone production and secretion by endocrine organs (pituitary and testes) initiates pubertal development. The increasingly **pulsatile GnRH secretion is delayed** in boys with CDP. To date it is not clear which neural, endocrine, or metabolic signal causes maturation of hypothalamic centers and the onset of puberty. Similarly, it is not clear why the activation of this mechanism is delayed in some children.

The duration and sequence of pubertal events, once puberty has started, is usually normal in boys with CDP. Pubertal development finally ends with complete sexual maturity and normal fertility. CDP may therefore be seen as an **extreme functional variant** of the onset of normal pubertal development. While CDP is not a disease, the delay in pubertal development may be a pressing psychological burden for the adolescent. CDP occurs as a **familial or sporadic** condition.

7.5.3 Clinical Picture

The children or adolescents present for two possible reasons. The first reason ist **short stature**. Height is decreased compared to age-related standards. Patients who have not yet reached pubertal age may belong to this subgroup. In these cases the diagnostic term of constitutional delay of growth and puberty (CDGP) is preferable. These children are usually seen in pediatric departments rather than by andrologists.

The second reason is **delay or arrest of pubertal development**. Patients of pubertal age, older than 14 years, belong to this subgroup. In addition to their lack of virilization these patients may present with short stature which adds to the psychological pressure these patients often feel. Short stature is due to a transitory partial growth hormone deficiency. Treatment with growth hormone is not indicated. It has to be stressed, however, that short stature is not an obligatory diagnostic sign in patients with CDP. CDP occurs in adolescents with body heights in all centiles.

Bone age, which serves as a measure of the individual's biological age, is always **retarded**. In extreme cases bone age retardation may reach five years. Height and pubertal stage are normal in relation to bone age. Overall, development is harmonic if related to bone age. However, it must be emphasized that most patients with CDP or CDGP **do not reach their genetic target height**. The later the pubertal growth spurt occurs in life, the less growth is achieved during the spurt. Patients with CDP or CDGP are likely to present with slightly eunuchoid body proportions owing to their prolonged prepubertal growth phase, which impairs spinal growth (Albanese and Stanhope 1994). This mild dysproportion often persists into adulthood.

7.5.4 Diagnosis

In addition to **anamnesis, growth curve** and complete physical examination, the radiographic determination of **bone age** of the left hand and wrist (including the ulnar and radial epiphyses) is the most important diagnostic procedure. Bone age is determined according to Greulich and Pyle (1959). CDP is the most likely diagnosis in the the event that clinical signs are harmonic and normal in relation to bone age. However, the **diagnosis of CDP can only be made after excluding all other possibilities**. Thus, it is important to exclude organic forms of hypogonadism such as Kallmann syndrome, multiple pituitary hormone deficiencies, hypercortisolism, syndromal diseases, malabsorption, and – in general – severe chronic diseases. Psychosocial deprivation and malnutrition may also lead to pubertal delay.

The major **diagnostic problem** is the **differentiation between CDP and idiopathic hypogonadotropic hypogonadism** (see Sect. 7.1). This differential diagnosis is important since different therapeutic options may arise and counselling of patients is different. **In both disorders basal gonadotropin levels and serum testosterone are low.** The response of LH and FSH in a standard **GnRH test** is also low. If a marked increase of LH is seen in the GnRH test (cut-off levels to be defined for each laboratory and each assay), the onset of pubertal development is imminent (Partsch et al. 1990).

The short-term **GnRH pump test** is an elegant diagnostic method as it imitates physiology. For diagnostic purposes pulsatile GnRH is given for 36 h. A standard GnRH test after 36 h of pulsatile stimulation ("priming") has relatively good diagnostic sensitivity and specificity (see Sect. 6.4.2, 7.1.4) (Partsch et al. 1985; Smals et al. 1984). In CDP patients the increase of LH is higher than in idiopathic hypogonadotropic hypogonadism patients. **The criterion for CDP is an increase of 3 IU/l LH following the standard GnRH bolus test.** The induction of LH and FSH secretion in patients with idiopathic hypogonadotropic hypogonadism warrants a stimulation time longer than 36 h. Despite numerous diagnostic tests, however, differential diagnosis between CDP and idiopathic hypogonadotropic hypogonadism can be made only after long-term follow-up in difficult cases.

7.5.5 Treatment

In most CDP patients spontaneous pubertal development starts before the age of 20 years. The **indication for treatment** is usually not the delay of puberty itself, but the **psychological pressure** caused by lack of virilization and/or short stature. There is some evidence that bone density may be compromised in later life in patients with CDP. Whether the mildly eunuchoid proportions in adulthood can be prevented by early treatment is not known to date. If the patient shows either clinical or biochemical signs of the beginning of pubertal development, therapeutic interventions should not be initiated. Intensive counselling and, in some cases, psychological help should be provided.

The treatment of choice for adolescents without signs of puberty is the intramuscular injection of **testosterone enanthate** at a dose of 250 mg every four weeks for three months (see Chap. 15). This treatment leads to the development of secondary sex characteristics and to a growth spurt. The acceleration of bone maturation is proportional to the gain in height age: there is no decrease in predicted final height (Bougnignon 1993). The effect of treatment should be documented in a standardized **growth chart**. Alternatively, oral testosterone undecanoate at a dose of 20–80 mg may be administered (Brown et al. 1995; Schmidt et al. 1998).

After cessation of treatment, spontaneous activation of the hypothalamic pulse generator and subsequent endogenous puberty occurs after three months in most patients. **Treatment can be repeated** if spontaneous puberty does not occur after the first treatment period. In the event that a patient with bone age > 13 years fails to show spontaneous pubertal development, it is likely that he has idiopathic hypogonadotropic hypogonadism. As an **alternative** to testosterone, **hCG** (1000 to 2000 IU/week i. m.) or **pulsatile GnRH** (see Sect. 7.1.5) can be given for three months. Theoretically, these treatment regimens have the advantage that testicular growth and spermatogenesis are stimulated. However, for achieving the goals of treatment in patients with CDP, hCG and pulsatile GnRH have no advantages.

7.6 Secondary GnRH Deficiency

7.6.1 Etiology and Pathogenesis

Any disturbance in the region of the diencephalon can also cause impairment of hypothalamic GnRH secretion. The localization and the extent of the damage determine the clinical picture; an isolated disturbance of GnRH secretion is rare.

Tumors in the region of the diencephalon (**craniopharyngiomas** or **meningiomas**) and **metastases** of other tumors can cause GnRH deficiency. **Granulomatous illnesses** such as sarcoidosis, histiocytosis, tuberculosis, neurolues or **hemochromatosis** can likewise lead to a hypothalamic dysfunction. **Fractures of the skull base, ischemic and hemorrhagic lesions** in the area of the hypothalamus, as well as **radiotherapy** of malignant tumors or metastases in the region of the nasopharynx, the central nervous system, the orbita and the skull can cause a dysfunction of the hypothalamus and/or pituitary gland (Constine et al. 1993).

Gastrointestinal illnesses such as Crohn's or celiac disease – even without distinctive gastrointestinal symptoms – can lead to pubertal delay (Cacciari et al. 1983). Significant **malnutrition** (malabsorption syndromes, tumor cachexia, anorexia nervosa etc.) and **chronic diseases** (sickle cell anemia, thalassemia, renal

Table 7.2. Inactivating GnRH receptor mutations. *ECL*, extracellular loop; *ICL*, intracellular loop; *TM*, transmembrane domain

Nucleic acid exchange	Amino acid position	Amino acid exchange	Localization	Authors
CAA to GGA	106	Q–R	ECL 1	De Roux et al. 1997
GCC to GAC	129	A–D	TM 3	Caron et al. 1999b
AGT to AGA	168	S–R	TM 4	Pralong et al. 1999
AGC to AGA	217	S–R	TM 5	De Roux et al. 1999
CGG to CAG	262	R–Q	ICL 3	De Roux et al. 1997 Laymann et al. 1998 Caron et al. 1999b
TAT to TGT	284	Y–C	TM 6	Laymann et al. 1998

failure etc.) can cause a hypogonadotropic disturbance (see Chap. 12). The probable cause of testicular dysfunction in these cases is a **dysfunction of hypothalamic GnRH secretion**. A similar mechanism may also cause pubertal delay in young athletes.

7.6.2 Clinical Picture

The clinical picture of the hypogonadism depends on the time of manifestation of the disorder (see Chap. 6, Table 6.1) and can be disguised by other symptoms. Any suspicion of a hypothalamic disturbance will emerge from the general clinical appearance.

7.6.3 Diagnosis

Diagnosis takes account of the anamnesis, a physical examination, endocrine investigations including stimulation tests to differentiate between hypothalamic and pituitary lesions and imaging diagnosis (nuclear magnetic resonance tomography).

7.6.4 Therapy

Therapy should primarily be **treatment of the cause of the underlying disease** (see Chap. 12). If this is not possible, **symptomatic treatment** is applied by **substitution of the missing hormones**.

7.7 Inactivating GnRH Receptor Mutations

7.7.1 Etiology and Pathogenesis

The GnRH receptor belongs to the group of G-protein coupled receptors and is localized in the cell membrane of anterior pituitary cells. The gene of the GnRH recep-

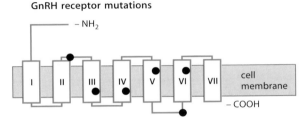

GnRH receptor mutations

● inactivating mutations

Fig. 7.7. Schematic display of the known inactivating GnRH receptor mutations (*red*)

tor has been localized on the long arm of chromosome 4 (Kottler et al. 1995). The gene has three exons and two large introns (Fan et al. 1994). **Inactivating mutations of the GnRH receptor** have recently been identified in several families as the cause of hypogonadotropic hypogonadism (Caron et al. 1999b; De Roux et al. 1997, 1999; Layman et al. 1998; Pralong et al. 1999; Table 7.2). The localizations of these mutations are shown in Fig. 7.7. Inheritance of these mutations is autosomal recessive; males and females can be affected. Compound heterozygosity is present in most patients described so far. The mutations lead to reduced or blocked signal transduction or binding of the receptor (Achermann and Jameson 1999).

7.7.2 Clinical Picture and Diagnosis

The **clinical picture** is quite **variable**. It ranges from complete hypogonadism in patients with bilateral cryptorchism, micropenis and very low serum levels of gonadotropins and testosterone to cases of partial hypogonadism with delayed and incomplete pubertal development. Patients with GnRH receptor mutations typically show an absent or blunted gonadotropin response during a **GnRH test**. Pulsatile GnRH treatment is without success (Caron et al. 1999b; De Roux et al. 1997, 1999; Layman et al. 1998; Pralong et al. 1999).

According to very preliminary data (few cases have been described so far), the proportion of GnRH receptor mutations is estimated as 2% among all patients with idiopathic hypogonadotropic hypogonadism without anosmia (Layman et al. 1998). In families with several affected patients, the probability of a GnRH receptor mutation increases to 7%.

7.7.3 Therapy

Patients with inactivating GnRH receptor mutations are completely or at least partially resistant to pulsatile GnRH stimulation. The therapy for induction of spermatogenesis is **administration of hCG/hMG or LH/FSH** (Pralong et al. 1999). Testosterone is administered when fertility is not desired (see Chap. 15).

7.8 Hypopituitarism

7.8.1 Etiology and Pathogenesis

The most frequent causes of pituitary insufficiency are **tumors (gonadotropin, prolactin, growth hormone, TSH, ACTH-secreting or endocrine-inactive adenomas) or metastases of the pituitary and the hypophyseal stalk**, as well as post-operative states and **radiotherapy** of the pituitary area. Likewise, **trauma**, infections, hemochromatosis and vascular disorders can lead to pituitary insufficiency.

Endocrine deficiencies are to be expected if more than 75% of the hypophyseal tissue is destroyed. A disturbance of testicular function caused by a lack of **LH** and **FSH** secretion is often the first sign of an acquired insufficiency. Subsequent decreases in other pituitary hormones (**TSH, ACTH, STH**) cause dysfunction of the thyroid gland, the adrenals and a reduction in growth. In addition, dysfunction of the neurohypophysis causes diabetes insipidus (**panhypopituitarism**).

7.8.2 Clinical Picture

The clinical symptoms are determined by the time at which the insufficiency is manifested (see Chap. 6, Table 6.1). **Prepubertal pituitary insufficiency** causes the **changes of body proportions** characteristic of hypogonadism; however, because of **growth-hormone de-**ficiency, the typical eunuchoid, tall stature is not seen. In addition to the other androgen deficiency symptoms, the clinical picture is determined by symptoms of **thyroid and adrenal dysfunction** and possibly **diabetes insipidus**. Puberty does not begin, or pubertal development is delayed and incomplete. Hypopituitarism **appearing after puberty** causes insufficiency of the thyroid gland and adrenal cortex, may cause diabetes insipidus and may lead to the typical symptoms of postpubertal androgen deficiency (see Chap. 6, Table 6.1).

7.8.3 Diagnosis

Diagnosis is made by imaging of the sella region, particularly by **nuclear magnetic resonance tomography**, examination of the **visual fields** and determination of **basal hormone levels** in the serum (LH, FSH, prolactin, TSH, ACTH, STH, thyroid hormones, cortisol, IGF-1) and the absence of a rise in pituitary hormone levels during the **combined pituitary stimulation test** [100 µg GnRH, 200 µg TRH (thyroid-stimulating hormone releasing hormone), 100 µg GRH (growth hormone releasing hormone), 100 µg CRH (corticotropin releasing hormone) intravenously; blood to be sampled before and 30, 60 and 90 minutes after injection of releasing hormones]. If a large pituitary tumor is suspected, pituitary stimulation tests are relatively contra-indicated because of possible complications such as acute tumor necrosis.

7.8.4 Therapy

If a **pituitary tumor** is responsible for the pituitary insufficiency, **neurosurgical removal** should usually be performed, which is preferably accomplished by the **trans-sphenoidal route** with protection of the healthy pituitary tissue. After surgery, regeneration of the remaining pituitary tissue is possible. Some tumors can be primarily **irradiated**. **Prolactinomas** (both micro- as well as macroprolactinomas) are treated primarily by **medical drugs** (see Sect. 7.9).

Substitution therapy of the absent hormones (cortisol, thyroid hormones, testosterone, possibly ADH) is required until restoration of pituitary function, if neurosurgical removal is not possible or if the pituitary is completely destroyed. Before puberty or in a boy who is not yet fully grown, growth hormone is given in addition. Infertility is treated by hCG/hMG injections (see Sect. 7.1.5 and Fig. 7.3, 7.4).

7.8.5 Hypopituitarism in Heritable Disorders of Pituitary Development

Congenital hypopituitarism is rare, but can be caused by mutations of transcription factor genes. These factors are important for pituitary development. A gene defect of the transcription factor Pit-1 leads to pituitary deficiency of growth hormone, prolactin and TSH, but **not** to hypogonadism. The gene defect of the **transcription factor PROP1** causes an additional deficiency of LH and FSH. The inheritance is autosomal recessive. The clinical appearance is variable. Short stature and hypothyroidism are predominant during the first years of life. Most of the patients experience spontaneous puberty; gonadotropin deficiency develops later in life (Deladoey et al. 1999; Flück et al. 1998). Hypogonadism is a constant symptom in adults (Rosenbloom et al. 1999). It has been suggested that familial aggregation and prolactin deficiency point to mutations in the PROP1 gene.

An important differential diagnosis of hypopituitarism during childhood is **septo-optic dysplasia** (Willnow et al. 1996). However, only one third of patients have the classical triad of optic nerve anomalies, agenesis of the septum pellucidum and pituitary hormone deficiency. A familial form of X chromosomal recessive panhypopituitarism is associated with variable degrees of mental retardation (Lagerström-Fermér et al. 1997).

7.9 Isolated LH or FSH Deficiency

Besides complete deficiency of both gonadotropins, as described in Sect. 7.7, **isolated LH deficiency (Pasqualini syndrome, 1950, "fertile eunuchs")** is observed in rare cases. In these patients there is a striking discordance between the clinical picture of hypogonadism and almost normal testicular volume. Testicular histology shows qualitatively preserved, quantitatively reduced spermatogenesis and atrophy of the Leydig cells. Endocrine investigations show decreased LH and normal FSH serum levels. Normal LH secretion by the pituitary after GnRH treatment indicates a **hypothalamic cause** of this disease (Hornstein et al. 1974). The administration of GnRH or hCG (LH activity) leads to normalization of the testosterone serum levels and to quantitatively normal spermatogenesis.

Inactivating mutations of the LH-β subunit are rare, only one patient has been identified so far. This patient presented with undetectable LH bioactivity, delayed puberty and small testicular volume. Testicular histology showed an arrest of spermatogenesis and absence of Leydig cells (Weiss et al. 1992). Long-term hCG treatment resulted in normal testicular volume, virilization and induction of spermatogenesis.

Occasionally **isolated FSH deficiency** has been described which led to decreased spermatogenesis, while LH activity and thus androgenization was normal (Maroulis et al. 1977). In these patients GnRH stimulation of the pituitary gland induces a normal FSH response and, therefore, proves the **hypothalamic cause** of the disease.

In rare cases, mutations of the FSH-β-subunit may cause an isolated FSH deficiency (Philip et al. 1998). So far, these mutations have been described in two patients with azoospermia.

7.10 Hyperprolactinemia

7.10.1 Etiology and Pathogenesis

The peptide hormone prolactin, which is produced in the anterior lobe of the pituitary gland, has no known physiological function in the adult male. The causes of hyperprolactinemia in man are multiple (Fig. 7.8).

Small increases of prolactin levels can be caused by **physical** or **psychological** "stress". In certain patients, even the atmosphere of the consulting room or the announcement of taking blood can cause an increase in prolactin levels.

> **Prolactin-secreting pituitary adenomas (prolactinomas)** are the most frequent cause of hyperprolactinemia. Prolactinomas can be divided into **microprolactinomas** (with a diameter up to 10 mm) and **macroprolactinomas** (Fig. 7.8). The latter are large, rapidly proliferating tumors that exceed the margins of the sella and can lead to the destruction of surrounding structures, particularly the optic nerves.

The basal level of prolactin is correlated, within broad limits, with the size of the adenoma. Malignant prolactinomas are extremely rare. Familial prolactinomas have also been described (Berezin and Karasik 1995), but in most cases prolactinomas occur sporadically.

Prolactin secretion by the pituitary is regulated by the suppressive effect of **dopamine** secreted by the hypothalamus (Fig. 7.8). Lesions of the hypothalamus or the hypophyseal stalk can, therefore, induce excessive prolactin secretion. **Pituitary tumors not secreting prolactin, craniopharyngiomas** and other **processes in the sella region** can also cause hyperprolactinemia. Primary hypothalamic disturbances can probably cause an **increased stimulation of the pituitary** by increased levels of **prolactin releasing factors** (Fig. 7.8), as is assumed for TRH, vasopressin and vasoactive intestinal polypeptides (VIP).

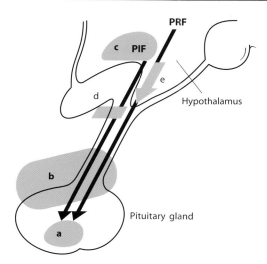

Fig. 7.8 a–e. Schematic diagram of possible causes of hyperprolactinemia: **a** prolactin-secreting tumor; **b** inhibition of transport of the prolactin-inhibiting factor (*PIF*, dopamine), e. g. by a suprasellar pituitary tumor; **c** destruction of the PIF-producing hypothalamic nuclei, e. g. by a tumor; **d** inhibition of the secretion or biological action of PIF by drugs; **e** increased secretion of hypothalamic prolactin-releasing factor (*PRF*)

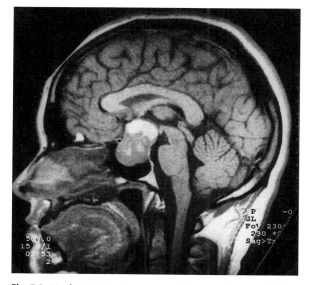

Fig. 7.9. Nuclear magnetic resonance image of a newly diagnosed macroprolactinoma

Drug-induced hyperprolactinemia is caused by the dopamine-antagonistic effects of the substances administered (e.g. butyrophenones, phenothiazines, imipramine), their interference with dopamine synthesis (e.g. α-methyldopa), the depletion of dopamine stores (e.g. reserpine) or the direct stimulation of prolactin synthesis and secretion (e.g. H_2-blockers, estrogens). Additional important causes for hyperprolactinemia are **chronic renal failure** and **hypothyroidism**.

Hyperprolactinemia can cause disturbances of male reproductive functions via various mechanisms. At the hypothalamic level, hyperprolactinemia can **impair pulsatile GnRH release**. As a consequence of suppressed LH and FSH levels, secondary gonadal insufficiency develops with low testosterone levels and suppressed spermatogenesis. Hyperprolactinemia does not cause simultaneous gonadotropin deficiency in all cases: sellar and suprasellar processes of different kinds can cause both hyperprolactinemia (Fig. 7.8) and a simultaneous blockade of GnRH flux to the gonadotropic cells of the pituitary.

The second, and clinically more important, mechanism of impaired testicular function due to hyperprolactinemia is the **displacement and destruction of gonadotropic cells of the pituitary by macroprolactinomas**, resulting in suppression of LH and FSH levels (see Sect. 7.8, Fig. 7.9). A direct inhibitory effect of prolactin on the testis has not yet been demonstrated.

7.10.2 Clinical Picture

Hyperprolactinemia in men is manifested clinically by signs of **androgen deficiency and infertility**. Primarily, some of the patients complain of **disturbances of libido and potency**, and may **rarely develop gynecomastia and galactorrhea**. Some men with documented hyperprolactinemia are free of symptoms and complaints. Processes in the sella region can cause additional symptoms according to location and size, e.g. headaches or visual field defects.

7.10.3 Diagnosis

Diagnosis is based on **increased prolactin serum levels**. For evaluation of hypophyseal function, the basal hormone levels (LH, FSH, TSH, ACTH, STH, thyroid hormones, cortisol, IGF-1; as described in Sect. 7.8.3) are measured and a combined pituitary function test (GnRH, TRH, GRH, CRH) is performed.

In stress-induced hyperprolactinemia the basal prolactin levels generally do not exceed twice the upper normal limit of 500 mU/l. Very high values (>5000 mU/l) are typical for a macroprolactinoma; serum levels, however, can be variable. In each case of repeatedly measured, significantly increased prolactin levels **nuclear magnetic resonance imaging** of the hypothalamus/pituitary region should be performed to check for a prolactinoma or other tumors which might cause hyperprolactinemia. Likewise, a **visual field examination** is performed if suprasellar expansion of the tumor is suspected.

The TRH test can be used for differentiation of a macroprolactinoma, but not of a microprolactinoma from stress-induced hyperprolactinemia (see Sect. 6.4.3).

7.10.4 Therapy

There is no need for treatment of stress-induced hyperprolactinemia. For therapy of prolactinomas the **dopamine agonist** bromocriptine (**Pravidel, Kirim**) is generally used. Because of the hypotensive effect of bromocriptine, therapy should begin with low doses given in the late evening just before the patient retires (1.25 mg/d). The dose is raised slowly and is distributed over the course of the day (morning – noon – evening), until prolactin levels become normal (Fig. 7.10). The decrease of prolactin will be accompanied by a diminution in size of the prolactinoma (Bevan et al. 1992). At the beginning of therapy, side-effects can appear as decreased blood pressure, fatigue, headaches or gastrointestinal disturbances; occasional long-term side-effects include headaches, dry nasal mucosa, and digital vasospasms upon exposure to cold.

In the event of bromocriptine intolerance, lisuride (**Dopergin, Cuvalit**) or metergoline (**Liserdol**) can be applied. Because of high efficacy and fewer side-effects, the long-lasting, **second generation dopamine agonists quinagolide** (**Norprolac**) and **cabergoline** (**Dostinex**), can be used initially (Ferrari and Crosignani 1995; De Rosa et al. 1998; Cannavo et al. 1999).

Today, **trans-sphenoidal excision of prolactinomas** is rarely indicated because of the effective drug treatments available (Saeki et al. 1998). The primary indication for neurosurgery or neuroradiotherapy is hyperprolactinemia caused by other tumors (Fig. 7.8).

Under effective therapy with dopamine agonists, normal LH pulsatility reappears and testosterone serum levels soon rise. **Persisting androgen deficiency** must be treated with adequate androgen substitution (see Chap. 15). At the beginning of dopamine agonist therapy, however, a "wait and see" approach can be taken according to the degree of androgen deficiency, or oral androgen therapy can be initiated in order to interfere with pituitary function as little as possible. If hypogonadism persists despite therapy, or if neurosurgery or neuroradiotherapy has been performed, resulting in a loss of pituitary function, adequate testosterone substitution therapy is necessary (see Chap. 15) in addition to substitution with thyroid hormones and cortisol (see

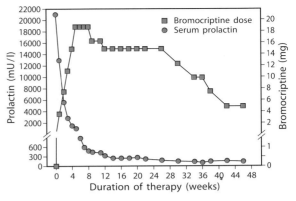

Fig. 7.10. Graphic display of prolactin serum levels during dopamine agonist therapy (*Pravidel®*) in a patient with a macroprolactinoma. After initial suppression of prolactin levels by high doses of Pravidel it is possible to reduce the dose slowly, while prolactin levels remain suppressed

Sect. 7.7). In patients with persistent gonadotropin suppression seeking paternity, hCG/hMG therapy can be initiated (see Sect. 7.1)

7.11 Gonadotropin-secreting Tumors

Gonadotropin-secreting pituitary tumors are relatively frequent (20–25 % of all pituitary tumors) (Snyder 1995) and are predominantly FSH-secreting tumors. Interestingly, in most cases the increased gonadotropin secretion causes no clinical symptoms. The patients, whose average age at manifestation is about 55 years, have usually undergone normal puberty and have children. The first clinical symptoms of these tumors are often caused by significant tumor growth, resulting in neurological symptoms and visual field defects.

Standard therapy for gonadotropin-secreting pituitary tumors is trans-sphenoidal surgery, which can be complicated, however, by large tumor size with extrasellar expansion. In view of the great effectiveness of dopamine agonist therapy for prolactinomas (see Sect. 7.9.4), drug therapy of gonadotropin-secreting pituitary tumors would be very desirable. Since GnRH stimulates gonadotropin secretion by pituitary tumors, a possible drug therapy is based on the suppression of GnRH activity. Using GnRH antagonist treatment over one year, a decrease in FSH secretion by such tumors has been achieved, but a significant reduction of tumor volume was not seen (McGrath et al. 1993).

7.12 References

Achermann JC, Jameson JL (1999) Fertility and infertility: genetic contributions from the hypothalamic-pituitary-gonadal axis. Mol Endocrinol 13:812–818

Albanese A, Stanhope R (1994) Pathogenetic mechanisms and management priorities in constitutional delay. In: Savage MO, Bourguignon JP, Grossman AB (eds) Frontiers in paediatric neuroendocrinology. Blackwell Scientific Publications, Oxford, pp 33–37

Baraitser M (1997) Cerebellar ataxia. In: The genetics of neurological disorders, 3rd edn. Oxford University Press, Oxford, pp 146–165

Barrio R, de Luis D, Alonso M, Lamas A, Moreno JC (1999) Induction of puberty with human chorionic gonadotropin and follicle-stimulating hormone in adolescent males with hypogonadotropic hypogonadism. Fertil Steril 71:244–248

Bassett JH, O'Halloran DJ, Williams GR, Beardwell CG, Shalet SM, Thakker RV (1999) Novel DAX-1 mutations in X-linked adrenal hypoplasia congenita and hypogonadotropic hypogonadism. Clin Endocrinol 50:69–75

Beales PL, Elcioglu N, Woolf AS, Parker D, Flinter FA (1999) New criteria for improved diagnosis of Bardet-Biedl syndrome: results of a population survey. J Med Genet 36:437–446

Berezin M, Karasik A (1995) Familial prolactinoma. Clin Endocrinol 42:483–486

Bevan JS, Webster J, Burke C, Scanlon MF (1992) Dopamine agonists and pituitary tumor shrinkage. Endocr Rev 13:220–240

Bourguignon JP (1993) Delayed puberty and hypogonadism. In: Bertrand J, Rappaport R, Sizonenko PC (eds) Pediatric endocrinology – physiology, pathophysiology, and clinical aspects. Williams and Wilkins, Baltimore, pp 404–419

Brown DC, Butler GE, Kelnar CJ, Wu FC (1995) A double blind, placebo controlled study of the effects of low dose testosterone undecanoate on the growth of small for age, prepubertal boys. Arch Dis Child 73:131–135

Budarf ML, Emanuel BS (1997) Progress in the autosomal segmental aneusomy syndromes (SASs): single or multi-locus disorders? Hum Mol Genet 6:1657–1665

Büchter D, Behre HM, Kliesch S, Nieschlag E (1998) Pulsatile GnRH or human chorionic gonadotropin/human menopausal gonadotropin as effective treatment for men with hypogonadotropic hypogonadism: a review of 42 cases. Eur J Endocrinol 139:298–303

Burgues S, Calderon MD (1997) Subcutaneous self-administration of highly purified follicle stimulating hormone and human chorionic gonadotrophin for the treatment of male hypogonadotrophic hypogonadism. Spanish Collaborative Group on Male Hypogonadotropic Hypogonadism. Hum Reprod 12:980–986

Cacciari E, Salardi S, Lazzari R (1983) Short stature and celiac disease: a relationship to consider even in patients with no gastrointestinal tract symptoms. J Pediatr 103:708–711

Cannavo S, Curto L, Squadrito S, Almoto B, Vieni A, Trimarchi F (1999) Cabergoline: a first-choice treatment in patients with previously untreated prolactin-secreting pituitary adenoma. J Endocrinol Invest 22:354–359

Caron P, Imbeaud S, Bennet A, Plantavid M, Camerino G, Rochiccioli P (1999a) Combined hypothalamic-pituitary-gonadal defect in a hypogonadic man with a novel mutation in the DAX-1 gene. J Clin Endocrinol Metab 84:3563–3569

Caron P, Chauvin S, Christin-Maitre S, Bennet A, Lahlou N, Counis R, Bouchard P, Kottler M-L (1999b) Resistance of hypogonadic patients with mutated GnRH receptor genes to pulsatile GnRH administration. J Clin Endocrinol Metab 84:990–996

Cassidy SB (1997) Prader-Willi syndrome. J Med Genet 34:917–923

Constine LS, Woolf PD, Cann D, Mick G, McCormick K, Raubertas RF, Rubin P (1993) Hypothalamic-pituitary dysfunction after radiation for brain tumors. N Engl J Med 328:87–94

Deladoey J, Flück C, Büyükgebiz A, Kuhlmann BV, Eblé A, Hindmarsh PC, Wu W, Mullis PE (1999) "Hot spot" in the PROP1 gene responsible for combined pituitary hormone deficiency. J Clin Endocrinol Metab 84:1645–1650

De Michele G, Filla A, Striano S, Rimoldi M, Campanella G (1993) Heterogenous findings in four cases of cerebellar ataxia associated with hypogonadism (Holmes' type ataxia). Clin Neurol Neurosurg 95:23–28

De Rosa M, Colao A, Di Sarno A, Ferone D, Landi ML, Zarrilli S, Paesano L, Merola B, Lombardi G (1998) Cabergoline treatment rapidly improves gonadal function in hyperprolactinemic males: a comparison with bromocriptine. Eur J Endocrinol 138:286–293

De Roux N, Young J, Misrahi M, Genet R, Chanson P, Schaison G, Milgrom E (1997) A family with hypogonadotropic hypogonadism and mutations in the gonadotropin-releasing hormone receptor. N Engl J Med 337:1597–1602

De Roux N, Young J, Braillard-Tabard S, Misrahi M, Milgrom E, Schaison G (1999) The same molecular defects of the gonadotropin-releasing hormone receptor determine a variable degree of hypogonadism in affected kindred. J Clin Endocrinol Metab 84:567–572

Dittrich B, Buiting K, Korn B, Rickard S, Buxton J, Saitoh S, Nicholls RD, Poustka A, Winterpacht A, Zabel B, Horsthemke B (1996) Imprint switching on human chromosome 15 may involve alternative transcripts of the SNRPN gene. Nat Genet 14:163–170

European Metrodin HP Study Group (1998) Efficacy and safety of highly purified urinary follicle-stimulating hormone with human chorionic gonadotropin for treating men with isolated hypogonadotropic hypogonadism. Fertil Steril 70:256–262

Fan NC, Jeung EB, Peng C, Olofsson JI, Krisinger J, Leung PC (1994) The human gonadotropin-releasing hormone (GnRH) receptor gene: cloning, genomic organization and chromosomal assignment. Mol Cell Endocrinol 103:R1–R6

Ferrari CPG, Crosignani PG (1995) Cabergoline: a new drug for the treatment of hyperprolactinaemia. Hum Reprod 10:1647–1652

Flück C, Deladoey J, Rutishauser K, Eblé A, Marti U, Wu W, Mullis PE (1998) Phenotypic variability in familial combined pituitary hormone deficiency caused by a PROP1 gene mutation resulting in the substitution of Arg → Cys at codon 120 (R120 C). J Clin Endocrinol Metab 83:3727–3734

Franco B, Guioli S, Pragliola A, Incerti B, Bardoni B, Tonlorenzi R, Carrozzo R, Maestrini E, Pieretti M, Taillon-Miller P, Brown CJ, Willard HF, Lawrence C, Persico MG, Camerino G, Ballabio A (1991) A gene deleted in Kallmann's syndrome shares homology with neural cell adhesion and axonal path-finding molecules. Nature 353:529–536

Georgopoulos NA, Pralong FP, Seidman CE, Seidman JG, Crowley WF, Vallejo M (1997) Genetic heterogeneity evidenced by low incidence of KAL-1 gene mutations in sporadic cases of gonadotropin-releasing hormone deficiency. J Clin Endocrinol Metab 82: 213–217

Gillessen-Kaesbach G, Gross S, Kaya-Westerloh S, Passarge E, Horsthemke B (1995) DNA methylation based testing of 450 patients suspected of having Prader-Willi syndrome. J Med Genet 32:88–92

Green JS, Parfrey PS, Harnett JD, Farid NR, Cramer BC, Johnson G, Heath O, McManamon PJ, O'Leary E, Pryse-Phillips W (1989) The cardinal manifestations of Bardet-Biedl syndrome, a form of Laurence-Moon-Biedl syndrome. N Engl J Med 321:1002–1009

Greulich WW, Pyle SI (1959) Radiographic atlas of skeletal development of the hand and wrist, 2nd edn. Stanford University Press, Stanford

Habiby RL, Boepple P, Nachtigall L, Sluss PM, Crowley WF, Jameson JL (1996) Adrenal hypoplasia congenita with hypogonadotropic hypogonadism: evidence that DAX-1 mutations lead to combined hypothalamic and pituitary defects in gonadotropin production. J Clin Invest 98:1055–1062

Hauffa BP (1997) One-year results of growth hormone treatment of short stature in Prader-Willi syndrome. Acta Paediatr Suppl 423:63–65

Hornstein OP, Becker H, Hofmann N, Kleißl HP (1974) Pasqualini-Syndrom ("fertiler Eunuchoidismus"). Klinische, histologische und hormonanalytische Befunde. Dtsch Med Wochenschr 99:1907–1914

Houchin LD, Rogol AD (1998) Androgen replacement in children with constitutional delay of puberty: the case for aggressive therapy. Bailliere Clin Endocrinol 12:427–440

Jeffcoate WJ, Laurance BM, Edwards CRW, Besser GM (1980) Endocrine function in the Prader-Willi syndrome. Clin Endocrinol 12:81–89

Kaisermann KB, Nakamoto JM, Geffner ME, McCabe ER (1998) Minipuberty of infancy and adolescent pubertal function in adrenal hypoplasia congenita. J Pediatr 133:300–302

Kallmann FJ, Schoenfeld WA, Barrera SE (1944) The genetic aspects of primary eunuchoidism. Am J Ment Defic 48:203–236

Kelch RP, Virdis R, Rappaport R, Greig F, Levine LS, New MI (1984) Congenital adrenal hypoplasia. Pediatr Adolesc Endocrinol 13:156–161

Kletter GB, Gorski JL, Kelch RP (1991) Congenital adrenal hypoplasia and isolated gonadotropin deficiency. Trends Endocrinol Metab 2:123–128

Kliesch S, Behre HM, Nieschlag E (1995) Recombinant human follicle stimulating hormone and human chorionic gonadotropin for induction of spermatogenesis in a hypogonadotropic male. Fertil Steril 63:1326–1328

Koeppen AH (1998) The hereditary ataxias. J Neuropathol Exp Neurol 57:531–543

Kottler M-L, Lorenzo F, Bergametti F, Commercon P, Soubrier C, Counis R (1995) Subregional mapping of the human gonadotropin-releasing hormone receptor (GnRH-R) gene to 4q between markers D4S392 and D4S409. Hum Genet 96:477–480

Lagerström-Fermér M, Sundvall M, Johnsen E, Warne GL, Forrest SM, Zajac JD, Rickards A, Ravine D, Landegren U, Pettersson U (1997) X-linked recessive panhypopituitarism associated with a regional duplication in Xq25-q26. Am J Hum Genet 60:910–916

Largo RH, Prader A (1983) Pubertal development of Swiss boys. Helv Paediatr Acta 38:211–228

Layman LC, Cohen DP, Jin M, Xie J, Li Z, Reindollar RH, Bolbolan S (1998) Mutations in gonadotropin-releasing hormone receptor gene cause hypogonadotropic hypogonadism. Nature Genet 18:14–15

Liu L, Chaudhari N, Corle D, Sherins RJ (1988) Comparison of pulsatile subcutaneous gonadotropin-releasing hormone and exogenous gonadotropins in the treatment of men with isolated hypogonadotropic hypogonadism. Fertil Steril 49:302–308

Liu PY, Turner L, Rushford D, McDonald J, Baker HW, Conway AJ, Handelsman DJ (1999) Efficacy and safety of recombinant human follicle stimulating hormone (Gonal-F) with urinary human chorionic gonadotropin for induction of spermatogenesis and fertility in gonadotrophin-deficient men. Hum Reprod 14:1540–1545

Maroulis GB, Parlow AF, Marshall JR (1977) Isolated follicle-stimulating hormone deficiency in man. Fertil Steril 28:818–822

McGrath GA, Goncalves RJ, Udupa JK, Grossman RI, Pavlou SN, Molitch ME, Rivier J, Vale WW, Snyder PJ (1993) New technique for quantitation of pituitary adenoma size: use in evaluating treatment of gonadotroph adenomas with a gonadotropin-releasing hormone antagonist. J Clin Endocrinol Metab 76:1363–1368

Meitinger T, Heye B, Petit C, Levilliers J, Golla A, Moraine C, Dalla Piccola B, Sippell WG, Murken J, Ballabio A (1990) Definitive localization of X-linked Kallmann syndrome (hypogonadotropic hypogonadism and anosmia) to Xp22.3: Close linkage to the hypervariable repeat sequence CRI-S232. Am J Hum Genet 47:664–669

Merke DP, Tajima T, Baron J, Cutler GB (1999) Hypogonadotropic hypogonadism in a female caused by an X-linked recessive mutation in the DAX1 gene. N Engl J Med 340:1248–1252

Meschede D, Horst J (1999) Neue Erkenntnisse zur Genetik des Kallmann-Syndroms und des Idiopathischen Hypogonadotropen Hypogonadismus. Geburtsh Frauenheilkd 59:381–385

Morrison IM, Reeve AE (1998) A catalogue of imprinted genes and parent-of-origin effects in humans and animals. Hum Mol Genet 7:1599–1609

Muscatelli F, Strom TM, Walker AP, Zanaria E, Récan D, Meindl A, Bardoni B, Guioli S, Zehetner G, Rabl W, Schwarz HP, Kaplan JC, Camerino G, Meitinger T, Monaco AP (1994) An unusual member of the nuclear hormone receptor superfamily responsible for X-linked adrenal hypoplasia congenita. Nature 372:672–676

Ohta T, Gray TA, Rogan PK, Buiting K, Gabriel JM, Saitoh S, Muralidhar B, Bilienska B, Krajewska-Walasek M, Driscoll DJ, Horsthemke B, Butler MG, Nicholls RD (1999) Imprinting-mutation mechanisms in Prader-Willi syndrome. Am J Hum Genet 64:397–413

Partsch CJ, Sippell WG (1989) Hypothalamic hypogonadism in congenital adrenal hypoplasia. Horm Metab Res 11:623–625

Partsch CJ, Hermanussen M, Sippell WG (1985) Differentiation of male hypogonadotropic hypogonadism and constitutional delay of puberty by pulsatile administration of gonadotropin-releasing hormone. J Clin Endocrinol Metab 60:1196–1203

Partsch CJ, Hümmelink R, Sippell WG (1990) Reference ranges for lutropin and follitropin in the luliberin test in prepubertal and pubertal children using a monoclonal immunoradiometric assay. J Clin Chem Clin Biochem 28:49–52

Pasqualini RQ, Burr GE (1950) Sindrome hypoandrogenico con gametogenesis conservada. Classification del la insufficiencia testicular. Rev Asoc Med Argent 64:6–19

Peter M, Viemann M, Partsch C-J, Sippell WG (1998) Congenital adrenal hypoplasia: Clinical spectrum, experience with hormonal diagnosis, and report on new point mutations of the DAX-1-Gene. J Clin Endocrinol Metab 83:2666–2674

Phillip M, Arbelle JE, Segev Y, Parvari R (1998) Male hypogonadism due to a mutation in the gene for the beta-subunit of follicle-stimulating hormone. N Engl J Med 338:1729–1732

Prader A, Labhart A, Willi H (1956) Ein Syndrom von Adipositas, Kleinwuchs, Kryptorchismus und Oligophrenie nach myoatonieartigem Zustand im Neugeborenenalter. Schweiz Med Wschr 86:1260–1261

Pralong FP, Gomez F, Castillo E, Cotecchia S, Abuin L, Aubert ML, Portmann L, Gaillard R (1999) Complete hypogonadotropic hypogonadism associated with a novel inactivating mutation of the gonadotropin-releasing hormone receptor. J Clin Endocrinol Metab 84:3811–3816

Quabbe HJ, Müller OA, Oelkers W, Willig RP (1993) Hypothalamus und Hypophyse. In: Deutsche Gesellschaft für Endokrinologie (ed) Rationelle Diagnostik in der Endokrinologie. Thieme, Stuttgart, pp 1–41

Rosenbloom AL, Almonte SA, Brown MR, Fisher DA, Baumbach L, Parks JS (1999) Clinical and biochemical phenotype of familial anterior hypopituitarism from mutations of the PROP1 gene. J Clin Endocrinol Metab 84:50–57

Rump P, Hamel BCJ, Pinckers AJLG, van Dop PA (1997) Two sibs with chorioretinal dystrophy, hypogonadotrophic hypogonadism, and cerebellar ataxia: Boucher-Neuhäuser syndrome. J Med Genet 34:767–771

Saeki N, Nakamura M, Sunami K, Yamaura A (1998) Surgical indication after bromocriptine therapy on giant prolactinomas: effects and limitations of the medical treatment. Endocr J 45:529–537

Sampson JR, Tolmie JL, Cant JS (1989) Oliver McFarlane syndrome: a 25-year follow-up. Am J Med Genet 34:199–201

Schmidt H, Knorr D, Schwarz HP (1998) Oral testosterone undecanoate for the induction of puberty in anorchid boys. Arch Dis Child 78:395

Schopohl J, Mehltretter G, von Zumbusch R, Eversmann T, von Werder K (1991) Comparison of gonadotropin-releasing hormone and gonadotropin therapy in male patients with idiopathic hypothalamic hypogonadism. Fertil Steril 56:1143–1150

Schwankhaus JD, Currie J, Jaffe MJ, Rose SR, Sherins RJ (1989) Neurologic findings in men with isolated hypogonadotropic hypogonadism. Neurology 39:223–226

Schwanzel-Fukuda M, Bick D, Pfaff DW (1989) Luteinizing hormone-releasing hormone (LHRH)-expressing cells do not migrate normally in an inherited hypogonadal (Kallmann) syndrome. Mol Brain Res 6:311–326

Seminara SB, Hayes FJ, Crowley WF (1998) Gonadotropin-releasing hormone deficiency in the human (idiopathic hypogonadotropic hypogonadism and Kallmann's syndrome): pathophysiological and genetic considerations. Endocr Rev 19:521–539

Smals AGH, Hermus ARM, Boers GHJ, Pieters GFF, Benraad TJ, Kloppenborg PWC (1994) Predictive value of luteinizing hormone releasing hormone (LHRH) bolus testing before and after 36-hour pulsatile LHRH administration in the differential diagnosis of constitutional delay of puberty and male hypogonadotropic hypogonadism. J Clin Endocrinol Metab 78:602–608

Snyder PJ (1995) Extensive personal experience: gonadotroph adenomas. J Clin Endocrinol Metab 80:1059–1061

Soussi-Yanicostas N, Hardelin JP, Arroyo-Jimenez MM, Ardouin O, Legouis R, Levilliers J, Traincard F, Betton JM, Cabanie L, Petit C (1996) Initial characterization of anosmin-1, a putative extracellular matrix protein synthesized by definite neuronal cell populations in the central nervous system. J Cell Sci 109:1749–1757

Spratt DI, Carr DB, Merriam GR, Scully RE, Rao PN, Crowley WF Jr (1987) The spectrum of abnormal patterns of gonadotropin-releasing hormone secretion in men with idiopathic hypogonadotropic hypogonadism: clinical and laboratory correlations. J Clin Endocrinol Metab 64:283–291

Takahashi T, Shoji Y, Haraguchi N, Takahashi I, Takada G (1997) Active hypothalamic-pituitary-gonadal axis in an infant with X-linked adrenal hypoplasia congenita. J Pediatr 130:485–488

von Werder K (1995) Alte und neue Therapieoptionen bei der Hyperprolaktinämie. In: Allolio B, Grußendorf M, Müller OA, Olbricht T, Schulte HM (eds) Syllabus des III. Intensivkurses für Klinische Endokrinologie. Bundesdruckerei, Neu-Isenburg, pp 108–115

Waldstreicher J, Seminara SB, Jameson JL, Geyer A, Nachtigall LB, Boepple PA, Holmes LB, Crowley WF (1996) The genetic and clinical heterogeneity of gonadotropin-releasing hormone deficiency in the human. J Clin Endocrinol Metab 81:4388–4395

Weiss J, Axelrod L, Whitcomb RW, Harris PE, Crowley WF, Jameson JL (1992) Hypogonadism caused by a single amino acid substitution in the beta subunit of luteinizing hormone. N Engl J Med 326:179–183

Willers B, Engelhardt L, Pelz L (1996) Sexual maturation in East German boys. Acta Paediatr 85:785–788

Willnow S, Kiess W, Butenandt O, Dörr HG, Enders A, Strasser-Vogel B, Egger J, Schwarz HP (1996) Endocrine disorders in septo-optic dysplasia (De Morsier syndrome) – evaluation and follow up of 18 patients. Eur J Pediatr 155:179–184

Young J, Rey R, Couzinet B, Chanson P, Josso N, Schaison G (1999a) Antimüllerian hormone in patients with hypogonadotropic hypogonadism. J Clin Endocrinol Metab 84:2696–2699

Young T-L, Penney L, Woods MO, Parfrey PS, Green JS, Hefferton D, Davidson WS (1999b) A fifth locus for Bardet-Biedl syndrome maps to chromosome 2q31. Am J Hum Genet 64:900–904

Zanaria E, Muscatelli F, Bardoni B, Strom TM, Guioli S, Weiwen G, Lalli E, Moser C, Walker AP, McCabe ERB, Meitinger T, Monaco AP, Sassone-Corsi P, Camerino G (1994) An unusual member of the nuclear hormone receptor superfamily responsible for X-linked adrenal hypoplasia congenita. Nature 372:635–641

CHAPTER 8

Disorders at the Testicular Level

8

E. Nieschlag · H. M. Behre · D. Meschede · A. Kamischke

8.1 Anorchia

Unilateral or bilateral absence of testicular tissue in genetic males is called anorchia. Anorchia has to be differentiated from partial or complete testicular atrophy, e.g. following torsion or orchitis, when, at least histologically, degenerated remains of a male gonad can be found. Anorchia can be congenital or acquired.

8.1.1 Congenital Anorchia

Bilateral congenital anorchia occurs only in one of 20,000 males. **Unilateral congenital anorchia** is about 4 times as frequent. Vascular and genetic disturbances, intrauterine infections, trauma or teratogenic factors are discussed as causes for the loss of one or both testes. A suspected abnormality in the sex-determining region of the Y chromosome, the SRY gene, could not be confirmed so far (Lobaccaro et al. 1993). Currently **intrauterine torsion** is favored as the most probable cause.

The morphological findings in bilateral congenital anorchia can be directly derived from the embryonic development of the male genital system. In the 8th week of pregnancy the testes developing from the undifferentiated gonadal system start to secrete anti-Muellerian hormone (AMH) and, only at a later stage, testosterone. If the testicular tissue is lost before testosterone production begins, the Muellerian ducts have regressed; however, the androgen-dependent differentiation of the Wolffian ducts as well as the masculinization of the urogenital sinus and the external genitalia have not yet started. If the testes originally present are destroyed after they have produced testosterone for a certain period, the androgen-dependent target organs of the urogenital tract are more or less completely differentiated towards the male phenotype (Josso et al. 1991).

Subjects with **bilateral congenital anorchia,** in whom the testes had produced AMH but no testosterone, present with the **phenotype of male pseudohermaphroditism** including female external genitalia. Neither gonads nor derivatives of the Muellerian ducts (oviducts, uterus, upper vagina) nor the Wolffian ducts (epididymis, ductus deferentis, seminal vesicles) can be found. If the testes have produced testosterone during embryonal development, the external genitalia are male and the Wolffian duct derivatives are developed. A small penis may indicate diminished androgen-dependent growth during fetal development. If left untreated, pubertal development will not start in patients with bilateral congenital anorchia and the typical phenotype of **eunuchoidism** develops. Since a single intact testis is functionally suffi-

cient, disorders of sexual differentiation and pubertal development do not occur in **congenital unilateral anorchia** although unilateral retention of Muellerian ducts can be present (depending on timing of testicular loss).

In patients with **congenital bilateral anorchia** testicular tissue cannot be demonstrated either by morphological or by endocrine techniques (see Sect. 6.5.4). FSH and LH serum levels are already elevated in children and rise to castrate levels from the age of puberty onwards. In contrast, testosterone is very low. For a **differential diagnosis** cryptorchidism must be ruled out (see Sect. 8.3). The **hCG-test** is used for differentiation (see Sect. 6.4.5). While a rise in serum testosterone can be measured in patients with cryptorchidism, the values remain low even after a 7-day period of stimulation in patients with bilateral anorchia (Davenport et al. 1995). In addition, AMH, which is lacking in anorchia, should be measured since it shows a higher sensitivity, but equal specificity compared to testosterone (Lee et al. 1997). In cases with suspected **unilateral** anorchia the absence of gonadal tissue must be ascertained by **imaging diagnostic procedures** (sonography, computer tomography, MRT) and if necessary by **exploratory surgery**, since non-descended and dysgenetic gonads have a high rate of malignant degeneration.

Unilateral anorchia does not require **therapy**. In phenotypically male patients with bilateral congenital anorchia **testosterone substitution** has to be implemented at the time of expected puberty (see Chap. 15). In phenotypically female patients estrogen substitution will be started. Intersexual external genitalia may be corrected by **plastic surgery**. For cosmetic reasons, testicular prostheses may be implanted into the scrotum. Infertility in bilateral anorchia cannot be treated.

8.1.2 Acquired Anorchia

Accidental Castration

Testes can be lost due to trauma, tumors, severe inflammation, torsion, surgical accidents (e.g. during herniotomy or orchidopexy) or surgical removal (e.g. because of a testosterone-dependent tumor such as prostate carcinoma) and very rarely after self-mutilation. The loss of one testis will be compensated for by the remaining testis if it is normal concerning fertility and testosterone production, and therapy will not be necessary. In cases of acute bilateral testicular loss it should be remembered that sperm may still be found weeks after the acute incident and cryopreserved for paternity unless the man has definitely completed his family (Fig. 8.1) (see Chap. 18).

The **clinical symptoms** of bilateral testicular loss depend on the time when testicular function is lost. Before puberty, testicular loss leads to the characteristic pheno-

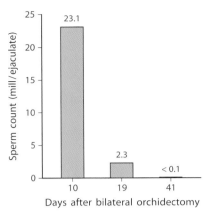

Fig. 8.1. Sperm in the ejaculate of a 15-year old boy following bilateral orchidectomy due to testicular torsion. Although several ejaculations had taken place, even 10 days after surgery (when the patient was first seen by us), enough sperm were present to make cryopreservation worthwile

type of eunuchoidism; after puberty it will lead to the phenotype of postpubertal testosterone deficiency (see Chap. 6, Table 6.1).

When both testes are lost, **testosterone must be permanently substituted** from the time of the expected beginning of puberty in order to induce pubertal development and in an adult immediately after testicular loss to maintain the various androgen-dependent functions. Testicular prostheses (usually silastic) may be implanted for psychological or cosmetic reasons.

Medical and Legal Castration

If the testes have been removed because of prostate carcinoma or as a legal prophylactic procedure in sexual delinquents, **testosterone** must certainly **not be substituted** since the elimination of its effect is the intended therapeutic purpose in these cases. In some countries castration is a legal procedure for sexual delinquency in order to avoid imprisonment. For example, in the Federal Republic of Germany 400 men were castrated between 1970 and 1980 on the basis of the "law for voluntary castration" (1969, amended 1973) (Wille 1991). In other countries this procedure is illegal. In some countries medical castration (e.g. by antiandrogens) is used instead but this is also controversial ethically. In Germany, surgical castration is currently not praticed nor is chemical castration applied. Instead, psychosocial treatment modalities are preferred.

Socio-Cultural Castration

Beyond medical purposes, castration has been and is still performed for socio-cultural reasons. Societies practicing polygamy have been known to employ castrates as **overseers (eunuchs as harem guards)** who may then have gained political influence. For example, at the Chinese imperial court castration consisting of amputation of penis, testes and scrotum without anesthesia was performed in adult men. These procedures were extremely painful and accompanied frequently by severe complications so that 25% of those undergoing this "treatment" did not survive. Since, however, lucrative positions were the possible rewards, many candidates underwent the risk (Wagenseil 1993; Mitamura 1992). The last castrate of the Chinese empire, terminated by revolution in 1912, Sun Yaoting, died at the age of 93 in 1996.

Castration before puberty maintains the high voice of boys so that in the adult **soprano and alto voices** with the acoustic volume of a male result. Such high-pitched voices were considered desirable among music-lovers. Prepubertal castrates belonged to casts of operas in the 17th and 18th century and in the Vatican choirs these voices could be heard until the early 20th century (Ortkemper 1993).

Roman physicians recommended castration for the treatment of leprosy and epilepsy; in the 17th century it was practised to cure gout and dementia. In the USA castration was practised for the treatment of the mentally handicapped until the early 20th century.

Castration has also been reported as self-mutilation for **religious reasons** since ancient times. The early church father Origines (186–254) is one of the most prominent examples. More recently, castration was practised in southern Russia among members of the **Scoptic sect** founded in the 18th century. The largest contemporary groups of castrates are the **Hijras** in India. They function as professional well-wishers at birth rites and receive considerable financial rewards. Several thousand of them exist.

Patients with acquired anorchia could (involuntarily) contribute to the question whether the **shorter life expectancy of men compared to woman** (Chap. 21, Fig. 21.1) may be caused by testosterone or the presence of testes, as has often been claimed. Astonishing little, however, is known about this "model". A retrospective analysis of the life expectancy of inmates of an institution for the mentally handicapped in the USA came to the conclusion that early castration may lead to a higher life expectancy (Hamilton and Mestler 1969). However, this may be explained by the preference for castration of physically active inmates whereas lack of mobility is the major predictor of shortened life expectancy among institutionalized men. In contrast, we could find no difference in the lifespan of intact and prepubertally cas-

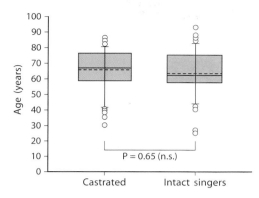

Fig. 8.2. Lifespan of castrated and intact singers from the 16th to 19th centuries. In each group 50 singers with similar birthdates were selected. Box and whisker plot: *solid line* = median, *dotted line* = average (Nieschlag et al. 1993)

trated singers from the 16th to the 19th century when analyzing their biographical data (Fig. 8.2) (Nieschlag et al. 1993b). Since neither the investigation of mentally handicapped nor historical analysis can be considered representative for the present normal population, these studies can only provide hints, while the question as such remains unresolved.

8.2 Polyorchidism

Supernumerary testes are a rare finding with little more than 100 cases reported in the literature. In most instances a third testis is found (**triorchidism**), predominantly on the left side. The most likely explanation for this condition is a transverse division or doubling over of the genital ridge caused by peritoneal bands in early embryonic development (4th to 6th week). The duplication may only concern the testis, but doubling of the epididymis and vas deferens may also be found (Leung 1988; O'Sullivan et al. 1995).

Most patients have no symptoms and the supernumerary testis may be discovered incidentally. Fertility may be normal. However, malignancies and torsions may occur in the third testis and require acute intervention. Most are discovered in association with hernias or because of maldescent. A third testis with epididymis and vas may be the rare cause of persistent fertility following vasectomy (Hakami and Mosari 1975).

In recent years sonography and magnetic resonance imaging have aided the diagnosis and may make surgical exploration for histological confirmation superfluous (Figler et al. 1996; Ghiacy 1996).

Therapeutic management must be decided on a case-to-case basis. While tumors and torsion require surgical removal, the testis may remain in situ in other cases.

Such cases should be followed by regular investigations including sonography for early discovery of a tumor.

In the medical literature polyorchidism was first documented in 1880 (Ahlfeld 1880). Historically, supernumerary testes have often been associated with extraordinary strength and sexual vigour of their bearers. Several such cases have been reported anecdotally. Of these, the Venetian admiral Bartolomeo Colleoni (1400–1475) achieved special fame ("colleoni" in Italian means "testes" and nowadays is spelled "coglioni") and in 1539 Philipp Count of Hesse (1504–1567) was granted permission by Martin Luther to take a second wife simultaneously because of an alleged third testis.

8.3 Maldescended Testes

8.3.1 Pathophysiology and Classification

About the end of the first trimester of early embryonic development the testes move from the region of the kidneys to the inner opening of the inguinal channel. During the last two months of gestation the testes descend from the position close to the inner opening of the inguinal channel into the scrotum. At the time of birth, testicular descent is normally completed and is a characteristic sign of maturity of a newborn. Descent may, however, come to a halt at various positions. According to the location of the testes, the following anomalies are differentiated:

- **Cryptorchidism:** The testis lies above the inner inguinal channel intraabdominally or retroperitoneally and can neither be seen nor palpated.
- **Inguinal testis:** The testis is positioned firmly in the inguinal channel (Fig. 8.3).
- **Retractile testis:** The testis lies at the orifice of the inguinal channel and can be pushed into the scrotum, but returns to the original position when released. In other cases the testis alternates its position spontaneously from the scrotum into the inguinal channel and back. This movement will also be induced by the cremasteric reflex when exposed to cold or during coitus.
- **Testicular ectopy:** The testis lies outside the normal route of descent, e.g. femorally or in the groin.

Retractile testes occur relatively frequently and rarely have pathological significance. The other anomalies of descent occur in about 0.5% of adult men. Mature male newborns show a prevalence of maldescended testes in

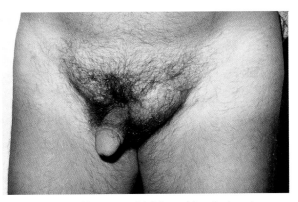

Fig. 8.3. 32-year old patient with bilateral inguinal testis

2–3%, however, spontaneous descent occurs in about 60% of these children within the first 3 months of life. Premature newborns have undescended testes in about 30%, however, in most cases the gonads assume a scrotal position within a few months. **Maldescended testes** occur about 5 times more frequently **unilaterally** than **bilaterally.**

In most cases the **etiology** of testicular maldescent is unclear, so that in 85% a so-called idiopathic maldescent is diagnosed. Presumably, the etiology is multifactorial. Since in most cases the incompletely descended testis has passed the inner opening of the inguinal channel, disturbances of inguinal scrotal descent are assumed which may, in addition to endocrine disturbances, be caused by defects in neurotransmitter secretion from a not fully matured genitofemoral nerve (Hutson et al. 1997).

Testicular maldescent is frequently found in patients with hypopthalamic – pituitary disturbances (see Chap. 7) or in patients with disorders of testosterone synthesis or testosterone action. Next to endocrine causes, anatomical abnormalities could be identified as causes of maldescent as well as reduced abdominal wall tension leading to lowered intraabdominal pressure (e.g. prune-belly syndrome, bladder exstrophy, omphalocele, gastroschisis). Maldescent is also frequently found in primary testicular disorders such als Klinefelter syndrome (see Chap. 8.9), Noonan syndrome (see Chap. 8.12) and in gonadal dysgenesis (see Chap. 8.15).

8.3.2 Infertility and Risk of Malignancy

Abnormal testicular location is associated with a disturbance of the germinal epithelium. Many men, even with unilaterally maldescended testis have **impaired fertility.** In our infertility clinic the percentage of patients with successfully treated or still existing maldescended testes

is 8.0% and thus significantly higher than the prevalence of 0.5% in the general male population.

Fertility-reducing alterations may occur very early and not – as once assumed – only at the time of puberty. Morphological alterations of the testis can be demonstrated even in the first years of life. Thus the maturation of gonocytes to A-spermatogonia as first step of postnatal spermatogenesis is disturbed (Huff et al. 1991). The longer the maldescent exists, the more pronounced the morphological alterations will be. In 163 men with a history of maldescended testes from our own fertility clinic who underwent biopsy, 28% showed moderate **hypospermatogenesis** and in two thirds a **Sertoli-cell-only syndrome** or **spermatogenetic arrest** was diagnosed. In 9 of these patients a **carcinoma in situ** or a **seminoma** was found. Maldescended testes usually do not show impaired endocrine function.

In addition to impaired fertility, patients with maldescended testes show an increased risk of **testicular tumors.** The risk of malignancy remains increased even in testes which are brought into the scrotum by orchidopexy as well as the contralateral, always-scrotal, testis. However, these testes are more accessible for diagnostic purposes after orchidopexy. In 2.8% of 599 men with maldescended testes a testicular tumor or a carcinoma in situ was histologically ascertained in one or both testes (Giwercman et al. 1993). The risk of developing a testicular tumor is 4–5 times higher in men with maldescended testes than in the general male population. It must be assumed that intrinsic congenital factors influence the potential for infertility and malignancy in the 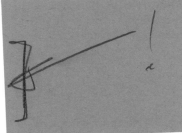 tralateral testis. Suc.....ear of life reduces the .....oller 1994).

.....testis should first be investigated with the patient standing. When the result of this palpation remains unclear, he should be reexamined in a recumbent position. Exposure to cold and stimulation should be avoided since they may induce the cremasteric reflex and retraction of the testes. Occasionally it may even be necessary to examine the scrotum after a warm bath. Testicular volume measured with an orchidometer or ultrasound should be recorded. Imaging sonography supports the diagnosis when the testis is in a still higher position. In bilateral cryptorchidism the hCG-test is essential for differential diagnosis if the baseline testosterone is in the castrate range (< 4 nmol/l). If testosterone rises under hCG-stimulation and confirms the existence of testicular tissue, the testes should be searched for by imaging diagnostic procedures such as CT or MRI.

8.3.4 Therapy

Testicular maldescent should be treated **as early as possible** (DGE 1991). If the testes do not descend by the end of the first year of life, **hormonal therapy** should be initiated. Either hCG or GnRH can be used. Up to the child's second birthday 500 IU **hCG** are administered **intramuscularly** at weekly intervals for 5 weeks. The dosage is increased to 1000 IU hCG per week after the second birthday and to 2000 IU hCG per week after the sixth birthday. Alternatively, **intranasal GnRH** (3 times daily one aerosol application of 200 µg in each nostril, total dose 1.2 µg per day) is administered over 4 weeks. The nasal GnRH therapy is better tolerated by the children, however, good compliance, including that of parents, and undisturbed mucosal absorption (i.e. absence of rhinitis) are prerequisites. Under hCG or GnRH therapy erections may occur, some pubic hair may grow, testicular volume may increase and the boys may appear more aggressive. These testosterone-dependent side-effects are reversible after the end of therapy. Success rates of 20–50% following hCG therapy and 0–78% following GnRH therapy have been reported but are controversial. A sequential combination of the two types of therapy is possible, but it is not fully established whether the success rates are increased. Additional administration of FSH does not improve therapeutic results (Hoorweg-Nijman et al. 1994). This underlines the role of androgens as the leading factor in testicular descent. The lower the testis is located prior to treatment and the younger the patient is (< or > 4 years) the higher the success of hormonal therapy will be (Pyörälä et al. 1995). HCG-induced testicular damage is not observed in humans (Kaleva et al. 1996).

If hormonal treatment does not induce testicular descent, **surgical orchidopexy** may be required. If, in addition to the maldescended testis, an inguinal hernia exists or if the testis is in ectopic position, surgical correction without prior hormonal treatment is warranted. Orchidopexy followed by GnRH analogue treatment has been found to result in better semen parameters in later adulthood (Hadziselimovic and Herzog 1997). Intraabdominal testes may be **autotransplanted** into the scrotum (Bukowski et al. 1995). This operation should be considered particularly in cases of bilateral cryptorchidism; it should be performed as early in childhood as possible. However, successful operations in adolescence and young adults have been reported. "Success" means correction of the location of the testis and maintenance of the endocrine function, while fertility will rarely be achieved in bilateral cryptorchidism. Orchidectomy should be a last resort if a testis cannot be repositioned to become palpable.

In adults hCG or GnRH therapy are useless. If orchidopexy is not or cannot be performed, regular check-ups – e.g. at annual or semi-annual intervals – for signs of malignancy are mandatory. Imaging sonography is of decisive importance in the framework of these preventive procedures to diagnose a malignancy early (see Chap. 6). The sonographic picture will influence the frequency of check-ups. Even successfully treated maldescended testes should be regularly palpated and investigated by ultrasonography because of the increased incidence of malignant degeneration. Finally, the patient should be instructed in regular self-palpation and should consult his physician if he encounters suspicious alterations.

The general **recommendation of early therapy** for maldescended testes is based on findings of alterations in testicular morphology which have been documented as early as the first years of life. Treatment shortly before or during puberty as practised in earlier times could not prevent testicular damage. It is now hoped but not proven that timely therapy will **reduce the incidence of infertility and malignancy**. However, since early treatment has been generally practiced for less than two decades and not enough patients have reached the stage when they want to father children, it cannot yet be ascertained that early treatment will indeed help to avoid infertility in patients with maldescended testes (Lee 1993). Only large-scale investigations of patients treated according to the new therapeutic scheme and who have reached reproductive age will clarify this question.

For adult infertile patients with a history of maldescended testes currently no rational therapy is available; as symptomatic treatment, techniques of assisted fertilization may be considered and applied (see Chap. 17).

8.4 Varicocele

8.4.1 Pathophysiology

> The term varicocele denotes a tortuous convoluted formation of the internal spermatic vein forming the pampiniform plexus in the scrotum.

The varicose alteration is favored by the extended free passage of the testicular vein in the retroperitoneum, by the lack of supporting muscle pump, by congenitally weak vessel walls or by an atonic cremaster muscle in part accompanying the spermatic vein. For many years it was assumed that the condition was caused by incompetence or aplasia of the spermatic venous valves. More recently conducted cadaver studies and angiographic investigations have revealed that men without varicocele may also lack valves (Wishahi 1991; Ergün et al. 1996). Probably because of hemodynamically unfavorable merging of the spermatic vein into the renal vein – the right spermatic vein leads directly into the v. cava inferior – a varicocele is found on the left side in about 95% of patients. When the internal spermatic vein is compressed by a neoplasm (e.g. a kidney tumor) one speaks of a **secondary varicocele.**

By just what mechanism varicocele influences fertility remains unclear. Various possibilities continue to be discussed: **reduced perfusion** of the affected testis because of increased venous pressure leading to atrophy with typical reduction of testicular volume; an **increase in scrotal temperature** or insufficient removal or **backflow of toxic substances** of renal origin. The hypothesis that a varicocele is nature's attempt to compensate for an otherwise damaged testis is also unproven.

8.4.2 Prevalence and Influence of Varicocele on Fertility

The **prevalence of idiopathic varicocele is high** with estimates varying greatly. This is in part due to the nature and origin of the study population examined. Beyond this, the diagnosis of varicocele remains partly subjective, all attempts to achieve objectivity notwithstanding. This applies above all to first and second degree varicoceles. In general, a prevalence of 15–20% is assumed in the male population. 17% of 3 million recruits for the German army, born between 1937 and 1945, were found to have a varicocele (Nöske and Weidner 1999). When, however, stricter diagnostic criteria were applied to sperm donors (Handelsman et al. 1998) and volunteers in clinical studies (Lemcke et al. 1996), a prevalence of 20% was found. It is generally assumed that the proportion of men with varicocele and disturbed fertility is even higher than that in the normal population. Here too estimates range up to 40%, depending on the composition of the investigator's population and it stands to reason that these estimates are higher due to referral bias when made by surgically orientated urologists than by endocrinologists. We found a varicocele in 16% of over 10,000 consecutive patients attending our institute (Table 5.2). This corresponds to statistics from other comparable centers of reproductive medicine. While this makes **varicocele the second most frequent pathological finding** after idiopathic infertility, it does not give any indication of the importance of the finding and whether is it really a cause of infertility at all.

In general, a certain degree of uncertainty surrounds the prevalence of varicocele in the normal population and in men attending a fertility clinic. There is urgent need for clarification. The situation is even less clear concerning the **influence of varicocele on fertility.** The varying frequency of varicocele observed in proven fathers and in patients attending the infertility clinic prompted some investigators to assume a connection between fertility and varicocele. The fact that varicocele does not exclude paternity, however, causes some investigators to deny this connection. This overlooks the complexity of a couple's fertility. Slight disturbance in one partner can usually be overcome by particularly good reproductive functions of the other. Only when disturbances in both partners coincide do problems arise (see Sect. 1.4). Investigations in fathers with and without varicocele suggest that varicocele may be associated with poor semen and hormone parameters (Nagao et al. 1986). Further, it is assumed that the connections between varicocele and testicular function are not static. Although initially fertility parameters may be largely normal, these are said to decline over the course of years, considerable individual variations notwithstanding (Chehval and Persel 1992). These results are based on rather small patient groups and in our own patient population we are not able to corroborate any increase in the prevalence of varicocele with the age of patients (for the proportion of patients with varicocele is just as high in those patients over 50 years as in 30-year old patients). **Thus to date there is no indisputable evidence that varicocele reduces fertility.**

8.4.3 Clinical Picture

Infertility observed with varicocele manifests itself in a spermiogram characterized by oligo-, astheno- or teratozoospermia, or a variable combination of these findings, without a causal connection necessarily existing between these conditions and varicocele. Varicoceles can also be found in azoospermic patients. Varicoceles may also be associated with increased FSH values, indicating **damage of the germinal epithelium** and a poor prognosis. It should be emphasized that not all men bearing a varicocele show decreased sperm parameters and impaired fertility. Some patients mention **feelings of pressure or sometimes pain** in the afflicted testis or in the scrotum which can worsen after longer periods of standing or sitting in unchanged position. Occasionally a varicocele can become so enlarged as to represent a **mechanical problem**, especially in the elderly.

8.4.4 Diagnosis

Careful **palpation** of the pampiniform plexus while the patient is standing is an important diagnostic measure. The **Valsalva maneuver** can provoke engorgement of the pampiniform plexus. Longstanding varicocele can also induce a **reduction in volume and consistency of the afflicted testis.** According to results from palpation the varicocele can be classified into three degrees of severity.

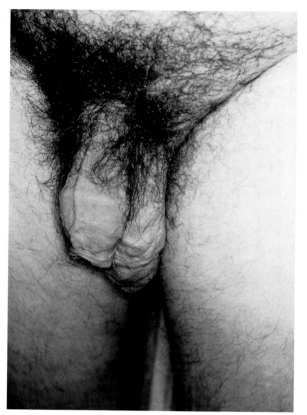

Fig. 8.4. 28-year old patient with grade III varicocele

- **Varicocele grade I:** Enlargement of the pampiniform plexus, only palpable following **Valsalva maneuver.**
- **Varicocele grade II:** Clearly **palpable** enlargement of the pampiniform plexus.
- **Varicocele grade III: Visible** enlargement of the pampiniform plexus (Fig. 8.4).

While grade III varicoceles are clinically easily identifiable, the diagnosis of low grade varicocele very much depends on the experience of the examiner. Moreover, palpation may be made more difficult by previous surgery, hydroceles or when the testis is positioned in the upper scrotum. In these cases, Doppler and **imaging sonography** is a valuable tool for corroborating diagnosis (Marsman and Schats 1994). Enlargement of the diameter of a varicose vein can also be objectified by sonographic imaging (see Sect. 6.3).

8.4.5 Influence of Therapy on Fertility

There is as little evidence that therapy improves fertility as there is a firm connection between a varicocele and disturbed fertility. Since the early 50s **ligation of the spermatic vein** has held a firm place among the therapies offered by andrologists to improve fertility in cases of varicocele. A review of 50 publications comprising 5471 patients showed an average pregnancy rate of 36% with a range of 0–50% after ligature of the spermatic vein (Mordel et al. 1990). The great variability is probably due to the size, composition and period of observation characteristic of very heterogenous populations. In general, the larger, more representative studies have been interpreted as suggesting that surgery has a beneficial influence on fertility. Thus, varicocele treatment represented an oasis of hope in the otherwise desolate landscape of ineffective medical treatments for male idiopathic infertility. The development of new **angiographic methods** for occlusion of the spermatic vein provided new avenues of treatment without altering the outcome.

However, not many efforts at **critical evaluation of invasive interventions** were completed, although several investigators indicated the urgency of the situation. The first of these studies concluded that in varicocele the pregnancy rate is roughly equal, both with and without treatment if only the female is adequately treated (Rodriguez-Rigau et al. 1978). However, the group of 24 patients treated was small and true randomization had not been carried out. A further study, likewise limited by the lack of a suitable control group, came to similar conclusions (Vermeulen et al. 1986). While both these studies were provocative, results were not convincing due to limitations of study design. Randomization was performed in a third study which again showed no improved pregnancy rates with varicocele treatment. Although 96 couples were followed up to 5 years after treatment or diagnosis, the pregnancy rate of 12% remained surprisingly low, suggesting that other factors may have interfered (Nielsson et al. 1979).

With this background and following the tenets of evidence-based medicine, several controlled studies on the effectiveness of therapy in varicocele were performed. These studies aimed not only at the physical effect of surgery (negative Valsalva maneuver), but along with semen parameters, especially considered the resultant pregnancy rates. Moreover, subgroups or strata were formed according to whether methods for occlusion of the spermatic vein were applied or not. An initial study concluded that invasive treatment of the spermatic vein increased chances of inducing a pregnancy within the following year (Madgar et al. 1995). The study is part of a larger WHO multicenter study which came to similar conclusions. This study comprised 238 couples and reg-

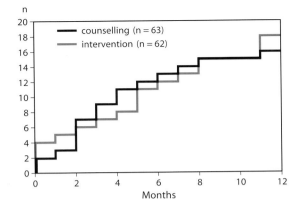

Fig. 8.5. Cumulative pregnancy rates over 12 months in 62 untreated varicocele patients and 63 patients treated surgically or angiographically (Nieschlag et al. 1998)

istered 35% pregnancies in the ligature group as opposed to 17% in the untreated group. However, because of massive criticism of the design this study failed to be published to date in a peer reviewed journal (Hargreave 1997) and its credibility remains doubtful. In contrast, we conducted a single-center study in which varicocele patients with occlusive treatment had the same pregnancy rates in the year following treatment as those not subjected to therapy (pregnancy rate of 29% of 62 couples as opposed to 25.4% of 63 couples) (Fig. 8.5) (Nieschlag et al. 1998). We found a slight temporary rise of testicular volume and of sperm concentration in treated patients. No difference was found between groups in duration of involuntary infertility. Female partners of patients inducing pregnancies were significantly younger than those failing to achieve pregnancy within 12 months (28.8 ± 0.6 versus 31.2 ± 0.3 years). As patients had been selected on the basis of comparable criteria, at first sight the results of these two studies seem contradictory. The patients in our study were seen every 3 months for examination and intensive counselling and the reproductive functions of the female partners were regularly checked by a gynecologist and, if necessary, optimized. In contrast, non-treated couples were not seen in the WHO study. It would be justified to conclude that treatment of infertile couples in which the male has a varicocele is not superfluous.

Our study allows the conclusion that regular and intensive examination and counselling of these couples is as effective in regard to pregnancy rates as interventive treatment of varicoceles.

8.4.6 Treatment Modalities

The above-mentioned studies show that **at present occlusion of the spermatic vein does not represent a proven modality for treatment of varicocele.** Further studies taking into consideration the placebo-effect of the physician's involvement and which may identify subgroups requiring treatment will be necessary to clarify these issues. Ideally such a study should include, in addition to a surgical group, a non-treated group and a placebo-group, a fourth sham-operated group. Owing to the risks of anesthesia and surgery, however, such a group would be unethical. Furthermore it is becoming increasingly difficult to recruit patients for such a study in view of the possibilities of assisted reproduction.

Considering these facts the Royal College of Obstetricians and Gynecologists (London) states: "There is insufficient evidence to recommend occlusion of the left internal spermatic vein in subfertile or oligozoospermic men with varicocele" (Templeton et al. 1998).

Notwithstanding, some physicians continue to consider a varicocele as a reason for intervention. In that event the **decision for treatment should be made according to the following criteria:**

- involuntary childlessness persisting at least one year,
- varicocele confirmed by physical and technical examinations,
- lower volume of the affected testis,
- subnormal semen parameters,
- FSH not elevated above the upper limit of normal,
- ovulation and tubal patency assured.

Before a decision for treatment is taken all investigations have to be performed at least twice within 4 to 12 weeks. Unresolved female reproductive functions, e.g. tubal patency not investigated or confirmed should further delay a decision for therapy. Varicoceles causing discomfort and pain or a mechanical problem because of size may require intervention independent of desire for paternity.

Once a decision in favor of active intervention has been made, surgical or angiographic procedures available today can be applied. All these procedures have the same goal, i.e. to interrupt the main branch(es) of the spermatic vein in order to divert the venus reflux into collaterals with intact venous valves.

Surgical Procedures

Surgical intervention is the classical procedure for varicocele treatment, ligating the internal spermatic vein. For the preferred **high ligation** an incision medial to the anterior iliac spine is made and the spermatic vein is ligated at a "high" location, i. e. close to where it merges into the renal vein.

For **low ligation**, access is made through a suprapubic incision on the left and each vein lying under the spermatic fascia is individually ligated. More recently, the spermatic vein has also been ligated **laparoscopically** and using microsurgery.

Therapeutic success is evaluated by detumescence of the venous plexus in the scrotum, a negative Valsalva maneuver and a lack of reflux documented by Doppler or ultrasonography. Almost 5 % of operations are technical failures by these criteria and in about 10 %, varicoceles reappear. On a long-term basis therapeutic success may be evaluated by increased testicular volume which can best be documented by ultrasonography and by improved semen parameters. Accidental ligation of the lymph vessels accompanying the spermatic vein may cause hydroceles to develop in about 5 % of all cases. Other post-operative sequelae such as epididymitis or hematomas occur at a low incidence of 1–3 %. Ultimately, success must be evaluated by the occurrence of pregnancy.

Angiographic Procedures

Attempts to clarify lack of success of surgical procedures by phlebography led to the development of angiographic occlusion of the spermatic vein. **Sclerosing of the spermatic vein** by hypotonic solutions injected directly into the vein was first introduced at the end of the 70s. This was followed by **angiographic occlusion** of the spermatic vein by locally **polymerizing tissue adhesives** or by **balloons or spirals** inserted into the vein. Usually, the lead catheter will be introduced from the right femoral vein under local anesthesia. Most recently, **antegrade sclerosing of the spermatic vein** has been practised, in which access to the vein is obtained from the scrotum. However, convincing improvements in pregnancy rates have not been reported (Schoeneich and Braendle 1994).

Complications resulting from disturbed lymph drainage seen after surgical procedures do not occur. The sclerosing agent used may, however, enter the testicular or renal area and thrombophlebitis, epididymitis, testicular atrophy and perinephritis may result. These disadvantages do not arise when embolization procedures using tissue adhesives are applied. The rate of recurrence is lower in embolization than in sclerosing. In a prospective, randomized study comparing a surgical method (high ligation) with an angiographic method (embolization with tissue adhesives) we were able to show that in a total of 71 patients both methods produced nearly identical pregnancy rates of 29 or 33 % respectively within 12 months (Nieschlag et al 1993a). The advantage of the angiographic method is that it can be performed on an outpatient basis avoiding hospitalization and general anesthesia. In addition, healthy patients appreciate the lesser amount of time required for the procedure.

8.4.7 Varicocele in Adolescence

Varicocele in adolescence raises the general question of prophylaxis. As cross-sectional and longitudinal observations show, varicocele develops concomitantly with testicular growth at puberty. Usually varicoceles do not exist before puberty. In 2470 boys aged 10–20 years grade I varicoceles were found in 18 %, grade II in 12 % and grade III in 5 % (Niedzielski et al. 1997). At the end of puberty the incidence of varicocele reaches a plateau. Several authors argue in favor of prophylactic ligature or occlusion of the spermatic vein, but adequate studies supporting this position are lacking. Reduced growth or volume of the afflicted testis relative to the contralateral organ has been documented as an indication of reduced circulation. Also morphological alterations of intratesticular vessels and germinal epithelium as seen in adults with varicocele have been described. Whether timely treatment will lead to long-term normalization and undisturbed fertility has not been proven. Short-term increases in testicular volume and in semen parameters have been observed (Laven et al. 1992). Rates of recurrence in long-term fertility studies are not known. In order to resolve the question of safety and efficacy of early varicocele treatment, studies lasting at least 10–15 years are necessary.

These circumstances argue in favor of a cautious position. A finding of varicocele does not automatically justify treatment. Initially, a careful physical diagnosis should be made. Care should specifically be taken to determine testicular volume exactly. As soon as possible, semen parameters should be investigated. Usually it is more difficult to convince parents of the necessity of this measure than sons. A 1–2 year period of observation should follow, during which the development of the varicocele, testicular volume and semen and hormone parameters are checked. Whether subnormal semen parameters can be correctly ascribed to incomplete pubertal development or to the varicocele can only be resolved at the end of puberty by controlled studies. If the varicocele is progressive, if testicular volume is clearly reduced and if semen parameters remain subnormal, treatment may be considered. A particularly enlarged varicocele representing a physical hindrance may indicate the need for timely intervention. After treatment, both physical findings and laboratory parameters should be checked at yearly intervals.

8.5 Orchitis

> Isolated inflammation of the testis (**orchitis**) is extremely rare and usually occurs in association with an inflammation of the epididymis (**epididymo-orchitis**).

Viral orchitis is most frequent. Mumps virus, Coxsackie virus, lymphocytic choriomeningitis (LCM) virus, Marburg virus, group B arbo virus, Dengue virus, varicella-zoster virus and various similar viruses can cause damage to the testes. The testes may become affected in cases of nephritis, prostatitis, vesiculitis or epididymitis caused by gonococci or unspecific bacteria, usually chlamydia. In children pneumococci and salmonella can cause **unspecific orchitis**. **Specific infections** (syphilis, tuberculosis, leprosy) no longer play a dominant role in most European countries. **Non-specific granulomatous** orchitis is rare and presumably of autoimmune origin. It usually affects older men with disturbed bladder function.

8.5.1 Clinical Picture and Diagnosis

When **mumps** occurs after puberty **orchitis** develops in about 25 % of patients; in about 1/3 of these cases both testes are afflicted. Usually, orchitis develops after parotitis occurs, but may also precede it. Isolated mumps orchitis without parotitis is rare, but it may also go unrecognized. The acute phase of infection is accompanied by painful testicular swelling, fever and generalized symptoms. Increased intratesticular pressure, resulting ischemia or the virus itself may lead to irreversible damage of spermatogenesis. Decreased Leydig cell function, present during the acute stage, is usually rapidly restored. When the parenchyma is badly damaged, postorchitic testicular atrophy with irreversible complete tubular sclerosis may result. Testes damaged by mumps orchitis are characterized by a firm consistency, in the ultrasound image the testicular parenchyma often appears inhomogeneous ("snow flurries"). The ejaculate is characterized by oligo(asthenoterato)zoospermia or azoospermia; FSH, as a marker for damaged germinal epithelium, is clearly elevated.

Orchitis caused by viruses or bacteria other than mumps usually produces much less severe effects. Usually, it is only possible to diagnose specific infections from the general clinical picture or by specific microbiological investigations.

8.5.2 Therapy

Vaccination against mumps in childhood may prevent orchitis as a complication ensuing from the infection.

Only **symptomatic treatment** is possible in **acute viral orchitis** and consists of elevating and cooling the scrotum and administering glucocorticoids for about ten days (60 mg prednisone daily followed by gradually decreasing doses). In addition, anti-inflammatory, antiphlogistic and antipyretic drugs may be useful adjunctive therapy. This usually produces rapid reduction of swelling and relief from pain. When IgM antibodies can be detected, therapy with α-interferon has been tried (Rüther et al. 1995). It is not clear to what extent this therapy may also improve testicular function. Administration of gammaglobulin preparations or mumps-immunoglobulins is controversial (Brinkmann and Brinkmann 1993). **Bacterial orchitis** is treated according to antibiotic sensitivity results from bacteria cultured from the ejaculate. During the acute phase of infection **sperm parameters** are suppressed, but may recover. Permanent infertility is also possible.

There is no therapy for disturbed testicular function following orchitis which is directed at improving semen parameters. Only methods of assisted reproduction may be considered (see Chap. 17). Even in azoospermic patients an attempt with TESE may be warranted as focal spermatogenesis may still be present. Any resulting androgen deficiency must be substituted with testosterone (see Chap. 15).

8.6 Germ Cell Aplasia (SCO Syndrome)

8.6.1 Pathophysiology

Germ cell aplasia does not represent a diagnosis but rather a characteristic histopathologic phenotype first described by Del Castillo et al. in 1947 which is sometimes referred to by his name.

> In **complete germ cell aplasia** the tubules, which are reduced in diameter, contain only Sertoli cells and no other cells involved in spermatogenesis (**Sertoli-cell-only syndrome = SCO syndrome**); the patients are infertile.
> In the **focal SCO syndrome** a variable percentage of tubules contain germ cells, but in these tubules spermatogenesis is often limited in both quantitative and qualitative terms.

About 30 % of our infertile patients in whom testicular biopsies were performed present with focal or complete

SCO syndrome. 8% of this group suffer from **bilateral SCO syndrome**. In view of the possibility of retrieving sperm from testicular tissue to be used in techniques of assisted reproduction the question arises how representative a testicular biopsy is. Under all circumstances the biopsied tissue must be screened most scrupulously before a firm diagnosis of complete SCO can be established. In such cases several biopsies must be prepared and investigated.

Testosterone production in the Leydig cells is only minimally affected so that patients are usually normally androgenized and only infertility prompts them to seek medical advice.

In **congenital germ cell aplasia** for some unexplained reason the germ cells do not migrate into or survive in the epithelium of the tubule. Microdeletions of the Y chromosome (see Sect. 8.13.2) represent an important genetic cause of the SCO syndrome (Foresta et al. 1998). The syndrome of germ cell aplasia can also be caused by severe **endogenous and exogenous damage**, such as **maldescended testes, irradiation, cytostatic drugs** and **viral infections**.

8.6.2 Clinical Picture and Diagnosis

Patients with the complete form of germ cell aplasia are always azoospermic; the focal SCO syndrome is characterized by **oligoasthenoteratozoospermia** of varying degrees but may also present with azoospermia. Usually **testicular volume** is reduced, but may be in the lower normal range (Fig. 6.2). **Testicular ultrasonography** may show inhomogeneities. **FSH** is generally elevated, with serum levels correlating positively with the degree of severity of germ cell aplasia (Bergmann et al. 1994). Determination of inhibin B, correlating negatively with the degree of testicular damage, may improve the diagnostic sensitivity, but also provides no certainty concerning the presence or absence of sperm in the biopsy (von Eckardstein et al. 1999).

Diagnosis can only be made by **testicular biopsy**, which should discriminate between total and focal SCO syndrome in view of ICSI. A testicular biopsy should therefore be planned as a diagnostic-therapeutic procedure including the possibility of TESE.

8.6.3 Therapy

There is no therapy for complete SCO syndrome leading to improvement of spermatogenesis. Nor can current knowledge increase the number of sperm produced by any residual functions. Pregnancies may be induced by homologous inseminations or IVF; in high-grade oligo-asthenoteratozoospermia success rates remain low. Therefore, in most cases ICSI possibly combined with

TESE provides symptomatic therapy (see above and Chap. 17).

8.7 Spermatogenic Arrest

8.7.1 Pathophysiology

> Spermatogenic arrest is the interruption of germ cell maturation leading from spermatogonia to sperm. Like the SCO syndrome, spermatogenic arrest is a histopathological phenomenon with many possible causes.

Spermatogenic arrest can occur **at the level of spermatogonia, primary or secondary spermatocytes or round spermatids**. Patients with fertility disturbances show a prevalence of spermatogenic arrest of about 4–30% of testicular biopsies according to the literature. In a series of 293 patients from our clinic undergoing diagnostic testicular biopsy, 23% showed spermatogenic arrest localized mostly at the level of primary spermatocytes. In almost one third of these patients the arrest was bilateral.

The reasons may be primarily genetic or may be traced to secondary influences. Primary genetic reasons occur in trisomy, in balanced-autosomal anomalies (translocations, inversions) or in deletions in the Y chromosome (Yq11) (see Sect. 8.13.2). Secondary factors such as toxic causes (radiotherapy, chemotherapy, antibiotics), heat or general diseases (liver or kidney insufficiency, sickle cell anemia) may be causative (Matin-du Pan and Campana 1993). In some patients with arrest at the round spermatid level the cAMP Responsive Element Modulator (CREM) is reduced or missing. Since CREM-negative spermatids do not develop further, the lack of this signal transduction factor is considered the cause of the arrest (Weinbauer et al. 1998).

8.7.2 Clinical Picture

Patients with complete arrest of spermatogenesis are **azoospermic**. In cases of partial arrest varying degrees of **oligoasthenoteratozoospermia** occur, but sperm production may be so low that azoospermia occurs and sperm can only be extracted from testicular tissue (TESE) (see Chap. 17). Testicular volume as well as FSH and inhibin B values may lie in their normal ranges, but may also be elevated or decreased, respectively.

8.7.3 Diagnosis

A definite diagnosis can only be made by **testicular biopsy**. Azoospermia and severe oligoasthenoteratozoospermia with normal FSH serum values and normal testicular volume require a testicular biopsy to distinguish arrest from obstruction of the excurrent ducts. In 15 % of our patients with suspected obstructive azoospermia we find considerable disturbances of spermatogenesis (either unilaterally or bilaterally).

8.7.4 Therapy

There is no known therapy for spermatogenic arrest. Attempts to increase sperm production have not been successful. For the application of techniques of assisted reproduction the statement in Sect. 8.6.3 referring to SCO syndrome is also relevant here.

8.8 Specific Structural Sperm Defects

Even in normal fertile men spermatozoa viewed by light microscopy show considerable morphological variability so that an unequivocal definition of a "normal" sperm cell is not without its problems (WHO 1999). In a minority of infertile patients it is possible to ascertain specific anomalies of sperm cell structure but often only with the help of electron microscopy (Dadoune 1988). It is possible to distinguish between head defects, which may occur with and without midpiece defects and tail defects. A normal sperm tail has 9 pairs of microtubules arranged concentrically around a central pair (9+2). The tubules of each pair are connected with each other by dynein arms and with the central pair by radial spokes (see Chap. 4) (Chap. 6, Fig. 6.13).

8.8.1 Globozoospermia

Globozoospermia is a structural disturbance of spermiogenesis in which the Golgi-apparatus is not transformed into the acrosome needed for fertilization of an egg cell. The ejaculated sperm lack the acrosomal cap so that they have round heads.

Such sperm are occasionally found in ejaculates of normal men, but in a few patients all sperm show this structural defect. This condition is classified as "globozoospermia". In some cases familial occurrence is observed, indicating a possible genetic cause. Considering the importance of the acrosome for the fertilizing process (see Chap. 4) it becomes clear that under natural conditions these sperm cannot interact with egg cells and cannot penetrate them. But they still can be microinjected into eggs, whereby the possibly aberrant genetic constitution of these morphologically mishaped sperm must be considered (Carrell et al. 1999).

8.8.2 9 + 0 Syndrome

This syndrome is characterized by a structural defect of the sperm tail. The central pair of microtubules is missing, leading to immotility (Neugebauer et al. 1990).

Only few cases have been described to date. One of 1000 patients of our infertility clinic could be identified as having this diagnosis. Usually all sperm are affected by this condition and show complete immotility. Occurrence in brothers indicates a genetic basis of this disorder.

8.8.3 Syndrome of Immotile Cilia

In this very rare disease a congenital defect in spermiogenesis causes a construction defect in the sperm tail. The dynein arms connecting the microtubules are absent and immotility results.

As the cilia of the respiratory epithelium may show the same structural features, afflicted patients often suffer from recurrent sino-respiratory infections. If a situs inversus and bronchiectasis are also present, it is called the **Kartagener syndrome.**

To date none of these specific structural defects could be completely explained by an **underlying molecular pathomechanism.** Transgenic mice have been developed whose sperm show the same structural defects as patients with immotile cilia, which provide a model to investigate the development of these defects (Merlino et al. 1991). Pedigree studies have provided convincing evidence that the syndrome of immotile cilia including the Kartagener syndrome is genetically determined; in most cases the disorder is autosomal recessive.

8.8.4 Clinical Picture

Structural sperm defects lead to infertility. A spermiogram often reveals terato- and/or asthenozoospermia despite normal sperm concentration. In addition, the immotile cilia syndrome is often accompanied by chronic bronchitis, rhinitis, sinusitis or otitis media.

8.8.5 Diagnosis

In **globozoospermia** the heads of normally motile sperm appear round when viewed in the light microscope. Notably disturbed motility in the presence of otherwise almost normal sperm parameters raises the suspicion of **9 + 0 syndrome** and the **immotile cilia syndrome**. In the latter case the **saccharine test** is used to screen for cilia dysfunction. The speed with which the beat of the cilia propels saccharine from the nose to the epipharyngeal space is measured. The disturbed cilia motility can be directly demonstrated in nasal mucosal cells. To differentiate between immotile, but viable, and dead sperm in the ejaculate the **eosin test** is used. Electron microscopy of the sperm tail confirms the diagnosis. FSH in serum is usually normal. The **Kartagener syndrome** is additionally diagnosed by an X-ray of the thorax.

8.8.6 Therapy

At the present time there is no causal therapy available. Pregnancies can be induced by microinjection of defect sperm into oocytes (Liu et al. 1995) (see Chap. 17).

8.9 Klinefelter Syndrome

8.9.1 Incidence and Etiology

> With a prevalance of 0.2 % of the male population the Klinefelter syndrome is the most frequent form of male hypogonadism.

It must be suspected that about half of the cases remain undiagnosed and untreated throughout life (Abramsky and Chapple 1997). In about 80 % of cases the disease is due to the **congenital numerical chromosome aberration 47,XXY**. The other 20 % are represented either by 46,XY/47,XXY mosaics, one or more additional Y chromosomes (e.g. 48,XXYY), higher-grade X chromosomal aneuploidies (48,XXXY; 49,XXXXY) or structurally abnormal X-chromosomes.

The numerical aberrations arise by **non-disjunction** either in the meiotic divisions during germ cell development or in early embryonic mitotic cell divisions. Incorrect meiotic divisions are predominant; in two thirds of cases non-disjunction derives from maternal oogenesis, one third from paternal spermatogenesis. Advanced maternal age seems to be a risk factor; a connection with the father's age has not been established (see Sect. 21.5). In contrast to many other aneuploidies, the Klinefelter syndrome is not associated with an increased rate of abortion and does not represent a lethal factor.

8.9.2 Clinical Picture

Patients with Klinefelter syndrome usually go unnoticed until after puberty so that often diagnosis is relatively late. **Prior to puberty** only discrete physical anomalies may be noticed, e.g. slightly reduced testicular volume or **long-leggedness**. A portion of the children have **learning difficulties** and their **verbal expressiveness** is limited. In the **adolescent and postpubertally** the syndrome is typically characterized by the constellation of **small firm testes and symptoms of androgen deficiency**. The testicular volume of an adult patient with a 47,XXY-karyotype is generally in the range of 1–2 ml, rarely over 4 ml. With extremely rare exceptions, patients with Klinefelter syndrome are **always infertile** (see below) (Fig. 8.6).

There is a great range of variations in the **degree of virilization**. Because of initially still normal serum androgen levels, about 60 % of patients have a penis of normal length. At the time of normal puberty characteristic skeletal proportions begin to develop. The patients are often of greater than normal height. In contrast to typical eunuchoid tall stature, the arm span seldom exceeds total body height; the **legs**, however, **are remarkably longer than the trunk** (lower height > upper height). After the age of 25 about 70 % of patients complain of **decreasing libido and potency**. Normal **beard** growth is present only in about one fifth of patients. As a result of reduced androgen production often **osteoporosis** develops and muscle strength declines (Horowitz et al. 1992). One third of patients have **varicose veins** of the legs leading to ulceration (Breit et al. 1984). Frequently **obesity**, reduced glucose tolerance and **diabetes mellitus** are observed.

During puberty bilateral painless **gynecomastia** of varying degrees develops in about half the cases. In contrast to earlier observations based on small patient numbers (Evans and Crichlow 1987), the risk of developing mammary carcinoma is not higher than in normal men (Hasle et al. 1995). This study based on 696 Danish Klinefelter patients also finds no increased risk for other malignancies except mediastinal non-seminomatous germ cell tumors, which occur preferentially at the age of 15 to 30 years. Histology shows terato- and chorioncarcinomas. The origin of the increased risk of a germ cell tumor is not clear. Emigration of dysgenetic germ cells and numerical chromosome aberrations per se are discussed as causes (Gohji et al. 1989).

The **intelligence** of some but not all Klinefelter patients is limited and deficits are observed in **verbal and cognitive abilities**. Some of the youths attract attention because of school difficulties and they fail to reach the

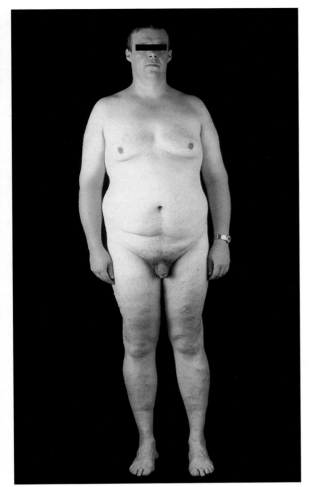

Fig. 8.6. 30-year old man with Klinefelter syndrome. Sparse virile hair pattern with horizontal pubic hairline, bilateral gynecomastia and bilateral testicular volume of 2 ml each, venous varicosities of both legs

tosterone deficiency including extreme osteoporosis. He had a devoted daughter who did not know she had been adopted.

8.9.3 Diagnosis and Therapy

A suspected diagnosis can usually be based on the combination of typical clinical findings. The most important of these are **very low testicular volume** (2–4 ml) and **firm consistency of the testes**. This can be differentiated from the softer atrophic testis where severe damage has occurred but only after full testicular development. Symptoms described above of varying degrees provide additional indications. Often **involuntary childlessness** provokes diagnosis. Often other symptoms such as **leg ulcers, osteoporosis** and **diabetes mellitus** lead to diagnosis if and when the possible underlying disease occurs to the physician.

In clinical routine the occurrence of **Barr bodies in a buccal smear** has proved to be a rapid and simple diagnostic method. Because of its relatively high percentage of error the procedure can only give indications and cannot replace mandatory chromosome analysis. **Chromosome analysis** performed in lymphocytes proves the diagnosis of a Klinefelter syndrome. Occasionally such analysis shows a normal male karyotype. In these cases karyotyping from skin fibroblasts or testicular biopsies may be used to confirm chromosome mosaicism.

Serum testosterone values are reduced in about 80% of patients with 47,XXY karyotype. On average estradiol is higher than in normal men. Simultaneously **SHBG** serum concentrations are elevated, causing a further reduction of biologically active free testosterone. Development of gynaecomastia depends on the ratio of estrogens to serum androgen levels. The gonadotropins **LH and FSH** are usually above normal levels. **FSH may be highly increased.**

An hCG-test will show reduced Leydig cell reserve capacity, a GnRH-test an extreme increase of the elevated gonadotropins. Neither test is necessary for routine diagnosis.

Practically all ejaculates from patients with 47,XXY karyotype show **azoospermia.** Very rarely can sperm be observed and the literature reports some exceptional cases of spontaneous paternity (e.g. Terzoli et al. 1992). As a rule **histological examination** of these small testes reveals **hyalinizing fibrosis** of seminiferous tubules, **absence of spermatogenesis** and relative **hyperplasia of the Leydig cells.** This picture is so reliable that testicular biopsy is not necessary for diagnosis. Single cases of germ cells and few sperm in testicular tissue have been observed in the past. Recently this prompted a search for sperm in testicular tissue from Klinefelter patients. In isolated cases it was possible to retrieve sperm by TESE-techniques (see Chap. 17) and to use them to fertilize egg

level of achievement or professional niveau of their families (Propping 1989; Ratcliffe 1994; Rovet et al. 1995). Compared with their classmates certain abnormal physical and psychological characteristics of the patients become obvious and they may become socially alienated. This may explain the fact that some Klinefelter patients become criminals. Higher-grade aneuploidy of the sex-chromosomes (48,XXXY etc.) is associated with outright mental retardation.

Klinefelter patients with **chromosome mosaics** (46,XY/47,XXY) may show very few clinical symptoms. Some of these patients are also subfertile.

On account of the lack of symptoms, patients may seek medical advice late in life, e.g. upon development of osteoporosis, or perhaps never. The oldest patients with a 47,XXY karyotype was first diagnosed at our institute at the age of 74 and showed full symptoms of severe tes-

cells and to induce pregnancies. The embryos show normal or aneuploid karyotypes which can be identified by preimplantation or prenatal diagnosis. The birth of normal children conceived in this manner has been reported (Staessen et al. 1996; Reubinoff et al. 1998). It must be emphasized that there are isolated cases and these techniques will not provide a larger number of Klinefelter patients with chances for fertility.

When testosterone serum levels are reduced, **substitution with testosterone** is necessary as described in Chap. 15. To avoid symptoms of androgen deficiency and its sequelae hormone replacement therapy should be initiated as early as possible.

> In particular Nielsen et al. (1988) could show that **early testosterone replacement** not only relieves biological symptoms such as anemia, osteoporosis, muscular weakness and impotence, but also leads to better social adjustment and integration. Testosterone replacement must be considered a **lifelong therapy** in Klinefelter patients to assure quality of life. The criteria set out in Chap. 15 should be followed for monitoring replacement therapy. Klinefelter patients will benefit from long-term testosterone preparations now being developed.

Usually gynecomastia is not influenced by hormone therapy. If it disturbs the patient, a plastic surgeon experienced in cosmetic breast surgery can perform a **mastectomy.**

In therapeutic terms **patients with a criminal record** represent a special case. According to their serum testosterone values and clinical symptoms they should be substituted. Because of the widely held belief that testosterone induces aggressive behavior, a cautionary stance seems advisable. Since, however, androgen deficiency may provoke social maladjustment, and "being different" and "trying to prove one's manhood" may be causes for criminal behavior, carefully supervised replacement therapy should be considered for these patients (Nieschlag 1992). In cooperation with psychiatrists and social workers we have had positive experience in a number of cases. For such patients replacement without exceeding upper normal values would be especially well suited.

Fig. 8.7. Schematic illustration of the abnormal meiotic X/Y-exchange leading to translocation of the testis-determining (SRY) gene on the X chromosome. This abnormal exchange occurs during meiosis in the XX male's father. *PAR* pseudoautosomal region (identical sequences on X and Y). *SRY* "sex determining region Y" gene; *RHS* recombination hot spot (location most favored for abnormal X-Y recombination).

8.10 XX Male Syndrome

> XX men with female karyotype (46,XX) are phenotypically male and have neither internal nor external female genitalia. This disorder shows a prevalence of 1:10,000 to 1:20,000.

This finding, which seems a paradox in a male individual, can be explained by the presence of genetic information specific to the Y chromosome appearing on one of two X chromosomes. Translocation of a DNA-segment from the Y to the X chromosome takes place during paternal meiosis. Among others, the testis-determining gene ("SRY" = Sex Determining Region Y) becomes attached to the X chromosome (Fechner et al. 1993) (see Fig. 8.7). The presence of the gene is sufficient to cause the initially indifferent gonad to develop into a testis. However, during translocation other essential genes responsible for the induction of spermatogenesis are lost, and so XX males are infertile. In addition to the SRY-positive XX men there is also a more rarely occurring SRY-negative variant. These patients are less virilized than SRY-positive men and show malformations of the genital organs such as maldescended testes, bifid scrotum or hypospadias.

The **testes are small** (1–2 ml) **and firm** as in Klinefelter patients, and, similarly, endocrine testicular function is often insufficient with **decreased serum testosterone** and elevated estrogen and gonadotropin levels. The semen is **azoospermic.** Fat distribution shows a female configuration; **bilateral gynecomastia** as well as an in-

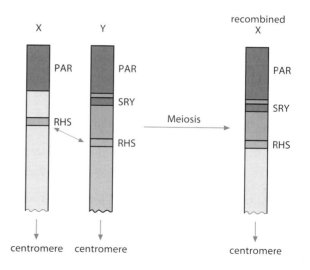

Light grey area: X-chromosome-specific sequences; *dark grey*: Y-chromosome-specific sequences. This X-Y exchange causes 75% of XX males. (According to Weil et al. 1994)

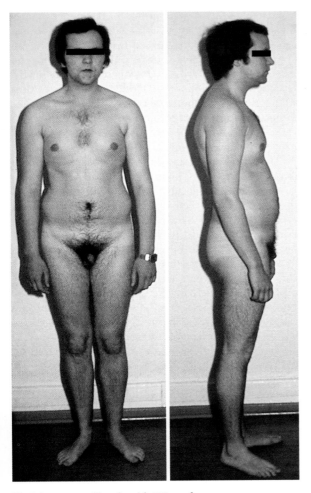

Fig. 8.8. 27-year old male with XX-syndrome

creased incidence of hypospadias (Fig. 8.8) are found. Patients have normal intelligence, while body size is smaller than that of normal men.

Infertility cannot be treated. In case of endocrine testicular insufficiency **testosterone replacement therapy** must be initiated (see Chap. 15).

8.11 XYY Syndrome

In clinical terms individuals with a 47,XYY karyotype are not remarkable. Considered as a group they are of **above average stature** and have larger teeth than men with a normal set of chromosomes. In contrast to Klinefelter patients, these men are fertile and their intelligence is normal. Therefore the finding of a 47,XYY karyotype should not be considered the cause of impaired fertility in an infertile male. The intelligence quotient (IQ) lies within the normal range, but on average 10 points below the mean of chromosomally normal men.

Much attention has been given to the finding that 47,XYY-individuals show criminal tendencies more often than other men, predominantly crimes of theft. However, this is probably an artefact due to selection bias. In this connection it must be stressed that the majority of 47,XYY men are fully normal in terms of behaviour and any stigmatisation on the basis of the karyotype must be avoided (Propping 1989). Children and adolescents with a 47,XY karyotype often cause problems due to impulsiveness, decreased frustration, decreased tolerance and maladjustments.

The chromosomal aneuploidy is caused by **non-disjunction in paternal meiosis.** Usually the finding is incidental, occurring when karyotyping has been undertaken for another indication. If in a 47,XYY man semen parameters are impaired, the same treatment as in idiopathic infertility is applicable. Children of 47,XYY men almost always have a normal karyotype. Nevertheless, to be safe, prenatal diagnosis should be offered, especially when pregnancy is induced by ICSI.

8.12 Noonan Syndrome

8.12.1 Incidence and Etiology

The Noonan syndrome is of genetic origin. Its prevalance is estimated at 1:1000 to 1:5000. The term "male Turner syndrome" formerly used was based on a certain overlap of the clinical picture with "true" Turner syndrome, which is characterized by the 45,X karyotype. As there is no common pathophysiological basis (e. g. chromosomal anomaly) and since female individuals may also be afflicted with this syndrome, the term "male Turner syndrome" is misleading and should no longer be used.

The disease occurs sporadically or in familiar aggregation (Sharland et al. 1993). An autosomal dominant mode of inheritance with incomplete penetrance and variable expressivity is well established. A gene responsible for Noonan syndrome has been mapped to the long arm of chromosome 12 between D12S84 and D12S366 (Jamieson et al. 1994).

8.12.2 Clinical Picture

There are no symptoms or findings pathognomonic for the Noonan syndrome, the overall impression leads to the diagnosis (Sharland et al. 1992). The disease occurs in men and women. **Well-proportioned short stature** is typical, with height often being below the third percentile. Growth is parallel to the percentile curves in the somatogram. Delayed or incomplete pubertal development, bone age delayed by an average of 2 years, disturbed testicular descent and reduced testicular volume may occur. Disturbed fertility is frequent in men (Elsa-wi et al. 1994). The impression of "typical Noonan" facial characteristics arises from mild ptosis, ocular hyper-telorism, low-set ears, broad nasal bridge and an anti-mongoloid palpebral slant. Other somatic anomalies such as short and broad neck up to the presence of pterygia, cubitus valgus, clinodactyly of the fifth fingers as well as a malformed sternum with pectus carinatum cranially and pectus excavatum caudally may occur. The most serious malformations are **congenital cardiac defects,** especially pulmonary valve stenosis and hypertrophy of the ventricular septum, which characterize 80% of patients and are documented by echocardiography. It is not widely appreciated that anomalies in the clotting system frequently occur, usually, however, without serious clinical symptoms. In contrast to former beliefs, mental retardation is rather an exception, but functionally significant disturbances in hearing and vision are also frequent. The combination of neurofibromatosis type I (von Recklinghausen disease) with Noonan syndrome signifies the neurofibromatosis Noonan syndrome (Meschede et al. 1993).

8.12.3 Diagnosis

The diagnosis of Noonan syndrome must be established clinically. History, physical examination and documentation of anthropometric data provide the clue data. Basal hormone status, a combined pituitary function test to establish differential diagnosis, as well as a clotting status are advisable. Proof of anomalies in the intrinsic system supports a suspected diagnosis of Noonan syndrome. Clinical chemistry, radiographic determination of bone age as well as echocardiography should be implemented.

8.12.4 Therapy

If pubertal development is delayed the same schedule should be followed as for constitutionally delayed puberty (see Chap. 7). Maldescended testes must be corrected early (see Sect. 8.3). Diagnosis and therapy of functionally significant heart defects and disturbed hearing and vision should be made as early as possible. It is important to inform the patient about the genetic basis of the disease; if offspring is desired, genetic counselling should follow.

8.13   Structural Chromosome Abnormalities

Aside from numerical chromosome abnormalities (e. g. Klinefelter syndrome), **structural chromosomal aberrations** constitute a separate category of pathological karyotypes which are important for the clinical andrologist. Structural anomalies of the sex chromosomes (gonosomes) are distinguished from anomalies of the autosomes. In addition, aside from the chromosomes involved in the anomaly, a further distinction between deletions, translocations, inversions etc. is made according to the mechanism that gave rise to the anomaly. When evaluating a structural chromosomal anomaly for clinical purposes, it must be kept in mind whether the **karyotype** is **balanced or unbalanced.**

The latter is the case when genetic material is missing or an excess is present in the "net balance" of the cell. For example, a deletion leads to an effective loss of a chromosomal segment and thus to an unbalanced karyotype. On the other hand, the genetic balance is maintained in a reciprocal translocation (counter exchange between two chromosomes); the karyotype is balanced.

Both balanced and unbalanced structural chromosomal anomalies can cause disturbances in the male reproductive system (Langer et al. 1990; De Braekelaer and Dao 1991; Van Assche et al. 1996; Meschede and Horst 1999). Almost all unbalanced karyotypes are associated with severe disturbances of general health, if they are at all compatible with the bearer's survival. Severe congenital physical and mental handicaps are the rule. In this regard, aberrant chromosomal findings of this kind play an important role in pediatrics and clinical genetics, but not in andrology. One exception are deletions of the Y chromosome. They may limit reproductive functions selectively, and are therefore of importance in reproductive medicine.

No causal treatment of chromosome abnormalities is yet available and somatic gene therapy now under development has no application here. Symptomatic treatment modalities such as assisted fertilization (see Chap. 17) can be applied in some infertile patients with chromosomal aberrations. However, success rates may be lower than in couples with normal karyotypes (Montag et al. 1997). It should also be considered that unbalanced karyotypes of the embryo may result from balanced parental chromosomal anomalies (Meschede et al. 1997). Genetic counselling should be obligatory to estimate the risk potential and prenatal diagnostic options.

8.13.1   Structural Abnormalities of Sex Chromosomes

An intact **Y chromosome** is essential for the normal structure and function of the male reproductive system (Sue 1994). The **SRY gene** is localized on its short arm and it influences differentiation of the embryonic gonad in the testicular pathway (see Sect. 8.10). In addition, the Y chromosome contains areas responsible for regular spermatogenesis. The long arm of the Y chromosome is of particular importance for spermatogenesis. Submicroscopic microdeletions on the long arm of the Y chromosome are dealt with in Sect. 8.13.2.

When speaking of **deletions of the Y chromosome**, those of the short and the long arm must be distinguished. If the entire short arm or its distal parts are lost, the patient will lack the SRY gene. The cascade of embryonic development will be disturbed at the level of gonadal differentiation. Clinically, a Turner syndrome-like phenotype with gonadal dysgenesis will result. If the deletion affects the long arm, the phenotype will be male and, depending on the size of the lost segment, spermatogenesis will be affected to varying degrees. A proximal euchromatic and a distal heterochromatic portion (chromosome band Yq12) are distinguished. The latter is variable from man to man and there are no active genes. Its loss is without negative consequences, although a very small Y chromosome is found upon analysis. The strong band of fluorescence, typical of the long arm of the Y chromosome, will be absent. If the deletion extends into the euchromatic area of the long arm, i. e. that bearing active genes (chromosome band Yq11), a severe disturbance of germ cell formation with azoospermia or marked oligozoospermia will result. Some of these patients show short stature and undervirilization as further pathological findings.

In addition to deletions and microdeletions, a series of further structural anomalies of the Y chromosome are known. **Pericentric inversions** are without consequence. An **isodicentric Y chromosome** is a more complex aberration nearly always occurring as a mosaic with a 45,X-cell line. The phenotype may be male, female or indeterminate. Patients with a male phenotype are usually infertile. **Reciprocal translocations** between the Y chromosome and one of the autosomes are rare. Mostly spermatogenesis is severely disturbed, several men with this karyotype are, however, fertile. **Translocations between the X and Y chromosomes** occur in several variations; often the karyotype is unbalanced. The correlation between karyotype and clinical presentation is complex. The phenotype may be male or female, fertility may be normal or disturbed. In some particular variants of X-Y-translocations physical and mental handicaps may occur.

The **X chromosome** contains numerous genes essential to survival. Every major deletion of this chromosome has a lethal effect in the male sex. The loss of a small segment of the distal short arm (Xp22-pter) is, however, compatible with life. The Xp22 contiguous gene syndrome is characterized by severe disturbances. Ichthyosis congenita, chondrodysplasia punctata, short stature, mental retardation as well as the **Kallmann syndrome** appear in variable combinations. The latter component, prompted by loss of the KAL-1-gene (see Chap. 7) affects about half of the patients. Translocations between the X chromosome and an autosome usually results in azoospermia or oligozoospermia. Conversely,

inversions of the X chromosome do not substantially affect male fertility.

8.13.2 Y Chromosome Microdeletions

The long arm of the Y chromosome contains at least three distinct regions, the integrity of which is essential for normal spermatogenesis (Vogt et al. 1996) (Fig. 8.9). The loss of one of these loci, designated as "azoospermia factors" (AZFa, AZFb, AZFc) and caused by spontaneous mutation in the paternal germ line, leads to severely disturbed fertility. The deleted regions are usually of submicroscopic dimensions and are known as **Y chromosomal microdeletions**. Their prevalence in azoospermic men lies between 5–10 % and between 2–5 % in cases of severe oligozoospermia (Simoni et al. 1997). Thus the deletions represent one of the quantitatively important causes of male infertility. Deletions of the AZFc region occur significantly more often than AFZa or AFZb. It remains unclear just which of these genes of the AZF region are indeed pathologically relevant as several exist as multiple copies which are homologous to a high degree (McElreavey and Krausz 1999). The socalled DAZ ("Deleted in Azoospermia") gene cluster in AFZc seems to be the most important.

Clinically the patients present with severely disturbed spermatogenesis; endocrine testicular function remains unaffected by the microdeletion. Testicular **histopathology** varies from complete or focal Sertoli-cell-only pattern to spermatogenic arrest or qualitatively in-

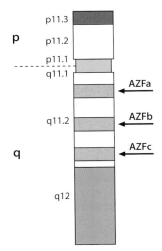

Fig. 8.9. Schematic representation of the 3 AZF loci ("azoospermia factors") on the long arm of the Y chromosome. *p* = short arm, q = long arm of the Y chromosome

tact but quantitatively severely reduced spermatogenesis. FSH values are normal or elevated.

Investigations using **specific molecular genetic** techniques are required for diagnosis. The test is based on the polymerase chain reaction (PCR) which enables certain selected marker sequences of the long arm of the Y chromosome of patient DNA to be amplified and analyzed (Kostner et al. 1998). This test should be performed in all men with severely disturbed spermatogenesis of unclear origin.

It can be used as a **screening procedure** in these patients without further selection. These tests are still in the process of refinement both technically and with respect to evaluation of their scientific contribution, including their cost-benefit-effectiveness. A first important step in this direction was the establishment of laboratory guidelines for the diagnosis of Y chromosome microdeletions (Simoni et al. 1999b).

A positive result of the analysis provides a causal explanation for the patient's disturbed spermatogenesis. Beyond this, the test also has **prognostic value**, as every son of such a patient will carry the paternal Y chromosome microdeletion and will probably inherit disturbed fertility (Kamischke et al. 1999). Genetic counselling is indicated for all carriers of Y chromosome microdeletions.

8.13.3 Structural Abnormalities of the Autosomes

Structural anomalies of the autosomes (chromosome pairs 1–22) may lead to disturbances of male fertility. Their prevalence among infertile men is about 1–2%. For reasons explained above only balanced karyotypes are relevant; for the detailed effects of unbalanced chromosome sets reference should be made to cytogenetic textbooks.

Balanced autosomal anomalies may interfere with the meiotic pairing of the chromosomes and thus adversely affect spermatogenesis. If, and to what extent, disturbed fertility may occur, can hardly be foreseen for individual cases, unlike gonosomal aberrations. The same balanced autosomal aberration can have a severe effect on spermatogenesis in one patient and none at all or only slightly so in another patient. Even between brothers with the same pathological karyotype results from spermiograms can differ widely. So far no clinical or laboratory parameter in an infertile male is known which reliably indicates the presence of an autosomal structural anomaly. Therefore, in cases of unclear azoospermia or severe oligozoospermia karyotyping is generally advised.

Often the non-specialist overinterprets the frequent, but functionally irrelevant **chromosomal polymorphisms of the autosomes,** believing them to be pathological. Some labs mention such polymorphisms in their cytogenic reports, sometimes failing to explain them sufficiently. Two particularly frequent findings of this type are small pericentric inversions of chromosome 9 and the enlargement of the pericentrometric heterochromatin of this chromosome (9qh+). These and similar findings have no pathological significance and should not be mentioned to the patient.

In contrast, **reciprocal and Robertsonian translocations** as well as **peri- and paracentric inversions** may have real pathogenic significance. The impact of a given chromosome anomaly of this kind on the spermiogram is impossible to predict for the individual case. However, since translocations and inversions are found much more often in infertile men than in unselected neonates, there is no doubt that a pathogenetic relation exists. The most frequent situation arising in clinical practice is that a translocation or inversion is found in a patient with a clearly pathological spermiogram, and the questions arises whether this is the underlying cause for disturbed spermatogenesis. The question will have to be answered positively if, after all due care, all other reasons for infertility have been excluded. In contrast to numeric chromosomal disturbances and structural anomalies of the gonosomes, autosomal structural aberrations tend to be associated with oligo- rather than with azoospermia.

Translocations and inversions usually represent cases of **familial chromosomal aberrations.** Often an infertile patient is the first family member in whom the aberration is identified. In such a situation a family study should be encouraged. This should begin with the patient's parents and, depending on results, be extended to include siblings, grandparents, etc. In this manner, often substantial number of relatives may be identified with the same chromosomal aberration as the index patient. It is important to ensure a family study as the presence of a translocation or inversion is often associated with a higher rate of abortion and, in some cases, the risk for the birth of a severely handicapped child. This also applies to the index patient, who may be pursuing treatment with assisted reproduction. Patients with balanced autosomal chromosomal anomalies require careful genetic counselling before they are admitted to an IVF or ICSI programme. Here the potential risks and suitable prenatal diagnostic measures must be discussed. In pre-implantation diagnosis using fluorescence in situ hybridization (FISH) the rate of chromosomally unbalanced sperm in men with autosomal structural aberrations can be estimated.

8.14 Persistent Muellerian Duct Syndrome (Oviduct Persistence)

If the Muellerian inhibiting hormone (MIH) or anti-Mueller-Hormone (AMH) is not produced at the time of fetal sex differentiation, the Muellerian ducts will fail to regress even in male individuals. Alongside male genitalia, Fallopian tubes and uterus develop from Muellerian ducts. Mutations in the AMH gene or the AMH receptor type II gene were described as causes (Imbeaud et al. 1996). As the function of the Leydig cells is not affected, masculine sexual differentiation and puberty takes its normal course. Testicular maldescent and disturbed fertility may, however, be observed. Usually, Fallopian tubes and uterus are coincidentially discovered during herniotomy or laparotomy, or not until autopsy. For therapeutic purposes, uterus and oviducts should be removed; care must be taken that the vasa deferentia, passing through the round ligament, not be injured.

8.15 Gonadal Dysgenesis

8.15.1 Definition

The concept of gonadal dysgenesis covers a group of disorders of genetic origin affecting gonadal differentiation (Berkowitz 1992). A synonym for gonadal dysgenesis is "**streak gonads**". They are characterized by the **absence of germ cells as well as the lack of Sertoli/granulosa cells**. Histologically, only stromal tissue is found.

Three major forms of gonadal dysgensis can be distinguished:

- Gonadal dysgenesis with 45,X karyotype (Turner syndrome),
- **pure gonadal dysgenesis** as well as
- **mixed gonadal dysgenesis**.

Pure gonadal dysgenesis is characterized by the presence of bilateral streak gonads, whereas the mixed form may have a unilateral streak gonad and contralaterally a more or less completely differentiated and descended testis.

8.15.2 Clinical Picture

Individuals with **pure gonadal dysgenesis** and a 46,XX karyotype are phenotypically female, but fail to develop sexually at the anticipated age of puberty. The clinical picture of individuals with true gonadal dysgenesis and 46,XY karyotypes (Swyer syndrome) is identical, occasionally partial virilization occurs at the expected age of puberty. A typical course of pure gonadal dysgenesis occurs in both XX and XY forms. Females with pure gonadal dysgenesis of the 46,XX-type sometimes have residual ovarian function which allows them to have menstrual cycles for a certain time. In some patients with 46,XY karyotype partial virilization of the external genitalia is present at birth.

Patients with **mixed gonadal dysgenesis**, most of whom bear a chromosomal mosaic of 45,X/46,XY-type, have intersexual genitalia. Uterus, vagina and oviducts are almost always present, the position of the testis is intra-abdominal, less often inguinal or scrotal. Breast development is rare. The degree of virilization of the external genitals shows considerable variability. Most of these patients are raised as females. The most typical symptoms of patients with a male phenotype are hypospadias and cryptorchidism, as well as androgen deficiency and azoospermia in later life. Growth pattern varies between eunuchoid, normal and Turner-like appearance.

8.15.3 Diagnosis

Aside from patients with established Turner syndrome the diagnosis of pure gonadal dysgenesis can only be ascertained by laparoscopy with gonadal biopsy. In pure gonadal dysgenesis with **46,XX karyotype** LH and FSH are elevated, while estrogens and gestagens are low. Sometimes gonadal dysgenesis occurs in a pedigree; however, mutations in the FSH receptor gene could only be traced in Finnish patients (Aittomäki et al. 1995). The endocrine findings in 46,XY patients are identical with those of the **46,XX variant**. In some patients a mutation of the SRY gene can be found.

In **mixed gonadal dysgenesis** gonadotropin levels are clearly increased, with LH usually less elevated than FSH. Testosterone is usually below normal for males, but above normal for females. Administration of hCG is often followed by a low, but significant testosterone increase. Laparoscopy always reveals at least vestiges of Muellerian ducts. Biopsies from intra-abdominal streak gonads almost always show only connective tissue similar to ovarian stroma with no indication of germ cells. Testicular biopsies have revealed single cases of precursor stages of germ cells, but absence of Sertoli cells and of Leydig cell hyperplasia. The karyotype has to be established. Because of phenotypically similar appearance pure gonadal dysgenesis should be considered for differential diagnosis. Moreover, anorchia or bilateral cryptorchidism should be considered as differential diagnosis.

8.15.4 Therapy

At the anticipated age of puberty adequate hormone replacement therapy must be initiated. In cases of intersexual genitalia, surgical correction should enable the affected child to grow up with an unambigious sexual identity. There is a high risk of neoplastic transformation (gonadoblastoma, seminoma, dysgerminoma, carcinoma in situ) for all patients with a cell line bearing a Y chromosome (Savage and Low 1990). For this reason, streak gonads should be removed surgically in cases where regular check-ups of gonads by ultrasonography are not possible. There is no therapy for infertility. In patients with pure gonadal dysgenesis, pregnancies have been successfully induced following IVF with donor egg cells.

8.16 Disturbance of Testosterone Synthesis: Male Pseudohermaphroditism

8.16.1 Definition

> Whereas true hermaphrodites possess both testicular as well as ovarian gonadal tissue, male pseudohermaphroditism is characterized by unambiguous male gonadal and chromosomal sex, but with female or intersexual internal and external genitalia.

Although these patients have testes, phenotypically they appear female – although to highly varying degrees – and consult the physician as females. Enzyme defects in testosterone biosynthesis as a cause for intersexual development are discussed below, whereas androgen receptor defects in the target organs which also lead to male pseudohermaphroditism are dealt with in Chap. 11.

8.16.2 Etiology

Disturbances of steroid biosynthesis from cholesterol can take place at every enzymatic step. These may lead to symptoms of mineral or glucocorticoid deficiency as well as to hypogonadism. Enzymatic defects in 20,22 desmolase (P450scc, cholesterol side chain cleavage enzyme), 3ß-hydroxysteroid dehydrogenase and 17α-hydroxylase which are involved in the synthesis of mineral- or glucocorticoids can also lead to congenital adrenal hyperplasia. Enzyme defects selectively affecting **testosterone biosynthesis** are the **17,20-desmolase-defect** (17, 20 lyase defect) and the 17ß-**hydroxysteroid-dehydrogenase-defect**. In pathogenetic terms an autosomal recessive mutation in the cytochrome p450$_{17\alpha}$-gene is responsible for both the 17,20-desmolase defect and the 17α-hydroxylase defect. The protein product of this gene (p450c17) has both 17, 20-desmolase as well as 17α-hydroxylase activity.

8.16.3 Clinical Picture

The spectrum of phenotypical variation is broad because of the many aspects of androgen-dependent development and ranges from almost **normal male genitalia** with **mild hypospadias** to formation of **female external genitalia with complete lower vagina, labia and clitoris** (Fig. 8.10). The **testes** are usually **inguinal**, but may also be located **intra-abdominally**, which makes clinical diagnosis especially difficult. The age of puberty often marks the onset of increasing **virilization**, as a consequence of which untreated patients may seek reorientation of their psycho-social gender. Most phenotypically female patients seek medical help because of **hirsutism** and **primary amenorrhoea**. It should be noted that several of the enzyme defects are associated with adrenal insufficiency or hypertension caused by mineral corticoid excess. Particularly in neonates and infants the adrenal dysfunction can cause an emergency situation.

8.16.4 Diagnosis

Patients with partial enzyme defects and with **low serum testosterone** levels can be diagnosed because of the accumulation of steroids proximal to the enzyme block. Determination of Δ4-**androstenedione**, possibly following hGC-stimulation, is of diagnostic relevance for 17ß-hydroxysteroid-dehydrogenase defects. As androgens are also estrogen precursors, the concentration of estradiol in serum is also reduced. Diseases of the androgen target organs (androgen resistence) must be excluded by differential diagnosis and screening the androgen receptor for mutations (see Chap. 11).

8.16.5 Therapy

The decision whether neonates are to be raised as girls or boys must be made on an individual basis and depends on the extent of ambiguity of the external genitalia. In addition to necessary surgical correction, sex hormone levels should be monitored closely at the time of expected puberty in order to initiate timely hormone replacement therapy. **Depending on the phenotype, lifelong estrogen or testosterone substitution is indicated** from the time of anticipated puberty. In male phenotypes, non-descended testes should be brought into the scrotum surgically; they should be palpated regularly and monitored by ultrasonography, because of the danger of tumor development. For the same reason, testes should be removed in patients who are brought up and continue their life as females.

For treatment of the possibly coexisting adrenal disturbances reference is made to textbooks of endocrinology.

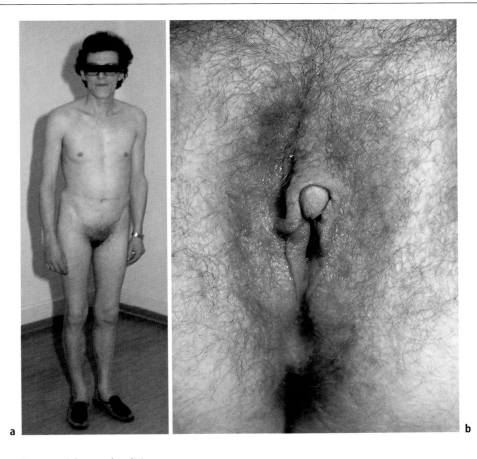

a
b

Fig. 8.10 a, b. Patient with male pseudohermaphroditism caused by 17β-hydroxysteroid-dehydrogenase defect in testosterone biosynthesis. The patient was raised as a girl and sought medical advice for primary amenorrhea without being diagnosed. Diagnosis was not made until the age of 29, when a herniotomy lead to the discovery of the intra-abdominal testes. Estrogen substitution therapy was implemented following gonadal exstirpation. **a** Full body view showing male proportions. **b** External genitalia showing "clitoris" hypertrophy and a vaginal introitus

8.17 Mutations of Gonadotropin Receptors

Specific receptors enable the gonadotropins LH and FSH to become effective in the Leydig or Sertoli cells (see Chap. 3). Mutations in the receptors cause functional alterations in these cells with drastic clinical consequences. Principally **inactivating mutations** must be distinguished from **activating mutations**. Whereas the former lead to a loss of function, the latter mutations cause constitutive i. e. autonomous activity of the target cells without the need for LH or FSH. An overview of the diseases caused by mutations of gonadotropin receptors is provided in Table 8.1.

Table 8.1. Clinical effects of gonadotropin receptor mutations in men

Inactivating LH receptor mutations	(depending on type of mutation) male pseudohermaphroditism, hypogonadism and delayed puberty, undervirilization and micropenis
Activating LH receptor mutations	Precocious puberty
Inactivating FSH receptor mutations	Infertility
Activating FSH receptor mutations	Intact spermatogenesis despite complete pituitary insufficiency

While investigations into the molecular biology of gonadotropin receptors have allowed highly interesting disease entities to be identified, they have not yet contributed much to the treatment of hypogonadism and infertility because of the rarity of these diseases.

8.17.1. Inactivating LH Receptor Mutations: Leydig Cell Hypoplasia

Leydig cell hypoplasia or Leydig cell agenesis is a very rare disease with an approximate incidence of 1:1,000,000, occurring only in the male sex with a limited autosomal recessive inheritance. The name of the syndrome, Leydig cell agenesis, is misleading as Leydig cells are present but are unable to develop because of an inactivating mutation of the LH receptor which fails to provide the necessary stimulation (Themmen et al. 1998).

The phenotype is highly dependent on the extent of intrauterine testosterone secretion. Consequently either 1. **a male phenotype with slight virilization and microphallus** or 2. **hypogonadism with delayed puberty** or 3. **male pseudohermaphroditism** (Fig. 8.11) develops. The various inactivating mutations in the LH receptor gene are described in Fig. 8.12 and Table 8.2. In a patient with hypogonadism and delayed puberty a mutation in exon 10 of the LH receptor was described which reacts to hCG but not to LH (Gromoll et al. 2000). Thus maternal hCG can stimulate intrauterine testosterone production and male sexual differentiation but postnatally the Leydig cells fail to respond to LH.

The possible appearance of the external genitalia ranges from an unremarkable female phenotype (Fig. 8.11) to intersexual genitalia to a predominantly male habitus with microphallus. In the mostly maldescended testes seminiferous tubules can be found. Leydig cells are not present or appear only in immature preliminary stages. Epididymides and deferent ducts are ususaly present, leading to the conclusion that local intrauterine testosterone production was sufficient for the anlage of these organs. Uterus, tubes or upper vagina are not found in these patients. In those cases where ambivalent genitalia did not lead to diagnosis, delayed puberty usually does.

In such cases basal hormone status, usually with normal FSH, elevated LH and low testosterone provides an initial diagnostic hint of the underlying defect. Depending on the type of LH receptor defect, hCG stimulates either no or a pronounced rise in testosterone. Diagnosis is confirmed by testicular biopsy showing Leydig cell hypoplasia or aplasia and by techniques of molecular biology revealing mutations of the LH receptor gene.

Differential diagnosis should especially differentiate the disease from male pseudohermaphroditism on the basis of testosterone synthesis defects, from the adreno-

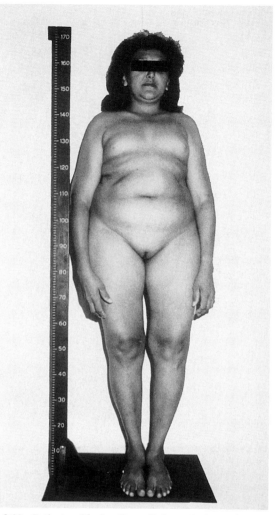

Fig. 8.11. Patient with Leydig cell hypoplasia and male pseudohermaphroditism caused by the LH receptor mutation described by Kremer et al. (1995). (Photograph kindly provided by Dr. A. Themmen, Rotterdam)

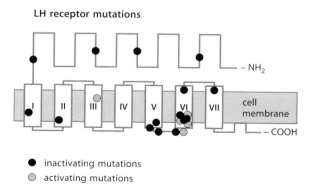

Fig. 8.12. Activating and inactivating mutations of the LH receptor

Table 8.2. Inactivating mutations of the LH receptor which can cause Leydig cell hypoplasia with male pseudohermaphroditism, undervirilization with micropenis or hypogonadism with delayed puberty. *ECD*, extracellular domain; *TM*, transmembrane domain

Exchange of nucleic acid	Amino acid position	Exchange of amino acid	Localization	Reference
Insertion between position 54–55	18	Insertion of 11 amino acids	ECD	Wu et al. 1998
TGT to CGT	131	C–R	ECD	Misrahi et al. 1997
Deletion of Exon 8	–	Deletion	ECD	Laue et al. 1996
Deletion of Exon 10	–	Deletion	ECD	Gromoll et al. 2000
GAA to AAA	354	E–K	ECD	Stavrou et al. 1998
TGC to TGA	545	C–Szup	TM 5	Laue et al. 1995
CGA to TGA	554	R–Szup	TM 5	Latronico et al. 1996
GCC to CCC	593	A–P	TM 6	Kremer et al. 1995
				Toledo et al. 1996
Deletion of nucleic acid 1822–1827	608–609	Deletion	TM 7	Latronico et al. 1998
TCT to TAT	616	S–T	TM 7	Laue et al. 1996
ATA to AAA	625	I–L	TM 7	Martens et al. 1998

genital syndrome, from 5α-reductase deficiency and from androgen receptor defects. Early gender assignment, with microsurgical support, is important. Depending on gender assignment, when the expected age of puberty is reached, lifelong substitution with estrogens or androgens must follow.

8.17.2 Activating LH Receptor Mutations

Activating LH receptor mutations lead to constitutive, LH-independent activity of the Leydig cells, causing **precocious puberty limited to male family members** and often becoming manifest before the fourth year of life. The syndrome is mentioned here for the sake of completeness; reference is made to reviews (e.g. Themmen et al. 1998) and to textbooks of pediatrics or endocrinology.

Activating LH receptor mutations are also described in the section dealing with **Leydig cell tumors** (see Sect. 8.19.4).

8.17.3 Inactivating FSH Receptor Mutations

Inactivating FSH receptor mutations may cause **infertility**. In Finland five males were identified bearing an autosomal recessively inherited Cys-189-Thr mutation of the FSH receptor. Although testicular volume was reduced, two males proved to be fertile, one was definitely infertile and the status of the other cases remained unclear (Tapanainen et al. 1997). It is not surprising that complete infertility was not observed, considering that spermatogenesis is guarded by a double safety mechanism through FSH and LH, and the fact that spermatogenesis can be maintained, albeit in reduced form, by LH stimulation alone (Nieschlag et al. 1999).

Wide screening for inactivating FSH receptor mutations revealed that these mutations are largely confined to the Finnish population (Jiang et al. 1998). However, the **FSH receptor shows polymorphism**, mostly affecting amino acid positions 307 (Thr or Ala) and 680 (Asn or Ser). These isoforms of the FSH receptor are equally distributed among fertile and infertile populations (Simoni et al. 1999a).

8.17.4 Activating FSH Receptor Mutations

Men with activating mutations of the FSH receptor are difficult to distinguish clinically as they have hardly any characteristic phenotypical traits. So far only one case has been described. This man had intact spermatogenesis despite complete hypophysectomy with loss of gonadotropins and required only testosterone substitution in order to achieve multiple paternity naturally. In his FSH receptor gene an exchange of amino acid Asp and Gly was found in position 567 which was responsible for the constitutive activation of the receptor (Gromoll et al. 1996) (Fig. 8.13).

FSH receptor mutations

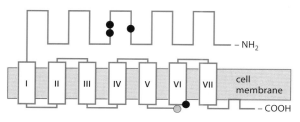

● inactivating mutations
○ activating mutations

Fig. 8.13. Activating and inactivating mutations of the FSH receptor

8.18 True Hermaphroditism

8.18.1 Definition and Etiology

> By definition **true hermaphrodites possess both testicular and ovarian tissue.** The gonads may consist of uni- or bilateral **ovotestes** with testicular and ovarian tissue. An ovary may also be present on one side and a testis on the other side or there may be combinations with ovotestis.

The exact incidence is not known, only several hundred patients have been described. The largest single series comprised 24 South Africans (Niekerk 1974). About two thirds of all patients have a 46, XX karyotype, 10% a 46, XY karyotype, the remaining patients show a chromosomal mosaic with at least one Y cell line. One patient observed by us showed a 46, XX/47, XXY-mosaic (Bergmann et al. 1989). Another patient showed a 45, X/46, X, idic (Y) mosaic. All patients reveal the "testis-determining factor" (TDF) on the Y chromosome, in whose presence the primary ambiguous gonads undergo differentiation into testes (McElreavey and Fellous 1997). The etiology of the disease is puzzling in patients with highly differentiated testicular tissue where no Y chromosome can be seen. Abnormal X to Y exchange during paternal meiosis is presumed to be the cause in some 46, XX patients in whom genetic material of Y chromosomal origin is found. In true hermaphrodites without detectable Y chromosomal material, X chromosomal or autosomal genes controlled by SRY are considered as the origin of this condition. The simultaneous occurrence of SRY-negative XX men and 46, XX hermaphroditism indicates an autosomal dominant mutation which may interfere with normal sexual differentiation to various extents.

8.18.2 Clinical Picture

Phenotypically, 90% of patients with true hermaphroditism show intersexual genitalia at birth. The remaining 10% have unambigious female or male external genitalia, 75% of the patients grow up as males. At the time of puberty, virilization takes place and gynecomastia develops. About half of phenotypic females menstruate and pregnancies have been reported in patients with a 46, XX or 46, XX/46, XY karyotype (first reported by Narita et al. 1975). About one quarter of the phenotypically male patients show cyclic hematuria, whereas ovulation in the ovotestis is taken for testicular pain. In the ovotestis normal spermatogenesis does not take place, whereas in the testes spermatogenesis is observed in about 10% of patients.

8.18.3 Diagnosis

Gonadotropins may be normal or elevated in patients with true hermaphroditism, the serum estrogen and progesterone concentrations depend on a possible ovarian cycle. Diagnosis is made on the basis of biopsy evidence of seminiferous tubules as well as follicle and ovarian stroma in the gonads. Karyotyping is essential in all cases. Diagnosis should differentiate true hermaphroditism from gonadal dysgenesis, forms of male pseudohermaphroditism, congenital adrenal hyperplasia and androgen resistance.

8.18.4 Therapy

In true hermaphrodites gender assignment should be made as early as possible and should be supported by plastic surgery of the genitalia if necessary. Neoplastic transformation occurs in about 10% of patients with a Y chromosome and in 4% of patients without a Y chromosome and is thus a much lower risk than in gonadal dysgenesis. Any decision in favor of excision of the gonads must consider the patients's fertility and hormonal status, along with karyotyping.

In phenotypically male patients with true hermaphroditism all ovarian tissue must be completely removed. In phenotypically female patients with true hermaphroditism all testicular tissue must be removed to avoid progressive virilization and because of the increased risk of tumors. If the gonads are not removed, close ultrasonographic monitoring is mandatory. If they are removed, lifelong estrogen or androgen hormonal replacement therapy must follow according to the phenotype after puberty.

8.19 Testicular Tumors

8.19.1 Incidence

A testicular tumor is the most frequent malignant disease in men between the ages of 25 and 40. It occurs most frequently in Caucasians and with lowest frequency in the black population. The incidence of testicular tumors has increased globally by a factor of 3 to 4 particularly during the last 4-5 decades. The highest rate of growth and total incidence is seen in Scandinavia, Germany, Poland, Switzerland and Hungary, with a doubling in incidence every 15-25 years (Adamai et al. 1997). The reasons for this increase are largely unknown. The incidence of testicular tumors varies between 0.7 (USA, black population) and 8.8 (Switzerland) newly reported cases per 100,000 men and year (Buetow 1995).

In addition to **geographic** and **ethnic factors** relevant for these tumors, a series of other **risk factors** is also known. The risk of testicular cancer/carcinoma in situ (CIS) is clearly elevated in men with **maldescended testes** (3%), a **contralateral testicular tumor** (5–6%), an **extragonadal germ cell tumor** (50%) and **gonadal dysgenesis** (up to 100%).

Several factors are probably responsible for an elevated incidence of testicular tumors in **infertility**. The highest incidence occurs at an age when involuntary childlessness becomes evident. Maldescent can lead to infertility as well as to increased risk of testicular cancer (see Sect. 8.3). More than other primarily non-testicular diseases, a testicular tumor can lead to **reduced fertility** (see Chapts. 13 and 18). Fifty percent of patients with a germ cell tumor have sperm concentrations below 10-15 million/ml (Petersen et al. 1998). Preexisting disturbances of spermatogenesis along with other causative factors are probably responsible. This is suggested by severely disturbed spermatogenesis seen in biopsies of the contralateral testis in unilateral germ cell tumors (Berthelsen and Skakkeback 1983). Testicular atrophy and sonographic inhomogeneities bear an increased risk for testicular tumors especially in patients with severe oligozoospermia (<3 million/ml) (Giwercman et al. 1997).

> Since the introduction of routine ultrasound examination of the testes we have found a testicular tumor **in one of 200 infertility patients.**

Fifty-nine percent of testicular cancers are germ cell tumors, with seminoma alone representing about half of the cases (Bosl and Motzer 1997). Leydig cell and Sertoli cell tumors represent only a fraction at the total. CIS is important as an obligatory precancerous stage of all germ cell tumors (with the exception of spermatocytic seminoma).

8.19.2 Carcinoma in situ

Carcinoma in situ (CIS) is considered an obligatory precancerous stage of a testicular tumor. It is defined as a typical neoplastic gonocyte which is distinguished from normal spermatagonia both morphologically and immunohistochemically and shares several morphological and immunohistochemical characterisitics with embryonic germ cells. Without therapeutic intervention almost all **CIS will develop into malignant germ cell tumors.** Both seminomas and non-seminomas may develop from a CIS. It is still unknown whether CIS arises during the course of development or whether it is congenital.

Both **clinical** and **diagnostic** presentation of CIS are heterogenous. Leading symptoms may be decreased seminal parameters along with an inhomogenous sonographic appearance of the testis (see Chap. 6). Diagnosis is only possible by testicular biopsy (fixed in Bouin's solution), followed by histological and immunohistological (P1AP, M2A, c-kit, 43–9F, TRA-1–60) tests. Tubules with CIS are normally distributed throughout the affected testis; few, many or all may be affected. Biopsies should always be performed bilaterally.

Therapy for CIS depends greatly on biopsy results. If only one side is affected, surgical **ablation** of the affected testis is the safest method. If the remaining testis is affected by CIS, local **irradiation** with 20 Gray (10 fractions of 2 Gy) is the method of choice, as it allows endocrine function to be maintained even when tubular function is lost (Bamberg et al. 1997; Giwercman et al. 1991). When chemotherapy is anticipated because of metastases or additional indications, irradiation should be delayed for 6 months after completion of chemotherapy, when a second biopsy should be performed for control purposes. Only if CIS persists should irradiation be carried out (Bamberg et al. 1997). Orchidectomy (loss of tubular and endocrine function) as well as delaying actions are only indicated in exceptional cases when only one remaining testis is affected. If both testes are affected, the one with the greatest damage should be removed and the other should be treated by local irradiation.

8.19.3 Germ Cell Tumors

Malignant cells of CIS can transform into both **seminoma** (with the exception of spermatocytic seminoma) and **non-seminoma** (Table 8.3), for which reason the same risk factors apply as for CIS. Seminoma and non-seminoma account for 95% of all testicular tumors (Bosl and Motzer 1997). Most seminoma reach their peak in the fourth decade of life, non-seminoma in the third. Almost all germ cell tumors and CIS have an isochromo-

Table 8.3. Histological classification of testicular tumors (from Bosl and Motzer 1997)

Germ cell tumors
  Seminoma
    (classic, anaplastic, spermatocytic)
  Embryonic carcinoma
  Teratoma
    (mature, immature)
  Chorion carcinoma
  Yolksac tumor
  Mixed germ cell tumor

Stromal tumors
  Leydig cell tumor
  Sertoli cell tumor
  Granulosa cell tumor

Mixed germinal cell/stromal tumors
  Gonadoblastoma

Paratesticular tumor
  Adenocarcinoma of the testis
  Mesothelioma

some on the short arm of chromosome 12 (iso-p12) as a specific chromosome marker (Bosl and Motzer 1997).

- In clinical **stage I** the germ cell tumor is limited to scrotal contents.
- In **stage II** lymphatic metastases are present below the diaphragm and are smaller than 2 cm (IIA), between 2–5 cm (IIB) or larger than 5 cm (IIC, bulky disease).
- Clinical **stage III** is characterized by lymphatic metastases above the diaphragm as extranodular metastases (Bosl and Motzer 1997).

The **clinical picture** of seminoma and non-seminoma is highly variable. Testicular pain and swelling may be present. Tumor growth may precipitate rapid decline of ejaculate parameters combined with altered testicular consistency. Compromised semen parameters may range from azoospermia to oligoasthenoteratozoospermia of various degrees. A sudden decline of semen parameters should always prompt thorough investigation of the testes. Bilateral development of gynecomastia is possible. Retroperitoneal lymph node metastases may contribute to development of varicocele and abdominal complaints.

When clinical symptoms arise, diagnosis is made by **palpation** and **sonographic investigation**. When tumors are small and at an early stage, palpation rarely indicates intratesticular events. Suspicion arises when sides differ and when alterations in consistency and volume are observed. Of those patients in our clinic in whom a testicular tumor was discovered only **less than one third had** a suspicious finding on the basis of palpation; the remainder were discovered exclusively with the aid of ultrasonography (see Chap. 6). Next to palpation, ultrasonography has become a preeminent tool for the diagnosis of testicular tumors. In ultrasound imaging, testicular tumors appear mostly inhomogenous with areas of increased or reduced echo density.

A further important role in diagnosis and therapy is played by the **tumor markers AFP and β-hCG** which are elevated in one to two thirds of germ cell tumors (especially in non-seminomas). Further markers are **placental alkaline phosphatase** (**PLAP**, only in seminomas) and **lactate dehydrogenase** (**LDH**) which correlate with the prognosis of metastasis stage and therefore complement the specific markers. Diagnostic certainty is achieved by **testicular biopsy** after inguinal severance of the spermatic chord.

As about half of the patients already have lymphatic metastases at the time of diagnosis, computer tomographic investigation of abdomen and thorax in layers of 10 mm is obligatory. Elective sonographic examination of the abdomen may be used for comparison in subsequent follow-up. CT of the skull and skeleton scintigraphy are only indicated if extensive metastases were found during previous examinations (Bamberg et al. 1997). A contralateral biopsy should be recommended to all patients with a testicular tumor to exclude the possibility of CIS.

Thanks to the establishment of multidisciplinary treatment concepts and the introduction of cisplatin to testicular cancer therapy, germ cell tumors have become a largely curable disease. The first therapeutic step is ablation of the testis on the affected side. When both testes are involved and when paternity is desired possibly only one side can be enucleated.

In addition to distinguishing pure seminoma from non-seminoma the clinical determination of disease stage is of great importance for further therapy. The following recommendations were made by German medical societies concerned with diagnosis and treatment of testicular tumors (Bamberg et al. 1997):

- For **stage I seminoma** standard therapy consists of irradiation of infradiaphragmatic para-aortal lymph nodes (26 Gy).
- In **stage II seminoma** infradiaphragmatic para-aortal and ipsilateral iliac lymph nodes are irradiated with 30 Gy (stage IIA) or 36 Gy (stage IIB).
- From **stage IIC** onward seminoma chemotherapy with cisplatin follows ablation.
- For **stage I non-seminoma** no uniform schemes exist so that along with nerve-sparing and thus ejaculation-protective retroperitoneal lymphadenectomy, observational strategy with intensive after-care, additional chemotherapy and risk-adapted procedures are practiced.

Table 8.4. Risk classification of the International Germ Cell Cancer Classification Group (Nach Bamberg et al. 1997)

Good risk (5 year survival rate 95 %)

Nonseminoma	Gonadal or retroperitoneal primary tumor and "low" markers and no pulmonary visceral metastases	Low markers: AFP < 1000 ng/ml and hCG < 1000 ng/ml (5000 IU/l) and LDH < 1,5 × upper limit of normal
Seminoma	Any primary site and any marker elevation and no pulmonary visceral metastases	Low markers: AFP < 1000 ng/ml and hCG < 1000 ng/ml (5000 IU/l) and LDH < 1,5 × upper limit of normal

Intermediate risk (5 year survival rate 80 %)

Nonseminoma	Gonadal or retroperitoneal primary tumor and "intermediate" markers and no pulmonary visceral metastases	Intermediate markers: AFP 1000–10000 ng/ml or hCG 1000–10000 ng/ml (5000 – 50000 IU/l) or LDH 1,5–10 × upper limit of normal
Seminoma	Any primary site and any marker elevation and nonpulmonary visceral metastases present (e.g. bone, liver, brain)	Intermediate markers: AFP 1000–10000 ng/ml or hCG 1000–10000 ng/ml (5000 – 50000 IU/l) or LDH 1,5–10 × upper limit of normal

Poor risk (5 year survival rate 50 %)

Nonseminoma	Mediastinal primary site or gonadal or retroperitoneal primary tumor with nonpulmonary visceral metastases present or high markers	High markers: AFP > 10000 ng/ml or hCG > 10000 ng/ml (50000 IU/l) or LDH > 10 × upper limit of normal

- For **stage IIA/B** nerve-sparing lymphadenectomy with or without additional chemotherapy or primary chemotherapy and later residual tumor resection is performed. (Also for stage IIC, for which primary surgery is considered obsolete).

For patients with advanced stages of disease, therapy plans follow the classification of the International Germ Cell Cancer Classification Group (Table 8.4). Patients with good or medium prognosis receive three cycles of PEB (cisplatin, etoposid, bleomycin). Patients with poor prognosis are treated with four cycles of PEI (cisplatin, etoposid, ifosfamid). Concerning therapy of relapses and residual tumors, reference is made to textbooks of oncology and urology.

Prior to bilateral orchidectomy, chemotherapy, testicular irradiation or retroperitoneal lymphadenectomy, patients must be given the possibility of cryopreserving their sperm to preserve fertility (see Chap. 18).

During therapy of testicular tumors, unilateral orchidectomy may cause a reduction of sperm concentration along with elevated FSH. If nerve-protective modified retroperitoneal lymphadenectomy is performed, 33 % of cases will show disturbed ejaculation (especially retrograde ejaculation) (Petersen et al. 1998). When irradiation is performed (Chap. 13), disturbed spermatogenesis may follow because of scattered rays affecting the remaining testis (ca. 1.7 Gy without, 0.5 Gy with gonad protection); this is mostly reversible (Greiner 1982; Hansen et al. 1990). The standard therapy of testicular tumors based on cisplatin almost always acutely causes azoospermia with elevated FSH. As for irradiation, precise prognosis of possible long-term effects of chemotherapy on spermatogenesis is not possible because of great individual variation. Dose, basal seminal values and duration of follow-up are among those factors influencing such variation. Most patients experience at least a partial recovery of spermatogenesis during the second to fourth year following cessation of chemotherapy. Patients receiving a cumulative total dose of more than 600 mg/m^2 cisplatin must reckon with permanent azoospermia or severe oligozoospermia (Petersen et al. 1998). Elevation of LH may follow ablation, irradiation or chemotherapy. Testosterone levels usually remain in the normal range. Should **testosterone deficiency** occur, testosterone must be substituted as after bilateral oridectomy (see Chap. 15).

8.19.4 Stromal Testicular Tumors with Endocrine Activity

Of the stromal tumors, the rarely occurring Leydig cell tumors and Sertoli cell tumors always show endocrine activity.

Leydig cell tumors are generally benign neoplasms and account for about 1–2% of all testicular tumors. They usually measure less than 5 cm. The larger they are, the greater the chance of malignancy. Prior to puberty they are almost always benign (Freeman 1986). Whereas before puberty they mostly produce androgens, thus leading to **precocious pseudopuberty**, after puberty they tend to produce estrogens.

Causes of Leydig cell tumors were long unknown. In recent times, however, activating mutations of the LH receptor in Leydig cell tumors were described in boys (Liu et al. 1999) as well as in adults (Fragoso et al. 1998). These arginine-to-cysteine (Arg 201 cys) or aspargine-to-histidine (Asp 578 his) mutations may cause tumor development.

In adult patients feminization occurs with a characteristic **triad of symptoms: gynecomastia, impotence and testicular tumor** (Chap. 11, Fig. 11.7).

Clinical symptoms, however, may be very discrete. The contralateral testis and the tissue surrounding the tumor may atrophy via feedback inhibition of the hypothalamic/pituitary function by estrogens. Spermatogenesis comes to a halt; the patient may be azoospermic or oligozoospermic. After removal of the afflicted testis (depending on the extent of the disease and possible desire for paternity, enucleation is also possible), symptoms usually disappear quickly. Malignancy occurs in about 10%; it cannot be established on the basis of histology of the Leydig cell tumor. When metastases are found, chemotherapy follows, as Leydig cell tumors are not radiosensitive (Freeman 1986).

Sertoli cell tumors are very rare and occur mostly in adolescents (Chang et al. 1998). They are almost always benign and may be associated with a Peutz-Jeghers syndrome. About 24% of patients with Sertoli cell tumors show signs of feminization because of increased estrogen production and symptoms seen in Leydig cell tumors (Gabrilove et al. 1980). Gynecomastia occurs in about 16% of patients with benign and in 60% of patients with malignant Sertoli cell tumors. Orchidectomy is the therapy of choice.

8.20 References

Abramsky L, Chapple J (1997) 47,XXY (Klinefelter syndrome) and 47,XYY: estimated rates of and indication for postnatal diagnosis with implications for prenatal counselling. Prenat Diagn 17:363–368

Adami HO, Arke O, Ekbom A (1997) Epidemiology of testicular cancer. In: Waites GMH, Frick J, Baker GWH (eds) Current advances in andrology (Proceedings of the VIth International Congress of Andrology). Monduzzi Editore, Bologna, pp 264–266

Ahlfeld F (1880) Die Missbildungen des Menschen. Grunow, Leipzig

Aittomäki K, Lucena JLD, Pakaranin P, Sistonen P, Tapanainen J, Gromoll J, Kashikari R, Sankila E-M, Lehväslaiho H, Engel AR, Nieschlag E, Huhtaniemi I, de la Chapelle A (1995) Mutation in the follicle-stimulating hormone receptor gene causes hereditary hypergonadotropic ovarian failure. Cell 82:959–959

Bamberg M, Schmoll HJ, Weißbach L (1997) Diagnostik und Therapie von Hodentumoren. Dtsch Ärztebl 94:c2050–2056

Bates SE (1991) Clinical applications of serum tumor markers. Ann Intern Med 115:623–638

Bergmann M, Behre HM, Nieschlag E (1994) Serum FSH and testicular morphology in male infertility. Clin Endocrinol 40:133–136

Bergmann M, Schleicher G, Böcker R, Nieschlag E (1989) True hermaphroditism with bilateral ovotestis: a case report. J Androl 12:139–147

Berkovitz GD (1992) Disorders of gonadal determination and differentiation. Semin Perinatol 16:289–298

Berthelsen JG, Skakkebaek NE (1983) Gonadal function in men with testis cancer. Fertil Steril 39:68–75

Bosl GJ, Motzer RJ (1997) Testicular germ-cell cancer. N Engl J Med 337:242–253

Breit R (1984) Lower leg ulcers in Klinefelter's syndrome. In: Bandmann HJ, Breit R (eds) Klinefelter's syndrome. Springer, Berlin Heidelberg New York, pp 71–79

Brinkmann B, Brinkmann OA (1993) Orchitis. In: Hertle L, Pohl J (eds) Urologische Therapie. Urban and Schwarzenberg, Munich, pp 454–455

Buetow SA (1995) Epidemiology of testicular cancer. Epidemiol Rev 17:433–449

Bukowski TP, Wacksman J, Billmire DA, Lewis AG, Sheldon CA (1995) Testicular autotransplantation: a 17-year review of an effective approach to the management of the intraabdominal testis. J Urol 154:558–561

Carrell DT, Emery BR, Liu L (1999) Characterization of aneuploidy rates, protamine levels, ultrastructure, and functional ability of round-headed sperm from two siblings and implications for intracytoplasmic sperm injection. Fertil Steril 71:511–516

Chandley AC, Cooke HJ (1994) Human male fertility – Y-linked genes and spermatogenesis. Hum Mol Genet 3:1449–1452

Chang B, Borer JG, Tan PE, Diamond DA (1998) Large-cell calcifying Sertoli cell tumor of the testis: case report and review of the literature. Urology 52:520–523

Chehval MJ, Purcel RN (1992) Deterioration of semen parameters over time in men with untreated varicocele: evidence of progressive testicular damage. Fertil Steril 57:174

Dadoune JP (1988) Ultrastructural abnormalities of human spermatozoa. Hum Reprod 3:311–318

Davenport M, Brain C, Vandenberg C, Zappala S, Duffy P, Ransley PG, Grant D (1995) The use of the hCG stimulation test in the endocrine evaluation of cryptorchidism. Br J Urol 76:790–794

De Braekeleer M, Dao TM (1991) Cytogenetic studies in male infertility: a review. Hum Reprod 6:245–250

Del Castillo EB, Trabucco A, de la Balze A (1947) Syndrome produced by absence of the germinal epithelium without impairment of the Sertoli or Leydig cells. J Clin Endocrinol 7:493

Deutsche Gesellschaft für Endokrinologie (DGE) (1991) Zur Therapie des Hodenhochstandes. Endokrinologie-Informationen, pp 20–22

Dieckmann KP (1993) Carcinoma in situ (testikuläre intraepitheliale Neoplasie) des Hodens. In: Hertle L, Pohl J (eds) Urologische Therapie. Urban and Schwarzenberg, Munich, pp 456–458

Dieckmann KP, Loy V (1993) Testicular intraepithelial neoplasia: the precursor of testicular germ cell tumors. Onkologie 16:61–68

Elsawi MM, Pryor JP, Klufio G, Barnes C, Patton MA (1994) Genital tract function in men with Noonan syndrome. Med Genet 31:468–470

Ergün S, Bruns T, Tauber R (1996) Die vaskuläre Organisation des Plexus pampiniformis beim Mann und ihre Bedeutung bei der antegraden Sklerosierung der Varikozele testis. Urologe A 35:463–467

Evans D, Crichlow RW (1987) Carcinoma of the male breast and Klinefelter's syndrome. Is there an association? CA Cancer J Clin 37:246–251

Fechner PY, Marcantonio SM, Jaswaney V, Stetten G, Goodfellow PN, Migeon CJ, Smith KD, Berkovitz GD (1993) The role of the sex-determining region Y gene in the etiology of 46,XX maleness. J Clin Endocrinol Metabol 76:690–695

Figler TJ, Olson MC, Kinzler GJ (1996) Polyorchidism and rete testis adenoma: ultrasound and MR findings. Abdom Imaging 21:470–472

Foresta C, Ferlin A, Garollo A, Moro E, Pistorello M, Barbaux S, Rossato M (1998) High frequency of well-defined Y chromosome deletions in idiopathic Sertoli cell-only syndrome. Hum Reprod 13:302–307

Forman D, Moller H (1994) Testicular cancer. Cancer Surv 19/20:323–341

Fragoso MC, Latronico AC, Carvalho FM, Zerbini MC, Marcondes JA, Araujo LM, Lando VS, Frazzatto ET, Mendonca BB, Villares SM (1998) Activating mutation of the stimulatory G protein (gsp) as a putative cause of ovarian and testicular human stromal Leydig cell tumors. J Clin Endocrinol Metab 83:2074–2078

Freeman DA (1986) Steroid hormone-producing tumors in man. Endocr Rev 7:204–220

Gabrilove JL, Freiberg EK, Leiter E, Nicolis GL (1980) Feminizing and non-feminizing Sertoli cell tumors. J Urol 124:757–767

Ghiacy S (1996) Case report: ultrasound diagnosis of polyorchidism. Br J Radiol 69:78

Giwercman A, von der Maase H, Skakkebaek NE (1993) Epidemiological and clinical aspects of carcinoma in situ of the testis. Eur Urol 23:104–114

Giwercman A, Clausen OPF, Skakkebaek NE (1988) Carcinoma in situ of the testis: aneuploid cells in semen. Br Med J 296:1762–1764

Giwercman A, Von der Maase H, Berthelsen JG, Rorth M, Bertelsen A, Skakkebaek NE (1991) Localized irradiation of testes with carcinoma in situ: effects on Leydig cell function and eradication of malignant germ cells in 20 patients. J Clin Endocrinol Metab 72:596–603

Giwercman A, Thomsen JK, Hertz J, Berthelsen JG, Jensen V, Meinecke B, Thormann L, Storm HH, Skakkebaek NE (1997) Prevalence of carcinoma in situ of the testis in 207 oligozoospermic men from infertile couples: prospective study of testicular biopsies. B M J 315:989–991

Gohji K, Goto A, Takenaka S, Arakawa S, Matumoto O, Hikosaka K, Kamidono S (1989) Extragonadal germ cell tumor in the retrovesical region associated with Klinefelter's syndrome. A case report and review of the literature. J Urol 141:133–136

Greiner R (1982) Die Erholung der Spermatogenese nach fraktionierter, niedrig dosierter Bestrahlung der männlichen Gonaden. Strahlentherapie 158:342–355

Gromoll J, Simoni M, Nieschlag E (1996) An activating mutation of the follicle-stimulating hormone receptor autonomously sustains spermatogenesis in a hypophysectomized man. J Clin Endocrinol Metab 81:1367–1370

Gromoll J, Eiholzer U, Nieschlag E, Simoni M (2000) Male hypogonadism caused by a homozygous deletion of exon 10 of the luteinizing hormone (LH) receptor: Differential action of human chorionic gonadotropin and LH. J Clin Endocr Metab 85:2496–2501

Hadziselimovic F, Herzog B (1997) Treatment with a luteinizing hormone-releasing hormone analogue after successful orchiopexy markedly improves the chance of fertility later in life. J Urol 158:1193–1195

Hakami M, Mosavy SH (1975) Triorchidism with normal spermatogenesis: an unusual cause for failure of vasectomy. Br J Surg 62:633

Hamilton JB, Mestler GE (1969) Mortality and survival: comparison of eunuchs with intact men and women in a mentally retarded population. J Gerontol 24:395–411

Handelsman DJ, Conway AJ, Boylan LM, Turtle JR (1984) Testicular function in potential sperm donors: normal ranges and the effects of smoking and varicocele. Int J Androl 7:369–382

Hansen PV, Trykker H, Svennekjaer IL, Hvolby J (1990) Long-term recovery of spermatogenesis after radiotherapy in patients with testicular cancer. Radiother Oncol 18:117–125

Hargreave TB (1997) Varicocele: overview and commentary on the results of the WHO varicocele trial. In: Waites GMH, Frick J, Baker GUH (eds) Current advances in andrology. Monduzzi, Bologna, pp 31–44

Hasle H, Mellemgaard A, Nielsen J, Hansen J (1995) Cancer incidence in men with Klinefelter syndrome. Br J Cancer 71:416–420

Hoorweg-Nijman JJG, Havers HM, Delemarre-van de Waal HA (1994) Effect of human chorionic gonadotrophin (hCG)/follicle-stimulating hormone treatment versus hCG treatment alone on testicular descent: a double-blind placebo-controlled study. Eur J Endocrinol 130:60–64

Horowitz M, Wishart JM, O'Loughlin PD, Morris HA, Need AG, Nordin BEC (1992) Osteoporosis and Klinefelter's syndrome. Clin Endocrinol 36:113–118

Hsu LYF (1994) Phenotype/karyotype correlations of Y chromosome aneuploidy with emphasis on structural aberrations in postnatally diagnosed cases. Am J Med Genet 53:108–140

Huff DS, Hadziselimovic F, Sayder III HM, Beyth B, Duckett JW (1991) Early postnatal testicular maldevelopment in cryptorchidism. J Urol 146:624–626

Hutson JM, Hasthorpe S, Heyns CF (1997) Anatomical and functional aspects of testicular descent and cryptorchidism. Endocr Rev 18:259–280

Imbeaud S, Belville C, Messika-Zeitoun L, Rey R, di Clemente N, Josso N, Picard J-Y (1996) A 27 base-pair deletion of the anti-Müllerian type II receptor gene is the most common cause of persistent Müllerian duct syndrome. Hum Molec Genet 5:1269–1277

Jamieson CR, van der Burgt I, Brady AF, van Reen M, Elsawi MM, Hol F, Jeffery S, Patton MA, Mariman E (1994) Mapping a gene for Noonan syndrome to the long arm of chromosome 12. Nat Genet 8:357–360

Jiang M, Aittomäki K, Nilsson C, Pakarinen P, Iitia A, Torresani T, Simonsen H, Goh V, Petterson K, de la Chapelle A, Huhtaniemi I (1998) The frequency of an inactivating point mutation (566C→T) of the human follicle-stimulating hormone receptor gene in four populations using allele-specific hybridization and time-resolved fluorometry. J Clin Endocrinol Metab 83:4338–4343

Josso N, Boussin L, Knebelmann B, Nihoul-Fékété C, Picard JY (1991) Anti-Müllerian hormone and intersex state. Trends Endocrinol Metab 2:227–233

Kaleva M, Arsalo A, Louhimo I, Rapola J, Perheentupa J, Henriksen K, Toppari J (1996) Treatment with human chorionic gonadotrophin for cryptorchidism: clinical and histological effects. Int J Androl 19:293–298

Kamischke A, Gromoll J, Simoni M, Behre HM, Nieschlag E (1999) Transmission of a Y chromosomal deletion involving the deleted in azoospermia (DAZ) and chromodomain (CDY1) genes from father to son through intracytoplasmic sperm injection. Hum Reprod 14:2320–2322

Kostiner DR, Turek PJ, Reijo RA (1998) Male infertility: analysis of the markers and genes on the human Y chromosome. Hum Reprod 13:3032–3038

Kremer H, Kraaij R, Toledo SPA, Post M, Fridman JB, Hayashida CY, van Reen M, Milgrom E, Ropers H-H, Mariman E, Themmen APN, Brunner HG (1995) Male pseudohermaphroditism due to a homozygous missense mutation of the luteinizing hormone receptor gene. Nat Genet 9:160–164

Kuhn JM, Mahoudeau JA, Billaud L, Joly J, Rieu M, Gance A, Archambeaud-Mouveroux F, Steg A, Luton JP (1987) Evaluation of diagnostic criteria for Leydig cell tumors in adult men revealed by gynaecomastia. Clin Endocrinol 26:407–416

Lange R, Michelmann HW, Engel W (1990) Chromosomale Ursachen der Infertilität beim Mann. Fertilität 6:17–28

Latronico AC, Anasti J, Arnhold IJP, Rapaport R, Menodonca BB, Bloise W, Castro M, Tsigos C, Chrousos GP (1996) Testicular and ovarian resistance to luteinizing hormone caused by inactivating mutations of the luteinizing hormone receptor gene. N Engl J Med 334:507–512

Latronico AC, Chai Y, Arnhold IJP, Liu X, Mendonca BB, Segaloff DL (1998) A homozygous microdeletion in helix 7 of the luteinizing hormone receptor associated with familial testicular and ovarian resistance is due to both decreased cell surface expression and impaired effector activation by the cell surface receptor. Mol Endocrinol 12:442–450

Laue L, Wu SM, Kudo M, Hsueh AJ, Cutler Jr GB, Griffin JE, Wilson JD, Brain C, Berry AC, Grant DB (1995) A nonsense mutation of the luteinizing hormone receptor gene in Leydig cell hypoplasia. Hum Mol Gen 4:1429–1433

Laue L, Wu SM, Kudo M, Bourdony CJ, Cutler GB, Hsueh AJW, Chan WY (1996) Compound heterozygous mutations of the luteinizing hormone receptor gene in Leydig cell hypoplasia. Mol Endocrinol 10:987–997

Laven JSE, Haans CF, Mali WPTM, te Velde ER, Wensing CJG, Eimers JM (1992) Effect of varicocele treatment in adolescents: a randomized study. Fertil Steril 58:756

Lee MM, Donahoe PK, Silverman BL, Hasegawa T, Hasegawa Y, Gustafson ML, Chang Y, MacLaughlin DT (1997) Measurements of serum Müllerian inhibiting substance in the evaluation of children with nonpalpable gonads. N Engl J Med 336:1480–1486

Lee PA (1993) Fertility in cryptorchidism. Adolesc Endocrinol 22:479–490

Lemcke B, Zentgraf J, Behre HM, Kliesch S, Nieschlag E (1996) Long-term effects on testicular function of high-dose testosterone treatment for excessively tall stature. J Clin Endocrinol Metab 81:144–152

Leung AK (1988) Polyorchidism. Am Fam Physician 38:153–156

Liu G, Duranteau L, Carel JC, Monroe J, Doyle DA, Shenker A (1999) Leydig cell tumors caused by an activating mutation of the gene encoding the luteinizing hormone receptor. N Engl J Med 341:1731–1736

Liu J, Nagy Z, Joris H, Tournaye H, Devroey P, van Steirteghem A (1995) Successful fertilization and establishment of pregnancies after intracytoplasmic sperm injection in patients with globozoospermia. Hum Reprod 10:626–629

Lobocarro J-M, Medlej R, Berta P, Belon C, Galifer R-B, Guthmann J-P, Chevalier C, Czernichow P, Dumas R, Sultan C (1993) PCR analysis and sequencing of the SRY sex determining gene in four patients with bilateral congenital anorchia. Clin Endocrinol 38:197–201

Loy V, Dieckmann KP (1993) Prevalence of contralateral testicular intraepithelial neoplasia (carcinoma in situ) in patients with testicular germ cell tumor. Eur Urol 23:120–122

Madgar I, Weissenberg R, Lunenfeld B, Karasik A, Goldwasser B (1995) Controlled trial of high spermatic vein ligation for varicocele in infertile men. Fertil Steril 63:120–124

Marsman JWP, Schats R (1994) Review: the subclinical varicocele debate. Hum Reprod 9:1–8

Martens JWM, Verhoef-Post M, Abelin N, Ezabella M, Toledo SPA, Brunner HG, Themmen APN (1998) A homozygous mutation in the luteinizing hormone receptor causes partial Leydig cell hypoplasia: correlation between receptor activity and phenotype. Mol Endocrinol 12:775–784

Martin-du Pan RC, Campana A (1993) Physiopathology of spermatogenic arrest. Fertil Steril 60:937–946

McElreavey K, Fellous M (1997) Sex-determining genes. Trends Endocrinol Metab 8:342–346

McElreavey K, Krausz C (1999) Male infertility and the Y chromosome. Am J Hum Genet 64:928–933

Merlino GT, Stahle C, Jhappan C, Linton R, Mahon KA, Willingham MC (1991) Inactivation of an epidermal growth factor receptor transgene whose product is overexpressed and comparmentalized during spermatogenesis. Genes Dev 5:1395–1406

Meschede D, Horst J (1999) Indikationen, Möglichkeiten, Grenzen und Perspektiven cytogenetischer Untersuchungen für die Reproduktionsmedizin. Med Genetik 11:365–368

Meschede D, Froster UG, Gullotta F, Nieschlag E (1993) Reproductive failure in a patient with neurofibromatosis-Noonan syndrome. Am J Med Genet 47:346–351

Meschede D, Louwen F, Eiben B, Horst J (1997) Intracytoplasmic sperm injection pregnancy with fetal trisomy 9p resulting from a balanced paternal translocation. Hum Reprod 12:1913–1914

Misrahi M, Meduri G, Pissard S, Bouvattier C, Beau I, Loosfelt H, Jolivet A, Rappaport R, Milgrom E, Bougneres P (1997) Comparison of immunocytochemical and molecular features with the phenotype in a case of incomplete male pseudohermaphroditism associated with a mutation of the luteinizing hormone receptor. J Clin Endocrinol Metab 82:2159–2165

Mitamura T (1992) Chinese eunuchs. The structure of intimate politics. Tuttle Company, Rutland, Tokyo

Montag M, van der Ven K, Ved S, Schmutzler A, Prietl G, Krebs D, Peschka B, Schwanitz G, Albers P, Haidl G, van der Ven H (1997) Success of intracytoplasmic sperm injection in couples with male and/or female chromosome aberrations. Hum Reprod 12:2635–2640

Mordel N, Mor-Yosef S, Margalioth EJ et al (1990) Spermatic vein ligation as treatment for male infertility. J Reprod Med 35:123–127

Nagao RR, Plymate SR, Berger RE, Perin EB, Paulsen CA (1986) Comparison of gonadal function between fertile and infertile men with varicoceles. Fertil Steril 46:930–933

Narita O, Manba S, Nakanishi T, Ishizuka N (1975) Pregnancy and childbirth in a true hermaphrodite. Obstet Gynecol 45:593–595

Neugebauer DCh, Neuwinger J, Jockenhövel F, Nieschlag E (1990) 9+0 axoneme in spermatozoa and some nasal cilia of a patient with totally immotile spermatozoa associated with thickened sheath and short midpiece. Hum Reprod 5:981–986

Niedzilski J, Paduch D, Raczynski P (1997) Assessment of adolescent varicocele. Pediatr Surg Int 12:410–413

Nielsen J, Pelsen B, Sornensen K (1988) Follow-up of 30 Klinefelter males treated with testosterone. Clin Genet 33:262–269

Nieschlag E (1992) Testosteron, Anabolika und aggressives Verhalten bei Männern. Dtsch Ärztebl 89:2967–2972

Nieschlag E, Behre HM, Schlingheider A, Nashan D, Pohl J, Fischedick AR (1993a) Surgical ligation vs. angiographic embolization of the vena spermatica: a prospective rendomized study for the treatment of varicocele-related infertility. Andrologia 25:233–237

Nieschlag E, Nieschlag S, Behre HM (1993b) Lifespan and testosterone. Nature 366:215

Nieschlag E, Hertle L, Fischedick A, Abshagen K, Behre HM (1998) Update on treatment of varicocele: counselling as effective as occlusion of the vena spermatica. Hum Reprod 13:2147–2150

Nieschlag E, Simoni M, Gromoll J, Weinbauer GF (1999) Role of FSH in the regulation of spermatogenesis: clinical aspects. Clin Endocrinol 51:139–146

Nilsson S, Edvinsson A, Nilsson B (1979) Improvement of semen and pregnancy rate after ligation and division of the internal spermatic vein: fact or fiction? Br J Urol 51:591

Nöske H-D, Weidner W (1999) Varicocele – a historical perspective. World J Urol 17:151–157

Ortkemper H (1993) Engel wider Willen: Die Welt der Kastraten. Henschel, Berlin

O'Sullivan DC, Biyani CS, Heal MR (1995) Polyorchidism: causation and management. Postgrad Med J 71:317–318

Petersen PM, Giwercman A, Skakkebaek NE, Rorth M (1998) Gonadal function in men with testicular cancer. Semin Oncol 25:224–233

Propping P (1989) Psychiatrische Genetik. Springer, Berlin Heidelberg New York, pp 307–315

Pyörälä S, Huttunen N-P, Uhari M (1995) A review and meta-analysis of hormonal treatment of cryptorchidism. J Clin Endocrinol Metab 80:2795–2799

Ratcliffe SG (1994) The psychological and psychiatric consequences of sex chromosome abnormalties in children, based on population studies. In: Poustka F (ed) Basic approaches to genetic and molecularbiolological developmental psychiatry. Quintessenz, Berlin, pp 99–122

Reubinoff BE, Abeliovich D, Werner M, Schenker JG, Safran A, Lewin A (1998) A birth in non-mosaic Klinefelter's syndrome after testicular fine needle aspiration, intracytoplasmic sperm injection and preimplantation genetic diagnosis. Hum Reprod 13:1887–1892

Rodriguez-Rigau L, Smith K, Steinberger E (1978) Relationship of varicocele to sperm output and fertility of male partners in infertile couples. J Urol 120:691–694

Rovet J, Netley C, Bailey J, Keenan M, Stewart D (1995) Intelligence and achievement in children with extra X aneuploidy: a longitudinal perspective. Am J Med Genet (Neuropsychiatr Genet) 60:356–363

Rüther U, Stilz S, Röhl E, Nunnensiek Ch, Rassweiler J, Dörr U, Jipp P (1995) Successful interferon-alpha therapy for a patient with acute mumps orchitis. Eur Urol 27:174–176

Savage MO, Lowe DG (1990) Gonadal neoplasia and abnormal sexual differentiation. Clin Endocrinol 32:519–533

Schoeneich G, Brändle E (1994) Therapiealternativherhalten bei idiopathischer Varicocele testis. Aktuel Urol 25:272–276

Schulze W, Thoms F, Knuth UA (1999) Testicular sperm extraction: comprehensive analysis with simulataneously performed histology in 1418 biopsies from 766 subfertile men. Hum Reprod 14:82–96

Sharland M, Burch M, McKenna WM, Paton MA (1992) A clinical study of Noonan syndrome. Arch Dis Child 67:178–183

Sharland M, Morgan M, Smith G, Burch M, Paton MA (1993) Genetic counselling in Noonan syndrome. Am J Med Genet 45:437–440

Simoni M, Gromoll J, Dworniczak B, Rolf C, Abshagen K, Kamischke A, Carani C, Meschede D, Horst J, Behre HM, Nieschlag E (1997) Screening for deletions of the Y chromosome involving the DAZ (Deleted in Azoospermia) gene in azoospermia and severe oligozoospermia. Fertil Steril 67:542–547

Simoni M, Gromoll J, Höppner W, Kamischke A, Krafft T, Stahle D, Nieschlag E (1999a) Mutational analysis of the follicle-stimulating hormone (FSH) receptor in normal and infertile men: identification and characterization of two discrete FSH receptor isoforms. J Clin Endocrinol Metab 84:751–755

Simoni M, Bakker E, Eurlings MCM, Matthijs G, Moro E, Müller CR, Vogt PH (1999b) Laboratory guidelines for molecular diagnosis of Y-chromosomal microdeletions. Int J Androl 22:292–299

Slaney SF, Chalmers, IJ, Affaar NA, Chitty LS (1998) An autosomal or X linked mutation results in true hermaphrodites and 46,XX males in the same family. J Med Genet 35:17–22

Staessen C, Coonen E, Van Assche E, Tournaye H, Joris H, Devroey P, Van Steirteghem AC, Liebaers I (1996) Preimplantation diagnosis for X and Y normality in embryos from three Klinefelter patients. Hum Reprod 11:1650–1653

Stavrou SS, Zhu YS, Cai LQ, Katz MD, Herrera C, Defillo-Ricart M, Imperato-McGinley J (1998) A novel mutation of the human luteinizing hormone receptor in 46XY and 46XX sisters. J Clin Endocrinol Metab 83:2091–2098

Tapanainen JS, Aittomaki K, Min J, Vaskivuo T, Huhtaniemi I (1997) Men homozygous for an inactivating mutation of the follicle-stimulating hormone (FSH) receptor gene present variable suppression of spermatogenesis and fertility. Nat Genet 15:205–206

Templeton A, Cooke I, Shaugh O'Brien PM (eds) (1998) Evidence-based fertility treatment. Royal College of Obstetricians and Gynecologists Press, London, p 399

Terzoli G, Simoni G, Lalatta F, Colucci G, Lobbiani A (1992) Fertility in a 47,XXY patient: assessment of biological paternity by deoxyribonucleic acid fingerprinting. Fertil Steril 58:821–825

Themmen AP, Martens JW, Brunner HG (1998) Activating and inactivating mutations in LH receptors. Mol Cell Endocrinol 145:137–142

Toledo SPA, Brunner HG, Kraaij, R, Post M, Dahia PLM, Hayashida CY, Kremer H, Themmen APN (1996) An inactivating mutation of the luteinizing hormone receptor causes amenorrhea in a 46,XX female. J Clin Endocrinol Metab 81:3850–3854

Van Assche E, Bonduelle M, Tournaye H, Joris H, Verheyen G, Devroey P, van Steirteghem A, Liebaers I (1996) Cytogenetics of infertile men. Hum Reprod 11 [Suppl 4]:1–26

Van Niekerk WA (1974) True hermaphroditism. Clinical, morphological and cytogenetic aspects. Harper and Row, New York

Vermeulen A, Vandeweghe M, Deslypere JP (1986) Prognosis of subfertility in men with corrected or uncorrected varicocele. J Androl 7:147–155

Vogt PH, Edelmann A, Kirsch S, Henegariu O, Hirschmann P, Kiesewetter F, Kohn FM, Schill WB, Farah S, Ramos C, Hartmann M, Hartschuh W, Meschede D, Behre HM, Castel A, Nieschlag E, Weidner W, Grone HJ, Jung A, Engel W, Haidl G (1996) Human Y chromosome azoospermia factors (AZF) mapped to different subregions in Yq11. Hum Mol Genet 5:933–943

von Eckardstein S, Simoni M, Bergmann M, Weinbauer GF, Gassner P, Schepers AG, Nieschlag E (1999) Serum inhibin B in combination with serum follicle-stimulating hormone (FSH) is a more sensitive marker than serum FSH alone for impaired spermatogenesis in men, but cannot predict the presence of sperm in testicular tissue samples. J Clin Endocrinol Metab 84:2496–2501

Wagenseil F (1933) Chinesische Eunuchen (Zugleich ein Beitrag zur Kenntnis der Kastrationsfolgen und der rassialen und körperbaulichen Bedeutung der anthropologischen Merkmale). Z Morphol Anthropol 32:415–468

Weil D, Wang I, Dietrich A, Poustka A, Weissenbach J, Petit C (1994) Highly homologous loci on the X and Y chromosomes are hot-spots for ectopic recombinations leading to XX maleness. Nat Genet 7:414–419

Weinbauer GF, Behr R, Bergmann M, Nieschlag E (1998) Testicular cAMP responsive element modulator (CREM) protein is expressed in round spermatids but is absent or reduced in men with round spermatid maturation arrest. Mol Hum Reprod 4:9–15

Wille R (1991) Kastration in Deutschland. Dt Ärztebl 88:95–96

Wishahi MM (1991) Anatomy of the venous drainage of the human testis: testicular vein cast, microdessection and radiographic demonstratin. A new anatomical concept. Eur Urol 20:154–160

WHO Laborhandbuch zur Untersuchung des menschlichen Ejakulats und der Spermien/Zervixschleim-Interaktion (1999). Übersetzung: Nieschlag E, Nieschlag S, Bals-Pratsch M, Behre HM, Knuth UA, Meschede D, Niemeier M, Schick A, 4th edn. Springer, Berlin Heidelberg New York

Wu SM, Hallermeier KM, Laue L, Brain C, Berry AC, Grant DB, Griffin JE, Wilson JD, Cutler GB Jr, Chan WY (1998) Inactivation of the luteinizing hormone/chorionic gonadotropin receptor by an insertional mutation in Leydig cell hypoplasia. Mol Endocrinol 12:1651–1660

CHAPTER 9

Diseases of the Seminal Ducts

9

H. M. BEHRE · E. NIESCHLAG · D. MESCHEDE

9.1 Infections of the Seminal Ducts

9.1.1 Etiology and Pathogenesis

Infections of the seminal ducts can lead to male infertility by different mechanisms. **Direct damage** is caused by microorganisms or their secretory products, while **secondary inflammation** is produced by increased numbers of activated leukocytes and an elevated secretion of lymphokines and monokines. In addition, increased formation of reactive oxygen species (ROS) can reduce the fertilization capacity of the spermatozoa (De Geyter et al. 1994; Comhaire et al. 1999; Weidner et al. 1999). Infections can also lead to **uni- or bilateral obstructions** of the seminal ducts, **formation of antibodies** against sperm and **dysfunction of ejaculation** (Purvis and Christiansen 1993; WHO 1999; Paschke et al. 1994a). Furthermore, an acute epididymitis can lead to infection of the testis **(epididymoorchitis).**

Whereas obstructive azoospermia caused by the classic venereal diseases, such as **gonorrhoea**, was formerly a common reason for male infertility among European men (i. e. before antibiotics became generally available), nowadays **Chlamydia trachomatis** and **Mycoplasma spp**, and particularly **Ureaplasma urealyticum**, as well as **gram-negative bacteria typical of urogenital infections** are the predominant microorganisms causing an infection of the seminal ducts (Paavonen and Eggert-Kruse 1999; Weidner et al. 1999). The infections are manifested along the seminal ducts (see Chap. 4, Fig. 4.1) in the forms of **urethritis, prostatitis, vesiculitis** or **epididymitis,** but can often present without clinical symptoms. **Balanitis** is without known influence on fertility. For **orchitis** see Sect. 8.5.

9.1.2 Clinical Picture and Diagnosis

Acute **epididymitis** is characterized by scrotal pain as well as local swelling and tenderness; it can cause fever and general malaise. Sonography of the scrotal content allows direct visualization of the epididymides, which are enlarged and hypo-echoic when inflamed. The testis can be involved in the process as epididymo-orchitis. The type of pathogen varies with the age of the patient. Among younger men infections are often caused by *Chlamydia trachomatis* and *Neisseria gonorrhoeae* (Weidner et al. 1999). *Escherichia coli, Pseudomonas aeruginosa* and typical bacteria for urinary tract infections are more common in older men. *Chronic epididymitis* with infiltrations, which occur in approximately 15% of patients, can eventually lead to scar formation in the tubules and thereby to obstruction. In these patients, extended diagnostics of infections, uroflowmetry and sonography are needed. When findings are pathological, diagnostic work-up can be completed by cystoscopy, voiding cystourethrography and manometry.

According to the National Institutes of Health (NIH; Nickel 1998), **prostatitis** is classified as follows:

- **Acute bacterial prostatitis** (category I: leukocytes and uropathogenic bacteria in expressed prostatic secretions).
- **Chronic bacterial prostatitis** (category II: leukocytes and uropathogenic bacteria in expressed prostatic secretions; chronic or recurrent infections).
- **Chronic abacterial prostatitis** (category IIIA: leukocytes in expressed prostatic secretions or ejaculate, no detection of uropathogenic bacteria; category IIIB: no leukocytes or uropathogenic bacteria in expressed prostatic secretions or ejaculate).
- **Asymptomatic inflammatory prostatitis** (category IV: leukocytes in expressed prostatic secretions or ejaculate, no clinical symptoms).

More than 10–15 leukocytes per high-power field (×1000) in expressed prostatic secretions or ≥3 leukocytes per high-power field in the urine after prostate massage can be considered as significant (Weidner et al. 1999). Only in case of purulent prostatic secretions is the **four-specimen test** for bacterial localization to be applied for further diagnostics.

Acute prostatitis can be diagnosed by acute febrile symptoms and the detection of the respective pathogens. A prostatic abscess is characterized by typical rectal palpation, positive urinary culture and an abscess cavity in transrectal ultrasonography (see Sect. 6.3.4). The diagnostics of **chronic prostatitis** can be difficult because of uncharacteristic rectal palpation. The main indications for diagnosis are the detection of leukocytes in urine, expressed prostatic specimens, and ejaculate. A chronic bacterial prostatitis is probable, if the number of pathogens in the urine is ten times higher after prostate massage compared to urine before (Nickel 1998). *Escherichia coli* is the most common pathogen in bacterial prostatitis (Weidner et al. 1999).

Inflammation of the seminal glands (**vesiculitis**) is not a distinct entity but appears clinically as male **adnexitis** or **prostatovesiculitis**. The symptoms of **prostatovesiculitis** can range from non-specific complaints in the perineal region to an acute clinical picture with high fever, purulent bacterial inflammation and abscesses. Tenderness to pressure and pasty consistency of the prostate and seminal gland can be found at rectal palpation. Hematospermia is a characteristic symptom (Mukelwitz et al. 1997; Furuya et al. 1999). Patients with prostatovesiculitis often show inhomogeneities or calcifications of the prostate, intraprostatic cysts, cysts of the ejaculatory ducts, and enlargements, asymmetries, disturbances of depletion and cysts of the seminal vesicles. In addition to clinical symptoms, increased numbers of leukocytes or pathogenic bacteria in the native ejaculate or after prostatic massage are typical for the diagnosis of prostatovesiculitis.

Patients with manifest **urethritis** complain of dysuria and urethral discharge, itching or pain. Redness of the glans and external orificium are typical. Infectious urethritis is often caused by *Neisseria gonorhoeae, Chlamydia trachomatis* and *Ureaplasma urealyticum* (Schiefer 1998). If urethral discharge is not present, the detection of granulocytes (≥15 per microscopic field at 400×) in the sediment of 3 ml of the first part of voided bladder urine is pathognomonic.

In infertile men inflammations of the seminal ducts are often **clinically silent**. Sometimes these patients have previously had infections of the urinary tract or **sexually transmitted diseases** (STD).

The suspicion of an infection of the seminal ducts has to be clarified by **microbiological investigations**. The microorganisms can be identified directly from the **ejaculate, prostate exprimate** or a **urethral swab**. A concentration of 1,000 colony forming units/ml ejaculate of gram-negative bacteria typical of urogenital infections or Ureaplasma urealyticum is significant (Ludwig et al. 1994; Weidner 1999). It must be emphasized, however, that the detection of Chlamydia trachomatis infection by culture is complicated by the presence of cytotoxic components of the seminal plasma. For this reason, the indirect proof of the infection by determination of IgA- or IgG-antibodies against chlamydia in seminal plasma has been widely used in the clinic. Studies applying direct detection of chlamydia-DNA by means of the polymerase chain reaction (**PCR**) show, however, no direct association between antibodies and the actual presence of microorganisms in the ejaculate (Dieterle et al. 1995). Therefore, PCR detection can be considered as more reliable in the diagnosis of chlamydia infections (Paavonen and Eggert-Kruse 1999).

If direct detection of microorganisms is not possible, an **increased leukocyte concentration (>1 million/ml ejaculate)** is often indicative of infection. The detection of granulocytes by peroxidase staining (see Sect. 6.5.2) is sufficient in most cases (Wang et al. 1994); however, an exact characterization of the leukocyte subpopulations and their level of activity is only possible by **immunocytology** (Wolff 1995). It should be noted, however, that leukocytospermia is not always associated with bacterial or viral infections (Trum et al. 1998). In addition to the determination of leukocytes, biochemical markers of inflammation (granulocyte elastase, complement factor C3, ceruloplasmin) have been used to detect infection of the seminal ducts. Increased concentration of **granulocyte elastase** (>600 ng/ml ejaculate) indicate infection (Ludwig et al. 1998).

Seminal duct infections can also lead to increased ejaculate viscosity, lower ejaculate volume, increased pH, as well as to decreased levels of the markers for accessory gland function in the ejaculate (e.g. α-**glucosidase** for the epididymis, **fructose** for the seminal vesicles, **zinc** for the prostate gland, see Sect. 6.5.3) (Comhaire et al. 1989; Cooper et al. 1990; WHO 1999).

In individual cases, diagnosis of an infection of the seminal ducts can be complicated, since neither normal leukocyte concentrations nor the failure to detect microorganisms in the ejaculate can categorically exclude an infection. Therefore, for practical reasons, the combination of a significant number of microorganisms and an increased leukocyte concentration in the ejaculate or the combination of one of these parameters with clinical symptoms is required for the diagnosis of an infection of the seminal ducts (WHO 1993).

9.1.3 Therapy

The therapy of an infection in the seminal ducts should be based on the respective microorganisms and the resistogram (Krieger 1995; Seligson et al. 1998). **Tetracyclines** are the drugs of choice for **Chlamydia trachomatis** infections (e. g. doxycycline 2×100 mg/d p.o. for 7–10 days). **Ureaplasma urealyticum** infections can be treated with **tetracyclines** (dosage as above) or **erythromycin** (2 g/d p.o. for 7–10 days). Because of a high co-infection with chlamydia trachomatis, **gonorrhea** is treated with **ofloxacin** (400 mg p.o. single dose), **ciprofloxacin** (500 mg p.o. single dose) or **cefixim** (400 mg p.o. single dose) **in combination with tetracyclines.** An uncomplicated **epididymitis** should be treated with **ceftriaxone** (250 mg i.m. single dose) **in combination with** 2×100 mg/d **doxycycline** p.o. for 10 days. **Gardnerella vaginalis** or **Trichomonas vaginalis** infections are treated with tinidazol (2 g p.o., single dose).

Acute, bacterial prostatitis is treated for 14 days with fluorochinolones (ciprofloxacin, ofloxacin) and in many instances with additional suprapubic tube urine drainage. Chronic bacterial prostatitis is treated with fluorochinolones for four weeks. If unsuccessful, patients should receive long-term therapy with 50 mg/d trimethoprim or nitrofurantoin for 3–6 months. Causal therapy of abacterial prostatitis is not possible.

Four to eight weeks after the completion of a course of antibiotic treatment the patients should be re-examined to test for therapeutic efficacy. It must be remembered, however, that antibiotics can temporarily lead to a deterioration of the ejaculate parameters and fertilization capacity (De Geyter et al. 1994) as a result of direct negative effects on spermatogenesis and sperm function (Schlegel et al. 1991).

The **simultaneous diagnosis and therapy of the female partner** is highly important for effective therapy of an infection of the seminal ducts, as otherwise "ping-pong"-infections between both partners may occur (see Chap. 14). Circumcision can be regarded as effective prevention of infections of the seminal ducts as well as HIV infections (Moses et al. 1998).

9.2 Obstructions of the Seminal Ducts

9.2.1 Etiology and Pathogenesis

Obstructions of the seminal ducts can occur in the epididymis and the deferent and ejaculatory ducts (see Fig. 4.1). In addition to congenital aplasia of the deferent duct and bilateral obstruction of the ejaculatory ducts, which is described separately in Sect. 9.3 and 9.4, and the rare Young syndrome (see Sect. 9.5), acute or chronic epididymitis or inflammations of the seminal vesicles and prostate gland can lead to obstruction (see Sect. 9.1, Table 9.1). Iatrogenic obstruction can be a complication arising from a herniotomy (particularly in childhood), from operations in the region of the ejaculatory ducts, and vasography of the seminal ducts with irritating contrast media. Sperm recovery from the epididymis [**PESA** (percutaneous epididymal sperm aspiration), more rarely **MESA** (microsurgical epididymal sperm aspiration)] or inadvertently performed incisions or biopsies of the epididymis lead, in most cases, to an iatrogenic obstruction. Bilateral vasectomy can be regarded as an acquired obstruction of the seminal ducts.

Recent investigations show that alterations in the region of the ejaculatory ducts can cause obstructions of the seminal ducts more frequently than formerly thought. Examples are utricular or intraprostatic cysts, in which external pressure can lead to obstruction of the ejaculatory ducts (see Fig. 9.1), or internal stenosis and cystic enlargements of the ejaculatory ducts (Pryor and Hendry 1991; Meacham et al. 1993) (see Sect. 9.4.5).

Table 9.1. Causes of obstruction in the seminal ducts

Epididymis	Acute or chronic epididymitis (past or present) (Accidental) incision or biopsy of the epididymis PESA (percutaneous epididymal sperm aspiration), MESA (microsurgical epididymal sperm aspiration) Young syndrome
Deferent duct	Aplasia/hypoplasia of the deferent duct and distal epididymis Vasectomy Vasography with irritant contrast media Herniotomy with accidental ligation of the deferent duct
Ejaculatory duct	Congenital cysts (utricular cysts), prostatic cysts, cysts of the seminal vesicles Infection Trauma Postoperative

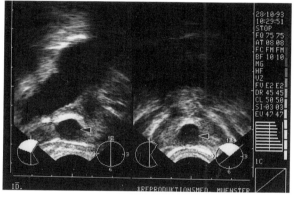

Fig. 9.1. Large utricular cyst (◄) with secondary obstruction of the ejaculatory ducts as demonstrated by transrectal ultrasonography

9.2.2 Clinical Picture

Complete bilateral obstruction of the seminal ducts leads to **azoospermia** and therefore to infertility. A **unilateral obstruction can be compensated completely** by the contralateral side, if this testis and seminal ducts are intact, and thus may remain symptomless. **Partial obstructions** on both sides can lead, according to the degree of obstruction, to a significant deterioration of the ejaculate parameters with severe oligo(asthenoterato)zoospermia.

If the obstruction is proximal to the ejaculatory ducts, the **ejaculate volume** generally remains normal, since the largest part of the seminal plasma originates from the seminal vesicles and prostate gland. A distal obstruction, however, leads to parvisemia (ejaculate volume < 2 ml).

9.2.3 Diagnosis

Obstructive azoospermia is the principal differential diagnosis of **normal testicular volume, normal FSH** in combination with **azoospermia** (see Fig. 6.9). Thickening and induration of the epididymis, and aplasia or hypoplasia of the deferent duct can be detected by palpation. **Ultrasonography** of the scrotal content allows direct imaging of the epididymis (see Sect. 6.3.1), while changes in the region of the prostate gland and seminal vesicles (infectious alterations, anomalies, cysts in the area of the ejaculatory ducts) are detected by transrectal ultrasonography (Fig. 9.1, see Sect. 6.3.4).

The most helpful variables for differential diagnosis of an obstruction are the **marker substances** for the **epididymis** (α-glucosidase), **seminal vesicle** (fructose) **and prostate gland** (zinc) in the seminal plasma (see Sect. 6.5.3). If a patient has a bilateral obstruction, marker substances secreted above the level of obstruction are not demonstrable in the ejaculate, while the levels of the markers secreted by organs distal to the obstruction are normal. Differential diagnosis can be difficult if the obstruction is unilateral or only partial. A **bilateral testicular biopsy** for the evaluation of spermatogenesis is recommended before any interventional therapy. This will allow identification of conditions such as spermatogenetic arrest, which can be found in patients with normal testicular volume and normal FSH, and an unsuccessful microsurgical reanastomosis attempt can be avoided.

9.2.4 Therapy

In patients with an obstruction of the seminal ducts and at least qualitatively normal spermatogenesis confirmed by histology, a **vasoepididymostomy** (epididymal obstruction) or a **vasovasostomy** (e. g. after vasectomy, see

Sect. 20.2) can be performed. The success of the operation as regards patency of the seminal ducts is dependent on the primary cause of obstruction, its duration and the surgical technique employed (Belker et al. 1991). In obstructive azoospermia, microsurgical techniques are superior to techniques of assisted reproduction regarding long-term pregnancy rates and costs and should be applied on first instance (Kolettis and Thomas 1997). The patient must be informed, however, that even if patency is re-established, fertility can remain reduced because of anti-sperm antibodies (see Sect. 9.7), and that a secondary obstruction can occur.

In principle, **microsurgical techniques** should be used for epididymo- or vasovasostomy because of higher patency rates. Preferably they should be performed in specialized centers, as the success rate clearly rises with the number of microsurgical operations per year performed by one operating team (Schlegel and Goldstein 1993).

Transurethral resection of obstructed ejaculatory ducts and cysts can lead to significant improvements in ejaculate parameters and pregnancy rates (Meacham et al. 1993).

If patency of the seminal ducts cannot be achieved, or microsurgery is contraindicated because of the anatomical conditions, direct microsurgical sperm aspiration from the epididymis (**MESA**) or sperm extraction from the testis (**TESE**) in combination with **assisted fertilization** [ICSI (intracytoplasmic sperm injection)] can be offered to the couple (see Sect. 17.5.2). Here, spermatozoa aspirated from the epididymis should, in parallel, be cryopreserved for a possible second ICSI attempt or if another pregnancy is desired in the future (see Chap. 18). Because of variability of anatomical structures, increased trauma and inferior efficacy, **fine needle biopsy or direct sperm aspiration from the testis or epididymis** should not be applied for sperm recovery (Ezeh et al. 1998; Sperling 1999; Tournaye 1999).

9.3 Cystic Fibrosis

9.3.1 Etiology and Pathogenesis

Cystic fibrosis (CF) is one of the most **common autosomal recessive disorders** in Caucasian populations, where it affects approximately one in 2,500 children. Until recently, only pediatricians were concerned with cystic fibrosis. Improved therapy allows increasing numbers of these patients to reach adulthood. The current mean life expectancy for Middle European CF patients has reached 30 years and is further increasing. While formerly fertility and parenthood could not be considered for individuals affected with CF, these issues are now gaining importance in the clinical management of the disorder.

Mutations in the CFTR gene are the basic cause of cystic fibrosis. The acronym CFTR is derived from "cystic fibrosis transmembrane conductance regulator", a name that points to the function of the CFTR protein as a membrane-bound ion channel. Extending over 230,000 base pairs and 27 exons, CFTR is a large gene. Since it was cloned in 1989 more than 800 different mutations have been characterized. Among patients of Middle European ancestry $\Delta F508$ is responsible for 70% of the CF alleles. This is a 3 base pair deletion resulting in the loss of a phenylalanine residue on the protein level. About 10 other mutations are responsible for a further 10–15% of CF alleles. All other mutations are exceedingly rare. Owing to the size of the gene and the highly heterogenous mutational spectrum, routine analysis characterizes only 85% of all CF alleles. There is a limited correlation between clinical phenotype and the type of mutation (Kerem and Kerem 1996). Probably other genes can modify the effects of CFTR mutations. This would explain the considerable clinical variability observed in patients with an identical CFTR genotype (Zielenski et al. 1999).

9.3.2 Clinical Picture and Diagnosis

The CFTR protein is strongly expressed in the **airway epithelia**, where it acts as a regulator of electrolyte transport. If the protein is deficient or dysfunctional because of a mutation, the bronchial secretions become abnormally viscous. Obstruction and bacterial colonization of the airways ensue, and progressive impairment of lung function and right ventricular failure develop as secondary complications. The pulmonary disease process usually determines the long-term course of cystic fibrosis. 85% of the patients have **pancreatic insufficiency**. Meconium ileus is a severe complication of CF in the newborn.

An **increased sweat chloride concentration** is the laboratory hallmark of cystic fibrosis (Stern 1997). Sweat secretion must be stimulated by local pilocarpin electrophoresis. To provide reliable results, the test needs to be carried out under strictly standardized conditions. Owing to its susceptibility to technical error, this diagnostic procedure should be performed only by laboratories with special expertise. A sweat chloride concentration of more than 60 mmol/l is diagnostic of CF. Borderline levels in the range from 40 to 60 mmol/l neither exclude nor confirm cystic fibrosis and are difficult to interpret.

Obstructive azoospermia is found **in more than 95%** of all men affected with CF. Most have a bilateral congenital occlusion of the proximal vas deferens or the epididymis (Kaplan et al. 1968). However, in some patients it is impossible to determine the exact level of the seminal duct obstruction (Wilschanski et al. 1996).

In typical cases the intrascrotal portion of the **vas is either totally absent or reduced to a cordlike structure** without a lumen. Mostly, the **epididymal corpus and cauda** are **hypo- or aplastic. The head of the epididymis,** not a derivative of the Wolffian ducts, is usually preserved and markedly **dilated.** Most men with CF have an **intact testicular parenchyma,** but nonspecific histological abnormalities are occasionally observed. These probably result from the long-term obstruction of the seminal ducts or the poor general health of these men. Sonography of the testes sometimes shows calcifications, cystic or hypoechogenic areas (Wilschanski et al. 1996). Aplasia of the deferent duct and epididymis is typically associated with **abnormalities of the seminal vesicles,** the latter being quite variable from patient to patient. Aplasia or hypoplasia, obstruction, dilatation and cystic degeneration may be observed. The seminal vesicle anomalies explain the almost universal finding of a **subnormal ejaculate volume.**

A small **minority of male CF patients** have **normal or only gradually impaired fertility.** They tend to have a **generally milder course of the disease.** Pancreatic function is often preserved, and the destruction of lung tissue proceeds at a slower pace than usual. Many of these patients are compound heterozygotes for the ΔDF508 and the 3849+10 kb C$\rightarrow$T mutations (Stern et al. 1995).

The **diagnostic work-up** of men with CF does not principally deviate from the standard procedures employed for other forms of obstructive azoospermia (see Sect. 7.2). Measurement of ejaculate volume, pH, and **fructose and α-glucosidase** concentrations (or other markers of seminal vesicle and epididymal function) is of particular importance. The vas deferens and epididymal malformations may be diagnosable by **scrotal palpation,** but this is not universally the case (Wilschanski et al. 1996). The ampullary vas deferens, the ejaculatory ducts and the seminal vesicles can be visualized by **transrectal ultrasound.** If treatment by assisted reproduction is considered, the integrity of spermatogenesis should be checked by **testicular biopsy.** This is not only of value for histology, but at the same time sperm can be extracted and cryopreserved. In fact, this therapeutic aspect is now a major reason for performing testicular biopsy (see below).

9.3.3 Therapy

As cystic fibrosis is an autsomal recessive disorder, it can recur in the offspring of CF patients only when the partner is also affected or heterozygous. While the former should be rare, asymptomatic carriership for CF is common in Caucasian populations. The heterozygote frequency ranges around 4–5%. For this reason, **CFTR gene mutation analysis** for the **female partners** of male cystic fibrosis patients is essential. If routine testing in the partner does not reveal a mutation and her family history is negative for cystic fibrosis, the residual risk for CF in offspring of the couple is only about 0.5%. On the other hand, the risk may be up to 50% if the partner tests positive for a CFTR mutation. The percentages given here are only applicable to patients of German ancestry. For individuals with another ethnic background the risk calculation must be modified, as both the prevalence and the spectrum of CFTR mutations show strong regional variation (Stuhrmann 1998).

Infertile couples in whom one of the partners is affected with CF should undergo **genetic counselling** prior to initiation of treatment. This also provides an opportunity to discuss the options of **prenatal diagnosis** (see Sect. 17.14). If an infertile couple desires treatment despite a significant recurrence risk for CF, this can be accepted as an autonomous decision (Meschede et al. 1997a). There is broad consensus that eugenic considerations should have no place in deciding about the fertility treatment for patients with heritable disorders. This notwithstanding, the physician is obliged to clarify the potentially grave implications for the health for the couple's children. In azoospermic patients with CF, **surgical reconstruction** of the seminal ducts is impossible. **Assisted reproduction** therefore represents the only workable option for these patients to have biological children. With microsurgical techniques, spermatozoa can be retrieved from the epididymis or directly from the testicular parenchyma (**MESA or TESE,** see Sect. 9.2) for subsequent **intracytoplasmic sperm injection (ICSI).** Conventional IVF is not advisable because of poor pregnancy rates.

9.4. Congenital Absence of the Vas Deferens

9.4.1 Etiology and Pathogenesis

Congenital bilateral absence of the vas deferens (CBAVD) occurs as an **isolated anomaly** or as **part of the systemic disease CF** (see Sect. 9.3) (De Braekeleer and Férec 1996; Meschede et al. 1998). Traditionally, these two variants have been treated as separate entities, which, from a clinical point of view, is still appropriate. However, molecular studies have clearly shown that most cases of "isolated" CBAVD represent a **minor variant of cystic fibrosis** and are caused by mutations in the CFTR gene (Dörk et al. 1997; Stuhrmann 1998).

Only a general outline of the complex **molecular pathology** of CBAVD can be given here. CFTR gene mutations are broadly classified into "severe" and "mild". While the former result in full-blown CF when present in the state of homozygosity, the latter are associated with less pronounced phenotypic abnormalities, such as chronic bronchitis. Apart from these mutations, a polymorphism in intron 8 of the CFTR gene plays an important role in the molecular pathology of CBAVD. The polymorphic sequence consists of either 5, 7 or 9 thymidine residues, also known as the 5 T, 7 T and 9 T alleles, respectively. While the 7 T and the 9 T alleles are functionally neutral, the 5 T allele interferes with the splicing of the CFTR mRNA (Rave-Harel et al. 1997). A high percentage of mRNA lacks exon 9, and it cannot be translated into active CFTR protein. From a functional perspective, the 5 T allele is similar to a "mild" mutation.

A valid rule of thumb is that patients with **full-blown CF** carry **two severe CFTR mutations**. In contrast, the most common genotypes of men with **CBAVD** are heterozygosity for a **severe and a mild mutation** or a **severe mutation and a 5 T allele**. An intensified molecular screen of the CFTR gene reveals two mutations or one mutation plus a 5 T allele in 75 % of men with CBAVD, a single mutation or 5 T allele in another 10 %, and no mutation or 5 T allele in 15 % (Dörk et al. 1997). Routine laboratory protocols have a somewhat lower yield of positive findings.

As indicated by molecular family studies and painstaking clinical analysis, 10 %–20 % of CBAVD cases are not due to CFTR gene mutations (Rave-Harel et al. 1995; Jarvi et al. 1998; Stuhrmann 1998). Notably, almost every patient with CBAVD and concomittant **renal anomalies** (unilateral aplasia, ectopy, horseshoe kidney) is mutation-negative. This is also true for men with CBAVD and normal ultrasound anatomy of the seminal vesicles and ampullary vas deferens. Obviously, congenital bilateral absence of the vas deferens is an **etiologically heterogenous** condition.

9.4.2 Clinical Picture and Diagnosis

The **anatomical abnormalities** of the genital tract and the ejaculate parameters are similar in CBAVD and cystic fibrosis (see Sect. 9.3.2). Azoospermic men carrying a CFTR mutation have a significantly **lower volume, pH and fructose concentration of the ejaculate** than fertile men or azoospermic patients without a detectable mutation (see Fig. 9.2) (Eckardstein et al. 2000).

Urinary tract anomalies have an increased prevalence in men with CBAVD and point to the disease variant not associated with CFTR mutations. A **renal ultrasound** should be performed routinely for all men with CBAVD.

Every second patient with CBAVD reports symptoms indicative of **mild upper airway disease**. Recurrent bronchitis and sinusitis is quite typical, as is a history of pneumonia in infancy or childhood. Importantly, a progressive worsening of the bronchopulmonary symp-

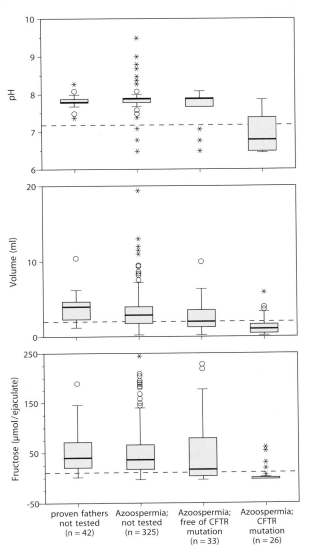

Fig. 9.2. PH (*upper panel*), volume (*middle panel*), and fructose concentration (*lower panel*) of the ejaculate in 42 proven fathers, 325 azoospermic patients, 33 azoospermic patients free of CFTR mutations and 26 patients with known CFTR mutations (Eckardstein et al. 2000)

toms does not occur. Occasionally signs and symptoms of maldigestion are reported, which may be due to mild pancreatic dysfunction. Some patients have somewhat elevated liver enzymes. The sweat chloride concentration may exceed the upper normal limit of 60 mmol/l, but this is not the rule (Meschede et al. 1995; Stuhrmann 1998; Dohle et al. 1999).

9.4.3 Therapy

As in cystic fibrosis, assisted reproduction for patients with CBAVD should be preceded by **genetic counselling**. CFTR mutation analysis in the female partner is of utmost importance. The risk for CF in children of the couple is usually low if the female partner has no detectable mutation. Otherwise, the risk for cystic fibrosis in any child of the couple may amount to 25–50%. The risk figures given here do not universally apply to all couples. Family history and ethnic background may modify them substantially (Stuhrmann 1998).

Sperm retrieval through **MESA** or **TESE** and **subsequent ICSI** is now the standard therapeutic approach to male infertility due to CBAVD (see Sect. 9.2. and 9.3). The pregnancy rates are not notably affected by the presence of a CFTR mutation (Schlegel et al. 1995; Silber et al. 1995).

9.4.4 Unilateral Absence of the Vas Deferens

Congenital unilateral absence of the vas deferens (CU-AVD) is compatible with **normal fertility**, and probably many cases never come to clinical attention. The diagnosis may be made accidentally on occasion of a vasectomy. However, unilateral vas deferens aplasia is occasionally found in men with abnormal semen parameters or even azoospermia. Strictly speaking, this condition should be referred to as unilateral "intrascrotal" vas deferens aplasia, as the distal parts of the vas are inaccessible to palpation. Many patients with CUAVD have a **contralateral obstruction of the seminal ducts** at a more distal level. Most patients from this particular group (azoospermia, unilateral vas deferens aplasia, more distal contralateral obstruction) carry **mutations of the CFTR gene**. In contrast, such mutations are rare among men with CUAVD who have a patent seminal duct on the other side. Similar to CBAVD, unilateral vas deferens aplasia is sometimes accompanied by **urinary tract anomalies**, most notably unilateral renal agenesis. These patients usually have no detectable mutation in the CFTR gene (Mickle et al. 1995).

9.4.5 Bilateral Obstruction of the Ejaculatory Ducts

The short intraprostatic segment of the vas deferens distal to the seminal vesicles is called the ejaculatory duct (see Chap. 4, Fig. 4.1). An obstruction at this level of the seminal ducts result in **azoospermia** and a **subnormal volume, pH and fructose content of the ejaculate**. Once CBAVD has been ruled out, this constellation is pathognomonic of ejaculatory duct obstruction. Transrectal ultrasound allows this abnormality to be visualized. The obstruction can be caused by accidental or iatrogenic trauma, infections, tumours, prostatic calcifications, or cysts (Pryor and Hendry 1991; Meacham et al. 1993; Werthman 1999). Patients may present with symptoms similar to acute or chronic prostatitis. Others report pain on ejaculation or hematospermia. The **surgical management** of ejaculatory duct obstruction must be tailored to the individual anatomical situation (Pryor and Hendry 1991; Meacham et al. 1993; Werthman 1999).

In some men with this disease none of the above mentioned etiologies is apparent. This probably represents a constitutional disorder, as substantiated by the finding of CFTR gene mutations in most of these patients (Meschede et al. 1997b). Apparently this form of ejaculatory duct obstruction is another **minor variant of cystic fibrosis**. Genetic diagnosis and counselling follow the procedures as for CBAVD.

An attempt at removing the obstruction by the transurethral route may be undertaken. If this fails (or as the primary therapeutic approach), surgical sperm retrieval with MESA or TESE with consecutive intracytoplasmic sperm injection is applicable.

9.5 Young Syndrome

9.5.1 Etiology and Pathogenesis

The combined occurence of **obstructive azoospermia** and **chronic sinobronchial disease** is the hallmark of Young syndrome (Young 1970). Although there may be similarities in presentation, it is clinically and etiologically distinct both from CF and congenital absence of the vas deferens (Handelsman et al. 1984).

Azoospermia in Young syndrome is caused by an obstruction in the middle segment in the epididymis, the lumen being occluded at this level by an **amorphous mass**. Several patients have been reported to have fathered children before the diagnosis was made, and biological parenthood was confirmed by genetic testing. This makes it likely that the occlusion develops over time in a primarily unobstructed epididymis, perhaps through inspissated secretions. Young syndrome is notable for the absence of structural abnormalities of the vas deferens, epididymis, and seminal vesicles. Volume and fructose content of the ejaculate are normal, another feature distinguishing this condition from CF and CBA-VD. Testicular palpation, biopsy, and measurement of FSH and the other reproductive hormones usually yield normal results. Quantitative electron microscopy shows that the sperm tails of men with Young syndrome more often than usual lack the central pair of microtubules, the radial spokes or the inner dynein arms. This may result in impaired ciliary and sperm tail function (Wilton et al. 1991).

9.5.2 Clinical Picture and Diagnosis

Patients affected with Young syndrome have a characteristic history of coughing, sputum production, and recurrent sinobronchitis since early infancy. These problems usually improve during adolescence. **Bronchiectases** are a frequent finding, but lung involvement does not progress as in CF. Pulmonary function tests may reveal some minor abnormalities. This does usually not have a perceptible effect on general physical fitness. Pancreatic function and sweat chloride levels levels are normal; again, in contrast to CF.

It is unclear whether Young syndrome has a genetic or an environmental basis. Some affected sibs have been reported, but familial aggregation is the exception rather than the rule. Because of the clinical similarities with CF, the CFTR gene (see Sect. 9.3) has been analyzed in men with Young syndrome. The largest study addressing this issue had a negative result (Le Lannou et al. 1995). However, other authors have occasionally demonstrated CFTR mutations in patients with Young syndrome (Hirsh et al. 1993; Wellesey and Schwarz 1998). Perhaps these were cases of atypical cystic fibrosis or CBAVD.

9.5.3 Therapy

Attempts at surgically deobstructing the seminal ducts have met with no or only temporary success. Sperm retrieval from the epididymis or testis by means of **MESA** or **TESE** and subsequent **intracytoplasmic sperm injection** are thus the therapeutic options of choice for patients who wish to have children.

9.6 Disorders of Liquefaction

The human ejaculate normally liquefies within 20 minutes after ejaculation. Non-liquefaction can cause infertility. Since the liquefaction of the ejaculate is an enzyme-dependent process for which – in addition to the release rate of phosphate and the levels of free reducing sugars – a peptidase and proteinase similar to collagenase are responsible, the addition of α-**amylase** (Vermeiden et al. 1989) or α-**chymotrypsin** (Freischem et al. 1983) to the ejaculate can lead to an increased pregnancy rate after insemination or IVF.

9.7 Immunological Infertility

9.7.1 Etiology and Pathogenesis

Meiotic and postmeiotic male germ cells express surface antigens that occur neither on somatic cells nor on premeiotic germ cells. During contact with immunocompetent cells, these antigens are recognized as foreign, and an autoimmune reaction can be initiated. Normally this reaction is prevented by the blood-testis barrier, which is formed by the Sertoli cells, and other immunoregulatory mechanisms (see Sect. 3.1.2). If the integrity of the blood-testis barrier is destroyed (e. g. by trauma, operation such as vasectomy, infection), **anti-sperm antibodies** can be produced. The association of anti-sperm antibodies with anti-nuclear and thyroglobulin-antibodies in serum suggests an "autoimmune disposition" of affected patients (Paschke et al. 1994b).

Anti-sperm antibodies can be detected in seminal plasma, either unbound or bound to spermatozoa, and in serum. In the ejaculate, **antibodies** of the **IgG- and IgA-class** are found almost exclusively, the latter are of particular clinical relevance. Anti-sperm antibodies can lead to infertility, as they impair sperm motility or reduce sperm penetration into the cervical mucus. Furthermore, they can interfere with the acrosome reaction and with sperm binding to the zona pellucida of the oocyte (Bandoh et al. 1992; Francavilla et al. 1997; Harrison et al. 1998; Hjort 1999).

9.7.2 Clinical Picture

The only clinical correlate for the existence of anti-sperm antibodies is otherwise unexplained **infertility**, which can be associated with normozoospermia or isolated astheno(terato)zoospermia (Fig. 9.3). **Vasectomized men** have a high prevalence of anti-sperm antibodies, which may increase following surgery. Therefore, anti-sperm antibodies in the ejaculate should be determined routinely after microsurgical reanastomosis of the vas. Previous **infections** (see Sect. 9.1) are of importance, since they can also lead to antibody formation.

9.7.3 Diagnosis

Sperm agglutinations in the fresh semen sample are suggestive of anti-sperm antibodies and may be caused by antibodies attached to spermatozoa. Their presence is determined by the direct **MAR test** (mixed antiglobu-

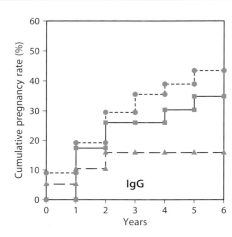
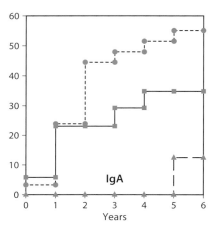

Fig. 9.3. Cumulative pregnancy rate in patients with anti-sperm antibodies. *Circles*, proportion of anti-sperm antibody coated sperm 10–49 %: *squares*, 50–90 %; *triangles*, >90 %. *Left panel*, IgG anti-sperm antibodies; *right panel*, IgA anti-sperm antibodies (Abshagen et al. 1998)

lin reaction test) (see Sect. 6.5.4), which should be the method of choice for anti-sperm antibody detection, being superior to other tests (e.g. the **immunobead test** or **tray agglutination test [TAT]**) because of its accuracy and biological relevance (Andreou et al. 1995). Due to high inter-assay variability, the detection of anti-sperm antibodies by the indirect MAR test is of minor clinical relevance (Bohring and Krause 1999).

Detection of anti-sperm antibodies does not always allow the diagnosis of immunological infertility. Immunological infertility is probable if **more than 50 % sperm are bound to IgG- or IgA-antibodies** (Abshagen et al. 1998; WHO 1999). A thorough diagnosis of possible seminal duct infections should be performed in MAR-positive patients, particularly if IgA-antibodies are detected (see Sect. 9.1). If a genital infection with more than 1 million/ml leukocytes in the ejaculate is present simultaneously, a repetition of the MAR test after successful antibiotic treatment is recommended (Paschke et al. 1994a).

The clinical significance of anti-sperm antibodies in the ejaculate or in the cervical mucus of the partner should be further clarified by sperm-mucus-interaction tests (see Sect. 6.6.2 and 14.2.4.5). Antibodies against sperm in the serum of either the man or the woman have no clinical relevance and, therefore, need not be determined (Kohl et al. 1992; Andreou et al. 1995).

Anti-sperm antibodies can also be detected by **flow cytometry** (Räsänen et al. 1992). This method is particularly suited for the diagnosis of immunological infertility, since IgG- and IgA-antibodies (and possibly other anti-sperm antibodies) can be determined simulta-

neously on individual spermatozoa. Dead sperm, which bind antibodies non-specifically, can be sorted out by flow cytometry, and thousands of sperm measured within a few seconds (Räsänen et al. 1992). Flow cytometry has the additional advantage that not only the presence of anti-sperm antibodies but also the exact number of the different types of antibodies on the surface of the spermatozoa can be determined (Räsänen et al. 1992). Whether a more exact diagnosis and more highly differentiated classification of immunological infertility will be made possible by flow cytometry and whether the sorting of antibody-bound and unbound sperm will lead to new therapeutic options for the infertile couple, has not yet been demonstrated by randomized clinical studies.

9.7.4 Therapy

Immunosuppressive therapy of immunological infertility with **corticosteroids** resulted in an improvement of the pregnancy rate in only 2 of 4 randomized studies (Table 9.2). Lengthy treatment seems to be required for the success of this therapy but this leads to corticosteroid-induced side-effects including significant decreases of bone mineral density in up to 60 % of the patients (Hendry et al. 1990; Sharma et al. 1995; Pearce et al. 1998). It has been shown by flow cytometry that corticosteroid therapy may only be effective on sperm with low numbers of attached anti-sperm antibodies (Räsänen et al. 1996).

Intrauterine insemination or **in vitro fertilization** are of minor efficacy in patients with anti-sperm antibodies (Vazquez-Levin et al. 1997), and additional corticosteroid therapy will not improve pregnancy rates (Lahteenmaki et al. 1995; Grigoriou et al. 1996). In patients with significant anti-sperm antibodies, intracytoplasmic sperm injection can be regarded as the therapy of choice (Clarke et al. 1997).

Table 9.2. Prospective, randomized studies with corticosteroids for treatment of immunological infertility in man

Author	Therapy	Observation time	Number of couples	Pregnancy rate (%)
Haas/Manganiello 1987	Verum Placebo	3 cycles	20 15	15 7 n.s.
Hendry et al. 1990	Verum Placebo (Cross-over design)	9 months	33 21	27 4 p<0.05
Bals-Pratsch et al. 1992	Verum Placebo (Cross-over design)	3 cycles	20 20	0 0
Omu et al. 1996	Verum No therapy	12–18 months	40 37	20 5 p<0.01

9.8 References

Abshagen K, Behre HM, Cooper TG, Nieschlag E (1998) Influence of sperm surface antibodies on spontaneous pregnancy rates. Fertil Steril 70:355–356

Andreou E, Mahmoud A, Vermeulen L, Schoonjans F, Comhaire F (1995) Comparison of different methods for the investigation of antisperm antibodies on spermatozoa, in seminal plasma and in serum. Hum Reprod 10:125–131

Bals-Pratsch M, Dören M, Karbowski B, Schneider HPG, Nieschlag E (1992) Cyclic corticosteroid immunosuppression is unsuccessful in the treatment of sperm antibody-related male infertility: a controlled study. Hum Reprod 7:99–104

Bandoh R, Yamano S, Kamada M, Daitoh T, Aono T (1992) Effect of sperm-immobilizing antibodies on the acrosome reaction of human spermatozoa. Fertil Steril 57:387–392

Belker AM, Thomas AJ, Fuchs EF (1991) Results of 1,469 microsurgical reversals by vasovasostomy study group. J Urol 145:505–511

Bohring C, Krause W (1999) The intra- and inter-assay variation of the indirect mixed antiglobulin reaction test: is a quality control suitable? Hum Reprod 14:1802–1805

Clarke GN, Bourne H, Baker HW (1997) Intracytoplasmic sperm injection for treating infertility associated with sperm autoimmunity. Fertil Steril 68:112–117

Comhaire FH, Vermeulen L, Pieters O (1989) Study of the accuracy of physical and biochemical markers in semen to detect infectious dysfunction of the accessory sex glands. J Androl 10:50–53

Comhaire FH, Mahmoud AM, Depuydt CE, Zalata AA, Christophe AB (1999) Mechanisms and effects of male genital tract infection on sperm quality and fertilizing potential: the andrologist's viewpoint. Hum Reprod Update 5:393–398

Cooper TG, Weidner W, Nieschlag E (1990) The influence of inflammation of the human male genital tract on secretion of the seminal markers alpha-glucosidase, glycerophosphocholine, carnitine, fructose and citric acid. Int J Androl 13:329–336

De Braekeleer M, Férec C (1996) Mutations in the cystic fibrosis gene in men with congenital bilateral absence of the vas deferens. Mol Hum Reprod 2:669–677

De Geyter C, De Geyter M, Behre HM, Schneider HPG, Nieschlag E (1994) Peroxidase-positive round cells and microorganisms in human semen together with antibiotic treatment adversely influence the outcome of in vitro fertilization and embryo transfer. Int J Androl 17:127–134

Dieterle S, Mahony JB, Luinstra KE, Stibbe W (1995) Chlamydial immunoglobulin IgG and IgA antibodies in serum and semen are not associated with the presence of Chlamydia trachomatis DNA or rRNA in semen from male partners of infertile couples. Hum Reprod 10:315–319

Dörk T, Dworniczak B, Aulehla-Scholz C, Wieczorek D, Böhm I, Mayerova A, Seydewitz HH, Nieschlag E, Meschede D, Horst J, Pander H-J, Sperling H, Ratjen F, Passarge E, Schmidtke J, Stuhrmann M (1997) Distinct spectrum of CFTR gene mutations in congenital absence of vas deferens. Hum Genet 100:365–377

Dohle GR, Veeze HJ, Overbeek SE, van den Ouweland AMW, Halley DJJ, Weber RFA, Niermeijer MF (1999) The complex relationship between cystic fibrosis and congenital bilateral absence of the vas deferens: clinical, electrophysiological and genetic data. Hum Reprod 14:371–374

Eckardstein von S, Cooper TG, Rutsch K, Meschede D, Horst J, Nieschlag E (2000) Seminal plasma characteristics as indicators of cystic fibrosis transmembrane conductance regulator (CFTR) gene mutations in men with obstructive azoospermia. Fertil Steril 73:1226–1231

Ezeh UI, Moore HD, Cooke ID (1998) A prospective study of multiple needle biopsies versus a single open biopsy for testicular sperm extraction in men with non-obstructive azoospermia. Hum Reprod 13:3075–3080

Francavilla F, Romano R, Santucci R, Marrone V, Properzi G, Ruvolo G (1997) Interference of antisperm antibodies with the induction of the acrosome reaction by zona pellucida (ZP) and its relationship with the inhibition of ZP binding. Fertil Steril 67:1128–1133

Freischem CW, Bordt J, Hanker JP, Schneider HPG, Nieschlag E (1983) Schwangerschaft nach Behandlung des Ejakulates mit α-Chymotrypsin wegen fehlender Liquefizierung. Geburtsh Frauenheilkd 43:490–491

Furuya S, Ogura H, Saitoh N, Tsukamoto T, Kumamoto Y, Tanaka Y (1999) Hematospermia: an investigation of the bleeding site and underlying lesions. Int J Urol 6:539–547

Grigoriou O, Konidaris S, Antonaki V, Papadias C, Antoniou G, Gargaropoulos A (1996) Corticosteroid treatment does not improve the results of intrauterine insemination in male subfertility caused by antisperm antibodies. Eur J Obstet Gynecol Reprod Biol 65:227–230

Haas GG, Manganiello P (1987) A double-blind, placebo-controlled study of the use of methylprednisolone in infertile men with sperm-associated immunoglobulins. Fertil Steril 47:295–301

Handelsman DJ, Conway AJ, Boylan LM, Turtle JR (1984) Young's syndrome. Obstructive azoospermia and chronic sinopulmonary infections. N Engl J Med 310:3–9

Harrison S, Hull G, Pillai S (1998) Sperm acrosome status and sperm antibodies in infertility. J Urol 159:1554–1558

Hendry WF, Hughes L, Scammell G, Pryor JP, Hargreave TB (1990) Comparison of prednisolone and placebo in subfertile men with antibodies to spermatozoa. Lancet 335:85–88

Hirsh A, Williams C, Williamson B (1993) Young's syndrome and cystic fibrosis mutation ΔDF508. Lancet 342:118

Hjort T (1999) Antisperm antibodies. Antisperm antibodies and infertility: an unsolvable question? Hum Reprod 14(10): 2423–2426

Jarvi K, McCallum S, Zielenski J, Durie P, Tullis E, Wilchanski M, Margolis M, Asch M, Ginzburg B, Martin S, Buckspan MB, Tsui L-C (1998) Heterogeneitiy of reproductive tract abnormalities in men with absence of the vas deferens: role of cystic fibrosis transmembrane conductance regulator gene mutations. Fertil Steril 70:724–728

Kaplan E, Shwachman H, Perlmutter AD, Rule A, Khaw K-T, Holsclaw DS (1968) Reproductive failure in males with cystic fibrosis. N Engl J Med 279:65–69

Kerem B, Kerem E (1996) The molecular basis for disease variability in cystic fibrosis. Eur J Hum Genet 4:65–73

Kohl B, Kohl H, Krause W, Deichert U (1992) The clinical significance of antisperm antibodies in infertile couples. Hum Reprod 10:1384–1387

Kolettis PN, Thomas AJ Jr (1997) Vasoepididymostomy for vasectomy reversal: a critical assessment in the era of intracytoplasmic sperm injection. J Urol 158:467–470

Krieger JN (1995) New sexually transmitted diseases treatment guidelines. J Urol 154:209–213

Lahteenmaki A, Rasanen M, Hovatta O (1995) Low-dose prednisolone does not improve the outcome of in-vitro fertilization in male immunological infertility. Hum Reprod 10:3124–3129

Le Lannou D, Jezequel P, Blayau M, Dorval I, Lemoine P, Dadabie A, Roussey M, Le Marec B, Legall JY (1995) Obstructive azoospermia with agenesis of vas deferens or with bronchiectasia (Young's syndrome): a genetic approach. Hum Reprod 10:338–341

Ludwig M, Kümmel C, Diemer T, Ringert RH (1994) Ejakulatinfektionen durch sexuell übertragbare Erreger. Urologe A 33:203–210

Ludwig M, Kümmel C, Schroeder-Prinzen I, Ringert RH, Weidner W (1998) Evaluation of seminal plasma parameters in patients with chronic prostatitis of leukocytospermia. Andrologia 30 [Suppl 1]:41–47

Meacham RB, Hellerstein DK, Lipshultz LI (1993) Evaluation and treatment of ejaculatory duct obstruction in the infertile male. Fertil Steril 59:393–397

Meschede D, Dworniczak B, Eigel A, Behre HM, Bergmann M, Schulze Everding A, Fischer R, Horst J, Nieschlag E (1995) Mutationsanalyse und genetische Beratung bei Männern mit kongenitaler Aplasie der Samenleiter. Fertilität 11:22–26

Meschede D, Nieschlag E, Horst J (1997a) Assisted reproduction for infertile couples at high genetic risk: an ethical consideration. Biomed Ethics 2:4–6

Meschede D, Dworniczak B, Behre HM, Kliesch S, Claustres M, Nieschlag E, Horst J (1997b) CFTR gene mutations in men with bilateral ejaculatory-duct obstruction and anomalies of the seminal vesicles. Am J Hum Genet 61:1200–1202

Meschede D, Dworniczak B, Nieschlag E, Horst J (1998) Genetic disorders of the seminal ducts. Biomed Pharmacother 52:197–203

Mickle J, Milunsky A, Amos JA, Oates RD (1995) Congenital unilateral absence of the vas deferens: a heterogenous disorder with two distinct subpopulations based upon aetiology and mutational status of the cystic fibrosis gene. Hum Reprod 10:1728–1735

Moses S, Bailey RC, Ronald AR (1998) Male circumcision: assessment of health benefits and risks. Sex Transm Infect 74:368–373

Munkelwitz R, Krasnokutsky S, Lie J, Shah SM, Bayshtok J, Khan SA (1997) Current perspectives on hematospermia: a review. J Androl 18:6–14

Nickel JC (1998) Prostatitis: myths and realities. Urology 51:362–366

Omu AE, al-Qattan F, Abdul Hamada B (1996) Effect of low dose continuous corticosteroid therapy in men with antisperm antibodies on spermatozoal quality and conception rate. Eur J Obstet Gynecol Reprod Biol 69:129–134

Paavonen J, Eggert-Kruse W (1999) Chlamydia trachomatis: impact on human reproduction. Hum Reprod Update 5:433–447

Paschke R, Schulze Bertelsbeck D, Bahrs S, Heinecke A, Behre HM (1994a) Seminal sperm antibodies exhibit an unstable spontaneous course and an increased incidence of leucocytospermia. Int J Androl 17:135–139

Paschke R, Schulze Bertelsbeck D, Tsalimalma K, Nieschlag E (1994b) Association of sperm antibodies with other autoantibodies in infertile men. Am J Reprod Immunol 32:88–94

Pearce G, Tabensky DA, Delmas PD, Baker HW, Seeman E (1998) Corticosteroid-induced bone loss in men. J Clin Endocrinol Metab 83:801–806

Pryor JP, Hendry WF (1991) Ejaculatory duct obstruction in subfertile males: analysis of 87 patients. Fertil Steril 56:725–730

Purvis K, Christiansen E (1993) Infection in the male reproductive tract. Impact, diagnosis and treatment in relation to male infertility. Int J Androl 16:1–13

Räsänen ML, Hovatta OL, Penttilä IM, Agrawal YP (1992) Detection and quantification of sperm-bound antibodies by flow cytometry of human semen. J Androl 13:55–64

Räsänen M, Lahteenmaki A, Agrawal YP, Saarikoski S, Hovatta O (1996) A placebo-controlled flow cytometric study of the effect of low-dose prednisolone treatment on sperm-bound antibody levels. Int J Androl 19:150–154

Rave-Harel N, Madgar I, Goshen T, Nissim-Rafinia M, Zaidni A, Rahat A, Chiba O, Kalman YM, Brautbar C, Levison D, Augarten A, Kerem E, Kerem B (1995) CFTR haplotype analysis reveals genetic heterogeneity in the etiology of congenital bilateral aplasia of the vas deferens. Am J Hum Genet 56:1359–1366

Rave-Harel N, Kerem E, Nissim-Rafinia M, Madjar I, Goshen R, Augarten A, Rahat A, Hurwitz A, Darvasi A, Kerem B (1997) The molecular basis of partial penetrance of splicing mutations in cystic fibrosis. Am J Hum Genet 60:87–94

Schiefer HG (1998) Microbiology of male urethroadnexitis: diagnostic procedures and criteria for aetiologic classification. Andrologia 30 [Suppl 1]:7–13

Schlegel PN, Goldstein M (1993) Microsurgical vasoepididymostomy: refinements and results. J Urol 150:1165–1168

Schlegel PN, Chang TSK, Marshall FF (1991) Antibiotics: potential hazards to male fertility. Fertil Steril 55:235–242

Schlegel PN, Cohen J, Goldstein M, Alikani M, Adler A, Gilbert BR, Palermo GD, Rosenwaks Z (1995) Cystic fibrosis gene mutations do not affect sperm function during in vitro fertilization with micromanipulation for men with bilateral congenital absence of vas deferens. Fertil Steril 64:421–426

Seligson RA, Pollack CV Jr, Section Editors, Talan DA, Moran GJ, Pinner RW (1998) Update on emerging infections: news from the Centers for Disease Control and Prevention. Ann Emerg Med 32:748–750

Sharma KK, Barratt CLR, Pearson MJ, Cooke ID (1995) Oral steroid therapy for subfertile males with antisperm antibodies in the semen: prediction of the responders. Hum Reprod 10:103–109

Silber SJ, Nagy Z, Liu J, Tournaye H, Lissens W, Férec C, Liebaers I, Devroey P, van Steirteghem AC (1995) The use of epididymal and testicular spermatozoa for intracytoplasmic sperm injection: the genetic implications for male infertility. Hum Reprod 10:2031–2043

Sperling H (1999) Operative sperm retrieval – the urological aspects. Urologe A 38:563–568

Stern RC (1997) The diagnosis of cystic fibrosis. N Engl J Med 336:487–491

Stern RC, Doershuk CF, Drumm ML (1995) 3849+10 kb C→T mutation and disease severity in cystic fibrosis. Lancet 346:274–276

Stuhrmann M (1998) Das klinische Spektrum von Fertilitätsstörungen durch Mutationen im CFTR-Gen. Reproduktionsmedizin 14:54–65

Trum JW, Mol BW, Pannekoek Y, Spanjaard L, Wertheim P, Bleker OP, van der Veen F (1998) Value of detection leukocytospermia in the diagnosis of genital tract infection in subfertile men. Fertil Steril 70:315–319

Tournaye H (1999) Surgical sperm recovery for intracytoplasmic sperm injection: which method is to be preferred? Hum Reprod 14(Suppl. 1):71–81

Vazquez-Levin MH, Notrica JA, Polak de Fried E (1997) Male immunologic infertility: sperm performance on in vitro fertilization. Fertil Steril 68:675–681

Vermeiden JPW, Bernardus RE, ten Brug CS, Statema-Lohmeijer CH, Willemsen-Brugma AM, Schoemaker J (1989) Pregnancy rate is significantly higher in in vitro fertilization procedure with spermatozoa isolated from nonliquefying semen in which liquefaction is induced by α-amylase. Fertil Steril 51:149–152

Wang AW, Politch J, Anderson D (1994) Leukocytospermia in male infertility patients in China. Andrologia 26:167–172

Weidner W, Krause W, Ludwig M (1999) Relevance of male accessory gland infection for subsequent fertility with special focus on prostatitis. Hum Reprod Update 5:421–432

Weiske WH (1994) Infertilität beim Mann: Diagnostik und Therapie. Thieme, Stuttgart

Wellesey D, Schwarz M (1998) Cystic fibrosis, Young's syndrome, and normal sweat chloride. Lancet 352:38

Werthman PE (1999) Disorders of ejaculation and ejaculatory duct obstruction. Infert Reprod Med Clin North Amer 10:517–537

WHO Laborhandbuch zur Untersuchung des menschlichen Ejakulats und der Spermien-Zervikalschleim-Interaktion (1999) Übersetzung von: Nieschlag E, Nieschlag S, Bals-Pratsch M, Behre HM, Knuth UA, Meschede D, Niemeier M, Schick A, 4th edn. Springer, Berlin Heidelberg New York

WHO Manual for the standardized investigation and diagnosis of the infertile couple (1993) Rowe PJ, Comhaire FH, Hargreave TB, Mellows HJ (eds). Cambridge University Press, Cambridge

Wilschanski M, Corey M, Durie P, Tullis E, Bain J, Asch M, Ginzburg B, Jarvi K, Backspan M, Hartwick W (1996) Diversity of reproductive tract abnormalities in men with cystic fibrosis. JAMA 276:607–608

Wilton LJ, Teichtahl H, Temple-Smith PD, Johnson JL, Southwick GJ, Burger HG, de Kretser DM (1991) Young's syndrome (obstructive azoospermia and chronic sinobronchial infection): a quantitative study of axonemal ultrastructure and function. Fertil Steril 55:144–151

Wolff H (1995) The biological significance of white blood cells in semen. Fertil Steril 63:1143–1157

Young D (1970) Surgical treatment of male infertility. J Reprod Fertil 23:541–542

Zielenski J, Corey M, Rozmahel R, Markiewicz D, Aznarez I, Casals T, Larriba S, Mercier B, Cutting GR, Krebsova A, Macek M, Langfelder-Schwind E, Marshall BC, DeCelie-Germana J, Claustres M, Palacio A, Bal J, Nowakowska A, Ferec C, Estivill X, Durie P, Tsui L-C (1999) Detection of cystic fibrosis modifier locus for meconium ileus on human chromosome 19q13. Nat Genet 22:128–129

CHAPTER 10

Disorders of Sperm Deposition

10

H. van Ahlen · L. Hertle

There are numerous functional and anatomical disturbances that can interfere with male sexuality. Purely mechanical disturbances of semen deposition due to anatomical features have to be differentiated from functional disturbances of libido and orgasm, from ejaculation disorders and the inability to achieve or maintain a rigid erection which allows penetration. While in the vast majority of cases disorders of orgasm are of psychological origin, disturbances of libido may be due to hormonal imbalance and can be a symptom of androgen deficiency. Further symptoms such as alterations of the secondary sexual characteristics or of semen volume point to organic origin. While functional disturbances of orgasm and libido fall into the realm of psychological and psychiatric or endocrinological therapy, this chapter deals mainly with disturbances of semen deposition and functional or organic impairment of erection.

10.1 Anatomical Penile Alterations

Congenital or acquired anatomical abnormalities of the penis may interfere with cohabitation and normal deposition of semen. These congenital anatomical variations especially include abnormal position of the urethral meatus (hypospadias/epispadias), but also, among acquired alterations, penile deviations due to Peyronie's disease which represents the most common clinical problem.

10.1.1 Hypospadias and Epispadias

In **hypospadias** the **urethra** does not extend to the glans and the meatus is situated on the **underside of the penis**. Depending on the severity of the abnormality, the meatus can be located at varying distance from the regular position somewhere between the glans and the perineum. In the majority of cases, **glandular**, **coronal** or **distal penile cases** are observed, severe **penoscrotal** or even **perineal forms** represent only a relatively small percentage.

In the vast majority of cases **surgical correction** with a distal advancement of the meatus within the first two years of life will allow normal sperm deposition. Therefore, patients with a straight penis and distal position and normal caliber of the meatus will experience no impairment of erection or fertility and the **hypospadias represents a cosmetic rather than a functional problem**. Mechanical problems, however, can result in cases with a chordee, resulting in ventral penile deviation during erection. Therefore, apart from optimization of the meatal position, complete resection of an existing chordee as part of the primary operation is essential in surgical correction of hypospadias. If surgery fails and the anatomical situation does not allow normal sperm deposition, **intrauterine insemination** appears to be the method of choice.

Epispadias is another congenital malformation of the urethra. The urinary meatus is located on the **dorsum of the penis** and often forms a **broad open urethral groove or cleft** in these cases. It is often part of a major genital abnormality and is regularly found in patients with bladder exstrophy. Epispadias will lead to severe dorsal deviation in the majority of cases which makes intercourse very difficult or even impossible. Cosmetically and functionally satisfactory surgical correction of this malformation requires a high degree of proficiency and postoperative results do not always meet the expectations of the patient.

In **epispadias cohabitation problems due to penile deviation often lead to disturbances of sperm deposition** because of the proximal position of the meatus. Should offspring be desired, insemination is the therapy of choice. Even after successful surgical correction of the mechanical components, disturbances of ejaculation due to anatomical malformation of the bladder neck are possible. In many cases insufficient closure of the bladder neck results in retrograde ejaculation, in other patients anejaculation is observed.

10.1.2 Phimosis

A phimosis is defined as a narrowing of the foreskin of the penis, mostly of congenital origin or acquired. Secondary forms usually follow infections, especially in patients with diabetes mellitus, severe balanitis or lichen sclerosus et atrophicus. Secondary phimosis due to scar tissue also occurs. In **complete phimosis** the foreskin cannot be withdrawn over the glans penis in the flaccid state. In **relative phimosis** this is only the case during erection and **paraphimosis** may occur (inability of the retracted foreskin to be repositioned over the glans with severe edema and strangulation of the glans penis resulting). In individual cases, uncorrected phimosis may impair semen deposition and cause infertility. The therapy of choice is usually surgical circumcision.

10.1.3 Penile Deviation

Penile deviations can be classified according to **congenital and acquired forms**. Insignificant deviations of the penis from the longitudinal axis are clinically uneventful and can be considered only cosmetic problems. **Surgical therapy is only indicated when cohabitation is mechanically impaired**, regardless of the cause for this penile deviation, or when pain occurs at erection or during intercourse. Clinical findings should be documented with polaroid photographs taken at three levels to give the urologist a three-dimensional view of the disorder.

Congenital Penile Deviation

These disorders represent an entity of their own based on **asymmetric corpora cavernosa** or their bony fixation. Clinically it leads to a **curvature of the penis**. This can be gradual or sharply angled, the deviation of the penis itself can point in any direction. In ventral deviations a relative shortening of the urethra (short urethra) or hypospadias can be the cause. While slight dorsal deviations are functionally without any significance, lateral and ventral deviations can severely **impair capability for cohabitation** and may prevent intercourse. The erectile capacity of these patients is usually not impaired.

Therapeutically, **surgical correction** is the only option in severe cases. The main principle is the relative shortening of the tunica albuginea and the convexity of the curvature. Relative shortening of the corpus cavernosum leads to elimination of the curvature. The most popular surgical method is the **corporal resection** as first described by Nesbit who excised one or more segments of the tunica albuginea and readapted the edges of the resulting defects (Nesbit 1954). Meticulous placement of segments and sutures enable not only lateral and ventral deviations to be corrected, but also slight torsion components. Alternatively, tapering techniques have been described, in which longitudinal parallel sutures with non-resorbable material are placed without previous excision of the tunica albuginea. The major advantage of this procedure is reduced surgical effort with shorter operating times. The main advantage of the original method described by Nesbit, however, is the formation of a very solid scar of the tunica albuginea which is not dependent on the stability of the suture material.

Postoperative results in these congenital deviations are very good; major complications are not observed if care is taken not to damage the structures of the dorsal nerves and vessels.

Acquired Penile Deviation

Secondary penile deviations can result from blunt trauma, bleeding into the corpora cavernosa after penile fractures, from urethral strictures and their treatment by urethrotomy or as a result of long-term cavernosal autoinjection therapy in patients with erectile dysfunction. In the majority of cases it is, however, due to **penile induration**, which is usually referred to as **Peyronie's disease**.

The disease is characterized by a localized and often progressive fibrosis at the borderline between cavernosal tissue and the tunica albuginea (Fig. 10.1a). Subsequent plaque formation is histologically preceded by a perivascular inflammatory reaction of which the etiology is still not completely clear. Possible immunological mechanisms are of major importance since cross-reacting antibodies against HLA B 27 were found in a high percentage of patients with Peyronie's disease.

Clinically the disease usually occurs in the fifth decade but has also been described in young men in their twenties. In its initial phase it is characterized by **pain during erection**. With spontaneous regression of the acute inflammatory reaction, pain usually subsides within approximately three months. Secondary to the consolidation of the inflammatory reaction, a progressive fibrosis with deposition of collagenous tissue is observed. Clinically this leads to palpable plaque formation. In approximately 15% of patients a simultaneous Dupuytren contracture of the **palmar aponeurosis** is seen. In up to 30% of cases ectopic calcification of plaques ensues with true bone formation of the penis (Fig. 10.1b). The majority of the plaques is situated at the dorsal aspect of the penis. They can, however, also occur on the lateral or relatively seldom on the ventral side. Depending on the extent and localisation of these plaques the insufficient elasticity of the tunica albuginea in the area of plaque formation will lead to **penile deviation**. This can attain varying degrees of severity and may lead to grotesque deviations which make sexual intercourse impossible. Involvement of the corpora cavernosa can lead to bandlike stricture and deformation of the penile shaft, causing insufficient engorgement of the distal corpora cavernosa with reduced rigidity or formation of a pseudojoint and consequent inability to perform intercourse.

The **spontaneous course** of the disease can be highly **variable** and often unpredictable. While initial pain at erection usually subsides without treatment after a certain period of time, there are no reliable anamnestic or clinical findings that allow the kind and extent of a later plaque formation or penile deviation to be predicted. The period up to final consolidation with a fixed clinical state of deviation usually extends over several months. In most cases the final extent of the deviation and the resulting subjective impairment of the patient or the part-

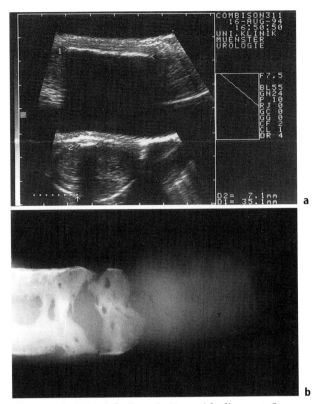

Fig. 10.1 a, b. Typical findings in Peyronie's disease. **a** Sonography of the penis with extensive dorsal plaque formation (> <) (*upper half* longitudinal, lower half transverse section). **b** Soft tissue X-Ray of the penis in the mammography technique with extensive ectopic calcifications

ner will determine further therapeutic strategy. In several cases spontaneous resolution of the plaques with straightening of the penis has been described even without any therapy at all.

Occasionally the disease has been diagnosed in its early inflammatory state due to pain in the flaccid state or under erection and because of a beginning induration of the penile shaft. **Diagnosis** is usually based on the finding of a palpable plaque during clinical examination. These plaques or progressive penile deviation usually prompt the patient to consult his physician. Additional investigations are usually not necessary for diagnosis, although they serve to objectify initial observations at a later point. Size may be determined by ultrasound, in cases with suspected calcifications an additional X-ray using mammography technique can be performed (Fig. 10.1 a, b).

Depending on clinical presentation therapy may consist of symptomatic antiphlogistic measures to relieve pain, oral or local drug therapy, radiation therapy or various surgical solutions (Moll 1992). In cases with minor pain and without significant deviation a purely symptomatic, conservative therapy is justified since in up to 30–50% of the patients spontaneous remission with straightening of the penis can be observed eventually. Of the various drugs tried, only potassium para-aminobenzoate (Potaba®) seems to have a significant influence on the clinical progression of the disease, as recent studies have shown. Intralesional injections of orgotein advocated earlier have been abandoned lately because of lethal allergic reactions. Injection therapy with Ca-antagonists/-steroids will at the most lead to pain reduction without proven effects on the plaque itself. Radiation therapy is especially successful in management of pain of early lesions; significant changes of the plaques or the deviation are not to be expected and severe fibrosis of the corpora cavernosa has been documented.

If, independent of etiology, penile deviation reaches an angle of more than 45°, thus either permitting intercourse only under severe pain, or not at all, surgical procedures are indicated. Generally the disease should come to a clinical standstill at least 3, or better, 6 months before surgery with no increase of penile deviation during this time. Otherwise the risk of postoperative recurrences with newly developing deviations is markedly increased. For most patients whose erectile capacity is not markedly impaired preoperatively, the above-mentioned correction with the Nesbit-technique or with other shortening procedures are the therapy of choice. Postoperative results are good, in most cases surgical shortening of the penis is without any clinical significance and deterioration of erectile function is not to be expected (Kelami 1985). In cases with extensive plaques due to Peyronie's disease excision of these plaques may appear desirable. A major problem of all plaque resections and patch techniques is the markedly increased incidence of postoperative erectile dysfunction. Better results may possibly be achieved by plaque wedging or resection and coverage with venous patches (Brock et al. 1993; Kim and McVary 1995a).

In cases with preoperatively impaired erectile capacity these surgical techniques will often lead to a straightening of the penis but erectile dysfunction will also increase. Apart from psychological factors and arterial problems, disturbances of the cavernosal occlusive mechanism or scarring of the corpora cavernosa especially can be involved. Thorough preoperative diagnosis should provide information on the causes underlying erectile dysfunction. Organic findings are usually so severe that primary implantation of a prothesis, in selected cases, combined with plaque incision, appears indicated. Only when the patient refuses such invasive measures but appears inclined to accept later injection therapy may deviation correction be warranted in very selected cases.

10.2 Erectile Dysfunction

Until recently disturbances of penile erection have often been regarded as psychogenic or of age-dependent physiological origin. The incidence of erectile dysfunctions is estimated to be up to **twice as high as that of the coronary heart disease**. Among 40 year-olds 5% complain of complete and 17% of moderate erectile dysfunction (Feldman et al. 1994). This underlines the enormous social and economical importance of a rational diagnostic workup and therapy of erectile dysfunction. New diagnostic procedures have revolutionized the understanding of physiology and pathophysiology of human penile erection and have contributed to reducing the taboos held by both physicians and patients. Contrary to earlier opinions, nowadays pathogenetically important organic disturbances are found in up to 50–80% of patients. One should, however, be aware of the fact that an accompanying psychological component is present in any patient with erectile dysfunction. With increasing knowledge about possible disturbances of penile erection, new organically oriented therapeutic options have been developed. The following sections deal with physiology, diagnostic workup and therapy of erectile dysfunction (ED).

10.2.1 Functional Anatomy

Arterial inflow of the penis is provided via the internal pudendal artery. Significant variations up to unilateral perfusion without any disturbances of erectile function have been described. A pelvic floor branch leaves the internal pudendal artery before the penile artery divides into the dorsal penile artery, the deep penile artery and the urethral artery (Fig. 10.2a).

The dorsal artery runs alongside the deep dorsal vein and the dorsal nerve between the deep penile fascia (Buck) and the tunica albuginea and perfuses the skin and the glans penis. In many patients there are anastomoses between these superficial vessels and the intracavernosal vasculature as well as the corpus spongiosum.

From the deep penile artery (arteria profunda penis) helix arteries branch off that are contracted in the flaccid state of the penis and show a three-dimensional corkscrew orientation. It is a characteristic feature of the vasculature of the human corpus cavernosum that these vessels drain directly into wide, communicating sinusoids. Between these helix arteries and the cavernosal veins there is only a very short arterial capillary bed.

This functions as a kind of arterial venous fistula, providing only minimal nutritive perfusion of the corpora cavernosa (CC) in the flaccid, non-erect penis with contracted arterial vessels.

The trabeculae of the **cavernous sinusoids** consist of smooth muscle cells covered with endothelium on the interior of the sinusoidal space. The intracavernous arteria helicinae and the draining veins run into these trabeculae. In contrast to the arteries, the **veins** (Fig. 10.2b) do not have their own musculature and their diameter is largely dependent on the tension of the trabeculae. These draining veins and intermedial veins join in a subtunical plexus from which the emissary veins arise. These emerge from the corpora cavernosa dorsally and laterally and join directly or via the venae circumflexae with the deep dorsal vein. Proximally they join the cavernous and crural veins, from which the latter form the internal pudendal vein. The superficial dorsal vein, similar to the dorsal artery, only drains the outer skin layers and the glans penis and sometimes forms a joint with the vena saphena magna.

The stability of the corpora cavernosa is guaranteed by the tunica albuginea and multiple septa that produce a fixed three-dimensional structure. Therefore, changes in the rigor of the cavernosal muscle cells will influence the whole system comprised of tunica albuginea, trabeculae and draining veins, and not only separate components. The septum penis is incomplete in humans so that clinically the corpora cavernosa represent a functional unit (Fig. 10.2).

The **innervation** of the penis is twofold and involves the autonomic and the somatosensory nerve system. Parasympathetic fibers arise from the sacral erection centre (S2–S4). Sympathetic fibers have their origin in the thoracolumbal area (Th12–L2) and run along the preaortal plexus into the plexus hypogastricus. Preganglionic parasympathetic fibers from the sacral erectile centre unite with sympathetic fibers from the plexus hypogastricus in the pelvic plexus and form the nervi cavernosi, which represent the autonomic innervation of the corpora cavernosa. These nervi cavernosi follow the pudendal arteries and enter the corpora immediately after running just laterocaudal to the apex of the prostate. This very exposed anatomical pathway explains the possible damage to penile innervation and arterial perfusion in patients with severe proximal urethal trauma or radical pelvic surgery.

Somatosensory innervation is represented by the dorsal penile nerve, a terminal branch of the pudendal nerve. Sensory afferent information reaches the dorsal roots of the sacral segments S2–S4, from there being conducted via the anterolateral spinothalamic pathways to the integrative medial preoptic area (MPOA). The pudendal nerve, however, also has efferent motoric fibers leading to the musculature of the pelvic floor, innervating the bulbocavernosal and the ischiocavernosal mus-

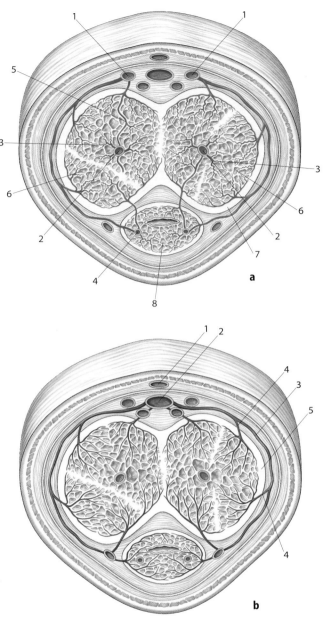

Fig. 10.2 a, b. Cross-section of the penis. **a** Arterial supply. *1* A. dorsalis penis; *2* A. profunda penis; *3* Helicene arteries; *4* A. urethralis; *5* Anastomoses between A. dorsalis and A. profunda penis; *6* Sinusoids of the corpora cavernosa; *7* Tunica albuginea; *8* Corpus spongiosum. **b** Venous supply. *1* V. dorsalis superficialis; *2* V. dorsalis profunda; *3* V. circumflexa; *4* V. emissaria

cles. During erection these compress the corpora cavernosa against the bony structure of the pelvis and thereby increase intracavernosal pressure.

10.2.2 Physiology of Erection

Hemodynamics

> Three **hemodynamic factors** are essential for erection (Fig. 10.3a, b):
> - intracavernosal **reduction of resistance** due to relaxation of the cavernosal muscle cells,
> - **increase of arterial inflow** by dilatation of the arterial vessels,
> - **restriction of venous outflow** by compression of intracavernosal and subtunical venous plexus.

Reduction of the tone of all muscular structures of the corpus cavernosum accompanied by relaxation of the sinoids results in increased arterial inflow. Clinically this correlates with increasing tumescence and elongation of the penis (Fig. 10.3a). In the venous system uninhibited drainage is reduced in the flaccid organ state by a marked decrease of the venous diameter. By the maximal extension of the cavernosal sinoids the venoles in the trabeculae and the emissary veins passing through the tunica albuginea are increasingly compressed. These changes finally lead to complete penile erection (Fig. 10.3b).

Hemodynamically **five erectile phases** can be distinguished (Table 10.1). The **latency phase** is characterized by a drop in intracavernosal pressure following stimulation of the nervi cavernosi. This is accompanied by an increase in arterial perfusion. Due to the elastic-fibromuscular structure of the corpora cavernosa this leads to elongation of the penis without any changes in intracavernosal pressure. During the **tumescence phase** increasing compression of the venous outflow slowly develops. When intracavernosal pressure is just below systolic blood pressure a plateau is established which is hemodynamically characterized by a steady state of arterial inflow and the only minimal venous outflow (**erection phase**). Maximal rigidity will be achieved by contraction of the pelvic floor muscles, allowing pressure inside the corpora cavernosa far in excess of systolic pressure (**rigidity phase**). When nervous impulses terminate, rigidity and tumescence will decrease (**detumescence phase**).

Neurophysiology

Clinically **three different types of erection** can be differentiated: reflexogenic, psychogenic and nocturnal erection. **Reflexogenic** erections are induced by direct stimulation of the genital area and are transmitted by the dorsal penile nerve. Intraspinally there is a transfer to efferent parasympathetic fibres (nervi erigentes). After

Fig. 10.3 a, b. Physiology of erection. **a** Contracted A. profunda penis (*1*) helicene arteries (*2*) and sinsuids in the flaccid state, unrestricted venous outflow of cavernosal blood via emissary veins (*3*). **b** During tumescence marked dilatation of the A. profunda penis and the sinsuids, elongation of the helicene arteries, compression of the intersinusoidal venules and mechanical occlusion of the subtunical emissary veins

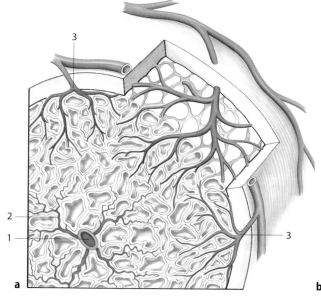

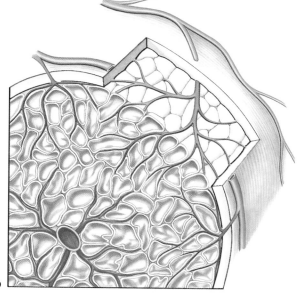

a   b

Table 10.1. The 5 phases of erection

I. Latency phase	Penile shaft elongation, constant intracavernosal pressure due to a decrease of the cavernosal resistance
II. Tumescence phase	Increase of tumescence and rigidity with increase of arterial inflow, cavernosal volume and intracorporal pressure
III. Erection phase	Completely elongated, pulsating penile shaft, stabilization of intracavernosal pressure at a plateau, 10–20 mmHg below systolic blood pressure; constant penile volume due to a reduction of the arterial inflow to baseline values
IV. Rigidity phase	Full tumescence and rigidity with intracorporal pressure that can clearly exceed systolic blood pressure due to the bulbo-cavernosus reflex; only minimal arterial inflow but complete venous occlusion
V. Detumescence phase	Loss of rigidity, decrease of penile volume and intracavernosal pressure with in- and outflow from the corpora cavernosa reaching baseline values

transformation in the pelvic plexus erection is induced via the cavernosal nerves. The somatic portion of the pudendal nerve induces contraction of the pelvic floor musculature with adequate rigidity. These pathophysiological circumstances explain the existence of normal reflexogenic erections in cases of supranuclear lesions of the spinal cord, while central perception can be maintained or abolished to a various extent in these patients.

Psychogenic erections occur when neurotransmitters, especially dopamine and nitrous monoxide (NO), are released following erotic stimuli in the central sexual centers. The signals are transmitted to the corpora cavernosa via activation of the parasympathetic nervous system and a signal transfer in the sacral erectile center, where NO and the vasoactive intestinal polypeptide (VIP) act as the main transmitters. Mainly inhibitory effects stem from the thoracolumbar erection center (TH 11/12–L 2/3). After signal transformation in the plexus hypogastricus the sympathetic fibers, along with the parasympathetic fibers in the nervi cavernosi, reach the penis. Here the sympathetic fibers reach the $\alpha 1$ receptors of the corpora cavernosa muscle cells or $\alpha 2$ receptors of the penile arteries. These have an inhibitory effect on smooth muscles of the erectile tissue of the penis. This is supported by clinical experience that penile erection may be absent even in the presence of high sympathetic tone.

Physiologically the corpora cavernosa are more under the influence of erection-inhibiting factors than erection-facilitating factors. This explains why the penis remains in a contracted i.e. flaccid state when at rest.

Nocturnal erections result from the day/night reversal and the parasympathetic tone which predominates during the night, leading to intermittent autonomic erections.

Local Control of Erection

Parasympathetic erection-facilitating nerve endings are largely of non-adrenergic, non-cholinergic nature. NO and VIP are the important transmitters. NO activates the membrane-bound guanylyl cyclase, causing cyclisation of 3'5' cyclic guanosine monophosphate (cGMP) from GTP. Along with 3'5'-cyclic adenosine monophosphate (cAMP) this second messenger is the most important transmitter, ultimately leading to increased calcium flux out of the cell and thence to muscle relaxation. The formation of cAMP is analogous to that of cGMP when membrane-bound adenylyl cyclase is activated by VIP. Both second messengers are subject to physiological metabolism by various phosphate diesterases, of which type III and type V are clinically relevant. These lead to a reduction of cGMP to 5'GMP or cAMP to 5'AMP, which are biologically inactive.

Sympathetic innervation follows largely via adrenergic $\alpha 1$ and $\alpha 2$ receptors, causing an increase of intercellular calcium levels and the contraction of muscle cells.

In addition, various local substances are synthesized in the penile erectile tissue which have largely inhibitory influence, e.g. prostanoids, endothelin and angiotensin. In addition, contrary to former opinion, local control of erection is influenced by testosterone. Thus a protracted testosterone deficiency causes a reduction of the NO-synthetase-containing nerve fibers and a continuous reduction in the number of smooth muscle cells by apoptosis.

10.2.3 Pathophysiology of Erection

Separately or in variable combinations psychogenic, vascular, neurogenic, hormonal or direct myogenic disturbances can cause **erectile dysfunction**. The development of new diagnostic procedures has revolutionized earlier opinions that in the vast majority of cases erectile dysfunction is of psychogenic origin. These new diagnostic procedures allow objectivity and quantitation of the various functions that are responsible for induction or maintenance of erection. However, the development of these diagnostic procedures led to the assumption that up to 80% of patients suffered from purely organic erectile dysfunctions, leaving psychogenic factors, which affect any patient with long standing erectile dysfunction, to go unobserved.

Psychogenic Erectile Dysfunction

Psychogenic stimuli such as sensory or mental stimuli can be very strong promoters of erection. Contrary reactions, especially fear or earlier traumatic experiences, can, on the other hand, impair erectile capability significantly and may lead to complete erectile dysfunction. In primary disturbances the reasons are often found in the social situation and upbringing. Secondary disturbances usually occur acutely and may be dependent on specific situations or partners. They are often accompanied by other characteristic sexual disturbances. Prognostically and therapeutically it is important to evaluate whether the disorder is characterized mainly by a reduction of libido or whether an initial erection cannot be maintained owing to fear of failure or other problems. Disturbances of libido may be derived from organic causes; in psychogenic impotence, however, they are usually a sign of partner problems and therefore have a relatively poor prognosis.

Vasculogenic Erectile Dysfunction

To induce a physiological erection two factors are mandatory: sufficient arterial influx into the cavernosal arteries and a competent cavernosal occlusion mechanism. Therefore **two kinds of vasculogenic erectile dysfunctions** can be differentiated, **those with reduced arterial inflow and those with disturbances of the cavernosal occlusion mechanism.**

> 50–80% of all organically caused erectile dysfunction is due to **arterial insufficiency of the penile vessels.**

In the majority of these cases patients have one or several of the well-known risk factors of arteriosclerosis such as severe nicotine abuse, arterial hypertension, diabetes mellitus or disturbances of lipid metabolism. Along with arteriosclerotic alterations, perineal trauma with injuries of the pudendal vessels or iatrogenic causes (vascular or pelvic surgery) have to be taken into account. Clinically purely arterial disturbances are characterized by diminished and delayed induction of erection after application of vasoactive substances. Symptoms usually develop over time and are generally not partner- or situation-dependent.

> **Disturbances of the cavernosal occlusion mechanism** can be due to various reasons:
> - congenital disturbances of venous drainage (ectopic veins),
> - morphological alterations of the smooth muscle cells of the corpora cavernosa with reduced ability for relaxation due to different pathological circumstances,
> - functional changes of the smooth muscle cells of the corpora cavernosa (disturbances of neurotransmitters or receptors),
> - morphological alterations of the tunica albuginea (age, Peyronie's disease, penile fracture),
> - pathological shunts between corpus cavernosum and glans penis/corpus spongiosum.

Ectopic veins are one of the very rare causes of primary erectile dysfunction. They can be corrected by a very simple surgical procedure by resecting the ectopic vein. Secondary venous and cavernosal erectile dysfunctions are usually due to alterations of the cavernosal tissue itself or the tunica albuginea. In most cases degenerative changes of these muscle cells with a replacement by connective tissue and fibroblasts and consecutive loss of elasticity are responsible for the incompetence of the cavernosal occlusion mechanism and the resultant increased venous drainage of the corpora cavernosa. Such changes are often observed in the presence of arterial insufficiency and show the same pathophysiological mechanisms well known from other organ systems. Extensive fibrosis can also be observed after priapisms or trauma. Impairment of the perfusion of the small intracavernosal vessels (small vessel disease) and simultaneous presence of morphological changes of the tunica albuginea lead to insufficient activation of the cavernosal occlusion mechanism by reduced filling of the corpora, which will in turn induce relative venous or cavernosal insufficiency.

The possibilities of functional impairment of the smooth muscle cells of the corpora cavernosa caused by reduced release or diminished contents of neurotransmitters, a competitive receptor blockage or quantitative disturbances of receptor status also have to be taken into account. In patients with diabetes mellitus a significantly reduced number of neurotransmitters could be demonstrated, as well as impaired relaxation capacity dependent on the endothelium and electrical stimuli. Competitive receptor blockage can also be caused by medication. Such competitive blockage can also be observed in patients with psychogenic erectile dysfunction when adrenergic tone prevents adequate relaxation of the smooth muscle cells of the corpora cavernosa. Morphological changes of the tunica albuginea (e.g. IPP) are much more frequent than functional or quantitative changes of intracavernosal receptors.

> Clinically patients present with an insufficient or extremely short erection with a rapid loss of primary rigidity, in advanced cases with complete erectile dysfunction. Many of these cases will be diagnosed as having a combination of reduced arterial perfusion and cavernosal insufficiency.

Neurogenic Erectile Dysfunction

Neurological disturbances on various levels of stimulation or its transmission can lead to erectile problems. Spinal lesions are among the most common causes. In approximately 95% of patients with supranuclear lesions reflexogenic erections are maintained, but only 25% of the patients with sacral lesions report normal psychogenic erections. This proves the dominant role of the sacral erection center compared to the thoracolumbal center.

Systemic diseases such as Morbus Parkinson, encephalitis disseminata, inflammatory or tumorous lesions display highly variable findings. In these cases erectile dysfunction is often a symptom of the imbalance between excitatory and inhibitory influences and clinical presentation can be very heterogenous. Peripheral neuropathies are usually observed in metabolic disorders such as **diabetes mellitus** and severe alcohol abuse. In diabetes mellitus **erectile dysfunction may be the primary manifestation**. Like vascular changes, neuropathy usually occurs with increasing duration of the disease and is only partly dependent on the quality of medical therapy. Reactive psychogenic disturbances due to major changes in lifestyle are a problem that is probably often overlooked.

Endocrine Erectile Dysfunction

The role of androgens in the regulation of erection is not clearly defined. Low serum testosterone levels are often associated with disturbances of libido and other functional sexual problems, reduced sperm production and reduction of nocturnal erections. However, complete rigid erections occur in infants and castrates (Greenstein et al. 1995). In hypogonadism, testosterone replacement will lead to a marked increase in nocturnal penile erections and libido; conversely, in patients with normal serum levels, substitution will not be beneficial compared to placebo (see Sect. 15.3.1).

Severe androgen deficiency is by definition correlated with low testosterone and only few cases of hypogonadism will be primarily diagnosed by the symptom of erectile dysfunction, despite the fact that androgen deficiency causes a decrease of NO-containing nerve fibers and apoptosis of smooth muscles, and consequently induces compromised signal transmission in the corpora cavernosa (see Sect. 6.4.4).

Altogether, endocrine factors are an essential etiological factor in erectile dysfunction, accounting for 2–5% of patients.

Drug-Induced Erectile Dysfunction

Different kinds of medication can play a significant role in the pathogenesis of erectile dysfunction. In most cases drugs will act on the central nervous system, influencing the hypothalamus-pituitary-gonadal axis, or on the autonomic nervous system. This concomittent drug action is best known from central and peripheral α- and β-sympatholytic drugs which will lead to disturbances of erection, ejaculation and libido to variable extents. In many cases, however, it remains unclear whether the disturbance of erectile function is due to the medication itself or to decreased blood pressure with insufficient circulatory reserve of the penile vasculature.

Psychotropic drugs including **tranquilizers** and **antidepressants** show strong sedative but also anti-cholinergic and anti-dopaminergic actions. Drugs influencing testosterone levels are either substances like **clofibrat** or H_2-blockers like **cimetidin**, but also **narcotic and hallucinogenic drugs**. **Alcohol abuse** will not only lead to polyneuropathy but will also induce a decrease in testosterone because of impaired liver function with a secondary increase in estrogen levels.

In many cases patients are dependent on various substances owing to different illnesses, making it very difficult to judge the effect of single drugs, for which therapeutic alternatives are not always available.

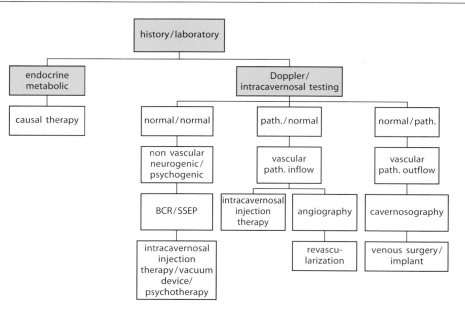

Fig. 10.4. Flow-chart for the diagnosis and principal therapeutic options for erectile dysfunction

10.2.4 Diagnostic Workup in Erectile Dysfunction

The complexity of the physiological process of erection and the multifactorial etiology of erectile dysfunction often necessitate an extensive diagnostic workup which cannot be dispensed with even in the age of oral therapeutics. The patient's history and a clinical examination provide the first important hints concerning the pathogenesis of an erectile problem. To evaluate further the individual cause of impotence it is usually necessary to choose those investigations from a variety of procedures that will lead to a sound diagnosis, taking into account the availability, objectivity and invasiveness, as well as time and economic aspects. All these will finally lead to a therapeutic decision that takes into account the individual etiology of the erectile dysfunction and the patient's personal preference. Therefore an established **differential diagnostic workup** will help to exclude or quantify organic factors in patients with erectile dysfunction (Fig. 10.4).

History and Clinical Presentation

Most often the first conversation will be the most important step towards a good patient-physician relationship. Often this first interview will give a decisive clue for classifying the sexual disturbance and can suggest further diagnostic and therapeutic procedures. It appears essential that this interview should be performed without undue disturbances (such as telephone calls) in a quiet and intimate setting without undue haste.

The general history usually covers **predisposing illnesses** possibly leading to arteriosclerosis, such as diabetes mellitus, arterial hypertension and disturbed lipid metabolism. Another factor of importance is **nicotine abuse**, which, apart from acute impairment of arterial perfusion, can lead to diminished occlusive function of the smooth musculature of the corpora cavernosa. The history should take note of **alcohol abuse** as well. In addition to cardiovascular disease, neurologic systematic diseases like epilepsy or multiple sclerosis should be inquired after, in patients with paraplegia the kind and extent of neurological deficits have to be worked up. Major pelvic surgery can interfere not only with penile perfusion, but also with innervation of the corpora cavernosa and therefore needs to be noted. This includes reconstructive vascular surgery. Depending on the kind and extent of the laceration, pelvic trauma can also interfere with penile perfusion and/or innervation. Very often **blunt trauma** to the perineum is only remembered if asked for explicitly.

A detailed **drug history** is essential since a number of widely used substances, especially anti-hypertensives and H_2-blockers or substances against fatty acid metabolism disorders may lead to disturbances of erectile function; conversely, cardiac medication can influence possible oral therapy.

Finally, the general history should also evaluate the social and psychological situation of the patient since latent depression may play an important role in temporary functional erectile dysfunction. An extensive sexual history provides first insights into the kind of sexual disturbance. Generally, disturbances of libido, erection and ejaculation have to be differentiated. The evaluation and interpretation of any clinical presentation should take into account all three aspects of sexuality.

Primary erectile dysfunction usually exists from puberty and in most cases is due to congenital vascular abnormalities. **Secondary erectile dysfunction** is characterized by onset after a period of normal sexual activity and normal erectile function. Often differential diagnosis requires a precise description of the kind of sexual disturbance. Erectile dysfunction as the primary subjective symptom is evaluated by questioning the quality of erection and frequency of intercourse. Frequency of intercourse diminishes with increasing age, a fact often not accepted by the patient. Therefore it is important to clarify how the patient would judge his personal situation before the onset of erectile dysfunction.

Discontinuous problems that occur in specific situations or with specific partners usually point towards mainly psychogenic etiology. The same would apply to problems that are only connected with intercourse, but where early morning and nocturnal erections are not impaired and where a rigid and full erection is observed during masturbation. Similarly, these problems are usually of functional, non-organic origin. A premature ejaculation will also point to a significant functional non-organic factor. These patients should be seen by an experienced psychotherapist or psychologist early in the course of evaluation and therapy. Psycho-sexual disturbances of development and partner problems should be an indication to **involve the partner in psycho-sexual evaluation**. Sexual deviations make consultation of a psychiatric colleague mandatory. Ultimately, however, a diagnosis of psychogenic or "idiopathic" impotence should be established only in patients in whom significant organic pathologies have been excluded.

Clinical Examination

The clinical examination pays special attention to the secondary sexual features and the genitalia. Obvious changes in hair distribution, body fat distribution and general constitution may indicate hypogonadism. Since a pronounced androgen deficiency is generally accompanied by testicular atrophy, evaluation of size and consistency of the testes is of great importance. Many cases of hypogonadism, including patients with Klinefelter syndrome, are diagnosed because of an erectile dysfunction presenting as a primary symptom. **Palpation of the penis** will reveal cases with induratio penis plastica (Morbus Peyronie), which can lead not only to penile deviation but also to erectile dysfunction. Congenital penile deviation, however, will not show any pathological findings at physical examination and can only be diagnosed during erection (photographic documentation).

Laboratory Tests

To exclude endocrine causes of erectile dysfunction primarily serum testosterone levels are necessary. In selected cases additional endocrinological parameters include LH, prolactin, estradiol and SHBG (see Sect. 6.4).

Other laboratory investigations should be restricted to those patients with special clinical indications. Patients with diabetes mellitus or disturbances of lipid metabolism should undergo evaluation of their present metabolic state.

Intracavernosal Testing with Vasoactive Substances

Even today the diagnostic workup of erectile dysfunction by **intracavernosal testing** with vasoactive substances plays a **central role** (Porst 1990). Injection of vasoactive substances usually enables a largely physiological erection to be induced. Thus, by eliminating nervous stimuli, vascular perfusion reserve and functional integrity of the smooth muscle cells of the corpora cavernosa, and therefore of the cavernosal occlusion mechanism, can be evaluated. By this procedure especially vascular disturbances can be evaluated or ruled out. The induction of a full rigid erection after small doses of vasoactive substances, however, will allow first insights into neurogenic or functional/psychogenic disturbances, especially when vasoactive testing is combined with other clinical investigations (Fig. 10.4).

Injection of vasoactive substances into the corpora cavernosa is performed after careful desinfection from a lateral position on either side with a 27G-insulin canula to exclude laceration of the dorsal nerves and vessels and the urethra. Owing to the anatomical connections between the two corpora, an even distribution of the drug is guaranteed. Additional compression at the base of the penis is usually not necessary (Fig. 10.5).

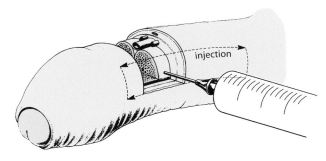

Fig. 10.5. Technique of intracavernosal injection

15 minutes after intracavernosal injection of vaso-active substance in a standing position the result of the test is evaluated with reference to tumescence and rigidity. Several different rating scales are available; in most cases the following will be used:

- E0: no visible reaction,
- E1: slight tumescence, no rigidity,
- E2: medium tumescence, no rigidity,
- E3: full tumescence, no rigidity,
- E4: full tumescence, medium rigidity (sufficient for intercourse),
- E5: full tumescence, full rigidity.

A reaction between E0 and E3 is considered a negative vasoactive test; the patient is classified as a non-responder. If, after injection of the vasoactive substance a rigid erection sufficient for intercourse (E4–E5) occurs, this is classified as a **positive test** and the patient will be declared a responder. In patients who need additional testing, this diagnostic phase can be the first opportunity for the patient to be instructed in basic techniques of drug handling for self-injection therapy.

Evaluation of intracavernosal vasoactive testing has to take into account not only the quality of the induced erection, but also the latency of the induction and the duration of the erection. The procedure and final result of the tests together provide important clues to the etiology of erectile dysfunction (Fig. 10.4):

- If during intracavernosal testing with a low dose of vasoactive substance the patient shows a rapid and continuing full rigid erection with normal Doppler sonography of the penile vessels, arterial disorder and venous/cavernosal insufficiency are virtually excluded. Vascular abnormalities are very unlikely and for differential diagnosis between neurogenic and psychogenic etiology of erectile dysfunction, a further neurological workup may be helpful.
- If the erection only occurs after prolonged latency of 15–30 minutes but the patient reaches a full rigid erection, a hemodynamically relevant **arterial reduction of penile perfusion** appears very likely. This can be documented by pathological results of Doppler sonography of the penile vessels.
- A **positive result** in vasoactive testing will practically exclude a relevant venous or cavernosal insufficiency as the cause of erectile dysfunction.

- A **negative result** in vasoactive testing correlates in over 90 % of cases with a venous/cavernosal insufficiency and an impairment of the cavernosal occlusion mechanism. Pharmacocavernosonography is necessary for further evaluation.

In routine diagnostic workup today prostaglandin E_1 (PGE_1) as vasoactive substance has replaced papaverine alone, or in combination with the α-adrenoceptor antagonist. Papaverine is an opium alkaloid. By blockage of the phosphodiesterase intracellular cAMP is increased and will lead to a release of calcium from the smooth muscle cells. The rationale for the use of α-adrenoceptor antagonists is the fact that the sympathetic tone is responsible for the flaccid resting state of the penis. Given alone they usually show a very limited clinical effect; in combination with papaverine or other drugs they facilitate the induction of an erection by reduction of the sympathetic tone and therefore a marked increase in the efficacy of other drugs.

Prostanoids in vitro have a different effect on the human cavernosal tissue. Under PGE_1 especially there is a marked relaxation of the human corpus cavernosum by an increase of intracellular cAMP via specific PGE_1 receptors. Additionally, PGE_1 in vitro inhibits the electrically-stimulated release of noradrenaline via presynaptic PGE_1 receptors which lead to a modulation of the endogenous sympathetic tone (Molderings et al. 1992). In vivo PGE_1 leads to strong vasodilatation. The substance is rapidly metabolized; degradation takes place mainly in the lung.

Generally, intracavernosal testing is possible with all of the above-mentioned vasoactive drugs. In addition to **papaverine** alone (Paveron®), the **combination of papaverine and phentolamine** (Androskat®) **and prostaglandin** E_1 (Viridal®, Caverjet®) is well established; the combination of all three substances is also used (**triple drug therapy**). Within the usual therapeutic dose range **prostaglandin** E_1 is the most potent monosubstance.

The efficacy of the various vasoactive substances can vary intra- and inter-individually concerning quality and duration of an erection. From the patient's history alone the effect of the drug is often not well predictable. Since the efficacy of the substances is usually proportional to the applied dose and an erection should not exceed 2–3 hours in duration even in primary testing, it is always advisable to start with a low initial dose. If this low initial dose proves to be insufficient to induce a complete erection, further testing with increased doses is necessary. There should be a gradual increase in dose, with a time interval between two injections of at least 24 hours.

Initial dosing and dose escalation for the various substances are:

- PGE_1 – 10; 20; 40 µg,
- Papaverine/phentolamine (30 mg + 1 mg/ml) – 0,5; 1; 2 ml.

Escalation of the dose of PGE_1 above 20 µg, however, has a beneficial effect in only 20 % of patients, since in most cases there will be a saturation of the intracavernosal receptors at a dose of 20 µg (Heyden et al. 1993).

Contraindications for intracavernosal vasoactive testing are:

- severe decompensated cardiovascular insufficiency,
- critical coronary heart disease,
- severe disturbances of liver function (papaverine),
- glaucoma (papaverine),
- pronounced benign hyperplasia of the prostate with increased residual urine (papaverine).

Anticoagulant therapy with cumarins, low molecular heparins or aspirin represent only relative contraindications since no increased rate of complications has been observed when these patients use vasoactive substances.

Adverse side-effects can occur:

- hematoma,
- intracavernosal pain,
- prolonged erections (3–6 h),
- priapism (>6 h),
- infections of the corpora cavernosa.

Pain in the glans is described by 10–80 % of the patients after papaverine/phentolamine during injection of the substance. This pain is usually of very short duration and subsides within a few minutes (Lue and Tanagho 1987). With PGE_1 10–40 % of patients complain of a very irritating feeling of increased intracavernosal pressure, in some patients severe pain may persist for several hours and even show a duration longer than the erection itself. In only about 2 % of these patients is this discomfort and pain so strong that it will prevent them from having intercourse. The cause of these complaints is unclear and a connection with various solvents is being discussed. With papaverine a slight reduction in blood pressure with dizziness is sometimes reported.

Complications of intracavernosal testing with vasoactive drugs are mostly small, insignificant hematomas that will resolve spontaneously and that do not require specific therapy. **Septicemic infections of the corpora cavernosa** are dangerous but extremely rare. The most important complications of intracavernosal testing with vasoactive substances, however, are **prolonged erections** and **priapism**. The borderline between a prolonged erection and priapism is not clearly defined and some authors classify 3–6 hours of full erection as prolonged. Such a situation usually requires no or limited therapeutic measures, depending on the substance used. Priapism is characterized by a duration of the artificial erection of more than 6 hours. Depending on the elapsed time and the consequent metabolic changes with acidosis in the corpora cavernosa the situation may lead to complete destruction of the smooth muscle cells with consecutive fibrosis. Irreversible damage is usually seen after priapism of more than 12 hours duration (Porst and van Ahlen 1989).

Therapy of choice is usually the puncture of the corpora cavernosa with drainage of 50–200 ml of cavernosal blood until marked arterialization of the cavernosal blood can be visually identified. After this α-sympathomimetic drugs will be applied in slowly escalating doses. The use of these substances should always be accompanied by close observation of blood pressure and cardiovascular function, since vital circulatory complications with hypertensive crisis may occur. The practice of administering prophylactic doses of nitroglycerine with the onset of drug-induced hypertension is well established.

Aside from lower effectiveness, the significantly greater frequency of prolonged erections and priapism occurring after papaverine or the combination of papaverine and phentolamine during the test and dose-finding phase of injection therapy has made PGE_1 the substance of choice (7 %). The reason for the markedly reduced incidence of priapism under PGE_1 may be the local intracavernosal metabolism of prostaglandin (van Ahlen et al. 1995).

When choosing a vasoactive substance, theoretically papaverine has the advantage of **very low cost**, combined with a comparatively high diagnostic risk. Aside from its limited efficacy, slow dose escalation may lead to an increased number of necessary injections.

Prostaglandin E_1 is by far more expensive, but because of its superior efficacy and broad therapeutic safety requires a low number of injections.

Doppler Sonography

To date **Doppler sonography of the penile vessels** remains a mandatory part of organically oriented diagnostics. As a **non-invasive, cost-effective method** it will pick up disturbances of the **arterial penile circulation** which are one of the most important etiological factors in the pathogenesis of erectile dysfunction. Only after the introduction of smooth muscle stimulation by intracavernosal injection of vasoactive substances did the systematic examination of the deep penile artery perfusing the corpora cavernosa become possible. In the flaccid state of the penis this artery has a very small diameter of approximately 0.5 mm, since most of the penile perfusion will be extracavernous. Therefore in a flaccid state visualization will be difficult even with high-resolution ultrasound of 8–10 MHz. Nowadays Doppler sonography should always be performed in combination with the application of vasoactive substances into the corpora cavernosa during vasoactive testing.

In earlier times most investigators tried to establish baseline findings on the dorsal penile artery and, if possible, also on the deep penile artery before application of vasoactive substances. Today most investigators will perform Doppler sonography only 5–10 minutes after injection of the vasoactive substances, with still increasing tumescence of the penis. Only an examination before induction of a full rigid erection will allow reliable judgement of the dilatatory capacity and the perfusion reserve of the examined vessel, since physiologically arterial perfusion will be markedly reduced after induction of phase III of the erection, when blood flow usually drops to baseline levels.

Purely acoustic judgement of the Doppler signal is clearly not adequate. Registration of the Doppler curve with a **c**ontinuous-**w**ave-Doppler (cw-Doppler) is a minimum technical requirement. Since the cw-Doppler will record all vessels within the Doppler signal it is essential to differentiate superficial branches of the dorsal penile artery from the cavernosal arteries. This is usually achieved by slight compression of the penile skin and by the different character of the recorded Doppler signal.

Evaluation of Doppler sonography usually takes into account the absolute height of the Doppler curve and the maximal perfusion velocity, as well as the relative increase compared to the base line examination just before application of the vasoactive substance. A broad pulse curve with reduced initial velocity and low amplitude are typical signs of insufficient arterial perfusion.

Duplex Sonography

In duplex sonography, which, like cw-Doppler sonography, is always combined with intracavernosal application of vasoactive substances, the penile arteries are examined by a **combination of conventional ultrasound and a pulsed Doppler**. This will allow the examiner to position the cursor and thereby the measuring point of the pulsed Doppler exactly inside the lumen of the investigated penile vessel, under direct visual control. Apart

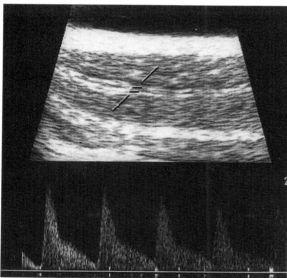

Fig. 10.6. Duplex sonography of the cavernosal artery after intracavernosal injection of 10 μg PGE₁. **a** Upper half: sonography of the corpus cavernosum of the cavernosal artery. The probe of the Doppler is positioned in the lumen of the cavernosal artery. Lower half: simultaneous registration of the pulsed Doppler curve. **b** Registration of the pulsed curve of the cavernosal artery with increased diastolic flow (*arrow*) as a possible indication of disturbed cavernosal occlusion

from a precise sonographic documentation of an isolated vessel, this allows highly precise registration of Doppler curves and thus makes measurements of arterial perfusion possible. Apart from changes in diameter of specific arteries, one can calculate systolic and diastolic velocities of blood flow (Fig. 10.6 a).

After injection of vasoactive substances a diameter of 1 mm of the cavernosal arteries together with visible pulsations of the vessel and a drug-induced dilatation by at least 75 % compared to the base line findings are regarded as normal values. Maximal blood flow velocity should be above 25 cm/second to exclude a major impairment of arterial circulation (Rhee et al. 1995).

Since blood flow velocity will increase physically in areas of stenosis, both flow velocity and diameter increase should always be taken into account when judging the arterial status of the penis. Maximal flow velocity as the only criterion has to be seen very critically. The measurement of blood flow itself in volume/time (ml/minute) has not found wide acceptance owing to considerable variation. The reliability of the examinations can be increased by an additional evaluation of the form of the Doppler curve and measurements of the systolic rising velocity. Short times below 110 ms reveal unimpaired dilatation capacity of the examined artery and documents the integrity of arterial perfusion (Oates et al. 1995). Increased diastolic flow velocities above 5 cm/second can be a hint for insufficient relaxation of the smooth muscle cells of the corpora cavernosa and for the existence of a cavernosal insufficiency with increased venous drainage (Hatzichristou et al. 1995) (Fig. 10.6 b).

Whereas a few years ago pulsed Doppler sonography hardly appeared widely applicable, owing to very high equipment costs, it has by now been established as a routine procedure. Nowadays it appears to be the **almost ideal screening investigation** for the evaluation of arterial perfusion and has replaced conventional cw-Doppler sonography almost completely. It is easy to learn and there is practically no additional effort compared to conventional Doppler. A combination of morphological and functional evaluation allows much better judgement of the functional perfusion reserve than would be possible with conventional Doppler sonography.

Another technical improvement of pulsed duplex sonography is **color-coded duplex sonography**. The ultrasound signals that are reflected from the moving erythrocytes are color-coded depending on flow direction and velocity so that arterial and venous vessels can be rapidly differentiated. This new technique not only allows quantitative measurements of flow velocity but also visualization of perfusion of the whole penile course of the vessel. Therefore different areas of the vessel can be recorded at the same time with visualization of blood flow into the helix arteries and into possible collaterals between superficial and deep arteries.

Penile Angiography

In the past angiography of penile arteries was often regarded as the gold standard in the evaluation of vascular disturbances. It is, however, a very invasive diagnostic procedure that is not without risk. Even the conventional cw-Doppler sonography under vasoactive stimulation, however, correlates in over 90 % with the results of selective angiography (Porst et al. 1988a). Since the technical progress of non-invasive, cheap and less time-consuming sonography, especially duplex sonography, angiography today is only indicated in a forensic setting or in patients with a primary erectile dysfunction with suspected congenital vascular dysplasia or malformation. Presurgical visualization of the internal pudendal artery and the inferior epigastric artery before reconstrucive vascular surgery remains a therapeutic indication.

Like Doppler sonography, angiography will only be reliable after intracavernosal injection of vasoactive substances. Since it will only provide morphological information in dubious cases, the hemodynamic relevance of these angiographic findings has to be cross-checked by duplex sonography.

Evaluation of Venous Drainage

In approximately 10 % of patients with erectile dysfunction even the highest doses and appropriate combinations of the usual vasoactive substances are not able to induce an adequate erection, intracavernosal pharmacon testing is negative and the patient is classified as a non-responder. Usually this situation is a sign of the incompetence of the cavernosal occlusion mechanism with increased drainage of venous blood from the corpora cavernosa, a phenomenon that has in the past often been classified as venous leakage.

The indication for quantification and visualization of the venous drainage from the corpora cavernosa must be judged carefully owing to the relatively high costs, invasiveness of the examination and limited therapeutic consequences. Therefore pharmacocavernosography should only be performed in cases with a history of incomplete or rapidly declining erections and when sufficient erection cannot be induced even under high doses of vasoactive substances. Positive test results will exclude clinically relevant venous or cavernosal insufficiency (Gall et al. 1989). The therapeutic consequence of cavernosometry and cavernosography is reconstructive vascular surgery or, in the majority of cases, implantation of penile protheses which are generally not accepted by a large number of patients.

The diagnostic workup of the cavernosal occlusive mechanism consists of two parts. It includes **intracavernosal pressure readings under the circumstances**

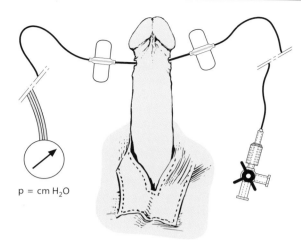

Fig. 10.7. Principle of cavernosometry and cavernosography

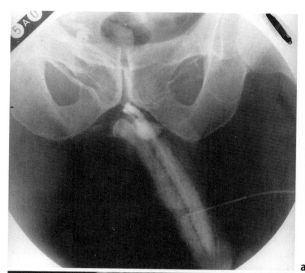

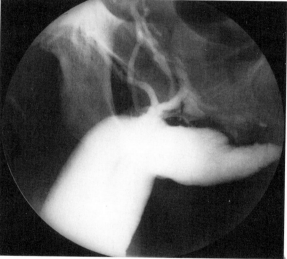

Fig. 10.8. Pathological findings in cavernosography. **a** Isolated insufficiency of the dorsal vein complex with minimal filling of the corpora cavernosa and rapid venous drainage of the applied contrast media via the V. dorsalis profunda. **b** Increased drainage via crural veins, which leave the corpora cavernosa dorsomedially

of an artificial erection following the infusion of saline under controlled flow rates. By means of a intracavernosal canula, saline is infused into the corpus cavernosum while a second canula continuously registers intracavernosal pressure. This part of the examination is called **cavernosometry** (Fig. 10.7).

Since adequate compression of the draining veins via the relaxed cavernosal sinoids is only achieved during increasing rigidity, nowadays the investigation is always performed with the use of vasoactive substances and is then classified as **pharmacocavernosography** (Stief et al. 1988). High doses of the vasoactive substances are necessary because the indication for pharmacocavernosography is a negative result in vasoactive testing. To achieve complete relaxation of the smooth muscles of the corpora cavernosa, additional small doses of vasoactive substances after an initial injection of a high dose may be necessary. New experimental data show that only a limited percentage of patients will reach this complete relaxation with a single dose of vasoactive substances (Hatzichristou et al. 1995).

In cavernosometry the infusion flow rate is reduced after a supersystolic pressure plateau has been reached. The flow rate/minute to maintain a defined intracavernosal pressure will be measured and is defined as the maintenance flow, one of the most important criteria in the evaluation of cavernosal compliance. A linear correlation of maintenance flow rates and intracavernosal pressures is an indication for complete relaxation of the cavernosal smooth muscles. Maintenance flow rates below 5 ml/minute are regarded as normal.

Another parameter that appears to be a relevant criterion in the evaluation of cavernosal occlusive function is the pressure decay time. After reaching a defined pressure plateau the intracavernosal infusion is stopped and the pressure decay is measured over a period of 30 seconds. Normally there is a slow linear decline of intra-cavernosal pressure. Exponentially dropping pressure values with a half-life of less than 1 minute and a pressure reduction of more than 50 mmHg within 30 seconds indicate a severe cavernous/venous disturbance.

In cases with increased maintenance flow rates the application of contrast medium can allow radiological documentation and localization of the venous leakage and the draining veins under direct visual control (cavernosography). Without previous vasoactive stimulation venous outflow from the corpora cavernosa shows great anatomical variability. In most cases the proximal corpus cavernosum will be drained by cavernosal veins while the drainage from the middle and distal parts of the corpora cavernosa will take place via the emissary veins and the circumflex veins into the superficial and deep dorsal veins. Ectopic veins which drain cavernosal blood directly into the femoral vein are relatively rare (Aboseif et al. 1989) (Fig. 10.8 a). In most cases of cavernosal insufficiency the increased drainage will be via physiological veins. Those types of insufficiency where the increased drainage appears via crural and cavernosal veins or via the glans penis and the corpus spongiosum especially will often prevent sufficient surgical therapy (Fig. 10.8b).

Complications of cavernosometry and cavernosography are often local hematomas which are usually resolved within a few days. Penile oedema after dislocation of the needles is a rare complication with correct positioning and sufficient length of the needles. Local infections of the corpora cavernosa have been described in the literature but are extremely rare so that routine antibiotic prophylaxis does not seem to be justified. In the event of local inflammatory changes of the penis the investigation should be postponed. Of course, allergies to the contrast medium can also occur with the use of non-ionic contrast media and have to be explained to the patient. In patients with cardiac insufficiency a critical fluid load will rapidly be reached in conventional dynamic cavernosometry. The introduction of pharmaconcavernosometry and cavernosography has reduced the necessary flow rates markedly and has thereby increased the safety of the investigation, especially in critical patients. In most patients, however, the indication for pharmaconcavernosography should be critically evaluated since therapeutic consequences of this invasive investigation are usually surgical.

Neurophysiological Investigations

From the patient's history, accompanying symptoms have to be questioned that might be an indication for **motory or sensory lesions** due to a neurologic disorder. Most of the systematic neurological diseases are already known and therefore easy to evaluate. The primary manifestation of a neurological disease by erectile dysfunction is extremely rare.

Clinically and electrophysiologically the most easily measurable reflex is the bulbus-cavernosus-reflex (BCR), which represents the nervous conduction between the penis and the sacral erectile center (S2–S4). A defined electrical impulse is applied via circular electrodes on the penile shaft and the reflex latency can be measured bilaterally via needle electrodes in the bulbocavernosal muscles (Porst et al. 1988b). Simultaneous registration of cortically evoked potentials is performed at known reference points at the scalp (somatosensory evoked potentials; SSEP). The absolute latency of the

BCR and differences between the two sides after repeated application of identical stimuli will provide information on the integrity of the short tracts between the penis and the sacral erectile spine. The potentials evoked are largely influenced by the patient's height which will allow the detection of disturbances of the long cerebrospinal tracts. Only a standardization of these diagnostic procedures made analysis of the somatosensory aspect of penile innervation, as well as of neurogenic erectile dysfunction, objectively possible (Kaneko and Bradley 1987; Lavoisier et al. 1989).

Another part of the efferent fibers belongs to the parasympathetic system, coming from the inferior hypogastric plexus and reaching the corpora cavernosa as the cavernosal nerve which inhibits the tonic activity of the smooth muscle cells. Direct diagnosis of lesions below the level of the pelvic floor has not been possible up to now. Indirect signs of disturbances of autonomous innervation are reduced urinary flow rates or impairment of bladder emptying without any other distinguishable cause. Direct measurement of the electrical activity of single smooth muscle cells of the corpus cavernosum (corpus cavernosum EMG, formerly also known as single potential analysis of cavernous electrical activity, "SPACE") is possible today (Stief 1993).

The interpretation of accumulated data, however, is difficult and often unclear, independent of the method of qualitative, semi-quantitative or computer-aided registration. Despite acceptable reproducibility, the diagnostic role of this procedure cannot yet be finally judged. Other indicators of disturbed sympathetic innervation can be a reduced or absent sympathetic skin reflex. In combined problems, but also in patients with normal somatosensory innervation and normal BCR, the sympathetic skin reflex is able to prove a neurogenic etiology in some patients and may be performed in selected cases (Dettmers et al. 1994).

As somatic and autonomic nerve fibers follow a separate anatomical course in some regions, iatrogenic or traumatic lesions can be the reason for certain patterns of damage. In many cases parasympathetic innervation can be very difficult to evaluate and therefore the patient's history and clinical data have to be given special attention. In forensic questions especially, anamnestic and clinical data need to be considered in addition to electrophysiological findings. In the face of elaborate and time-consuming diagnostics the lack of therapeutic relevance has diminished the importance of all these procedures.

Nocturnal Penile Tumescence and Rigidity Measurements (NPT)

In normal males there are 3–5 erection phases of 20–30 minutes' duration which occur physiologically during the rapid eye movement phase of sleep. On the assumption that psychological factors do not influence this type of erection, measurement of nocturnal penile erections has long been regarded as the reference method for differentiating organic and psychogenic erectile dysfunction (Davis-Joseph et al. 1995).

While investigations in sleep laboratories are very personnel and time-intensive, nowadays several different methods for registering nocturnal penile erections are available. Simple methods like the stamp test or the snap-gauge device only allow judgement of achieved tumescence and are therefore suitable for a rough estimation that does not include penile rigidity. With the **registration of nocturnal penile erections** by a Rigiscan®, changes in tumescence can be measured continuously and separately at the tip and the base of the penis and can be correlated with relative rigidity, which is the most relevant parameter concerning ability for penetration. Sensitivity and specificity of the method are, however, much lower than has been previously assumed and the findings can only be interpreted in conjunction with other organically oriented investigations. Since nocturnal penile tumescence measurements will register the quality of penile erections, but not the quality of nocturnal sleep, the results of these tests cannot be used in patients with sleep disturbances. Different medications and psychogenic psychiatric disturbances like depression can interfere with nocturnal erections. Also, with increasing age and in patients with hypogonadism, the number and rigidity of nocturnal erections is markedly reduced. In several neurological systematic diseases like multiple sclerosis nocturnal erections can be maintained, but psychogenic and refluxogenic erections can still be severely impaired, making intercourse impossible (Morales et al. 1990).

Owing to the low sensitivity and specificity and the high costs of the apparatus, the method is not suited to routine diagnostic work-up. It rather plays a role in forensic questions and in the evaluation of post-operative or post-traumatic erectile dysfunction, especially if isolated lesions of the autonomous innervation (nervi cavernosi) are questions under discussion.

Even in cases with pathological organic findings often clear-cut cause-and-effect relationships cannot be established so that diagnoses, which may appear to be scientifically founded, should be considered with caution and initially as a working diagnosis. It is not infrequent that patients without clinical manifestation of erectile dysfunction will show organic findings comparable to those found in patients with pronounced symptoms. Furthermore, few cases have only a single cause. In the majority of cases several factors are involved in the etiology of erectile dysfunction, so that not only a multidisciplinary approach but also an adequate therapeutic strategy should be aimed for. Despite revolutionary developments in the therapeutic sector, even today thorough diagnostic classification is mandatory.

10.2.5 Therapy of Erectile Dysfunction

Generally, therapy of erectile dysfunction can be classified into conservative, non- or minimal invasive and surgical treatment forms. Conservative methods include the various psychologically orientated treatments, transcutaneous topic and oral pharmacological efforts and the application of external vacuum devices. Injection therapy can be classified as minimally invasive.

Psychological Treatment

Strictly speaking, psychological treatment really begins with the initial evaluation of the patient and the discussion of his sexual disturbance. In many cases with short-term, non-fixated sexual disturbance without any relevant organic deficit only a few conversations will be sufficient. It is not infrequent that one of the main problems is a completely unrealistic, exaggerated expectation concerning sexual capacity, often produced or worsened by public media. The patient's attitude concerning his sexuality should be questioned. His own expectations and fear of failure should be clarified and the physiology of human erection should be explained. In many patients it has proven extremely helpful to explain the biochemical connections between fear of failure and increased sympathetic tone on the one hand, and a functional erectile problem on the other. Such counselling should prompt the patient and his partner to analyze their relationship. The aim of psychological counselling and treatment should not be limited to therapy of erectile dysfunction, but should also try to improve communication within the partnership.

In recent years classical psychodynamic therapies have been largely replaced by sexual therapeutic methods. Sexual therapy again relies on experience from other treatment forms such as couple therapy, family therapy or behavioural therapy. Overcoming fear of failure is one of the most important aspects of sexual therapy, as promulgated by Masters and Johnson (Masters and Johnson 1970). To reach this aim, the couple will usually be asked to refrain from coitus for a limited period of time, which will help to limit these fears of failure. One of the main aims of the therapy is to produce an atmosphere free of tension and fear and to promote and develop non-coital sexual practices. In most cases this alone will lead to a significant improvement of communicative ability and of the partner relationship. In most cases it is beneficial to involve both partners in the therapeutic process. Longstanding disturbances, additional severe problems in the partnership or a marked loss of libido have an unfavorable prognosis.

The results of sexual therapy as a causal therapeutic intervention in psychogenic erectile dysfunction are very good and reach success rates of approximately 90 % when therapy is of adequate duration. In many cases the involvement of the partner can be understood as one of the main reasons for such excellent results. The treatment, however, is very time-consuming and often numerous sessions are necessary which may be one of the main reasons for poor compliance. Problems of practicability result not only from the great investment in time, but from insufficient availability of adequately trained sexual therapists in many European countries.

Psychologically oriented therapy should not only be performed for purely psychogenic disturbances, but should also be discussed and offered to the patient if the origin of his erectile dysfunction is mainly organic. It is rare that erectile disturbances are of single cause and even in patients with a severe organic finding, especially if longstanding, psychogenic components are rarely absent. On the other hand, patients with erectile dysfunction of mainly psychogenic origin may benefit from an additional organically oriented treatment. Recent studies have clearly demonstrated the highly beneficial effect of such combined treatment, often either in conjunction with injection or vacuum therapy (Hartmann and Langer 1993).

Hormone Therapy

Generally, hormonal therapy should be limited to those patients with erectile dysfunction of endocrine origin. In the absence of other organic or psychogenic factors, a severe androgen deficiency is present when testosterone values are below 12 nmol/l. Values in the low normal range or slightly below should first be checked. The initiation of testosterone substitution is not justified on the basis of one isolated measurement. Since androgen substitution is not superior to placebo when serum testosterone is normal, hormone therapy without proven deficit has to be regarded as obsolete. When, however, testosterone values are repeatedly subnormal, it must be considered that testosterone is a decisive conditioning factor for central, but also for peripheral intracavernosal signal transduction on which NO synthetase depends (see also technique of testosterone substitution, Chap. 15).

In hyperprolactinemia slight stress-induced elevations of the serum levels should be ruled out by repeated measurements. Pharmacological causes for elevated prolactin levels should be excluded and in patients with a prolactinoma, treatment with a dopamine antagonist should be initiated (see Sect. 7.10).

Topical Therapy

Various substances potentially facilitating erections have been used on the penis. **Nitroglycerine** is one of the most thoroughly investigated substances for diagnostic and therapeutic use. Nitroglycerine paste increases arterial perfusion to a limited extent and facilitates erection under visual stimulation; its efficacy in improving cohabitation and patients' ability for sexual intercourse has not yet been proven. The use of condoms in this therapy is obligatory since severe headaches may be induced in the patient and in the partner. Generally, the efficacy of nitroglycerine has to be classified as limited or marginal. A positive effect on erection can only be expected in patients with psychogenic problems or minimal reduction of arterial perfusion: in patients with severe impairment of penile circulation they do not represent a reasonable therapeutic option.

Various attempts with external application of prostaglandin gel have been as disappointing as the use of gels containing papaverine.

The main cause for the insufficiency of the various substances and preparations is the inadequate local resorption through the tunica albuginea into the corpus cavernosum. So far all efforts to overcome this problem have been without success.

Intraurethral application of prostaglandin E_1 can avoid the problem of local resorption, at least in part. Using a one-time applicator 500–1000 µg can be instilled in the penile urethra. MUSE, commercially available since 1998, has the advantage of simple needle-less application (Padma-Nathan et al. 1977). Despite doses of 500–1000 µg its effectiveness is not comparable to intracavernosal use of vasoactive substances. The main side-effect is a considerable burning sensation in the urethra. No reliable data are available concerning local complications with long-term use of excessive doses. The dropout rate after 15 months (ca. 75 %) was very high. The high dose of PGE_1 makes condom use obligatory if the partner is pregnant.

Oral Therapy

The introduction of highly effective substances, particularly oral medication, has revolutionized therapy of erectile dysfunction. Preparations with a central mode of action (yohimbine, apomorphine) can be distinguished from those with peripheral effects (yohimbine, phentolamine, sildenafil).

Yohimbine is the substance most thoroughly evaluated. Different prospective, randomized studies demonstrate a success rate of about 30 % in patients with psychogenic erectile dysfunction and in those without severely compromised arterial perfusion. The main mode of action is based on central and peripheral α2 adrenolytic effects (Ernst and Pittler 1998; Vogt et al. 1997). It becomes fully effective after about 4–8 weeks. 3×5 to 3×10 mg daily are required. Alternatively "on demand" therapy can be administered one hour before intercourse. Since the side-effects are relatively low, it is **suitable as a primary treatment option** for patients with no or only minor organic disturbances and who reject more invasive methods.

Of those substances with a central mode of action **trazodone** is well investigated. In some cases it causes priapism, although therapeutic effectiveness tends to be inadequate at a dose of 100 to 200 mg. Because of its antidepressive effect it is suitable for psychogenic cases.

Great expectations are placed in **apomorphine**, currently under development. This substance has been known for a long time and affects central dopamine receptors. In its original galenic form its use in men was limited by its short half-life and severe gastrointestinal side-effects with frequent vomiting. Altered formulation with sublingual application seems to have improved its tolerability while maintaining its therapeutic potential for erectile dysfunction treatment (Heaton et al. 1995). Data from clinical trials in Canada show efficacy rates of up to 60% with 4–6 mg apomorphine. Although effectiveness with placebo was relatively high (over 30%) considerable therapeutic potential is assumed. Moderate or severe nausea occurred in just under 20%, severe nausea with vomiting was hardly observed. Side-effects disappear with longer use. In the USA the substance is in the process of approval; phase III studies are in progress in Europe.

Exogenous and endogenous opiates have shown pronounced inhibitory effects on sexual functions in animals and humans. Stress factors lead to a physiological stimulation of the endogenous opiate system and the tonic hyperactivity of the central opiate system may be responsible for erectile dysfunction in a selected number of patients. Placebo-controlled investigations with the **opiate antagonist naltrexone** show a limited efficacy of the drug in selected patients without relevant organic deficit (Fabbri et al. 1989; van Ahlen et al. 1995). The effectiveness of the substance is not sufficient.

The well-known adrenolytic effect of α-receptor blockers led to trials with oral **phentolamine** (Vasomax®), a nonselective α1–α2-receptor blocker with mainly peripheral effects. It is applied ca. one hour before intercourse. The results of different international phase II multicenter trials vary considerably. While in Germany doses of up to 60 mg were no more effective than placebo, in the USA licensing bodies found its effectiveness was greater, reaching responder rates of up to 48% with 80 mg, as opposed to 22% responders with placebo. Because of increased adrenergic tone the substance is promising in men over 50. Side-effects seen in trials are slight. The substance should be suitable for patients with psychogenic disturbances and increased fear

of failure (increased sympathetic tone) as well as slight disturbances of arterial perfusion.

In the past few years revolutionary changes in the therapy of erectile dysfunction, accompanied by hitherto unheard of journalistic attention, resulted when the first oral phosphodiesterase inhibitor was introduced. Physicians of all specializations suddenly became acknowledged experts on erectile dysfunction and healthy men became patients overnight, unfortunately in some cases not without lethal consequences.

To date the **phosphodiesterase type V inhibitor sildenafil** (Viagra®) has become available. Its mechanism of action is based on a biochemically caused modulation of the relaxation of smooth muscle cells. A parasympathetic erection-inducing nervous impulse leads to the release of NO at the endothelial cells of the cavernosal tissue. By activation of guanylyl cyclase guanosine triphosphate and second messenger cGMP are metabolized. As shown in Sect. 10.2.2, cGMP leads to relaxation of smooth muscle cells by depletion of intercellular calcium. By inhibiting local phosphodiesterase, sildenafil leads to reduced metabolism of cGMP, which accumulates in the cavernosal tissue and thus impairs relaxation of the smooth musculature of the corpora cavernosa, resulting in improved erection (Fig. 10.9). Thus the effectiveness of sildenafil depends on the transmittal of a nervous impulse via an intact peripheral reflex system, on the presence of sufficient amounts of NO in erectile tissue and on adequate sexual stimulation.

Phosphodiesterase is an enzyme present in many tissues of the body. In erectile tissue types III to V predominate. Type III and IV inhibit the metabolism of cAMP in smooth muscle cells, Type V concentrates on cGMP. **Sildenafil is a highly selective phosphodiesterase type V inhibitor** which has only slight effects on other types of receptors. These crossreactions, however, are the basis for several of the observed side effects.

The substance displays excellent effectiveness in erectile dysfunction of various etiologies. It achieves success rates of up to 75% in patients with organically caused dysfunction, up to over 80% in patients with predominantly psychologically caused disturbances. It is not surprising that success rates of over 80% are reached in large-scale studies in paraplegic patients with intact reflexes. In patients with arterial hypertonus and other vascular disturbances the substance has excellent results. As to be expected, lower effectiveness is observed in patients with diabetes mellitus and latent or clinically manifest polyneuropathy in whom signal transduction is disturbed and in whom diminished transmittal occurs in the course of the disease. The effectiveness of 45% after radical prostatectomy heralded in initial publications can only be achieved when nerve-protective surgery is carried out (Zippe et al. 1998). Even if effectiveness rates of up to 80% with sildenafil can be achieved in a small series, if nerve-protective surgery

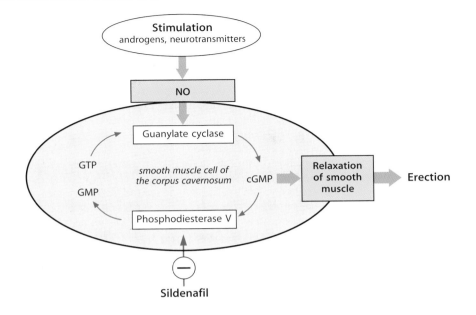

Fig. 10.9. Mechanism of action of sildenafil on the smooth muscle of the corpora cavernosa. Following stimulation NO activates the guanylyl cyclase and cGMP is released causing relaxation of smooth muscle. Phosphodiesterase deactivates cGMP. Inhibition of the phosphodiesterase by sildenafil leads to increased cGMP levels and thereby erection is enhanced. (From Rolf and Nieschlag 1998)

was not possible, the substance is only rarely effective. Especially for the diabetic patient, and for those with postoperative erectile disturbances, self-injection therapy remains the most effective therapeutic option, even after the introduction of oral therapy.

Sildenafil is rapidly absorbed after oral ingestion. When taken on an empty stomach, maximum plasma concentrations are reached after 30 minutes. Therapeutic plasma levels are maintained for about 4 hours. During this time an erection can be induced, given adequate stimulation. From the clinical point of view it has proved important to stress the necessity of appropriate stimulation, as an adequate erection is not an automatic pharmacologically induced process, as in self-injection therapy. The dose required depends on the underlying cause. In psychogenic erectile dysfunction 25–50 mg are usually entirely adequate; in organic disturbances it can be increased up to 100 mg. The duration of effective plasma concentrations increases with higher doses. Clinically this correlates with an extension of the time during which an erection can be induced. The effectiveness of the substance, however, can only be increased by 10 %

per dose stage, in total ca. 25 %. For this reason, as with other modalities, stepwise dose-finding and adjustment is recommended to avoid side-effects. True tachyphylaxis was not yet observed, even if dose adjustment was soon necessary. Conversely, an improvement in the quality of an erection under sildenafil was not observed after a 6-month therapy interval, as can occur in self-injection therapy.

The **spectrum of side-effects** results from the effect of phosphodiesterase on other parts of the body and from interaction with other phosphodiesterase isoenzymes. As phosphodiesterase type V occurs in relatively high concentrations in vessels of the nasal cavity and the central nervous system, **flu-like symptoms with slight headache, nasal congestion and flushed face** can frequently occur. Slight **gastrointestinal complaints** are not unusual. Effect on **blood pressure** is slight, with a decrease of systolic and diasystolic pressure. Interaction with phosphodiesterase type VI of the retina leads to **disturbed color perception** with slight blue/green shifts, **increased light sensitivity** and **blurred vision**. This side-effect is partly dose-dependent and occurs in only ca. 2 % of cases at a dose of 50 mg. At 100 mg 11 % report these effects; when raised to 200 mg side effects increased to 40 %. On the basis of available clinical and experimental data it is assumed that these accompanying effects are no cause for concern. **In patients with retinitis pigmentosa sildenafil should not be prescribed because of a genetic defect of the phosphodiesterases in the retina.**

As sildenafil was developed primarily as a medication for angina pectoris and as an alternative to nitrate therapy, it carries only few cardiovascular risks. As a general rule, the moderate decrease in blood pressure of

5–10 mmHg is clinically insignificant. Experience to date with **hypertonic patients and various antihypertensive medication** shows unchanged effectiveness of the substance when compared with other patient populations. Cardiac side-effects are not to be expected as phosphodiesterase type V is not active in the heart itself, so that contractability and pulse frequency are not influenced. Recent investigations show that the side-effect profile with antihypertensive mono- or combined therapy with up to 3 antihypertensive medications is not altered (Kloner et al. 1999). Conversely, sildenafil is contraindicated with simultaneous use of nitrates or NO medication. This derives from the substance's mode of action, as nitrates and NO donators affect the same target in vessel musculature, i.e. cGMP. While nitrates and limosidonin clearly increase intracellular concentrations of cGMP, metabolism is inhibited by sildenafil, leading to a potentiation of nitrates and NO donators in the circulation. Blood pressure can fall by as much as 40–50 mmHg and thus trigger longlasting syncope-like conditions.

> For this reason **sildenafil therapy is strictly contraindicated in patients with coronary disease or patients under nitrate or NO therapy.** As more than 100 different nitrate and NO preparations are currently available, a detailed drug anamnesis is absolutely necessary prior to sildenafil therapy. Conversely, a patient receiving a nitrate preparation must be prohibited from taking sildenafil. In cardiovascular emergencies the patient must be asked about possible previous sildenafil use.

It can be assumed that about $1/3$ of the deaths reported in connection with sildenafil can be ascribed to the interaction between it and nitrate and NO donors. In a proportion of these lethal cases death occurred during intercourse. Whereas data for intraurethral therapies such as MUSE or self-injection show that these treatments did not lead to a higher mortality rate during sexual activity, no certain data are yet available for sildenafil. In a meta-analysis of 11 placebo-controlled studies Conti et al. (1999) found the rate of severe cardiovascular events was not higher in coronary patients not using nitrates but using Viagra (7%) (placebo = 10%).

As performing sexual intercourse involves no higher exertion (average of 3–4 metabolic units [METS]) than other daily activities such as brisk walking or moderate gardening, the treatment of erectile dysfunction, regardless of the therapy modality, does not represent an incalculable risk. A consensus recently published by British experts pointed out that **for patients with low cardiovascular risk** (controlled blood pressure, slight stable angina pectoris, coronary heart disease following successful revascularization by stent and bypass), no additional cardiological investigations are necessary. In **moderate cardiovascular risk** (several risk factors, latent cardiac insufficiency [stage I or II, NYHA] moderately severe angina pectoria) cardiological diagnosis should be performed by stress ECG. A peak load of 150 watts or more with no sign of coronary ischemia presents no cardiological contraindication to erectile dysfunction therapy, regardless of the modality.

> For **patients with high risk** (unstable angina pectoris, decompensated cardiac insufficiency, uncontrolled hypertonus) erectile dysfunction therapy should not be carried out until the cardiac condition has been stabilized (Jackson et al. 1999).

In summary, the introduction of modern orally effective medication has produced a dramatic change in the therapeutic possibilities for erectile dysfunction. The effectiveness of the available substances and those under development varies greatly. Successful oral treatment of a broad spectrum of psychogenic and organic erectile dysfunction is possible. At the present time sildenafil is by far the most effective oral substance, nearly comparable to self-injection therapy, still considered the gold standard. Because of its mode of action and the unavoidable contraindications, oral therapy will not completely replace other treatment forms.

External Devices

The principle of **venous restriction by compression** at the base of the penis has long been known. Different commercially available rings have been designed to reduce venous drainage at the penis basis and to facilitate erection. These rings are only beneficial in patients with intact arterial perfusion, mostly young patients with primary erectile dysfunction. Since many cases of cavernosal insufficiency and incompliant cavernosal occlusion mechanism are combined with pronounced impairment of arterial perfusion and secondary degeneration of the smooth musculature, the use of penis rings is very limited as a monotherapy.

External vacuum devices have been successfully used for many years. The various available systems differ mainly in respect to a pump mechanism and the design of the restriction **rings** and bands. The devices consist of a plastic cylinder which is placed over the penis. A vacuum is established in the cylinder with a manual or battery power pump which leads to increasing engorgement of the penis, and to a state very similar to a physiological erection. To prevent premature drainage of blood from the corpora cavernosa and therefore to allow sexual intercourse, a penile ring or restricting rubber

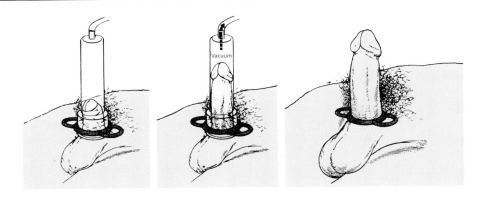

Fig. 10.10. Principle of vacuum devices. (With kind permission of the Osbon Company)

band is placed at the penis base after full tumescence has been achieved (Fig. 10.10).

While erection rings are only applicable in patients with adequate arterial perfusion, vacuum pumps can be used universally in patients with any kind of erectile dysfunction. In the majority of these patients, vacuum devices will be able to induce a sufficient erection and rigidity to allow intercourse. This includes patients with severe vascular problems. There may be a limited efficacy of vacuum systems in patients with pronounced intercavernosal scarring, which may be present after longterm injection therapy, priapisms of excessive duration or after explantation of infected protheses. In Peyronie's disease with severe angulation of the penis the use of vacuum devices may sometimes be impossible for purely mechanical reasons.

The main advantages of vacuum systems are that they are practically free of side-effects, even in longterm treatment (Witherington 1989). The induced erection, however, is distinguishably different from the normal physiological erection. In general the quality of the erection with respect to rigidity is not always completely satisfying: while in a normal erection only the corpora cavernosa will show enlargement, the entire penile tissue will show a venous enlargement distal to the restriction ring when a vacuum pump is used. This can lead to **petechial bleeding** and **ecchymoses** of the penile skin with subjective **sensations of coldness** and **numbness**. Additionally, **edemas** can be observed in some patients. For these reasons, manufacturers of the vacuum systems usually instruct the patients **not to use the restricting bands or rings for more than 30 minutes**.

Another typical problem with the use of vacuum devices is insufficient rigidity in the corpora cavernosa proximal to the restricting band which may lead to severe instability at the base of the penis. Ejaculatory problems are not infrequent. They can be caused by mechanical compression of the urethra, but functional causes due to insufficient precoital stimulation are also very common.

The acceptance of vacuum systems varies considerably and is cited as reaching 85% in American investigations (Cookson and Nadig 1993). In Germany acceptance is considerably less and strongly dependent on whether the patients respond to other forms of therapy (Derouet and Zehl 1990; Wechsel et al. 1993). For patients for whom oral or injection therapy is insufficient, the vacuum pump is the much more attractive alternative to venous or implant surgery. Younger patients especially will often refuse vacuum systems owing to their technical aspects and limitations of integrating it into their personal sexuality. In older patients with longstanding partnerships, with slow progressive or postoperative erectile dysfunction, the acceptance of vacuum devices is usually much better. Patients who have adopted this therapy often show better compliance in longterm use than patients undergoing injection therapy. Among the reasons for terminating the use of vacuum devices is often the loss of "cosmetic" acceptance, mostly by the patient himself rather than by the partner, insufficient efficacy of the vacuum system concerning rigidity, recurrent pain and subcutaneous hematomas or waning interest in sexual activity.

Injection Therapy

The intracavernosal application of vasoactive substances has not only become established for diagnostic purposes, but also for therapy. It is, indeed, one of the most important therapeutic options in organic erectile dysfunction. Injection therapy can be offered to all patients, especially those with normal or pathological arterial inflow but with intact cavernosal occlusion mechanism. Patients with neurogenic disturbances are especially suited for this type of treatment since causal therapy is not available, because of morphologically intact penile and cavernosal tissue and normal circulatory situation. Furthermore, only very small doses of vasoactive substances are needed to induce sufficient erections. As an alternative, application of the new oral substances can be considered, which in the case of sildenafil also has a success rate of over 80 %. The use of a vacuum device can be an excellent alternative; primary implantation of penile protheses is usually refused by the often young patients.

Even in patients with erectile dysfunction of arterial origin, therapy is usually effective. As pointed out in the chapter on diagnostic work-up, the reaction to vasoactive substances in this patient population is usually characterized by a delayed onset of action. When the cavernosal occlusion mechanism, however, is intact, practically all of these patients will achieve a full erection after a latency time. Therefore, injection therapy at individually adapted dosage is one of the most widely applied forms of treatment in vascular erectile dysfunction. In the meantime oral therapy has also become an acceptable treatment for this patient population. Only in selected cases are revascularization and penile protheses alternatives which are discussed separately.

For patients with mainly psychogenic erectile dysfunction, injection therapy as well as the use of orally effective substances can be very useful adjuvant options, accompanying psychologically oriented treatment. In these patients injection therapy can show a beneficial effect on the overall outcome and may reduce duration of treatment significantly. Such additional treatment will give the patient greater security, and will help to reduce fear of failure, especially in patients with refractory or longstanding psychogenic disturbances. Such a strategy can, however, be problematic for psychological reasons and close consensus between the physicians involved is particularly necessary in these patients. Patients without demonstrable organic deficits have to be clearly alerted to potential complications and side-effects of injection therapy.

Patients with cavernosal insufficiency are unsuited to injection therapy because, owing to the underlying pathophysiological mechanism, they will not react adequately to the injection of vasoactive substances. Because of the dual mechanism of action some of these patients will respond to sildenafil. If other invasive surgical options are refused, the application of a vacuum system or the combination of various therapy forms can be considered.

> From the medical point of view, autoinjection therapy appears to be suitable for the majority of patients with organic causes of erectile dysfunction. However, certain criteria should be fulfilled:
> - adequate patient selection,
> - cooperative, reliable patient,
> - adequate follow-up,
> - experience in dealing with possible side-effects.

Autoinjection therapy should only be offered to patients with a current sexual partner and who, apart from their proven organic origin of erectile dysfunction, have proved to have sufficient manual dexterity and intellectual capability. In physically handicapped patients with reduced vision or extreme adipositas the patient will not be able to perform controlled injections himself. The indication must be reevaluated. In these cases, the application of the vasoactive substance by the partner can be discussed. In all patients regular follow-up is mandatory due to the possible severe side-effects of this medication. The physician himself should be experienced in the treatment of acute complications like priapism, and close cooperation with a local hospital department for these rare circumstances is usually advisable.

> The contraindications for autoinjection are similar to those that apply to the diagnostic use of vasoactive substances:
> - decompensated cardiac and circulatory insufficiency,
> - intellectual incompetence,
> - lacking compliance,
> - severe psychiatric disorder,
> - sexual deviation.

Many authors will regard this kind of therapy as not indicated in patients without an existing partnership or with sexually transmitted diseases. These questions, especially whether an HIV patient with erectile dysfunction for whom the vacuum system and other non-invasive therapeutic options have proven inadequate, or were refused by the patient, can and should be treated with intracavernosal injections, certainly have to be decided on an individual basis. Anticoagulant medication like cumarin or aspirin does not represent a contraindication since an increased complication rate can be excluded in this often well-motivated and disciplined patient population if adequate compression at the site of injection is guaranteed.

The injection technique is equivalent to that when applying vasoactive substances as a diagnostic procedure. The whole length of the penis can be used and the patient should be instructed to change injection sites. This may reduce the risk of plaque formation at the tunica albuginea or the formation of localized corporal fibrosis.

Principally, two different forms of injection therapy are possible and have become established:

In **periodic interval therapy** the vasoactive substance is injected at fixed intervals by the physician or the patient himself in a previously tested dose. The application interval is usually 1 to 2 weeks. For this kind of application patients with residual erectile function and only a minor reduction of arterial perfusion are suitable. Patients with psychogenic impotence also often show marked improvement of the symptoms with increased activity of the smooth muscle cells even in the treatment-free interval. This effect has not been demonstrated for oral substances.

In **cavernosal autoinjection therapy** the patient injects the vasoactive substances himself at home, according to his own demand. This therapy is especially suitable for patients with neurogenic or other severe organic erectile dysfunction, especially patients with diabetes mellitus or post-surgical erectile dysfunction. Informed written consent about potential hazards and complications of the treatment is mandatory and intensive pre-treatment instructions on the preparation of the substances and the use of the injections is essential. As soon as the patient masters these tasks he can be integrated into an autoinjection programme with a recommended fixed dose and application interval. Regular routine follow-up visits should also be carried out.

The dosage of the vasoactive substances is dependent on their efficacy. An erection duration of 30–60 minutes is advisable and sufficient. As in the case of diagnostic use of vasoactive substances, dosage will be increased in small steps after initial testing to evaluate the correct therapeutic dose with a minimal risk of priapism. Often the reaction to a defined drug dose is much better under home conditions, so that in many cases the dose can be reduced by up to 30 %. On the one hand, this results from stabilization and other accompanying psychological effects caused by positive experiences following injection therapy. On the other hand, it is probably due to better compliance of the cavernosal vessels and smooth muscle cells. Moreover, an additive effect of pharmacological stimulation and sexually induced androgen neurotransmitter release occurs when the injection of the vasoactive substance is performed under home conditions.

Autoinjection therapy requires great patient discipline concerning constant dosage and application interval. In cases where an injection does not produce an adequate erection a second injection on the same day should be strictly avoided because of the danger of prolonged erection and priapism. With reliable patients the incidence of priapism, which represents a considerable risk of up to 10 % during the diagnostic use of substances even with careful patient selection, will not pose a major problem during long-term therapy (Porst and Weller 1989). Nevertheless, patients should be thoroughly informed about the possibility and potential hazards of such drug-induced priapism. Under PGE$_1$ prolonged erections usually subside spontaneously due to the short half-life of the substance and local metabolism (van Ahlen et al. 1994).

The worst long-term complication of autoinjection therapy is localized or generalized fibrosis of the corpora cavernosa. The main cause of local fibrosis may be the

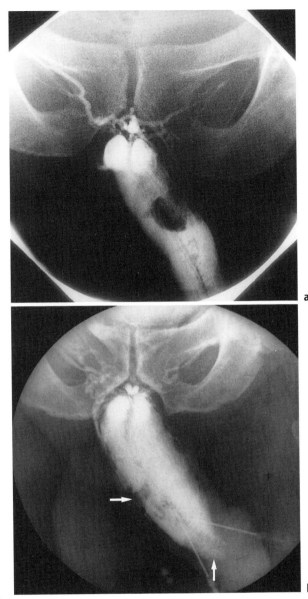

Fig. 10.11 a, b. Cavernosal fibrosis after autoinjection therapy. **a** Extensive local fibrosis with a filling defect in cavernosography; clinically palpable induration and penile angulation. **b** Diffuse fibrosis with a lateral filling defect in the midportion of the corpora (*arrow*) as well as a marked narrowing of the distal corporal tips (*arrow*). Marked pathological venous outflow with clinical signs of cavernosal insufficiency

recurrent microtrauma by the needle at the injection site, resorption of small local hematomas or toxic reactions, often seen in erections of long duration due to overdosing of the vasoactive substance. The formation of small nodules is clinically without consequences in most cases. During a 3-month treatment pause these changes are usually completely reversible. In severe fibrosis of the tunica albuginea or with a localized intracavernosal scarring with insufficient cavernosal relaxation capability penile deviation can ensue. The worst complication is generalized fibrosis of the corpora cavernosa due to chronic use. Such fibroses are reversible only in about half the patients, even if therapy is stopped immediately (Fig. 10.11). Animal experiments have shown that the incidence of such fibroses varies, but can occur with all vasoactive substances. Histologically, the initial alterations are seen in a pronounced hypertrophy of the smooth muscle cell, later converting to increased intracellular filaments and considerable intracavernosal fibrosis. The incidence of such an event is especially high with papaverine, because of which the substance is no longer used. A combination of papaverine with phentolamine seems to be tolerated much better, as is PGE_1. The hypothesis that the low pH of papaverine (pH 2.7) might be the main reason for scarring of the cavernosal tissue has been ruled out on the basis of blood gas analysis and systematic investigations on the use of solutions with different osmolarity and pH. Probably toxicity specific to the various substances is responsible.

At present a combination of vasoactive intestinal VIP and phentolamine available in injection form and awaiting approval as Invicorp® is well tolerated. Highly effective and comparable to PGE_1, it appears to have hardly any side-effects; longterm results with this solution are, however, not yet available.

Apart from substance-specific differences there is a clear-cut correlation between these toxic fibroses and the frequency and duration of intracavernosal injections. Therefore the patient should be advised to limit the number of injections to 2 per week regardless of the vasoactive substance used. The necessity of increasing the dosage of a given drug in injection therapy does not indicate tachyphylaxis of the substance used, but is usually accompanied by deterioration of the cavernosal tissue or the pre-existing disturbance.

This treatment is well accepted by the patient and his partner. Approximately 20% of the potential users will refuse this kind of therapy because they do not approve of intracavernosal injections. Drop-out rates under therapy amount to about 30–50%. In most cases this is either due to reduced efficacy of the drugs or increasing loss of sexual interest and deterioration of the partner relationship.

The exceedingly rare but potentially hazardous complications of autoinjection therapy make a multifactorial organic diagnostic work-up mandatory before therapeutic application of vasoactive drugs. The indication should therefore be evaluated very carefully and all requirements concerning informed consent must be fulfilled. All potential patients should be thoroughly informed in writing about possible complications, especially infections and progressive iatrogenic deterioration of the corporal tissue with consecutive fibrosis and complete loss of erectile capability. Regular follow-up examinations are mandatory.

Autoinjection therapy, however, still represents an indispensible option in erectile dysfunction. It is technically uncomplicated and can be rapidly learned by the patient. The main advantage is widereaching stimulation of the normal physiologic erection with a maximum of therapeutically achievable rigidity. After injection of the vasoactive substance an erection sufficient for intercourse is induced after a short latency period. With correct dosage this erection regresses spontaneously after ejaculation. In contrast to a physiological erection, however, there is no reaction of the glans and the corpus spongiosum.

It has proven effective to start patients with only slight perfusion disturbances and/or severe psychogenic symptoms on interval therapy. Increased arterial perfusion will often lead to an improved condition of the corporal tissue or will improve the sensitivity of spontaneous erections even in the injection-free interval. Not infrequently these patients will even observe complete normalization of erectile capability and anamnestic and physical findings will have improved after 8–10 injections so that further treatment is not necessary. If this improvement does not occur and the patient continues to be dependent on vasoactive substances, he may be enrolled in a self-injection programme. Patients with neurogenic erectile dysfunction or who have severely disturbed arterial perfusion should be directly treated by self-injection therapy.

In certain patient populations (diabetes mellitus, postsurgical dysfunction) cavernosal self-injection will certainly continue to be important, since up to 90% of the patients can be helped when all methods are applied. Moreover, in severe organically caused cases various oral and vasactive substances can be combined. The future will bring new developments.

The relative acceptance of this method has changed considerably since the introduction of highly effective oral substances.

Surgical Treatment

Even if non-invasive therapeutic forms available today offer very effective treatment options, a large number of patients would prefer surgical correction of organic factors to regain undisturbed sexuality free from the use of any auxiliary measures. This understandable desire on the part of the patient can justify surgical measures even when other, less invasive therapeutic options are generally available. Only surgery on the penile vessel offers the patient the possibility of reachieving physiological erections without acute intervention. Here proven organic deficits are a basic requirement for the indication of any kind of surgical therapy. Surgical possibilities can be classified into separate operations on the venous system in patients with increased venous drainage of the corpora cavernosa, into reconstructive vascular surgery in cases of arterial disease and into prothetic implants in patients with otherwise untreatable erectile dysfunction and specific indications. Altogether since the introduction of orally effective substances, indications for surgery have decreased and, for practical purposes, no longer play any role in prothetic implantation.

Venous Surgery. Typically patients with cavernosal insufficiency will react insufficiently to drug as well as to injection therapy, nor will vacuum devices be successful in all patients.

The basic principle of all surgical procedures is to increase the venous drainage resistance. Patients with congenital primary erectile dysfunction due to an ectopic vein are especially good candidates for this type of surgery. Simple surgical resection of this vessel leads to correction of the underlying cause and will abolish the clinical symptoms. Similar success may be achieved in the very rare cases of penile fracture with a fistula with secondary communication between the corpus cavernosum and the corpus spongiosum. Here, spongiolysis with closure of the fistula may treat this problem causally.

In all other patients surgical strategy will consist of a radical resection of all accessible drainage pathways that have previously been documented by pharmacocavernosography. In most cases, the superficial and deep dorsal veins are resected with ligation of all circumflex veins at the penile base. The operation is simple and serious complications are practically never observed. Disappointing long-term results with success rates of approximately 25–30%, especially in patients with drainage of the crural veins, lead to the propagation of a much more radical venous resection (Lewis 1990). Ligation of these proximal veins, however, will only be possible after division of the ligamentum suspensorium penis which in a percentage of patients will be followed by edema and often by persisting pain and disturbances of cutaneous sensitivity. Furthermore, a number of patients will report a considerable shortening of the penis (Kim et al. 1995b). Unfortunately, even these much more radical operations have not been able to improve the poor postoperative results with success rates of only 30% after 1–2 years of observation. The same applies to plication of the proximal crurae, the ligation of the internal ileac vein or the retrograde radiological embolization of penile veins with success rates of only up to 30%.

A completely different approach is the arterialization of the deep dorsal vein. This procedure was first inaugurated by Virag for the vascularization of arterial disturbances. It is supposed to increase blood flow to the penis and the corpora cavernosa itself and significantly increase the drainage resistance in the venous system (Virag et al. 1981). Whether this concept, requiring much greater surgical effort, will lead to an improvement of post-operative success rates has never been verified since controlled studies are lacking.

In view of the pathogenetically highly heterogenous patient population with considerable diagnostic inconsistencies it is not surprising that initial hopes for venous surgery could not be fulfilled in the long run. Notwithstanding improved technical possibilities, accompanying arterial problems often become evident (Hatzichristou et al. 1995). In many cases, they are the primary cause of cavernosal insufficiency. In cases with simultaneous severe arterial problems and cavernosal insufficiency, venous surgery alone is not very promising. Whether arterial revascularization is able to halt degenerative changes in the corpora cavernosa or even improve these changes is unclear.

In the vast majority of cases venous surgery represents a symptomatic therapy and does not treat the underlying pathomechanism of insufficient cavernosal occlusion at the level of the corpora cavernosa and the tunica albuguinea: it will therefore not be able to treat the cause of a clinical symptom. Therefore, in the long run even with successful resection of draining veins, the formation of new collaterals is predetermined. On the other hand, it cannot be excluded that after primary success of the operation progressive deterioration of the underlying clinical process will lead to later recurrence of symptoms.

It is unclear whether any prognostic criteria exist allowing the surgeon to predict possible success rates. While some authors have used pharmacocavernosometry and pharmaco-cavernosography (Aboseif et al. 1989) to demonstrate a connection between postoperative results and the severity of a demonstrable leakage, other authors could not see any correlation between these findings and postoperative results (Kim and McVary 1995b). Clinical experience shows that with maintenance flow rates of more than 100 ml/min even a temporary restoration of erectile capability will not be achieved by venous surgery. Possibly CC-EMG may be of prognostic help (Stief et al. 1994).

Although venous surgery has lost much of its previous importance during the last few years, it should not be overlooked that a few patients who do not react to other therapy or who fail to achieve good erections with a vacuum device will benefit from this minimal surgical procedure, especially if there is no concomittant arterial problem and venous drainage via the proximal crural veins can be dispensed with.

Revascularization Surgery. Vascular problems are the most common cause of erectile dysfunction. It appears only logical to make any effort to increase arterial perfusion in the penile musculature in order to restore physiological erection without any auxillary method. The main aim of all revascularization surgery is therefore optimization of corporal perfusion which may be compromised by arterial obstruction. Direct revascularization of the corpora cavernosa, in which the inferior epigastric artery is anastomosed directly to the tunica albuguinea and the corpora cavernosa, suffers from an increased rate of postoperative priapisms and rapid spontaneous closure of the anastomosis. These complications result from the higher flow rates that will regularly lead to hyperplasia with consecutive fibrosis and secondary shunt obstruction and from the poor blood outlet into the corpora cavernosa itself. For an anastomosis between the inferior epigastric artery and the dorsal penile artery a free vascular lumen at the bifurcation of the A. penis is necessary. This allows increased perfusion in the cavernosal artery via a retrograde perfusion of the dorsal penile artery. In cases of bilateral obstruction of the cavernosal artery, arterialization of the deeper dorsal vein is an alternative. It is supposed to increase blood flow to the corpora cavernosa by retrograde perfusion of the emissary veins. These surgical techniques are said to have success rates between 20% and 50%.

The most recent commonly used surgical method is an anastomosis of three vessels (between the inferior epigastric artery, dorsal artery and deep dorsal vein), which combines the principles of the previously mentioned procedures (Hauri 1984). The arterio-venous fistula leads to a decrease in outflow resistance in the arterial part of the anastomosis and results in a considerable increase in flow rates. At the same time this three-vessel anastomosis leads to increased resistance in the venous part. The success rate of this operation is between 30 and 70%. The main complication is a glans hyperemia which can be seen in up to 20% of the patients. This results from increased arterial perfusion of the glans, can occur up to 2 years after the operation and is clinically associated with congestion edema, meatal stenosis and necrosis, in severe cases, even with glans necrosis. The symptoms can be so pronounced that a distal subcoronal ligature of all superficial veins will not be sufficient and closure of the arterio-venous fistula will be necessary.

Up to very recently, indications for revascularization surgery continued to be unclear. For many years no coherent opinion emerged whether the operation should be performed in patients with cavernosal insufficiency, metabolic disorders such as diabetes mellitus or posttraumatic erectile dysfunction. MRT evidence indicates that revascularization surgery in its various modifications does not lead to an effective increase in perfusion of the corpora cavernosa itself. This pathophysiological background makes all kinds of reconstructive operations questionable (Sohn et al. 1992). Very possibly time-consuming penile re-

vascularization is indicated only in patients in whom a pronounced decrease in arterial perfusion can be documented and collaterals between the superficial and deep penile arteries can be demonstrated (Wegner et al. 1995).

The uncertain pathophysiological mechanism leading to disappointing surgical results in some studies as well as the sometimes considerable complications of the various methods have greatly reduced the optimism initially associated with this therapeutic option and lately it has played only a minor role.

Prothesis Surgery. Prothesis surgery is offered independently of the pathogenesis of erectile dysfunction as a primary therapeutic option and is well accepted by patients in Germany. In practically all cases **it represents the final therapeutic option.**

In most instances, it is offered to patients who do not or no longer react adequately to other forms of therapy or who absolutely refuse them. In vascular disturbances autoinjection therapy has usually been performed, but is no longer accepted by the patient or his partner or may have led to severe corporal fibrosis. In neurogenic erectile dysfunction the application of vasoactive drugs may have induced recurrent priapisms and in a small number of patients, the development of a retracting penis which makes the use of condoms extremely difficult. For such patients a penile implant may be indicated. Another indication may be erectile dysfunction after radical tumour surgery in the pelvis. In the vast majority of cases, the indication for a penile implant is cavernosal insufficiency failing to respond to therapy.

Modern prothetic surgery goes back to the fundamental developments of Scott (1973) and Small and Carrion (1975). All the different types of prothesis available to date derive from these prototypes. Apart from several semi-rigid flexible protheses, a large variety of different hydraulic implants is available (Fig. 10.12). The implantation of semi-rigid flexible protheses is technically uncomplicated and due to their simple construction, mechanical problems are rare. However, postoperative results are cosmetically and functionally unsatisfactory since the penis will have a constant size and tumescence at all times. Mechanical implants with improved cosmetic aspects and activation/deactivation by means of an internal tension mechanism represent further developments.

Hydraulic implants can be classified into different groups. In the single-piece prothesis a defined, very small amount of fluid is transferred between an outer and inner chamber. This prothesis allows only very limited changes in penile rigidity. The size of the penis in the activated and non-activated status is constant so that compared to semi-rigid implants cosmetic improvements are similar. In the multipiece hydraulic implants the greater transferrable fluid volume allows a considerably better cosmetic result. Here the patient himself can

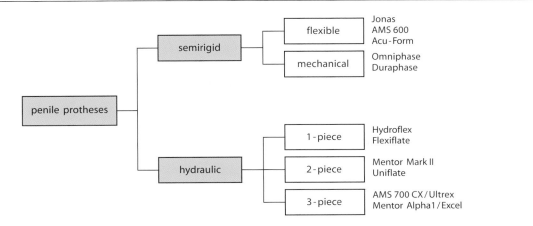

Fig. 10.12. Various penile implants

control tumescence and detumescence. As may be expected, two-piece protheses in which pump and reservoir are integrated into one functional unit will give slightly inferior results, both cosmetic and functional, than three-piece models due to the relatively small transfer volume. The usual three-piece implants in general use will show an increase in diameter only with increasing rigidity due to a unidirectional dilatatory capacity. The development of bidirectional elastic materials enables real increases in penile length to be reached in the activated status. The major advantage of these complex and expensive implants is the functional principle which is very similar to the physiological erection. By means of a scrotal pump fluid is transferred from the intraperitoneal or extraperitoneal paravesical reservoir into the corpora cavernosa. Practically on demand, an enlargement of the penis which is very similar to a natural erection with an increase not only in rigidity, but also in penile growth and length can be imitated (Fig. 10.13).

For implant acceptance not only optimal longitudinal rigidity, but also sufficient flexibility in rest is the most important point. If permanent pressure on the tissue is reduced the danger of local pressure lesions with perforation of the prothesis proximately or distally may be diminished. This risk is especially high in paraplegic patients with reduced sensitivity and trophic problems due to the underlying disease. Another typical complication, especially with semi-rigid protheses is the so-called Concorde-phenomenon when the insufficiently perfused glans is ventrally dislocated. The increased mobility of the glans may produce significant clinical problems for the patient and increase the risk of a distal perforation.

The reliability of hydraulic implants has been significantly improved over the last 10 years so that mechanical defects occur in only 5–10 % of implants (Grein et al.

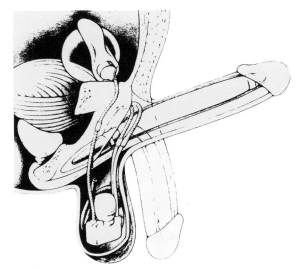

Fig. 10.13. General function of 3-piece hydraulic implants in flaccid state and erection (with kind permission of AMS Pfizer Company)

1989). Altogether the most serious complication in implant surgery is infection. The rate of this in primary operations will be between 2–4 %; in revision surgery in diabetic patients it may reach 15–20 %. In most cases, normal cutaneous bacteria play a major role (staphylococcus aureus). Clinically, these implant infections can present with very different symptoms, late infections can manifest even months after the primary operation and not infrequently fever and leukocytosis will be a major symptom. Due to the fact that bacteria invade the silicon substance and reside within the wall of the implant, antibiotic treatment is usually not successful so that in the vast majority of such cases removal of the whole implant is necessary. Taking together major and minor postoperative complications, even in large series the rate of later revisions 5 years after primary surgery has to be judged as approximately 20–30 %.

The acceptance of penile implants is very high in patients with good indications. Subjective satisfaction rates of 80 % in both partners can be reached after longer follow-up which is astonishingly high. However, it presumes that prior to surgery both partners will be extensively informed about the possibilities, but also about the limitations of such an implant. Counselling should include the fact that implantation of a penile prothesis will not result in normal erections. Both partners have to be well aware of the fact that even with the new bidirectionally expandable implants, the penis will often be relatively thinner and slightly shorter than before the occurrence of erectile dysfunction. The additional gain in length made possible by new materials is clinically less spectacular than in the demonstration model. Since with all implants there is only a prothetic augmentation of the corpora cavernosa and not of the glans, in contrast to a normal physiological erection the glans will remain small and soft, which is sometimes experienced as a definite drawback by some patients and partners. Apart from these organic factors both partners have to be aware that a penile implant will not be able to improve or rescue an inadequate partner relationship.

10.3 Ejaculation Disorders

Ejaculation is a complex event characterized by the emission of the semen and seminal plasma, which consists mainly of seminal vesicle fluid, into the prostatic urethra, the simultaneous closure of the bladder neck and the expulsion of the ejaculate. Emission and closure of the bladder neck are phenomena that are under sympathetic control by the thoraco-lumbar-segments TH9-L3, whilst the expulsion of the semen is transmitted by a reflex from the pudendal nerve.

10.3.1 Anejaculation and Retrogarde Ejaculation

Disturbances of semen transportation and emission of the ejaculate i.e, **anejaculation or aspermia** have to be differentiated from transport disturbances within the urethra or **retrograde ejaculation.** Of great clinical importance are functional disturbances like **premature ejaculation.** Apart from intact innervation with sequential contraction of the involved organs, quantitative and adequate production of seminal fluid is important for normal ejaculation. The primary absence of an ejaculation during normal orgasm points to an obstructive problem of emission and insufficient production of seminal plasma or to insufficient closure of the bladder neck with retrograde ejaculation.

In secondary loss of ejaculation a possible cause in the patient's history has to be searched for. Prostate and bladder neck surgery are typical reasons for retrograde

ejaculation. Retroperitoneal lymphadenectomy for testicular cancer, pelvic surgery, an aortofemoral bypass or sympathectomies can lead to a disturbance of the autonomic innervation of the bladder neck and the ductus deferens, and mainly to loss of ejaculation. Pharmacological causes (alpha-blockers) and neurological diseases also have to be excluded. A spontaneous loss of ejaculation is sometimes a symptom of diabetic polyneuropathy or can be observed in secondary post-infectious obstructions of the ejaculatory duct. Any process interfering with innervation of the bladder neck and ductus deferens or the seminal vesicles can cause a loss of emission or ejaculation disturbances. Differential diagnosis can rule out androgen deficiency which would lead to insufficient production of seminal plasma and possibly to a loss of emission.

In all patients lacking ejaculation or with a very low ejaculate volume the primary question is whether there appears to be a **loss of emission** or **retrograde ejaculation.** Diagnostically **transrectal sonography** and **microscopic investigations of the postcoital or postmasturbatory urine** are most important. Transrectal sonography will show anatomic variations in the seminal vesicles such as aplasias or ectasias with dilations of the ductus deferens. Obstructions are possible on all levels from the vas deferens to the ejaculatory duct. The most common causes are congenital, cystic or secondary postinflammatory obstructions of the ejaculatory duct which will typically lead to dilatation of the seminal vesicle and the ductus deferens. Sonographically detectable cysts of the ejaculatory duct can be opened by transurethral resection. Patency may be determined in ambiguous cases. This should be performed with inert dyes since radiological visualization, which in the past was often carried out using contrast media, always bears the risk of secondary obstruction. The demonstration of more than 15 sperm per field in postcoital urine sediment has to be regarded as a proof of retrograde ejaculation.

Therapeutically, pharmacological treatment can be tried. This applies to patients with **retrograde ejaculation** as well as to those with **anejaculation** who may in rare cases progress to retrograde ejaculation. The therapy of choice is direct or indirect sympathomimetic substances (**Gutron**® 3–4 × 25–50 mg/day or the tricyclic antidepressive **imipramin** 2×25 g/day). The aim of this therapy is to increase adrenergic tone and to achieve a better contraction of the vas deferens and the bladder neck. The effects of this therapy can be increased if drugs are taken over a number of consecutive days (Kamischke and Nieschlag 1999). In retrograde ejaculation it is possible to retrieve sperm from postmasturbatory urine to be used for **assisted fertilization** after preparation (see Chap. 17).

In complete loss of emission, there is the possibility of **transrectal electrostimulation.** This will induce antrograde or retrograde ejaculation in the vast majority of patients. Success rates of 90% in patients with lymphadenectomy and 75% with paraplegic symptoms have been reported in the literature (Denil et al. 1992; Ohl et al. 1991; Kamischke and Nieschlag 1999).

10.3.2 Premature Ejaculation

Premature ejaculation (ejaculatio praecox) is characterized by the inability of the patient to control the time of ejaculation in a way that allows his partner to reach orgasm. Very often this problem is initially articulated by the female partner. There is no uniform concept concerning the pathogenesis of this disturbance and in the vast majority of cases an underlying functional problem exists.

Therapeutically, a **local anesthesia**, often in the form of a gel, is applied to the glans or introduced into the anterior urethra. It is only partially effective. Better results can be reached with the use of **chlomipramine** (25–50 mg in the evening) (Colpi et al. 1991). This medication is perhaps effective due to an increase of the sensoric threshold in the genital region and this may allow better control of ejaculation. Today the standard therapy is still the "**squeeze technique**", which was originally introduced by Masters and Johnson. Just prior to the onset of ejaculation, a firm squeeze in the region of the frenulum for 3–4 sec will slightly reduce the erection and depress the urge for ejaculation. With increasing practice the man will learn to control his erection and the time of ejaculation much better (Masters and Johnson 1970). The success rate of this method is reported to be approximately 95% (Lorence and Madakasira 1992).

10.4 References

Aboseif SR, Breza J, Lue TF, Tanagho EA (1989) Penile venous drainage in erectile dysfunction. Anatomical, radiological and functional considerations. Br J Urol 64:183–190

Brock G, Nunes L, von HB, Martinez PL, Hsu GL, Lue TF (1993) Can a venous patch graft be a substitute for the tunica albuginea of the penis? J Urol 150:1306–1309

Colpi GM, Fanciullacci F, Aydos K, Grugnetti C (1991) Effectiveness mechanism of chlomipramine by neurophysiological tests in subjects with true premature ejaculation. Andrologia 23:45–47

Conti CR, Pepine CJ, Sweeney M (1999) Efficacy and safety of Sildenafil Citrate in the treatment of erectile dysfunction in patients with ischemic heart disease. Am J Cardiol 83:29C–34C

Cookson MS, Nadig PW (1993) Long-term results with vacuum constriction device. J Urol 149:290–294

Davis-Joseph B, Tiefer L, Melman A (1995) Accuracy of the initial history and physical examination to establish the etiology of erectile dysfunction. Urology 45:498–502

Denil J, Ohl DA, McGuire EJ, Jonas U (1992) Treatment of anejaculation with electroejaculation. Acta Urol Belg 60:15–25

Derouet H, Zehl U (1990) Die Behandlung der erektilen Dysfunktion mittels Vakuumsaugpumpen (EHS). Urologe A 32:312–315

Dettmers C, van Ahlen H, Faust H, Fatepour D, Tackmann W (1994) Evaluation of erectile dysfunction with the sympathetic skin response in comparison to bulbocavernosus reflex and somatosensory evoked potentials of the pudendal nerve. Electromyogr Clin Neurophysiol 34:437–444

Ernst E, Pittler MH (1998) Yohimbine for erectile dysfunction: a systematic review and meta-analysis of randomized clinical trials. J Urol 159:433–436

Fabbri A, Jannini EA, Gnessi L, Moretti C, Ulisse S, Franzese A, Lazzari R, Fraioli F, Frajese G, Isidori A (1989) Endorphins in male impotence: evidence for naltrexone stimulation of erectile activity in patient therapy. Psychoneuroendocrinology 14:103–111

Feldmann HA, Goldstein I, Hatzichriston DG, Krane RJ, McKinlay JB (1994) Impotence and its medical and psychosocial correlates: results of the Massachusetts Male Aging Study. J Urol 151:54–61

Gall H, Sparwasser CH, Stief CG, Bahren W, Scherb W, Holzki G (1989) Diagnostik der venösen Insuffizienz bei erektiler Dysfunktion: vergleichende Untersuchungen von Cavernosographie und Dopplersonographie. Urologe A 28:48–53

Greenstein A, Plymate SR, Katz PG (1995) Visually stimulated erection in castrated men. J Urol 153:650–652

Grein U, Noll F, Schreiter F (1989) Behandlung der erektilen Dysfunktion mit Penisprothesen. Urologe A 28:266–270

Hartmann U, Langer D (1993) Combination of psychosexual therapy and intrapenile injections in the treatment of erectile dysfunctions: rationale and predictors of outcome. J Sex Educ Ther 19:1–12

Hatzichristou DG, Saenz de Tejada I, Kupferman S, Namburi S, Pescatore ES, Udelson D, Goldstein I (1995) In vivo assessment of trabecular smooth muscle tone, its application in pharmaco-cavernosometry and analysis of intracavernous pressure determinants. J Urol 153:1126–1135

Hauri D (1984) Therapiemöglichkeiten bei der vaskulär bedingten erektilen Impotenz. Aktuel Urol 15:350–354

Heaton JPW, Morales A, Adams MA, Johnston B, El-Radhidy R (1995) Recovery of erectile function by the oral administration of apomorphine. Urology 45:200–206

Heyden Bv, Donatucci CF, Marshall GA, Brock GB, Lue TF (1993) A prostaglandin E1 dose-response study in man (see comments). J Urol 150:1825–1828

Jackson G, Betteridge J, Dean J, Hall R, Holdright D, Holmes S, Kirby M, Riley A, Sever P (1999) A systematic approach to erectile dysfunction in the cardiovascular patient. Int J Clin Pract 53(6): 445–451

Jackson JA, Waxman J, Spiekerman AM (1989) Prostatic complications of testosterone replacement therapy. Arch Intern Med 149:2365–2366

Kamischke A, Nieschlag E (1999) Treatment of retrograde ejaculation and anejaculation. Hum Reprod Update 5:448–474

Kaneko S, Bradley WA (1987) Penile electrodiagnosis: penile peripheral innervation. Urology 30:210–213

Kelami A (1985) Congenital penile deviation and straightening of the penis using the Nesbit-Kelami technique. Urol Int 40:267–268

Kim ED, McVary KT (1995a) Long-term follow up of treatment of Peyronie's disease with plaque incision, carbon dioxide laser plaque ablation and placement of a deep dorsal vein patch graft. J Urol 153:1843–1846

Kim ED, McVary KT (1995b) Long-term results with penile vein ligation for venogenic impotence. J Urol 153:655–658

Kloner R (1999) Safety of sildenafil citrate in men with erectile dysfunction taking multiple antihypertensive agents. AJH 12:37A

Lavoisier P, Proulx J, Courtois F, De CF (1989) Bulbocavernosus reflex: its validity as a diagnostic test of neurogenic impotence. J Urol 141:311–314

Lawrence S, Madakasira S (1992) Evaluation and treatment of premature ejaculation: a critical review. Int J Psychiatry Med 22:77–97

Lewis RW (1990) Venous surgery for impotence. Urol Clin North Am 15:115–121

Lue TF, Tanagho EA (1987) Physiology of erection and pharmacological management of impotence. J Urol 137:829–836

Masters WH, Johnson VE (1970) Human sexual inadequacy. Little Brown, Boston

Molderings GJ, van Ahlen H, Göthert M (1992) Modulation of noradrenaline release in human corpus cavernosum by presynaptic protaglandin receptors. Int J Impotence Res 4:19–25

Moll V (1992) Therapie kongenitaler und erworbener Penisdeviationen. In: Derouet H (eds) Erektile Funktionsstörungen. Springer, Berlin Heidelberg New York, pp 152–157

Morales A, Condra M, Reid K (1990) The role of nocturnal penile tumescence monitoring in the diagnosis of impotence: a review. J Urol 143:441–446

Nesbit RM (1954) The surgical treatment of of congenital chordee without hypospadias. J Urol 72:1178–1180

Oates CP, Pickard RS, Powell PH, Murthy LNS, Whittingham TAW (1995) The use of duplex ultrasound in the assessment of arterial supply to the penis in vasculogenic impotence. J Urol 153:354–357

Ohl DA, Denil J, Bennett CJ, Randolph JF, Menge AC, McCabe M (1991) Electroejaculation following retroperitoneal lymphadenectomy. J Urol 145:980–983

Padma-Nathan H, Hellstrom WJ, Kaiser FE, Labasky RF, Lue TF, Nolten WE, Norwood PC, Peterson CA, Shabsigh R, Tam PY (1997) Treatment of men with erectile dysfunction with transurethral alprostadil. Medicated Urethral System for Erection (MUSE) Study Group. N Engl J Med 336:1–7

Porst H (1990) Diagnostic use and side effects of vasoactive drugs – a report on over 2100 patients with erectile failure. Int J Impotence Res 2 [Suppl 2]:222–223

Porst H, Weller S (1989) Vasoaktive Substanzen bei erektiler Dysfunktion (ED) – Ergebnisse einer Umfrage und Literaturübersicht. Urologe B 29:10–14

Porst H, van Ahlen H, Köster O, Schlolaut KH (1988a) Vergleich von Papaverin-induzierter Doppler-Sonographie und Angiographie in der Diagnostik der erektilen Dysfunktion. Urologe A 27:8–13

Porst H, van Ahlen H (1989) Drug-induced priapism – a report of experiences in 101 cases. Urologe 28:84–87

Porst H, Tackmann W, van Ahlen H (1988b) Neurophysiological investigations in potent and impotent men. Assessment of bulbocavernosus reflex latencies and somatosensory evoked potentials. Br J Urol 61:445–450

Rhee E, Osborn A, Witt M (1995) The correlation of cavernous systolic occlusion pressure with peak velocity flow using color duplex Doppler ultrasound. J Urol 153:358–360

Rolf C, Nieschlag E (1998) Sildenafil (Viagra®) bei erektiler Dysfunktion: effektive Behandlung mit beachtenswerten Wechselwirkungen. Dtsch Med Wochenschr 123:1356–1361

Scott FB, Bradley WE, Timm GW (1973) Management of erectile impotence: Use of implantable inflatable prothesis. Urology 2:80–82

Small MP, Carrion HH (1975) A new penile prothesis for treating impotence. Contemp Surg 7:29

Sohn M, Sikora RR, Bohndorf KK, Wein B, Zabelberg U, Jakse G (1992) Objective follow-up after penile revascularisation. Int J Impotence Res 4:73–84

Stief CG (1993) Diagnostik und Therapie der erektilen Dysfunktion. Internist 34:767–774

Stief CG, Benard F, Diederichs W, Bosch R, Lue TF, Tanagho EA (1988) The rationale for pharmacologic cavernosonography. J Urol 140:1564–1566

Stief CG, Djamilian M, Truss MC, Tan H, Thon WF, Jonas U (1994) Prognostic factors for the postoperative outcome of penile venous surgery for venogenic erectile dysfunction. J Urol 151:880–883

van Ahlen H, Peskar BA, Sticht G, Hertfelder HJ (1994) Pharmacokinetics of vasoactive substances administered into the human corpus cavernosum. J Urol 151:1227–1230

van Ahlen H, Piechota HJ, Kias HJ, Brennemann W, Klingmüller D (1995) Opiate antagonists in erectile dysfunction: a possible new treatment option. Eur Urol 28:246–250

Virag R, Zwang G, Dermange H, Legman M (1981) Vasculogenic impotence: a review of 92 cases with 54 surgical operations. Vasc Surg 15:9–15

Vogt HJ, Brandl P, Kockott G, Schmitz JR, Wiegand MH, Schadrack J (1997) Double-blind, placebo-controlled safety and efficacy trial with yohimbine hydrochloride in the treatment of nonorganic erectile dysfunction. Int J Impot Res 9:155–161

Wechsel HW, Strohmaier WL, Wilbert DM, Bichler KH (1993) Erweiterung des Therapiespektrums durch das Erektionshilfesystem (EHS). Urologe B 33:19–21

Wegner HEH, Andresen R, Knispel HH, Banzer D, Miller K (1995) Evaluation of penile arteries with color-coded duplex sonography: prevalence and possible therapeutic implications of connections between dorsal and cavernous arteries in impotent men. J Urol 153:1469–1471

Witherington R (1989) Vacuum constriction device for management of erectile impotence. J Urol 141:320–322

Zippe CD, Kedia AW, Kedia K, Nelson DR, Agarwal A (1998) Treatment of erectile dysfunction after radical prostatectomy with Sildenafil Citrate (Viagra). Urology 52:963–966

CHAPTER 11

Disorders of Androgen Target Organs

11

D. Meschede · H. M. Behre · E. Nieschlag

In this chapter, as throughout this volume, we classify diseases according to where they originate, i. e. in which organ or physiological system. All disease entities dealt with under Sect. 11.1–11.2 have in common, to variable degrees, impaired action of androgens in their target organs. Gynecomastia represents an exception; this disorder will be discussed here more for reasons of clinical convenience rather than according to strictly nosological criteria.

Some of the diseases described below were formerly summarized under the category of "intersexuality". Because of the vague and discriminating character of this term we prefer not to use it.

11.1 Androgen Resistance

The term "androgen resistance" characterizes a group of disorders all caused by the impaired action of androgens at their target tissues. Table 11.1 summarizes these conditions. We follow the most widely accepted classification system which distinguishes between complete and incomplete testicular feminization and the Reifenstein syndrome. In clinical practice the phenotypes of these disorders may be less well demarcated than the orderly classification suggests. For the individual patient it may be problematic to classify him or her according to one of the well-defined entities. More recent classification systems take the clinical heterogeneity of androgen resistance states into consideration. The scheme proposed by Quigley et al. (1995) recognizes seven degrees of severity, and Sinnecker et al. (1997) distinguish five main categories and ten subcategories. Since neither of these systems has become generally accepted, we continue to refer to the above mentioned classic system.

The biochemistry of testicular androgens and the androgen receptor is covered in Chap. 3. Here, we discuss this topic only to the extent that is immediately relevant to the understanding of the clinical issues.

> Androgen resistance can be defined as a state where androgens do not induce the expected physiological effects at their target tissues even though they are present in sufficient quantities.

Table 11.1. Disorders with different degrees of androgen resistance. (WD Wolffian ducts, T testosterone, E_2 estradiol; ↑ markedly elevated, (↑) elevated)

Disorder	External genitalia and breasts	Internal genitalia and gonads	Hormones[a]	Fertility	Psychosexual identity
Testicular feminization, complete form	Female genitalia; breasts fully developed	No derivates of WD; abdominal, inguinal or labial testes without spermatogenesis	T normal or ↑; E_2↑; LH↑; FSH normal or (↑)	Infertile	Female
Testicular feminization, incomplete form	Female genitalia with clitoral hypertrophy and partial labial synechiae; fully developed breasts	Derivates of WD rudimentary; abdominal, inguinal, or labial testes without spermatogenesis	T normal or ↑; E_2↑; LH↑; FSH normal or (↑)	Infertile	Female
Reifenstein syndrome	Genitalia intersexual; gynecomastia	Development of derivates of WD variable; testes mostly inguinal, no spermatogenesis	LH↑; T, E_2, FSH normal or (↑)	Infertile	Usually male, sometimes female
Prepenile scrotum bifidum with hypospadias	Male genitalia; prepenile scrotum bifidum, hypospadias	Spermatogenesis impaired	LH und T normal or (↑), FSH (↑)	Infertile or reduced fertility	Male

a The hormonal levels are given in comparison to the normal range in healthy males

Disregarding exogenous factors (such as certain drugs with antiandrogenic properties), androgen resistance is always due to dysfunction of the **androgen receptor (AR)**, which constitutes the essential link between steroid hormone and cellular response. All disorders of the androgen receptor are genetic in nature and are ultimately caused by abnormalities of the **androgen receptor gene**. The extremely heterogeneous spectrum of mutations has been characterized by studies involving several hundred patients (Quigley et al. 1995; Hiort et al. 1996, 1999). Deletions of the entire gene, the loss of several exons, deletions or insertions of a few base pairs, splice site mutations as well as various nonsense and missense point mutations in the coding region have been described.

DNA analysis has assumed a firm place in the routine clinical workup of androgen resistance states even if the mutation causing the disorder cannot always be identified in all patients. The practical value of identifying a mutation is also diminished by the fact that patients with an identical alteration of the AR gene may present with distinctly different phenotypes (Rodin et al. 1996). Nevertheless, limited correlations between mutation type and clinical presentation are apparent: complete or partial deletions of the AR gene, nonsense and splice site mutations tend to cause severe forms of androgen resistance. Missense point mutations leading to the exchange of a single amino acid in the receptor protein can cause complete as well as only partial androgen resistance.

Improved molecular genetic diagnostic techniques have displaced **androgen-binding studies**, formerly the diagnostic standard. The technique is based on the measurement of androgen-receptor binding in fibroblasts recovered from a genital skin biopsy. Pathological results fall into three classes: (1) complete lack of androgen binding to the receptor ("receptor negative androgen resistance"); (2) androgen-receptor binding that is quantitatively abnormal, but qualitatively normal; (3) qualitatively abnormal androgen binding, e. g. lower binding affinity or increased thermolability. In some patients with clinically obvious androgen resistance, androgen-binding studies produce completely unremarkable results ("receptor-positive androgen resistance"). "Receptor-negative" patients present with the clinical picture of testicular feminization. Aside from this, there are no reliable correlations between the results of androgen-binding studies and the clinical phenotype.

When patients with normally functioning androgen receptors are given the steroid stanozolol, SHBG serum levels decline. This mechanism is disturbed in androgen receptor defects, correlating in severity with the degree of androgen resistance. This phenomenon is exploited in the so-called **SHBG test**. Over a period of 3 days 0.2 mg/kg body weight stanozolol is applied daily (evenings). SHBG is measured prior to and 5, 6, 7 and 8 days after the beginning of the test. If the lowest value fails to fall below 63% of the basal value, a disturbance of the androgen receptor is evident (Sinnecker et al. 1997).

11.1.1 Testicular Feminization

Testicular feminization is the most severe form of androgen resistance. We distinguish a **complete** from an **incomplete form**. Among genetically male newborns the former has a prevalence of about 1 in 50,000; the latter is markedly rarer. Patients with testicular feminization have a 46,XY karyotype, i. e. they are genetic males. In contrast to the milder forms of androgen resistance that will be discussed later (Sect. 11.1.2, 11.1.3 and 11.1.4), these individuals have a female outward appearance. It is therefore appropriate to refer to them as "women" with testicular feminization. This also corresponds to their psychosexual orientation, which is unambiguously female. These patients often primarily consult a gynecologist, if the diagnosis was not established previously by a pediatrician.

Complete Form of Testicular Feminization

All signs of androgen action are absent in the complete form of testicular feminization. The external genitalia appear normally female. The vagina ends blindly and may be shortened. As the production and action of anti-Muellerian hormone (AMH) is normal (cf. Chap. 4), in individuals with testicular feminization the Muellerian ducts have regressed. This explains the absence of a uterus and Fallopian tubes. The gonads may be in an abdominal, inguinal or more rarely in a labial position.

During childhood surgery for an inguinal hernia the diagnosis of testicular feminization is often made almost incidentally. In fact, testicular feminization is one of the major differential diagnoses to be considered in a girl with bilateral **inguinal hernias**. The gonads have the histologic characteristics of testes, but spermatogenesis does not develop. With progressive age adenoma-like changes are found with increasing frequency. Whether these represent hyperplasia or true adenomas is an unclarified issue. The nodular structures, which may grow to an impressive size and can be confused with malignant ovarian tumors, are composed of cells both from the germinal and the interstitial testicular compartments. In most cases Sertoli cells predominate. The issue of gonadal malignancies in testicular feminization will be covered in the section "Therapy".

With estrogens circulating in sufficient quantities the distribution pattern of the adipose tissue, muscle bulk and development of the **breasts** are as in normal women. If the testes are still *in situ*, estrogens are derived from direct gonadal secretion plus peripheral conver-

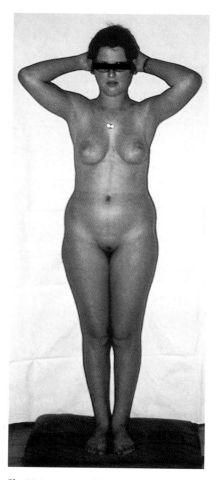

Fig. 11.1. 23-year-old patient with testicular feminization. Note normal female appearance of breasts and absence of axillary and pubic hair

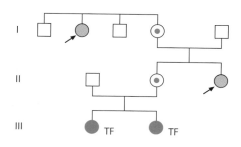

Fig. 11.2. Pedigree of a family with testicular feminization. The diagnosis was first established in the two index patients symbolized by solid circles. When the family history was taken, it became evident that an aunt and a great-aunt (*pink circles* marked by *arrows*) could not have children and never had menstrual bleedings. For these individuals the diagnosis of testicular feminization can be presumed with great confidence. Mother and grandmother of the index patients are obligatory carriers (indicated by *dot* in the pedigree symbol) of the gene defect. Phenotypically male family members are symbolized by *squares*

sion from androgens. In gonadectomized patients estrogens need to be substituted externally. The patients are usually taller and have larger teeth than average normal women, an effect ascribed to the action of Y chromosomal genes. In both sexes, the development of sexual hair is critically dependent on androgenic stimuli; patients with testicular feminization have **no or very scant pubic and axillary hair**. This conspicuous clinical sign is most valuable diagnostically (Fig. 11.1).

Testicular feminization is associated with **primary amenorrhea** and intractable infertility. Amenorrhea is often the presenting complaint that leads to the establishment of physician contact and ultimately to the correct diagnosis. Patients of postpubertal age have markedly elevated LH serum levels, while FSH is only moderately elevated or can even be normal. The testosterone concentration is within or even above the normal range for men, and estradiol levels are higher than in males. Prepubertal children usually have normal LH and testosterone serum levels.

The diagnosis is established in a multistep process. The first suspicion usually arises during the clinical workup for unexplained amenorrhea or with the chance finding of testicular tissue in an inguinal hernia. By demonstrating the discrepancy between genetic and phenotypic sex, **karyotyping** provides essential guidance for further diagnostic studies. In addition to comprehensive **endocrine testing (including an hCG test in prepubertal patients), DNA analysis** is required to meet present standards. The SHBG test also can provide valuable information. In contrast, androgen-binding studies are no longer obligatory. Some patients with testicular feminization have reduced activity of the enzyme 5α-reductase (Imperato-McGinley et al. 1982). The physiologic basis of this phenomenon is unclear, but it must be taken into account to distinguish testicular feminization from the primary 5α-reductase 2-deficiency in the condition termed perineoscrotal hypospadias with pseudovagina (cf. Sect. 11.2).

Testicular feminization is inherited in an **X chromosomal recessive** fashion. Only genetically male individuals can be affected, while women may act as asymptomatic carriers. Upon specific questioning the family history is positive in about two of three cases. Affected relatives are to be expected exclusively in the maternal line. A typical pedigree is shown in Fig. 11.2. The index patients have two maternal relatives who never menstruated and remained involuntarily childless.

Taking a meticulous family history is not only important from a diagnostic point of view. Parents of affected children have to be advised that in further pregnancies the recurrence risk amounts to 25%. Often other family members may also be at risk for having children affected with testicular feminization. We therefore recommend genetic counselling for any family where a first case of testicular feminization is diagnosed.

Just how the diagnosis of testicular feminization is to be communicated to the patient is subject to controversy.

> Disclosure of the diagnosis, including the fact that the gonads contain testicular cells and that the karyotype is male, can have disastrous consequences for the woman's self-image.

For this reason many physicians, ourselves included, until recently felt that full disclosure should not be made. In the meantime we tend towards a more individualized course of action which takes into consideration the patient's age, psychic constitution and the degree to which the patient is already aware of her condition. Under certain circumstances complete disclosure can be justified. In such cases it is important that the patient understands that in her case androgens cannot achieve their biologic effects and that therefore the pivotal step in sexual differentiation proceeded not in a male but in a female direction.

Therapy. Testicular feminization carries a high risk for development of a **gonadal malignancy**. According to Scully (1981) the cumulative incidence of gonadal malignant tumours surpasses 30% up to the age of 50 years. Therefore, the indication for **surgical removal of the testicular tissue** is absolute.

The optimal timing for gonadectomy is a contended issue. In our opinion, the advantages of gonadectomy at the earliest possible age prevail against later surgery at age 16 to 20 years. It appears that the risk for malignant transformation before the twentieth year of life is low, but such an event can never be excluded with absolute certainty. In addition, the operation may be less traumatic for a child than for an adolescent. Even when the diagnosis is not disclosed, girls of the latter age group will experience the loss of their "ovaries" and ability to have children much more consciously. Advocates of late removal of the gonads stress the fact that the girls may undergo spontaneous puberty under the influence of estrogens secreted directly from the gonads and derived from peripheral conversion. This is certainly a point to be considered, but nevertheless we see more advantages in early rather than late gonadectomy.

Once the age of expected puberty is reached (or if the gonads are removed thereafter), **estrogen substitution** treatment must be initiated. The modalities of this treatment do not deviate from estrogen replacement therapy for other indications. Usually, no other therapy is necessary. Women with testicular feminization are fully adapted to the female role and can have a normal marital life. Psychotherapeutic support may be valuable for patients who were confronted with the diagnosis or who have problems coping with their intractable infertility (see Chap. 19).

Incomplete Form of Testicular Feminization

In the spectrum of androgen resistance states the incomplete form of testicular feminization occupies an intermediate place. It therefore ranges between the complete form on one hand and Reifenstein syndrome on the other hand. The phenotype is predominantly female, but even at birth signs of mild virilization are present, and these may increase by the time of puberty.

Genital examination in affected children shows a mild degree of **clitoral hypertrophy** and partial synechiae between the labia. The masculinization of the external genitalia can increase when puberty occurs, but it may also remain unchanged. In contrast to the complete form, in the incomplete form of testicular feminization sexual hair is normally developed. Another important distinguishing criterion is that derivatives of the Wolffian ducts are present. Although the epididymides, vasa deferentia, and seminal vesicles are hypoplastic, they can be unequivocally demonstrated during surgical exploration. The previous points aside, there are no major other differences between complete and incomplete forms of testicular feminization in terms of clinical presentation, endocrinology, or molecular genetics. Endocrine substitution therapy is conducted along the same lines as in the complete form. An important point favoring early gonadectomy is the possibility of increasing virilization at the time of puberty.

11.1.2 Reifenstein Syndrome

Patients with Reifenstein syndrome are more virilized than individuals with testicular feminization, but less so than men who have a normally functioning androgen receptor (see Sect. 11.1.5). There is no single pathognomonic clinical or laboratory finding defining this disorder, but rather the overall impression of an intermediate grade of undervirilization will suggest the diagnosis of Reifenstein syndrome.

The external genitalia may have more resemblance to either the normal male or female anatomy, but there is always some degree of ambiguity. **Perineoscrotal hypospadias** is the most characteristic finding, but milder degrees of hypospadias, possibly combined with a **bifid scrotum**, are also compatible with the diagnosis. The penis is small, and the hypoplastic **testes** are usually found in an inguinal, less frequently in a scrotal or abdominal position. While pubic and axillary hair are normally developed, androgen-dependent hair at other body sites tends to be scant. Quite typically, **gynecomastia** develops around puberty (Fig. 11.3).

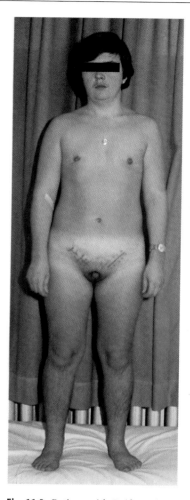

Fig. 11.3. Patient with Reifenstein syndrome. The scars from mastectomy and removal of the inguinal testes are easily visible. A malignant tumor was present in the right testis. Note the small phallus (the perineoscrotal hypospadias is not visible on this photograph)

Semen analysis in Reifenstein syndrome reveals **azoospermia**, and there is no effective therapeutic approach to this patient group's infertility. While Muellerian structures (uterus, Fallopian tubes) are notably absent, epididymides, vasa deferentia and seminal vesicles may be developed to a variable degree.

Endocrine findings resemble those in testicular feminization: serum levels of testosterone and FSH are normal or slightly elevated, and LH clearly exceeds the normal range. Androgen-binding studies most frequently show qualitative defects or a partial quantitative reduction of hormone binding. In some cases completely absent or normal androgen binding was observed.

As Reifenstein syndrome is so variable at the clinical level, **therapy** needs to be tailored quite individually to every single patient. Psychosexual orientation is usually male, and treatment aims at enhancing the male attributes of the phenotype. Hypospadias, cryptorchidism, gynecomastia and other anatomical anomalies are amenable to surgical correction. There are no sufficiently validated data concerning the risk of gonadal malignancy in Reifenstein syndrome. Cryptorchid testes should either be brought into the scrotum or entirely removed if orchidopexy proves impossible. Testes that are in a scrotal position should be regularly examined by palpation and ultrasound to pick up malignant changes as early as possible. The patient should be instructed in techniques of self-examination. The gonadal status should be checked by a physician at least once a year, and intervals of six months may even be more appropriate.

Non-gonadectomized patients with Reifenstein syndrome are not deficient in androgens, and therefore the value of additional supplementation with exogenous androgens is unclear. No unequivocal positive proof of beneficial effects of such an endocrine therapy has been brought forward yet. If the patient specifically requests it, it may be justifiable to give such treatment a try under the close supervision of a specialist. A certain degree of additional virilization may possibly be attained (Price et al. 1984). If orchidectomy cannot be avoided, supplementation with exogenous androgens becomes mandatory. The principles of this treatment are laid out in Chap. 15.

11.1.3 Prepenile Scrotum bifidum with Hypospadias

In this variant of androgen resistance the bifid scrotum is located anterior to the penis, and additionally there is severe hypospadias (Fig. 11.4). Cryptorchidism may be another associated finding. Spermatogenesis is severely compromised. While body proportions are unremarkable, decreased sexual hair, lack of voice change, and impotence may be observed. Gynecomastia does not occur. In one family with three affected brothers the binding capacity of the androgen receptor was clearly subnormal. Testosterone supplementation did not result in an improvement of the signs of undervirilization and androgen resistance (Bals-Pratsch et al. 1990).

11.1.4 X-Linked Spinal and Bulbar Muscular Atrophy (Kennedy Disease)

X-linked spinal and bulbar muscular atrophy (SBMA; Kennedy disease) is another disorder caused by dysfunction of the androgen receptor. The mode of inheritance is **X-linked recessive**. Thus, only men can be affected, while women may act as asymptomatic carriers. As in testicular feminization and Reifenstein syndrome, the primary cause of the disorder is a **mutation in the**

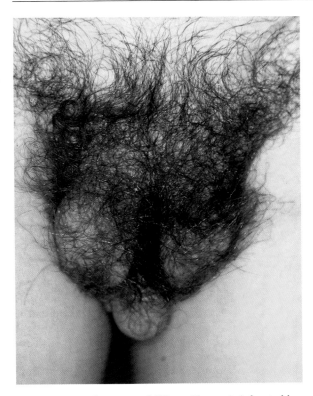

Fig. 11.4. Prepenile scrotum bifidum. The penis is located behind the scrotum. Hypospadias is not visible on this photograph

androgen receptor gene. However, the underlying type of mutation is specific for SBMA and does not occur in association with the diseases discussed above (Sect. 11.1.1–11.1.2; La Spada et al. 1991). This particular type of mutation is designated as expansion of a triplet repeat sequence.

The first exon of the androgen receptor gene contains a repetitive sequence of tandemly arranged **CAG triplets**. The number of these triplets is a polymorphic molecular trait and varies from person to person. In healthy individuals the number of CAGs ranges from 9 to 36, in patients affected with SBMA from 38 to 62. As the two ranges do not overlap, measuring the CAG repeat length is a highly specific diagnostic test.

The CAG repeat is translated into the amino acid sequence of the receptor protein, with every CAG coding for a glutamine residue. The stretch of polyglutamine is located in the N-terminal portion of the receptor protein that functions as an activator of genes under androgen control. This activating function is compromized both qualitatively and quantitatively in receptor proteins with an abnormally long stretch of polyglutamines. Through various mechanisms the integrity of spinal and bulbar motoneurons is curtailed by androgen receptor proteins with expanded polyglutamine sequences (Mer-

ry et al. 1998). This explains why in SBMA these neurons degenerate slowly, leading to the clinically observed neurologic deficits.

Clinical onset of the disease usually lies between the 20th and 40th year of life, but may occur later, even up to the age of 60 years (Harding et al. 1982). Slowly developing progressive neurological deficits are usually the presenting complaint when the patient first contacts the physician. **Muscle cramps** triggered by exercise and involuntary **muscle twitches** are typical for SBMA and may represent the initial symptom. Consecutively, **weakness** of the proximal muscle groups, especially in the lower extremities, becomes manifest. Later in the course of the disease muscle weakness and atrophy spread to the shoulders, the face and the more distal parts of all extremities. Progression tends to be slow, and the disease usually has a course over several decades. In advanced stages of SBMA bulbar symptoms such as dysarthria and dysphagia may become prominent.

Endocrine abnormalities usually become manifest after neurological symptoms. More than half the patients with SBMA develop **gynecomastia**. The **testes atrophy** with resulting impairment of sperm production and secondary **infertility**. More than 70 % of affected individuals already have children when the testicular dysfunction becomes clinically manifest. LH and FSH levels are frequently elevated, but this is not an obligatory finding. Only one of three patients with SBMA has subnormal serum testosterone concentrations (Harding et al. 1982; Arbizu et al. 1983). Another endocrine disorder encountered not infrequently is **diabetes mellitus** or subclinical glucose intolerance.

Upon **neurological examination** the most notable findings are weak or absent tendon reflexes and muscular atrophy, weakness and fasciculations. Electromyogram and histology point to a neurogenic basis of the muscular atrophy. Motor nerve conduction velocities are normal or only slightly reduced. Sensory nerve conduction velocities are subnormal, but this finding is without a clinical correlate. Serum levels of the muscle enzyme **creatine kinase** are moderately elevated, usually not exceeding the upper normal range by more than the factor five. It may be difficult to differentiate SBMA clinically from other slowly progressive neuro- and myopathies. A positive **family history** may sometimes provide a clue. Diagnosis should always be made objective by demonstrating the typical mutation in the androgen receptor gene (Kreß et al. 1993).

There is **no causal treatment** for this disorder. All therapeutic measures are symptomatic and should be tailored to the specific problems the individual patient presents with. We are not aware that treatment with exogenous androgens has been tried in men with SBMA. Apart from a few cases with an unfavorable clinical course, life expectancy in SBMA is normal or only slightly diminished.

11.1.5 Minimal Forms of Androgen Resistance

In the eighties the existence and high prevalence of minimal forms of androgen resistance were postulated on the basis of androgen-binding studies (Aiman and Griffin 1982; Morrow et al. 1987). These forms featured in the literature as "infertile male syndrome" (IMS) and "undervirilized fertile male syndrome" (UFMS). These terms were meant to signify very mild androgen resistance states resulting exclusively in oligozoospermia or azoospermia (IMS) or a slightly undervirilized male habitus with normal fertility (UFMS). In our experience IMS and UFMS never played a role in clinical andrology. Nor have techniques of DNA analysis, which have become very efficient, shown any notable prevalence of androgen receptor gene mutations in patients unremarkable except for a pathological spermiogram.

> We thus consider the entities IMS and UFMS superfluous in the nosology of androgen resistance states and suggest that they no longer be used.

As described in Sect. 11.1.4, in normal men there is a repetitive sequence comprising between 9 and 36 **CAG units in exon 1 of the AR gene**. According to several authors, men with disturbed fertility feature a slightly higher average number of CAG triplets in this sequence than do fertile controls (Dowsing et al. 1999). However, this finding has not been universally confirmed (Lundberg Giwercman et al. 1998). In view of this and of the fact that none of the androgen receptor genes of the infertile men exceeded the length of the normal CAG sequence of 9 to 36 units, the pathophysiologic and clinical relevance of these postulated minimal repeat expansions should be viewed sceptically. Routine analysis of this CAG sequence in men with unexplained disturbances of spermatogenesis is not warranted according to present knowledge.

11.2 Perineoscrotal Hypospadias with Pseudovagina

Perineoscrotal hypospadias with pseudovagina (PHP) is another disorder caused by an impairment of the physiologic action of androgens. However, the basic abnormality is located in androgen metabolism and not in androgen-receptor interaction. The principles of androgen physiology and metabolism have been laid out in Chap. 3. The reader is reminded that a major part of the biologic effects of testosterone is mediated via its metabolite **dihydrotestosterone** (DHT). All clinical manifestations of PHP result from a deficiency of DHT in its target cells of the genital tract. The basic biochemical defect lies in the conversion of testosterone to DHT by the enzyme (steroid) 5α-reductase 2 (Imperato-McGinley et al. 1974; Griffin et al. 1995). Therefore, an alternative designation for PHP is **5α-reductase 2 deficiency**.

In any karyotypically male newborn with ambiguous genitalia this disorder should be considered in the differential diagnosis. Typically, the external genitalia in infants with PHP have a female appearance with **clitoral hypertrophy**. Some newborns may be more virilized, so that the **gender assignment** is **male**. In any case, **scrotal or perineal hypospadias** is an obligatory finding. Contrary to testicular feminization the **gonads** are always in an **extra-abdominal** position, either in the inguinal region or in the labia or scrotum, respectively. PHP is further distinguished from testicular feminization in that the derivatives of the Wolffian ducts (epididymis, vas deferens, seminal vesicles) are present. The prenatal preservation and development of these structures depends on the presence of testosterone and not DHT. The anatomy of the derivative structures of the embryonic **urogenital sinus** is variable. The urogenital sinus per se may have persisted, or there may be a separate vaginal orifice. Such a **pseudovagina** ends blind, as the derivatives of the Muellerian ducts (upper third of the vagina, uterine cervix and body, Fallopian tubes) have not formed. The development of the prostate is strongly dependent on the presence of DHT. Thus, in PHP only a rudiment of this organ can be found in a position dorsal to the urethra. The derivatives of the Wolffian ducts end in the pseudovagina or the urogenital sinus.

Patients affected with PHP are mostly reared as girls, but they are **genetic males** (karyotype 46,XY). At the time of expected puberty there is no menarche and thelarche, and marked **virilization** develops. The patients often convert spontaneously to the male gender role. There are no reports so far about men with PHP having fathered children. In all cases that have been studied spermatogenesis was severely compromised.

Recent studies show that the clinical presentation does not always correspond to the classical phenotype described above. 5α-reductase 2 deficiency may occasionally become manifest as isolated hypospadias or penile hypoplasia.

The **family history** may be helpful in the diagnostic process. As PHP is an **autosomal recessive** disorder, additional cases mostly likely occur among the sibs of the index patient. The disease occurs more frequently in consangineous matings. The parents, who are heterozygotes, are clinically healthy. Interestingly, the same is true for genetically female individuals (e.g. sisters of affected men) homozygous for the enzyme deficiency. Obviously, the lack of 5α-reductase 2 does not adversely affect female sex differentiation.

Endocrine determinations are of utmost importance for diagnosis (Grumbach and Conte 1992). However, in children hormonal parameters measured under basal conditions are of little value. In this age group an **hCG stimulation test** must be undertaken to provoke the endocrine aberrations that are present under basal conditions in pubertal and postpubertal patients. The most specific indicator of 5α-reductase 2 deficiency is an **abnormally high testosterone/DHT ratio** which is above 50 in the classical phenotype; the upper normal level is 16. Serum testosterone levels are usually normal or slightly elevated, DHT levels moderately subnormal or in the lower normal range. Probably the DHT measurable in serum is produced by the enzyme 5α-reductase 1, which is active in extragenital tissues. Serum estrogen levels are normal, and LH and FSH concentrations are either normal or elevated.

The gene for 5α-reductase 2 (SRDSA2) is located on chromosome 2. Numerous different **mutations** of this gene have been characterized, mostly point mutations, and in a few cases deletions of the entire coding region (Wilson et al. 1993; Sinnecker et al. 1996). Along with the testosterone/DHT ratio direct **DNA analysis** is the choice diagnostic tool in patients suspected of having PHP.

The **activity of the enzyme 5α-reductase 2**, formerly measured in cultured fibroblasts from genital skin has lost ground to the highly efficient DNA analysis. Both endocrine parameters and enzyme studies in fibroblasts may indicate reduced activity of 5α-reductase 2 in some patients with testicular feminization (Imperato-McGinley et al. 1982). This finding is suspected of representing an epiphenomenon. The underlying mechanism is unknown.

Treatment of PHP depends on the patient's age, his psychosexual orientation, and the degree of virilization already attained. In any case **treatment** must be **tailored to the particular needs** of the individual patient. Sometimes it may be preferable to maintain female gender assignment, **remove the gonads, surgically correct the external genitalia** and initiate **estrogen replacement therapy.** Especially when virilization is already marked (in infancy or adolescence) the opposite therapeutic approach can be indicated: to enhance surgically the **male attributes of the genitalia** and treat with **testosterone** or DHT. Experience with this latter form of hormonal treatment is still limited, and it is recommendable to involve a specialist both in the general planing of the therapy and its supervision.

11.3 Estrogen Resistance

In connection with the discussion of target organ resistance to androgens, a recently characterized condition caused by estrogen resistance should be mentioned (Smith et al. 1994). The patient described in this report had eunuchoid body proportions and was 204 cm tall, with longitudinal growth still not completed at the age of 28. Bone age was 15 years, and bone density was extremely subnormal. However, the degree of virilization was fully appropriate, and a testicular volume of 20 to 25 ml was measured. Molecular studies revealed a homozygous mutation in the estrogen receptor gene, explaining the state of estrogen resistance.

This case illustrates the physiologic importance of estrogens in males. Quite surprisingly, only the bone is adversely affected by the state of estrogen resistance, and the role of estrogens in the functional maturation of this tissue is obviously prominent (Faustini-Fustini et al. 1999). The report contained no information as to the fertility status of the patient.

While in the above mentioned case estrogen effects were blocked by a defect of the hormone receptor, in two other patients with very similar clinical symptoms estrogen synthesis was compromised by a deficiency of the enzyme cytochrome 450 aromatase. Substitution therapy with estrogens led to rapid skeletal maturation (Carani et al. 1997).

11.4 Gynecomastia

Gynecomastia does not represent an independent nosological entity, but an ambiguous finding calling for clinical interpretation. Androgen action is impeded only in some cases and often no other endocrine basis for the abnormality can be detected. Therefore, the discussion of gynecomastia in this chapter is justified more for reasons of clinical convenience than from a strictly nosological point of view.

11.4.1 Pathophysiology

Mammary tissue is present in children of both sexes. Whether or not a breast develops from this anlage depends primarily on the endocrine situation. The basic determinant of breast development is the **balance between androgenic and estrogenic stimuli**. A hormonal milieu where estrogens prevail while there is little androgenic activity induces the unfolding and differentiation of mammary tissue. Conversely, the gland does not develop to any major degree when androgens prevail over estrogens. In adult men the molar ratio of plasma testosterone to plasma estradiol usually ranges at about 300 to 1. Any marked deviation from this ratio, be it through diminished androgens or increased estrogens, can stimulate the previously inactive mammary tissue to proliferate and thus lead to the development of gynecomastia. The various causes of androgen deficiency and excessive estrogen levels will be discussed below.

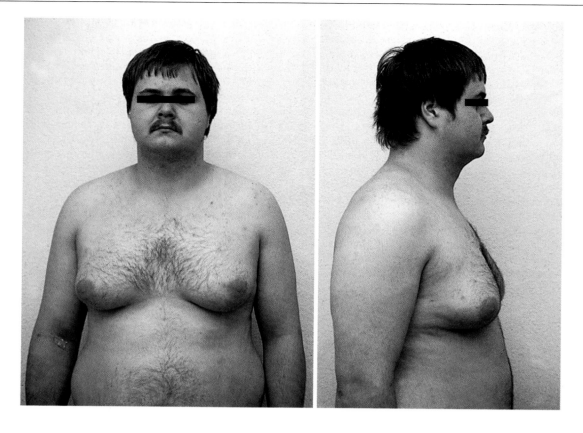

Fig. 11.5. Marked "idiopathic" gynecomastia. Apart from obesity no other factors contributing to breast development could be ascertained. In addition to the firm glandular tissue bilateral fat deposits were palpable

Even in the presence of normal or supranormal amounts of circulating androgens, gynecomastia can result when the action of androgens is blocked at the receptor level (see preceding sections). Prolactin does stimulate lactation, but at most it is of secondary importance for the development of mammary tissue. Thus, hyperprolactinemia unaccompanied by other endocrine deviations rarely induces gynecomastia. If, however, excessive prolactin levels lead to endocrine hypogonadism, gynecomastia and even galactorrhea may well occur. Medical disorders such as renal failure and some drugs may induce gynecomastia even though the androgen-estrogen ratio remains unaltered. The mechanism underlying the proliferation of mammary tissue in these cases is unclear.

In at least 50 % of patients presenting with gynecomastia no underlying cause can be found. Therefore, even a most diligent diagnostic workup often does not provide a diagnosis more specific than "**idiopathic gynecomastia**" (Fig. 11.5).

11.4.2 Clinical Examination

The two most immediate points to be clarified by physical examination are whether or not there is pathology at all and if so, whether one is dealing with gynecomastia or lipomastia. With careful palpation some glandular tissue can be made out in many men. As the demarcation between the normal and the mildly pathologic is hard to define, it will often be left to subjective clinical judgement whether the diagnosis of gynecomastia is made.

It is important to differentiate between gynecomastia and simple **lipomastia**. In particular obese men often have substantial deposits of adipose tissue in the pectoral region. Palpation usually allows differentiation of gynecomastia from lipomastia, and in cases of doubt, ultrasound may be helpful. Not rarely, gynecomastia is either strictly unilateral or more pronounced on one than on the other side. The cause for the asymmetry usually is obscure. The degree of gynecomastia can be estimated on a semiquantitative basis using the Tanner grading system for breast development:

- I: prepubertal,
- II: breast bud stage,
- III/IV: advanced stage of development,
- V: mature breast of an adult female.

Physical examination must not be restricted to the pectoral area. The general degree of virilization must be determined (see Chap. 6), and the patient should be specifically asked about symptoms suggestive of androgen deficiency (reduced libido or potency, reduced level of energy, decreasing beard growth).

> Palpation of the testes and (optionally) scrotal sonography should be an integral part of the diagnostic workup in gynecomastia. The physician must maintain a high index of suspicion as to the possibility of an endocrine active **testicular tumor** (see Sect. 8.19). Simultaneous loss of libido and potency can be considered as almost pathognomic.

Physical examination should also include a search for signs of **systemic disease** (hepatic, renal, syndromes).

11.4.3 Laboratory Investigation

The scope of laboratory investigations (endocrine, clinical chemistry) should be tailored to the specific clinical situation of the individual patient. If gynecomastia is mild and non-progressive or if adolescent gynecomastia is a very likely diagnosis there is no need for extensive endocrine investigations. Usually, determination of LH, FSH, estradiol and testosterone levels will suffice (Bowers et al. 1998). In less straightforward cases the basic laboratory workup should include testosterone, estradiol, SHBG, LH, FSH, prolactin, TSH, β-hCG, alpha-fetoprotein, renal and hepatic function tests. Other special investigations such as dynamic hormonal testing, karyotyping, or DNA-analysis may be useful depending on the individual case. The patient must be specifically asked about use of pharmaceutical and illegal drugs and alcohol consumption.

11.4.4 Physiologic Gynecomastia

The patient's age is a major factor determining the clinical interpretation of gynecomastia. In newborns, adolescents and senescent men a minor degree of breast development is usually not to be regarded as pathologic ("**physiologic gynecomastia**"). Mammary tissue may be easily palpable in male newborns, a sequel of stimulation by placentally transferred maternal estrogens. This is a finding that regresses spontaneously after some time.

Adolescent gynecomastia (Mahoney 1990) is another condition which usually does not require treatment. Often it can be considered as a normal variant. Careful palpation reveals some glandular tissue in up to 40% of

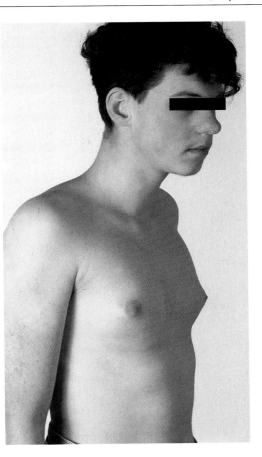

Fig. 11.6. Adolescent gynecomastia in a 16-year-old boy

male adolescents which by itself is not a pathologic finding. The degree of glandular proliferation may be more pronounced, however, and thus become a cosmetic and psychological problem for the affected individual (Fig. 11.6).

An endocrine or systemic disorder must not be overlooked, and in cases of more than very minor adolescent gynecomastia a limited diagnostic workup is recommendable. Mostly, a physical examination and measurement of basal levels of testosterone, estradiol, LH, and FSH is sufficient. There are no consistent hormonal endocrine deviations in adolescent gynecomastia. It is important to gain an impression of the overall androgenization of the patient. Adolescent gynecomastia develops after the onset of puberty. Thus, gynecomastia in a child or adolescent who shows no other signs of pubertal development must raise the suspicion of an endocrine problem, most notably a hormone-producing tumour.

Adolescent gynecomastia regresses spontaneously in most cases, but it may also persist to a variable degree. This is termed **persistent adolescent gynecomastia**. Indeed, this is one of the most frequent diagnoses among adult men presenting with gynecomastia. The condition can be confidently diagnosed if gynecomastia has occurred during adolescence, has shown no progression since, and if no other symptoms indicating an endocrine or other general medical problem have developed.

Men of **advanced age** often display gynecomastia to a minor degree. Here, systemic medical disorders have a high prevalence, and many such patients use drugs that can have an impact on the endocrine system. Minor deviations of the androgen-estrogen ratio may be observed (see Chap. 21). This is another patient population where the distinction between the normal variant and a mildly pathological finding is often hard to make. An individualized approach taking into account the general medical situation appears most sensible in addressing gynecomastia in elderly men.

11.4.5 Disorders with Gynecomastia

In this section we discuss the most important pathological forms of gynecomastia. Many of these disorders are covered more extensively in other chapters of this book. Table 11.2 lists the more frequent causes of gynecomastia, as well as some rare differential diagnoses that are not discussed in the text.

The first consideration in a patient with gynecomastia should be an endocrine disorder. Almost all conditions associated with **androgen deficiency** or **impaired androgen action** can present with gynecomastia. Pathological breast development is a frequent, albeit not an obligatory finding in men with **Klinefelter syndrome**. In contrast, outright gynecomastia is fairly untypical of **Kallmann syndrome** and **idiopathic hypogonadotropic hypogonadism**, but a mild degree of proliferation of glandular tissue may sometimes be observed. The frequency and degree of gynecomastia in other androgen deficiency states of testicular or hypothalamic-pituitary origin is variable. The diagnostic approach to and differential diagnosis of endocrine hypogonadism is laid out in detail in Chap. 7-9.

As patients with **testicular feminization** appear as normal females, it would be odd to speak of gynecomastia in this clinical situation, although from a strictly pathophysiological viewpoint this would be correct. The **Reifenstein syndrome** (Sect. 11.1.2), **X-linked spinal and bulbar muscular atrophy** (Kennedy disease; Sect. 11.1.4), and **perineo-scrotal hypospadias with pseudovagina** (Sect. 11.2) commonly feature gynecomastia.

Supranormal estrogen levels can induce gynecomastia. The estrogens may be derived from direct gonadal or adrenal biosynthesis or from peripheral conversion of androgens. Primarily estrogen-secreting **tumors of the testes** (Leydig or Sertoli cell tumors; Fig. 11.7) and the **adrenals** (especially carcinomas) are rare, but represent an

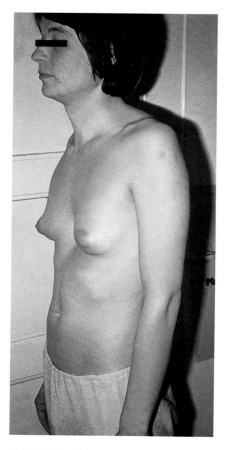

Fig. 11.7. Significant gynecomastia in a 22-year-old man that had developed over a couple of weeks and caused pain and tension. The gynecomastia was caused by a Leydig cell tumor and regressed completely after removal of the neoplasm

important differential diagnosis in patients with gynecomastia. Excessive estrogen production can be secondary to stimulation by increased hCG levels. Testicular teratomas, chorioncarcinomas, and embryonal carcinomas as well as extragonadal tumors, especially of lung and liver, are to be considered as potential sources of hCG.

The enzyme **aromatase** converts the androgens androstenedione and testosterone to estrone and estradiol, respectively. Supranormal estrogen production can occur if the substrates of this enzyme, especially androstenedione, are available for enzymatic conversion in higher than normal amounts. This is the case with **congenital adrenal hyperplasia** (21-hydroxylase deficiency) and **adrenal androgen-secreting tumors**. A rare hereditary form of gynecomastia is caused by an increased activity of the aromatase enzyme. In this condition plasma androgen levels are normal, but the rate of enzymatic conversion to estrogens is ten times higher than usual. The exact molecular basis for this abnormality is un-

Table 11.2. Differential diagnosis of gynecomastia

Pseudo-gynecomastia	Lipomastia Mammary tumor
Physiological gynecomastia	Gynecomastia of the newborn Adolescent gynecomastia Gynecomastia in senescence
Pathological gynecomastia	Idiopathic gynecomastia Persistend gynecomastia of adolescence Familial gynecomastia (no cause evident)
Disorders with a primary endocrine basis	Klinefelter syndrome XX male True hermaphroditism Kallmann syndrome Idiopathic hypogonadotropic hypogonadism Hyperprolactinemia Hyperthyroidism Congenital adrenal hyperplasia Adrenomyeloneuropathy Reifenstein syndrome X-linked spinal and bulbar muscular atrophy (Kennedy disease) Myotonic dystrophy Perineoscrotal hypospadias with pseudovagina Increased aromatase activity in peripheral tissue 17-Ketosteroid reductase deficiency 3β-Hydroxysteroid dehydrogenase deficiency
Endocrine active tumors	Malignant testicular tumor Leydig/Sertoli cell tumor of the testis Aromatase-producing testicular tumor in Peutz-Jeghers syndrome Tumor of the adrenal cortex Ektopic hCG production by a malignant tumor (especially lung, liver, kidney)
Androgen deficiency due todisorders of testicular parenchyma	Infectious orchitis Granulomatous orchitis Congenital anorchia Orchidectomy
Systemic disorders	Hepatic disease Renal disease Malnutrition Weight gain after period of malnutrition
Pharmaceutical and addictive drugs	Amphetamines Antineoplastic agents Calcium channel blockers Cimetidine Diazepam Digitalis Estrogens Flutamide Human chorionic gonadotropin Inhibitors of angiotensin-converting enzyme Isoniazid Ketokonazole Marihuana Methyldopa Metronidazole Opiates and opioids Penicillamins Reserpine Spironolactone Tricyclic antidepressants

known. The disorder is inherited in an autosomal dominant or X-linked recessive fashion (Berkovitz et al. 1985).

It has been speculated that accelerated conversion of androgens to estrogenic compounds may selectively occur in the glandular tissue of the breast. There is some indirect evidence for this hypothesis (Sasano et al. 1996), but currently definitive proof substantiating such a pathophysiological mechanism is wanting. This is also true for the unproven (but plausible) assumption that the sensitivity of the glandular tissue for estrogenic stimuli may vary from man to man and could be increased in patients with gynecomastia. Some cases of **familial gynecomastia** might be explained on this basis.

Untreated **hyperthyroidism** can induce increased estrogen production in men. Simultaneously SHBG is increased so that free bioavailable testosterone decreases. Probably it is a deviation from the normal androgen-estrogen ratio that leads to manifest gynecomastia in about one third of male patients with hyperthyroidism. Chronic hepatic or renal disease can also be accompanied by gynecomastia. The androgen-estrogen ratio may be abnormal, but not necessarily so.

In patients with medical disorders and gynecomastia it may be difficult to differentiate between the effects of the disease itself and the drugs used to treat it. A vast number of **drugs** can cause gynecomastia. Table 11.2 summarizes the generic names of those most relevant in this regard (Thompson and Carter 1993). Some of these drugs interfere with testosterone biosynthesis. The antifungal agent ketokonazole exerts a highly specific inhibiting activity of this kind, while the impairment of testosterone synthesis by antineoplastic drugs is an unspecific expression of their general toxicity. Other substances, e. g. cyproterone acetate, can block the androgen receptor. Drugs with opoid activity interfere with hypothalamic-pituitary function and thence induce secondary endocrine hypogonadism.

Estrogens and estrogen-like substances can also be absorbed from the intestine (food) or through the skin (cosmetics) and can induce gynecomastia. Phytoestrogens must also be considered in this context. Vaginal estrogen therapy (creams) can cause contamination of the partner during intercourse and can cause gynecomastia. There is the impressive case of a cook at a chicken grill with massive gynecomastia who was in the habit of eating the necks of the chickens which had been implanted with estrogens for castration, or the case of the embalmer who applied estrogen-containing lotions to corpses and failed to use protective gloves (Finkelstein et al. 1988). Even perverse practices must not be overlooked, as a 46 year-old man demonstrated, who regularly drank the urine of his female sex partners who used estrogen medication (Vierhapper and Nowotny 1999).

Tumors of the mammary gland are a rarity in men. As their clinical consequences are potentially grave, this possibility must always be taken into account in the differential diagnosis. Although unilateral gynecomastia is usually a transient stage in the development of bilateral gynecomastia, one-sided breast development must always raise the suspicion of a **mammary carcinoma** (O'Hanlon et al. 1995). Androgen and estrogen receptors are found in a large percentage of mammary carcinoma tissue but seem to show only little correlation with diagnosis, therapy and prognosis (Pich et al. 1999). There have been several reports about the occurrence of **breast cancer** in men with mutations of the androgen receptor gene (Wooster et al. 1992). It is unclear so far whether this represents a mere coincidence or whether such patients are really at increased risk for a malignant breast tumor. Contrary to earlier assumptions there is no greater incidence of breast cancer in Klinefelter patients, who almost always have gynecomastia, than in the general male population (see Sect. 8.9). As mutations in the BRCA2 gene were found in a high proportion of men with breast cancer, a genetic predisposition must be assumed (Csokay et al. 1999).

A painless and firm swelling in a subareolar or somewhat more excentric position should alarm the physician to the possibility of breast cancer. If clinically there is any doubt about the dignity of the lesion one should not hesitate to biopsy. It is beyond the scope of this text to discuss in more detail diagnosis and therapy of breast cancer in the male. The reader is referred to reviews (e. g. Crichlow and Galt 1990) and textbooks of oncology.

11.4.6. Therapy

The therapeutic approach to gynecomastia depends on several factors. The underlying cause, the objective degree of gynecomastia, the patient's subjective embarrassment by the abnormality, and the spontaneous course that the lesion is expected to take, all need to be considered. Quite frequently, no treatment at all is warranted, e. g. in cases with a very discrete degree of gynecomastia, if the patient does not feel handicapped by the abnormality, or if spontaneous remission is likely. The latter is true for most patients with adolescent gynecomastia. But even if the condition is harmless from a medical point of view, it may be onerous for the patient. Feminized appearance can lead to teasing and reduced self-confidence. As the patient is unwilling to disrobe in public, he will exclude himself from activities such as swimming and athletics, leading in turn to isolation and a lack of sexual contacts and consequent personality alterations and loss of quality of life. The physicians' guidance and care is especially required when no satisfactory diagnosis and treatment can be offered.

If the condition can be ascribed to an underlying disorder, treatment will be primarily directed at the basic problem. In this vein, correcting hyperestrogenism or testosterone deficiency may well lead to regression of gynecomastia if this was the underlying cause. However, this approach is not always successful. If proliferation of the glandular tissue has reached more than a minor degree, regression of gynecomastia may not be complete even though the disorder that has triggered it was treated. In longstanding gynecomastia **fibrosis** of the glandular tissue develops, and this also makes a complete spontaneous or therapy-induced regression unlikely.

Several endocrinologially active drugs (e.g. testosterone, dihydrotestosterone, danazole, testolactone, clomiphene, tamoxifen [Braunstein 1993]) have been tried to treat gynecomastia in patients without a distinct hormonal problem. The success rates in these mostly uncontrolled studies varied markedly. For the time being, the therapeutic value of such pharmaceutical interventions must be considered as unproven. As the rate of side-effects is low, the antiestrogen tamoxifen (10 mg twice a day) may be given a try even in patients with "idiopathic" gynecomastia. The earlier such therapy is tried, the greater its success seems to be, especially before fibrosis of mammary tissue occurs. If, after three months of this treatment, no improvement has occurred or if the patient desires primarily a surgical correction, we refer him for **gynecomastectomy**. The surgeon should have special experience with this operation (Courtiss 1987), as the cosmetic results can otherwise be more unsatisfactory than the preoperative status. Unattractive scars with irregular contours or keloid formation may result, the area may have a sunken appearance or the nipples may be asymmetrical (Colombo-Benkmann et al. 1998).

> It is wise not to be overzealous in arranging an immediate gynecomastectomy. Every patient must have undergone a complete diagnostic workup, and it is recommendable to observe the spontaneous clinical course for some time before a surgical correction is undertaken. Otherwise, the operation may ablate an abnormality which is only a symptom of another underlying disorder.

The case of a patient with a Leydig cell tumor may be taken as a warning example against an overzealous surgical approach to gynecomastia. Here, gynecomastia had developed rapidly and was corrected by surgery. However, due to this course of action the basic disorder went unrecognized for several months. The gynecomastia would have regressed spontaneously after removal of the testicular tumor.

11.5 Androgenetic Alopecia (Baldness)

11.5.1 Epidemiology and Pathophysiology

Androgenetic alopecia (**baldness**) is the most frequent form of alopecia and can affect both men and women. Among Caucasians every second male develops alopecia in the course of his lifetime. It is much less prevalent and less severe among Asians, Africans and native Americans. Widely prevalent but without real pathological implications, **alopecia can be considered a physiological event.** Young men are especially irritated by its occurrence, suffer from reduced self-image and seek treatment.

Hair grows continuously throughout life. Hair follicles proceed through a periodic growth cycle whose timing depends upon localization. Following the active growth phase (**anagen phase**) there is a brief phase of regression (**catagen phase**) which gives way to a resting phase (**telogen phase**). Thereafter the hair falls out. Normally the anagen phase lasts ca. three years and the telogen phase lasts only 100 days, so that the ratio of anagen to telogen hair is 9:1. Daily hair loss amounts to 100 hairs. In androgenetic alopecia the **anagen phase is shortened**, with a corresponding shift in the ratio of anagen to telogen hair. In addition, a **progressive miniaturization of hair follicles and terminal hair** occurs.

A precondition for the development of androgenetic alopecia is intact testicular function and androgen action. Testosterone is converted to 5α-DHT and can become effective only in this form (5α reductase type 2). A higher density of androgen receptors in the hair follicles of men with androgenetic alopecia was found (Randall 1998).

11.5.2 Diagnosis

Androgenetic alopecia begins with a **bitemporal loss of hair** in late adolescence or early adulthood and is generally tolerated as a typical androgen effect. Further development varies as to severity and localization, which can best be described according to the **categories** drawn up by Hamilton (1942) and Norwood (1975) (see Fig. 11.8). As it is an inherited autosomal dominant trait (Bergfeld 1995) the family history is of particular importance. Hyperthyroidism, malignomas and systemic diseases such as hepatopathies, iron deficiency anemias and diabetes mellitus, which may be associated with hair loss, must be excluded. However, in these diseases alopecia tends to be diffuse. High doses of vitamin A (over 50,000 IE) and cholesterol-lowering medication as well as thallium and mercury intoxication can lead to rapid hair loss. Special hormonal investigations are of little diagnostic help.

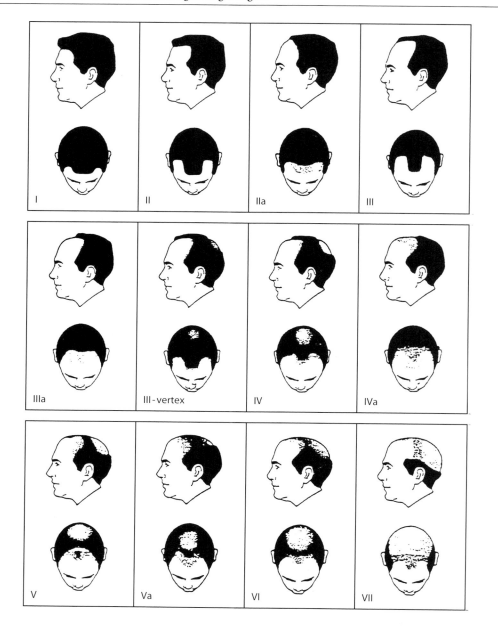

Fig. 11.8. The Hamilton-Norwood classification of androgenetic alopecia (Norwood 1975)

11.5.3 Therapy

As androgenetic alopecia is not a disease per se, in principle it requires no therapy. **Psychological guidance** with emphasis on **baldness as a sign of virility** is often sufficient. However, often the patient's suffering makes him turn to preparations whose efficacy is not proven, much to the advantage of the cosmetic industry. Some patients try to find relief by wearing toupets and wigs. Autologous hair transplants can be effective, but scars on the scalp can remain visible and the treatment is expensive.

It has long been known that **prepubertal castration** prevents male-pattern baldness (Hamilton 1942). Similarly, in genetically predisposed patients with delayed puberty androgenetic alopecia does not develop until treatment begins, as testosterone levels rise. **Antiandrogens** also counteract male-pattern baldness. These measures, however, are unacceptable because of the accompanying effects of hypogonadism.

By a specific inhibition of the 5α-reductase type 2 further progression of alopecia can be prevented and greater hair density can be achieved. **Finasteride**, licensed for treatment of benign prostate hypertrophy is presently being used under the name Propecia®. Controlled studies have demonstrated its effectiveness (Kaufman et al. 1998).

Minoxidil®, originally developed as an antihypertensive drug, was shown to increase hair growth within 4–6 months, as earlier controlled studies showed. After discontinuation of both preparations the original conditions return.

11.6 References

Aiman J, Griffin JE (1982) The frequency of androgen receptor deficiency in infertile men. J Clin Endocrinol Metab 54:725–732

Arbizu T, Santamaria J, Gomez JM, Quilez A, Peres Serra J (1983) A family with adult spinal and bulbar muscular atrophy, X-linked inheritance and associated testicular failure. J Neurol Sci 59:371–382

Bals-Pratsch M, Schweikert H-U, Nieschlag E (1990) Androgen receptor disorder in three brothers with bifid prepenile scrotum and hypospadias. Acta Endocrinol 123:271–276

Bergfeld WF (1995) Androgenetic alopecia: an autosomal dominant disorder. Am J Med 98:95S–98S

Berkovitz GD, Guerami A, Brown TR, MacDonald PC, Migeon CJ (1985) Familial gynecomastia with increased extraglandular aromatization of plasma carbon$_{19}$-steroids. J Clin Invest 75:1763–1769

Bowers SP, Pearlman NW, McIntyre RC Jr, Finlayson CA, Huerd S (1998) Cost-effective management of gynecomastia. Am J Surg 176:638–641

Braunstein GD (1993) Gynecomastia. N Engl J Med 328:490–495

Carani C, Qin K, Simoni M, Faustini-Fustini M, Serpente S, Boyd J, Korach KS, Simpson ER (1997) Effect of testosterone and estradiol in a man with aromatase deficiency. N Engl J Med 337:91–95

Csokay B, Udvarhelyi N, Sulyok Z, Besznyak I, Ramus S, Ponder B, Olah E (1999) High frequency of germ-line BRCA2 mutations among Hungarian male breast cancer patients without family history. Cancer Res 59:995–998

Colombo-Benkmann M, Buse B, Stern J, Herfarth C (1998) Surgical therapy of gynecomastia and its results. Langenbecks Arch Chir Suppl Kongressbd 115:1282–1284

Courtiss EH (1987) Gynecomastia: analysis of 159 patients and recommendations for treatment. Plastic Recon Surg 79:740–753

Crichlow RW, Galt SW (1990) Male breast cancer. Surg Clin North Am 70:1165–1177

Dowsing AT, Yong EL, Clark M, McLachlan RI, de Kretser DM, Trounson AO (1999) Linkage between male infertility and trinucleotide repeat expansion in the androgen-receptor gene. Lancet 354:640–643

Faustini-Fustini M, Rochira V, Carani C (1999) Oestrogen deficiency in men: where are we today? Eur J Endocrinol 140:111–129

Finkelstein JS, McCully WF, MacLaughlin DT, Godine JE, Crowley WF (1988) The mortician's mystery: gynecomastia and reversible hypogonadotropic hypogonadism in an embalmer. N Engl J Med 318:961–965

Griffin JE, McPhaul M, Russell DW, Wilson JD (1995) The androgen resistance syndromes: Steroid 5α-reductase 2 deficiency, testicular feminization, and related disorders. In: Scriver CE, Beaudet AL, Sly WS, Valle D (eds) The metabolic and molecular bases of inherited disease, vol II, 7th edn. McGraw Hill, New York, pp 2967–2998

Hamilton JB (1942) Male hormone stimulation is prerequisite and an incitant in common baldness. Am J Anat 71:451

Harding AE, Thomas PK, Baraitser M, Bradbury PG, Morgan-Hughes JA, Ponsford JR (1982) X-linked recessive bulbospinal neuronopathy: a report of ten cases. J Neurol Neurosurg Psychiatry 45:1012–1019

Hiort O, Sinnecker GHG, Holterhus P-M, Nitsche EM, Kruse K (1996) The clinical and molecular spectrum of androgen insensitivity syndromes. Am J Med Genet 63:218–222

Hiort O, Holterhus P-M, Sinnecker GHG, Kruse K (1999) Androgenresistenzsyndrome – Klinische und molekulare Grundlagen. Dtsch Ärztebl 96:A686–692

Imperato-McGinley J, Guerrero L, Gautier T, Peterson RE (1974) Steroid 5α-reductase deficiency in man: an inherited form of male pseudohermaphroditism. Science 186:1213–1215

Imperato-McGinley J, Peterson RE, Gautier T, Cooper G, Danner R, Arthur A, Morris PL, Sweeney WJ, Shackleton C (1982) Hormonal evaluation of a large kindred with complete androgen insensitivity: evidence for secondary 5α-reductase deficiency. J Clin Endocrinol Metab 54:931–941

Kaufman KD, Ohlsen EA, Whiting D et al (1998) Finasteride in the treatment of men with androgenetic alopecia (male pattern hair loss). J Am Acad Dermatol 36:578–589

Kreß W, Grimm T, Müller CR (1993) Molekulargenetische Diagnostik bei der X-chromosomal rezessiven bulbospinalen Muskelatrophie (Typ Kennedy). Med Genetik 5:269–270

La Spada AR, Wilson EM, Lubahn DB, Harding AE, Fischbeck KH (1991) Androgen receptor gene mutations in X-linked spinal and bulbar muscular atrophy. Nature 352:77–79

Lundberg Giwercman Y, Xu C, Arver S, Pousette A, Reneland R (1998) No association between the androgen receptor gene CAG repeat and impaired sperm production in Swedish men. Clin Genet 54:435–436

Mahoney CP (1990) Adolescent gynecomastia. Differential diagnosis and management. Ped Clin North Am 6:1389–1404

Merry DE, Kobayashi Y, Bailey CK, Taye AA, Fischbeck KH (1998) Cleavage, aggregation and toxicity of the expanded androgen receptor in spinal and bulbar muscular atrophy. Hum Mol Genet 7:693–701

Morrow AF, Gyorski S, Warne GL, Burger HG, Bangah ML, Outch KH, Mirovics A, Baker HWG (1987) Variable androgen receptor levels in infertile men. J Clin Endocrinol Metab 64:1115–1121

Norwood OT (1975) Male pattern baldness: classification and incidence. South Med J 68:1359–1365

O'Hanlon DM, Kent P, Kerin MJ, Giren HF (1995) Unilateral breast masses in men over 40: a diagnostic dilemma. Am J Surg 170:24–26

Pich A, Margaria E, Chiusa L, Candelaresi G, Dal Canton O (1999) Androgen receptor expression in male breast carcinoma: lack of clinicopathological association. Br J Cancer 79:959–964

Price P, Wass JAH, Griffin JE, Leshin M, Savage MO, Large DM, Bu'Lock DE, Anderson DC, Wilson JD, Besser GM (1984) High dose androgen therapy in male pseudohermaphroditism due to 5α-reductase deficiency and disorders of the androgen receptor. J Clin Invest 74:1496–1508

Quigley CA, De Bellis A, Marschke KB, El-Awady MK, Wilson EM, French FS (1995) Androgen receptor defects: historical, clinical, and molecular perspectives. Endocr Rev 16:271–321

Randall VA (1998) Androgens and hair. In: Nieschlag E, Behre HM (eds) Testosterone: action, deficiency, substitution, 2nd edn. Springer, Berlin Heidelberg New York, pp 169–186

Rodien P, Mebarki F, Mowszowicz I, Chaussain J-L, Young J, Morel Y, Schaison G (1996) Different phenotypes in a family with androgen insensitivity caused by the same M780I point mutation in the androgen receptor gene. J Clin Endocrinol Metab 81:2994–2998

Sasano H, Kimura M, Shizawa S, Kimura N, Nagura H (1996) Aromatase and steroid receptors in gynecomastia and male breast carcinoma: an immunohistochemical study. J Clin Endocrinol Metab 81:3063–3067

Scully RE (1981) Neoplasia associated with anomalous sexual development and abnormal sex chromosomes. Pediat Adolesc Endocr 8:203–217

Sinnecker GHG, Hiort O, Dibbelt L, Albers N, Dörr HG, Hauß H, Heinrich U, Hemminghaus M, Hoepffner W, Holder M, Schnabel D, Kruse K (1996) Phenotypic classification of male pseudohermaphroditism due to steroid 5α-reductase 2 deficiency. Am J Med Genet 63:223–230

Sinnecker GHG, Hiort O, Nitsche EM, Holterhus P-M, Kruse K, German Collaborative Intersex Study Group (1997) Functional assessment and clinical classification of androgen sensitivity in patients with mutations of the androgen receptor gene. Eur J Pediatr 156:7–14

Smith EP, Boyd J, Frank GR, Takahashi H, Cohen RM, Specker B, Williams TC, Lubahn DB, Korach KS (1994) Estrogen resistance caused by a mutation in the estrogen-receptor gene in a man. N Engl J Med 331:1056–1061

Thompson DF, Carter JR (1993) Drug-induced gynecomastia. Pharmacotherapy 13:37–45

Vierhapper H, Nowotny P (1999) Gynaecomastia and raised oestradiol concentrations. Lancet 353:640

Wilson JD, Griffin JE, Russell DW (1993) Steroid 5α-reductase 2 deficiency. Endocr Rev 14:577–593

Wooster R, Mangion J, Eeles R, Smith S, Dowsett M, Averill D, Barrett-Lee P, Easton DF, Ponder BAJ, Stratton MR (1992) A germline mutation in the androgen receptor gene in two brothers with breast cancer and Reifenstein syndrome. Nature Genet 2:132–134

CHAPTER 12

Testicular Dysfunction in Systemic Diseases

D. J. HANDELSMAN

12.1 Background

> Systemic illness has major effects on the testis although these have not always been sufficiently recognized. The clinical management of any medical disorder should include careful consideration of the effects of illness and its treatment on male reproductive function (including fertility, androgenic status and sexual function).

This will prevent patient dissatisfaction with their medical care if their management is too narrowly focussed on the presenting disease and neglects the patient's often unstated, but nevertheless deeply felt, expectations relating to his **reproductive health**.

12.2 Mechanisms of Reproductive Disruption by Systemic Diseases

The clinical manifestations of androgen deficiency and/or infertility depend at which epoch of life it begins, its severity and its chronicity. Prenatal androgen deficiency leads to various degrees of incomplete development of male internal and external genitalia varying from complete absence of masculine sexual development to various degrees of hypospadias, gynecomastia and/or cryptorchidism. Pubertal androgen deficiency is manifest as delayed puberty and virilization. Postpubertal androgen deficiency may present with the well known classical features of androgen deficiency in adults (see Chap. 6). At each epoch, the expression of androgen deficiency is quite variable. Not being life threatening, it is often underdiagnosed in adult life. Such under-recognition is particularly likely when the relatively subtle effects of androgen deficiency are overshadowed by a major systemic illness with more dramatic clinical features. Most classical features of androgen deficiency, apart from hot flushes in castrate men, are manifestations of prolonged, moderate to severe androgen deficiency. In contrast, defects in spermatogenesis are only recognized after puberty when spermatogenesis has usually developed so that infertility can be identified.

Most severe systemic nongonadal illness or trauma such as **burns, myocardial infarction, traumatic or surgical injury,** and **acute critical illness** (Woolf et al. 1985; Dong et al. 1992) depress testicular function as evidenced by low total and free testosterone levels, unchanged immunoreactive inhibin levels, decreased or mildly increased immunoreactive gonadotropin levels with low bioactive LH levels and abolition of pulsatile LH secretion (Woolf et al. 1985; Semple et al. 1987; Dong et al. 1992). Such **transient biochemical androgen deficiency (secondary hypogonadism)** is so common that it should be considered a normal accompaniment of severe acute or chronic illness. The impact of diminished anabolic status on morbidity is unclear and controlled clinical studies of androgen replacement therapy in this setting are lacking (Liu and Handelsman 1998). Secondary hypogonadism is even more frequent than hypothyroidism (historically once misnamed the "sick euthyroid" syndrome) as different facets of reversible, functional hypopituitarism due to systemic nongonadal illness.

Testicular function is depressed by common features of systemic illness such as **cytokines, fever** (Kandeel and Swerdloff 1988), **weight loss** and **chronic illness or catabolism** (Handelsman and Staraj 1985) and distinguishing between these effects is difficult. Extremes of nutrition influence testicular function but **male reproductive function is more robust than the female reproductive system** during catabolic states such as undernutrition, trauma and extreme physical exertion. **Strenuous physical exercise** has minimal effects on testicular function and spermatogenesis among elite athletes (Bagatell and Bremner 1990) but extreme physical exertion causes profound inhibition of testicular androgen secretion (see Chap. 15).

Anorexia nervosa is rare in males but then causes profound inhibition of testicular endocrine function (Buvat et al. 1983). The effects of moderate undernutrition or selective dietary micronutrient deficiencies (e. g. vitamins, cofactors) on human testicular function are less clear.

Obesity inhibits testicular endocrine function but effects on spermatogenesis have not been reported. Total and free testosterone and SHBG levels decrease; estradiol levels are increased, while gonadotropin levels remain unchanged, reflecting a widespread defect in hypothalamic function in obesity (Iranmanesh et al. 1991). The principal pathogenic mechanism may involve functional hyposomatotropism and/or insulin resistance causing a decline in hepatic SHBG secretion which lowers circulating testosterone levels. These hormonal changes are not accompanied by overt clinical features of androgen deficiency and are reversed by weight reduction. Moderate obesity has little overt effect on male reproductive

function but may contribute to the decline of hypothalamus and pituitary testicular function in ageing men (Gray et al. 1991).

Age is a crucial modifier of testicular response to systemic illness (see Chap. 21). The maturing hypothalamic pituitary testicular axis has heightened susceptibility, making adolescents particularly vulnerable to delayed puberty during chronic illness. Aging men exhibit decreased testosterone levels while SHBG and gonadotropin levels increase, changes which are markedly accentuated by the coexistence of chronic illness and/or its treatment. These changes reflect alterations in hypothalamic function including loss of diurnal testosterone rhythm, alterations in pulsatile LH secretion and sensitivity to both negative steroidal feedback and opioids as well as testicular changes such as progressive decreases in testis size, cell content and spermatogenesis.

Drugs may impair androgen action through numerous distinct and sometime multiple mechanisms including (i) decreasing LH secretion (eg opiates), (ii) inhibiting steroidogenic enzymes (eg aminoglutethimide, ketoconazole), (iii) increased testosterone metabolism (eg barbiturates, anticonvulsants and other hepatic enzyme inducers), (iv) androgen receptor antagonists blocking testosterone action (eg cimetidine, spironolactone, cyproterone acetate) or (v) acting as physiological antagonists of androgen action (estrogenic effects of digoxin, drug induced hyperprolactinemia). Very few therapeutic drugs, however, have had their potential effects on the human male reproductive system studied in detail.

Smoking has modest effects on spermatogenesis, sperm function and male fertility in otherwise healthy men (Stillman et al. 1986) but reversal after smoking cessation is not well established. Chronic heavy **alcohol** intake has multiple, cumulative effects on the male reproductive system due to direct, irreversible testicular toxicity (Villalta et al. 1997) as well as indirect toxic effects (eg nutritional, hepatoxicity). The effects of recreational drugs such as marijuana, cocaine and opiates on testicular function are not well understood; few studies have been reported and none are well controlled for confounding effects of undernutrition, multiple drug usage, psychological and socioeconomic factors.

Disruption of spermatogenesis can lead to infertility through reduction in either the number and/or function of ejaculated sperm. The intense cellular and DNA replication of the germinal epithelium makes it singularly susceptible to cytotoxines such as ionising irradiation, cytotoxic drugs (notably alkylating agents), other therapeutic agents (eg some antibiotics) and occupational or environmental exposures (see Chap. 13). Such agents cause all degrees of hypospermatogenesis from reversible depression to permanent ablation. As spermiogenesis forms the morphological basis for sperm function, interruption at this stage of spermatogenesis can produce hypofunctional (infertile) sperm.

12.3 Specific Diseases and Disorders

12.3.1 Renal Diseases

Chronic renal failure causes prominent disturbances of testicular function largely through aberrant hypothalamic regulation of pituitary gonadotropin secretion and secondary testicular effects (Handelsman 1985; Handelsman and Dong 1993). Gonadal dysfunction in uremia is manifest as delayed puberty in adolescents and as testicular atrophy, hypospermatogenesis, infertility, impotence and/or gynecomastia in men.

Most disturbances begin prior to inception of dialysis and deteriorate during **maintenance peritoneal or hemodialysis** but can be fully reversed by successful **renal transplantation**.

Inhibition of both spermatogenesis and steroidogenesis accompanied by modest to minimal reflex increases in gonadotropins (particularly with newer, more specific immunoassays; Samojlik et al. 1992) together with testicular histological features are indicative of a functional hypogonadotropic state (Handelsman and Dong 1993). Gonadotropin clearance rates are markedly reduced in uremia but net LH production rate fails to rise significantly which, together with defects in pulsatile LH secretion and aberrant hypothalamic opiatergic regulation of gonadotropin secretion (Handelsman and Dong 1993), reflect the predominance of aberrant hypothalamic regulation in the pathogenesis of human uremic hypogonadism. Although clinical and biochemical features of biochemical androgen deficiency are present in chronic uremia (Handelsman 1985; Handelsman and Dong 1993), controlled studies of androgen replacement therapy are lacking.

Acute **renal failure** is accompanied by decreased testosterone levels with minimal changes in gonadotropin or SHBG levels and preserved responses to GnRH stimulation also consistent with hypothalamic (secondary) hypogonadism that is reversed following recovery of renal function. Recent experimental studies confirm the predominance of alterations in hypothalamic regulation of pituitary gonadal function in the pathogenesis of uremic hypogonadism. Experimental subtotal nephrectomy in rats causes testicular dysfunction and infertility which is principally due to aberrant neuroendocrine regulation of GnRH secretion.

A triad of features involved, namely, inhibition of GnRH secretion, hypersensitivity to negative testicular feedback and resistance to naloxone, has been termed **ontogenic regression** (Handelsman and Dong 1992; Handelsman and Dong 1993).

The only effective treatment for uremic testicular dysfunction is a well functioning **renal transplant** in contrast to **dialysis**, which fails to correct or aggravates testicular dysfunction.

Claims that adjuvant treatments including suppression of hyperprolactinemia, zinc supplementation or erythropoetin improve testicular function have not been confirmed in well-controlled studies. Conventional immunosuppressive regimens involving prednisone, azathioprine, cyclosporin A and rapamycin appear to have minimal clinically significant effects on human testicular function.

12.3.2 Liver Diseases

Acute liver disease including **hepatitis** causes marked increases in circulating SHBG levels resulting in reflex increases in gonadotropin and sex steroid secretion to maintain testicular testosterone output and tissue androgen supply. The pathophysiological significance of such transient biochemical disturbance during acute illness is unclear.

Chronic liver failure is associated with prominent features of hypogonadism including infertility, impaired spermatogenesis, testicular atrophy, gynecomastia, reduced body hair and sexual dysfunction.

Testosterone production rate is decreased leading to lower circulating total and free testosterone levels although the concomitant increases in circulating SHBG levels with a consequential fall in testosterone clearance rate conceals the severity of the androgen deficiency. Despite subnormal testosterone levels, gonadotropin levels remain in the low to normal eugonadal range with diminished pulsatile LH secretion, emphasizing the importance of hypothalamic dysregulation in the pathogenesis of hypogonadism in chronic liver disease.

Men with alcoholic liver disease exhibit higher gonadotropin levels in the older radioimunoassays. More sensitive and specific dual site immunoassays reveal more consistently lowered gonadotropin levels, especially in men with severe hepatic failure and coma in whom gonadotropin levels are markedly reduced.

As **alcohol** is the most common cause of chronic liver failure in affluent societies, the usual clinical features of chronic liver disease are an amalgam of clinical manifestations due to chronic liver disease per se and chronic alcoholic toxicity. Apart from direct alcohol toxicity on the testis (Villalta et al. 1997), the major pathogenic factors for reproductive effects of liver disease are the loss of hepatic parenchyma and portocaval shunting (leading to cerebral dopamine excess) but their relative roles remain to be clarified.

Testosterone administration improves sense of well being, increases serum proteins and reduces edema without serious adverse effects (Puliyel et al. 1977; Kley et al. 1979; Gluud et al. 1981) but long-term benefits, particularly using noninjectable testosterone formulations which eliminate risk of injection site bleeding, remain to be demonstrated.

Men with **chronic active hepatitis** requiring immunosuppression have essentially normal spermatogenesis despite **azathioprine** doses of up to 150 mg daily (Lange et al. 1978). Little information is available about semen parameters in other chronic liver diseases. The testicular endocrine dysfunction (Handelsman et al. 1995) and the consequences of the partial androgen deficiency on the prostate (Jin et al. 1999) are proportional to the severity of the underlying liver disease and are reversed by successful **liver transplantation**.

Systemic **iron overload** due to either genetic or acquired posttransfusional **hemochromatosis** often causes hypogonadotropic hypogonadism due to pituitary iron deposition causing relatively selective damage to gonadotropes. **In more advanced disease**, the additional effects of **cirrhosis and diabetes** further highlight the clinical presentation of androgen deficiency. This disorder frequently presents with progressive androgen deficiency in middle-aged men and is readily amenable to androgen replacement therapy or, if fertility is required, gonadotropin therapy. The hypogonadism is rarely reversed by iron desaturation from venesection and/or iron chelation except in younger (< 40 yr) men (Cundy et al. 1993). **Testosterone replacement therapy** is often necessary and effective both symptomatically (Kley et al. 1992) and in restoring bone density loss due to androgen deficiency (Diamond et al. 1991). Gonadotropin induction of spermatogenesis is particularly effective in genetic **hemochromatosis** as the onset of gonadotropin deficiency follows a normal puberty while pulsatile GnRH therapy is ineffective since gonadotropin secretion cannot be induced (Wang et al. 1989). Earlier diagnosis by genetic and family screening should prevent the development of overt clinical manifestations of iron overload from genetic hemochromatosis.

Puberty is delayed in regularly transfused children with β-**thalassemia** (Wang et al. 1989) and prepubertal onset of iron chelation therapy enhances pubertal maturation, presumably by preventing **pituitary siderosis** (Bronspiegel-Weintrob et al. 1990).

12.3.3 Respiratory Diseases

Chronic sinopulmonary infections (recurrent bronchitis, bronchiectasis, chronic sinusitis and/or otitis media) are associated with infertility due to **Young syndrome**, **cystic fibrosis** (CF) and **dyskinetic cilia syndromes** (including **immotile cilia** and **Kartagener syndrome**).

Both Young syndrome and CF have obstructive azoospermia which is due to congenital absence of the vas deferens in CF whereas in Young syndrome the epididymis and vas deferens are anatomically intact but the epididymis becomes obstructed intraluminally by inspissated secretion (Handelsman et al. 1984). In contrast, the excurrent ductular system and sperm output are normal in dyskinetic cilia syndromes but sperm are immotile due to defects in axonemal function (Neugebauer et al. 1990), although rare variants of the dyskinetic cilia syndromes lacking respiratory disease, with cilial defects restricted to lungs or sperm or with ductular obstruction, have been described.

Classical CF is also associated with **delayed puberty** attributable to both chronic illness and suboptimal nutrition from exocrine pancreatic dysfunction. Congenital aplasia of vas deferens has recently been recognized as a primarily genital variant of CF with at least 50 % of afflicted men of European descent being heterozygous for the ΔDF508 deletion mutation of the CFTR gene (Anguiano et al. 1992). Since obligate heterozygotes for the CF mutation (ie fathers of CF children) have normal or increased fertility and normal sperm output (Handelsman, unpublished), the other CFTR allele must bear another, less common mutation of the CFTR gene (Patrizio et al. 1993). What determines the clinical pattern of disease (CF vs CAV) remains an intriguing biological puzzle (see Chap. 9).

Obstructive **sleep apnea** is associated with sexual dysfunction and lowered testosterone levels without reflex rise in gonadotropin levels indicative of a central hypogonadotropic mechanism (Grunstein et al. 1989). These effects are not due to the associated obesity alone and are reversed by mechanical maintenance of upper airways patency without weight loss (Grunstein et al. 1989). The relative contributions of hypoxia and sleep fragmentation to this central hypogonadism remain to be clarified. Testosterone administration can precipitate obstructive sleep apnea in some predisposed obese men (Sandblom et al. 1983) by blunting ventilatory drive and/or chemoreceptor sensitivity (Matsumoto et al. 1985); changes in upper airway dimensions or patency seem unlikely as causes (Schneider et al. 1986).

Asthma is associated with pubertal delay due to chronic illness and systemic corticosteroid therapy but has no reported effects on postpubertal male reproductive function apart from lowered circulating total testosterone levels due to glucocorticoid induced decreases in SHBG levels.

Emphysema due to α_1-**antitrypsin deficiency** is associated with normal testicular function and fertility and the late onset of severe symptoms may explain the unusually high prevalence of this deleterious genetic disease which presumably fails to impair genetic "fitness" due to the manifestations of illness being delayed until after reproductive age.

12.3.4 Malignant Diseases

The common malignancies of male reproductive life that are medically treated with curative intent include testicular (teratoma, seminoma) and hematological (Hodgkin and non-Hodgkin lymphoma) tumors and sarcomas.

Treatment with combination chemotherapy and/or therapeutic irradiation virtually always causes azoospermia and infertility.

The duration of azoospermia and the degree and rate of spermatogenic recovery varies according to the regimen used from full (eg cisplatinum/vinblastine/bleomycin for teratoma), partial (eg combination chemotherapy for sarcoma) and dose dependent (eg pelvic irradiation with testicular shielding for seminoma) reversibility over several years after treatment to essentially irreversible sterilisation (eg MOPP for Hodgkin disease (Whitehead et al. 1982); whole body irradiation for bone marrow transplantation). The testis is exceptionally sensitive to ionising irradiation (see Chap. 13) with single doses of 20 rads (cGy) causing azoospermia and time to recovery being proportional to dose (Rowley et al. 1974). In contrast to other tissues, dose fractionation enhances spermatogonial killing (Meistrich and van Beek 1990).

In principle, spermatogenic damage could be prevented by less toxic regimens, by cytoprotective therapies, or circumvented by sperm cryostorage (see Chap. 18) or autologous germ cell transplantation (Schlatt 1999). In men with Hodgkin disease the otherwise inevitable sterilization from a standard course of MOPP may be avoided by using fewer cycles of MOPP (da Cunha et al. 1984) or using the ABVD regimen (doxorubicin, bleomycin, vinblastine, dacarbazine), which has equal therapeutic efficacy but less spermatogenic toxicity than MOPP (Viviani et al. 1985). Effective testicular shielding can greatly reduced testicular dosage during pelvic irradiation but the scatter doses (typically ~2% of dose) still well exceed the threshold for spermatogenic damage (<0.5% of dose). Experimental hormonal cytoprotection treatments using either steroids and/or GnRH analogs to inhibit testicular function during chemotherapy have shown only limited promise in experimental models (Crawford et al. 1998) or preliminary human studies (Kreuser et al. 1993).

Moderate testicular dysfunction is frequent in men with malignant disease even prior to cytotoxic treatment and the contributions of fever, weight loss, diagnostic procedures or cytokines are hard to differentiate. Pretreatment testicular dysfunction is one constraint on sperm cryopreservation although most men are able to cryostore sperm if they wish. Sperm cryopreservation for men without completed families represents a cost effective, psychologically reassuring preparation for re-covery from treatment. As a form of fertility insurance only limited use of cryostored material in artificial insemination or male factor IVF/ICSI may be expected and ongoing appropriate followup, including appropriate advice on contraception, prognosis for cure and semen analysis, is required to determine whether to discard or continue sperm cryostorage (see Chap. 18).

12.3.5 Neurological Diseases

Genetic Disorders

Myotonic dystrophy, the commonest inherited muscle disease of adults, is associated with reduced fertility, testicular atrophy, hypospermatogenesis, elevated gonadotropin and low or normal testosterone levels.

The testicular defect has no relationship with severity, duration or treatment of the muscular disease nor does pharmacological testosterone therapy improve muscular strength despite increasing muscle mass (Griggs et al. 1989; Vazquez et al. 1990). The relationship of testicular dysfunction to the causative mutation, a polymorphic expansion of tandem CTG triplet codon repeats (>35) in the 3' untranslated region of the myotonin protein kinase gene, is unknown (Mastrogiacomo et al. 1996).

The genetic basis of **Kennedy disease** (late onset, X linked recessive bulbospinal muscular atrophy) has been identified as a variable increase in numbers of CAG triplet repeats in the first exon of the androgen receptor in a region coding for its nonbinding, N terminal domain (La Spada et al. 1991). This leads, by an unexplained mechanism, to late onset androgen resistance including gynecomastia and testicular atrophy. The disease severity and age of onset is correlated with the number of tandem CAG triplet repeats (La Spada et al. 1992) and with defects in androgen receptor binding (Warner et al. 1992) but the pathogenesis of the neurotoxicity and its relationship to the androgen receptor mutations remains unknown.

The **fragile X syndrome**, the most common familial cause of mental retardation and which explains the male excess in mental institutions, is associated with moderate mental retardation, dysmorphic features and macroorchidism. The macroorchidism is manifest after puberty and the testes have normal function (Cantu et al. 1976) but are enlarged in all dimensions, possibly due to prenatal lymphangiectasis. Macroorchidism (>40 ml) is a useful screening test for the fragile X syndrome within institutions but it is not invariably associated with mental retardation or the fragile-X locus and the syndrome is rare among infertile men with megalotestes (Meschede et al. 1995). The genetic basis involves a region of unstable DNA which acquires excessive multiple copies of the CCG triplet codons (>200 vs 6–60 on the normal

X chromosome) leading to abnormal methylation and inactivation of the FMR1 gene, but the pathogenesis of the phenotype remains unknown. The reason that these three diseases with heritable unstable DNA replication all manifest testicular and neurologic dysfunction remain unclear.

A variety of other rare genetic neurological disorders involving multiple congenital defects are associated with hypogonadotropic hypogonadism, presumably due to defective neural circuitry involving the hypothalamic GnRH neurons and/or their pulse generator (see Chap. 7). These syndromes include the **Prader-Labhart-Willi syndrome** of mental retardation, hypotonia, short stature and obesity caused by deletions or uniparental disomy of chromosome 15 (Nicholls 1993), the **Laurence-Moon-Biedl syndrome** of retinitis pigmentosa, obesity, mental retardation and polydactyly or other dysmorphic features, **Friedreich's and other cerebellar ataxia syndromes, multiple lentigines syndrome, steroid sulphatase deficiency** (X-linked congenital icthyosis) and other rare congenital neurological syndromes (**Moebius, RUD, CHARGE, Lowe, Martsolf, Rothmund-Thompson, Borjeson-Forssman-Lehman**) (Rimoin and Schimke 1971). Such patients may require androgen replacement although social factors usually dictate that fertility requiring gonadotrophin induction of spermatogenesis is rarely requested.

Acquired Disorders

Temporal lobe epilepsy is associated with hypogonadism and sexual dysfunction which usually responds to anticonvulsant therapy, but a minority require additional androgen replacement therapy. Other forms of epilepsy per se do not appear to be associated with abnormal testicular endocrine function although low free testosterone levels and hyposexuality are common in anticonvulsant treated epileptics (Fenwick et al. 1985; Isojarvi et al. 1989). Anticonvulsants increase hepatic SHBG secretion leading to decreased metabolic clearance rate for testosterone together with increases in total testosterone and gonadotropins while free testosterone levels are decreased. Sperm output remains normal but morphology and motility are impaired during long term treatment with phenylhydantoin (Schramm and Seyfeddinpur 1980). Although testosterone has antiseizure effects in experimental animal models, no controlled clinical studies of the effects of androgen administration on seizure control or androgenic status have been reported.

Spinal cord damage from trauma or neurological disease causes testicular dysfunction depending in severity on the level and extent of spinal cord interruption. Testicular function is disrupted by aberrant thermoregulation, recurrent ascending urinary tract infections from bladder catheterisation and neurogenic dysfunction and iatrogenic factors (diagnostic irradiation, drugs). Impotence is predominantly due to interruption of neural pathways controlling erection and emission while libido remains appropriate for age. Conservation of sexual function depends upon the level and extent of the spinal injury. Hypospermatogenesis and testicular atrophy is usually observed in men with long-term spinal injuries but fertility may be preserved by timely sperm cryopreservation using electroejaculation coupled with assisted fertilization.

Head injuries may cause gonadotropin deficiency due to disruption of the pituitary portal bloodstream and/or pituitary infarction following basal skull fractures.

12.3.6 Gastrointestinal Diseases

Celiac disease is associated with subfertility, impaired sperm output, morphology and motility together with elevated blood testosterone and gonadotropin levels which are reversible upon dietary improvement of the gluten enteropathy. This distinctive endocrine pattern is suggestive of acquired androgen resistance; however, detailed studies of androgen receptor function or action (Farthing and Dawson 1983) are lacking.

Inflammatory bowel disease is often associated with impaired spermatogenesis but testicular endocrine function is unaffected (Farthing and Dawson 1983). Hypospermatogenesis is common in **Crohn's disease** possibly related to fever, chronic illness and/or nutritional status (Farthing and Dawson 1983). Similarly men with **ulcerative colitis** taking salazopyrine exhibit impaired spermatogenesis, sperm function and male fertility (Cosentino et al. 1984). Routine use of salazopyrine for both acute and preventative maintenance therapy early in the course of **ulcerative colitis** in other countries has precluded studies of testicular function in untreated men to determine the extent of effects of ulcerative colitis per se. Semen parameters improve in patients switching from salazopyrine to 5-aminosalicylic acid (Zelissen et al. 1988); patients who have not completed their families should be treated with the latter drug.

Peptic ulceration has no reported effects on testicular function, although treatment with the H_2 receptor blocker cimetidine impairs testicular function by androgen receptor antagonism unrelated to its H_2 receptor blocking activity (Knigge et al. 1983). These effects are not observed with ranitidine and other H_2 receptor blockers or other anti-acid drugs.

12.3.7 Hematological Diseases

Hemoglobinopathies (including **sickle cell anemia** and **thalassemias**) are associated with delayed puberty while transfusion-induced iron overload leads to acquired gonadotropin deficiency functionally similar to that of genetic hemochromatosis (see Sect. 12.3.2). **Iron deficiency anemia** has no recognised effects on testicular function but men with **sickle cell anemia** have reportedly poor spermatogenesis (Agbaraji et al. 1988). **Megaloblastic anemia** from folate or vitamin B_{12} deficiencies inhibits DNA replication in the marrow and might cause arrest of the germinal epithelium; however, no reports of spermatogenesis among men with megaloblastosis are available to examine this hypothesis, presumably reflecting the paucity of vitamin B_{12} or folate deficiency in young nonalcoholic men in developed countries. **Hemophilia** is associated with a striking reduction in male fertility (Francis and Kasper 1983) although whether this is explained fully by voluntary restraint of fertility is unclear as no studies of testicular function in hemophiliacs are available.

12.3.8 Endocrine Diseases

Thyroid disease influences male reproductive function (Jannini et al. 1995) with the most striking effects manifest through changes in circulating SHBG levels (Ford et al. 1992). Thyroid hormones stimulate hepatic SHBG synthesis so **hyperthyroidism** increases circulating SHBG levels and **hypothyroidism** causes low SHBG levels and these changes are reversed by normalization of thyroid hormone levels (Kumar et al. 1990). The rise in SHBG decreases the testosterone clearance rate, resulting in increased total testosterone, estradiol and gonadotropin levels. The net effect on overall tissue androgen action remains unclear. Clinical features include gynecomastia and reduced sexual function in a minority of cases. Spermatogenesis is depressed in thyrotoxicosis (O'Brien et al. 1982) and long standing hypothyroidism of prepubertal onset but is little affected by postpubertal hypothyroidism (de la Balze et al. 1962).

Hypercortisolism from any cause can inhibit testicular function at multiple levels of the HPT axis leading to a reduction in circulating testosterone and gonadotropin levels which is reversed by interruption of the exposure to excessive glucocorticoids (Luton et al. 1977). The degree to which androgen deficiency contributes to the catabolic state and symptoms of sexual dysfunction and weakness during hypercortisolism is unclear. The mechanisms involve multiple levels of the HPT axis including inhibition of hypothalamic GnRH secretion, of GnRH stimulated pituitary LH secretion and of LH stimulation of Leydig cell testosterone biosynthesis.

The effects of diabetes on male reproductive function are primarily due to neuropathic and vascular complications of diabetes causing erectile and/or ejaculatory dysfunction (Dunsmuir and Holmes 1996). Direct effects on testicular function are less evident.

12.3.9 Immune Diseases

Autoantibodies to spermatozoa develop in about 70 % of men after vasectomy but have no apparent deleterious effects on general health (Petitti 1986) although they may inhibit sperm function and fertility after vasectomy reversal (Linnet et al. 1981). Sperm autoantibodies are observed in 5 to 10 % of nonvasectomised infertile men who also have an increased prevalence of other organ specific autoantibodies (see Chap. 9). Immune complexes of unknown significance have been observed in seminiferous tubular basement membranes of infertile men.

Most **autoimmune diseases** have a marked (> 5 : 1) female predominance (e. g. systemic lupus erythematosus, chronic active hepatitis, chronic biliary cirrhosis) which remains unexplained and testicular involvement in immune disease is unusual apart from **polyarteritis nodosa** where testicular biopsy may be diagnostic. **Rheumatoid arthritis** causes prolonged depression of testosterone levels during flares of disease activity with spontaneous recovery during remission (Cutolo et al. 1991). Testicular endocrine function is normal in men with **ankylosing spondylitis** (Gordon et al. 1986), **systemic lupus erythematosus** (Stahl and Decker 1978) or **osteoarthritis** (Spector et al. 1988). Treatment of immunological diseases with cytotoxic drugs may lead to severe, dose dependent and sometimes irreversible spermatogenic damage typical of alkylating agents.

Autoimmune orchitis (see Chap. 8) is a rare component of the organ specific autoimmune cluster and **autoimmune hypophysitis** causing isolated gonadotropin deficiency or panhypopituitarism is also uncommon (Obermayer-Straub and Manns 1998). **Amyloidosis** of the testis causing macro-orchidism is rare, occurring mostly in secondary systemic amyloidosis but massive primary infiltration has been reported (Handelsman et al. 1983).

12.3.10 Infectious Diseases

Systemic infections often influence testicular function even without causing orchitis (see Chap. 8). Many mechanisms are involved, including the effects of fever (including effects of tumor necrosis factor-α and cytokines), weight loss and chronic catabolism. The net effects depend on the severity and duration of the infection. A characteristic example is the testicular dysfunction that is common in **AIDS** reflecting the stage of clinical disease and/or its treatment (Raffi et al. 1991). Spermatogenic damage is almost universal at postmortem (de Paepe and Waxman 1989) whereas testicular endocrine function (Villette et al. 1990) and spermatogenesis (Crittenden et al. 1992) are unaffected in asymptomatic, HIV seropositive men but deteriorate with clinical status and treatment (Handelsman and Staraj 1985). Similar effects would be expected with comparable severe and/or chronic systemic infections such as tuberculosis (Post et al. 1994) or sleeping sickness (Petzke et al. 1996).

12.3.11 Cardiovascular Diseases

Hypertension is associated with lowered circulating total and free testosterone levels (Hughes et al. 1989) and antihypertensive medications further lowers testosterone levels (Suzuki et al. 1988) which may explain the inverse epidemiological association (independent of age and obesity) between blood pressure and testosterone levels (Khaw and Barratt-Connor 1988). Such small decreases in blood testosterone levels are insufficient to account for the disproportionately high prevalence of erectile dysfunction in treated hypertensive men. This presumably reflects both more advanced atherogenesis and hemodynamic factors rather than hormonal effects of antihypertensive medication (Jaffe et al. 1996).

There is a strong association between **atherosclerotic cardiovascular disease** and erectile dysfunction. In addition to the classical Leriche syndrome, there is a high prevalence of known and undiagnosed cardiovascular disease (angina, ischemia, infarction, thrombotic stroke, peripheral vascular insufficiency) among men with organic erectile dysfunction (see Chap. 10). This forms an important pathological basis of the most frequent form of organic erectile dysfunction. In addition, the interaction with nitrate therapy for cardiovascular disease creates the most serious adverse effect of sildenafil in treatment of erectile dysfunction. There is also evidence that atherosclerosis is an important determinant of the testicular degeneration in aging men.

12.3.12 Dermatological Diseases

Psoriasis is associated with impaired spermatogenesis which correlates with the extent and severity of the disease rather than with methotrexate or corticosteroid treatment (Grunnert et al. 1977).

12.4 Therapeutic Implications

Teleologically, the evolutionary significance of reversible inhibition of reproductive functions during acute or chronic illness is not clearly understood. Many common features observed in the underlying physiological mechanisms employed by mammals during puberty, seasonality, undernutrition, catabolic states and systemic illness have led to the term "ontogenic regression" to describe the common underlying mechanism (Handelsman and Dong 1992).

> Ontogenic regression refers to the orderly regression of reproductive function in a fashion that permits facile recrudescence when more favorable environment prevails. This mechanism may have evolved to defer reproductive activity until more favorable circumstances prevail for species propagation.

In this setting, the long spermatogenic cycle time requires prolonged periods to regress to infertile levels. This may have necessitated a speedier inhibition of fertility which is brought about by the inhibition of sexual function through withdrawal of androgen secretion. This latter adaptive mechanism, ideal for short periods, may, however, become deleterious during prolonged, nonfatal illness. In these circumstances prolongation of ontogenic regression may lead to tissue effects of androgen deficiency superimposed on the effects of the underlying disease. This is analogous to the damaging effects of autoimmunity which, in a corruption of necessary immune function, leads to damage to body systems.

The therapeutic implications of gonadal dysfunction during nongonadal systemic diseases vary from minimal to potentially major (Liu and Handelsman 1998). They depend on the exact manifestations of the gonadal dysfunction, its chronicity and severity. At minimum, systemic illness may alter routine tests of testicular function which may interfere with evaluation for infertility or other andrological disorders. The value of androgen supplementation to rectify the partial androgen deficiency associated with chronic medical illness is not well established. Certain specific instances of disease-related androgen deficiency such as bilateral orchidectomy or acquired hypogonadism due to iron overload warrant androgen replacement as causes of classical androgen deficiency. In many transient illnesses such as febrile infectious episodes, acute accidental or surgical trauma, the hypothalamic response to systemic illness with its attendant acute androgen deficiency has no known lasting effect on general health and well being.

> Despite the transient reductions in androgen secretion in such settings, the presently available evidence does not justify testosterone therapy. In more prolonged chronic medical illness leading to persistent and sustained lowering of androgen levels or during severe prolonged catabolic states, such as critical illness, there may be a plausible rationale for testosterone replacement therapy.

This would aim to reduce long-term morbidity from sustained androgen deficiency causing loss of bone and muscle mass. Convincing evidence from properly placebo-controlled randomized clinical trials to justify such treatment is, however, lacking. Uncontrolled and short term studies during the 1960's did suggest that androgen supplementation initially augmented anabolic status; however, this response was not sustained during prolonged treatment. Although testosterone supplementation cannot be recommended at present, well designed clinical trials to evaluate such interventions are feasible and desirable.

> Infertility is an increasingly common presenting problem among men with chronic medical illnesses.

These include men with kidney transplants who can now expect prolonged survival with good quality of life and, increasingly, among men with heart, liver or marrow transplants in whom prolonged survival is increasingly possible. Following many successful organ transplants, impaired reproductive function due to organ failure is often improved or normalized. In addition, most men now survive cancer treatment of testicular tumors, hematological malignancies or sarcomata but are effectively cured of their malignancy at the cost of sustained, severe and often irreversible testicular damage. In these men, counselling about the likelihood of spermatogenic recovery, contraceptive advice as well as appropriate application of assisted reproductive techniques such as pretreatment sperm cryostorage, insemination or male factor IVF/ICSI may be required and should be provided sympathetically. Difficult psychosocial and ethical decisions may be faced regarding the responsibilities of parenthood with limited life expectancy, risks of paternally-mediated malformations and post-mortem insemination. The advent of autologous germ cell transplantation may add further options for fertility insurance to the medical care of men facing impaired reproductive function as a predictable side-effect of life-saving medical therapies.

Sexual dysfunction including impotence is a common feature of aging and most chronic diseases which accumulate in older men. Androgen deficiency is an easily defined and rewardingly treated cause of sexual dysfunction but is relatively rare (see Chap. 15).

12.5 References

Agbaraji VO, Scott RB, Leto S, Kingslow LW (1988) Fertility studies in sickle cell disease: semen analysis in adult male patients. Int J Fertil 33:347–52

Anguiano A, Oates RD, Amos JA, Dean M, Gerrard B, Stewart C, Maher TA, White MB, Milunsky A (1992) Congenital bilateral absence of the vas deferens: a primarily genital form of cystic fibrosis. J Am Med Assoc 267:1794–1797

Bagatell CJ, Bremner WJ (1990) Sperm counts and reproductive hormones in male marathoners and lean controls. Fert Steril 53:688–692

Bronspiegel-Weintrob N, Oliver NF, Tyler B, Andrews DF, Freedman MH, Holland FJ (1990) Effect of age at the start of iron chelation therapy on gonadal function in beta-thalassemia major. N Engl J Med 323:713–719

Buvat J, Lemaire A, Ardaens K, Buvat-Herbaut M, Racadot A (1983) Profile of gonadal hormones in 8 cases of male anorexia nervosa studied before and during weight gain. Ann Endocrinol 44:229–234

Cantu JM, Scaglia HE, Medina M, Gonzalez-Diddi M, Moranto T, Moreno ME, Perez-Palacios G (1976) Inherited congenital normofunctional testicular hyperplasia and mental deficiency. Hum Genet 33:23–33

Cosentino MJ, Chey WY, Takihara H, Cockett ATK (1984) The effects of sulphsalazine on human male fertility potential and seminal prostaglandins. J Urol 132:682–686

Crawford BA, Spaliviero JA, Simpson JM, Handelsman DJ (1998) Testing the gonadal regression-cytoprotection hypothesis. Cancer Res 58:5105–5109

Crittenden JA, Handelsman DJ, Stewart G (1992) Semen analysis in human immunodeficiency virus infection. Fertil Steril 57:1294–1299

Cundy T, Butler J, Bomford A, Williams R (1993) Reversibility of hypogonadotrophic hypogonadism associated with genetic hemochromatosis. Clin Endocrinol (Oxf) 38:617–620

Cutolo M, Balleari E, Giusti M, Intra E, Accardo S (1991) Androgen replacement therapy in male patients with rheumatoid arthritis. Arthritis Rheum 34:1–5

da Cunha MF et al (1984) Recovery of spermatogenesis after treatment for Hodgkins disease: limiting dose of MOPP chemotherapy. J Clin Oncol 2:571–577

de la Balze FA, Arrillaga F, Mancini RE, Janches M, Davidson OW, Gurtman AI (1962) Male hypogonadism in hypothyroidism: a study of six cases. J Clin Endocrinol Metab 22:212–222

de Paepe ME, Waxman M (1989) Testicular atrophy in AIDS: a study of 57 autopsy cases. Hum Pathol 20:210–214

Diamond T, Stiehl D, Posen S (1991) Effects of testosterone and venesection on spinal and peripheral bone mineral in six hypogonadal men with hemochromatosis. J Bone Mineral Res 6:39–43

Dong Q, Hawker F, McWilliam D, Bangah M, Burger H, Handelsman DJ (1992) Circulating inhibin and testosterone levels in men with critical illness. Clin Endocrinol (Oxf) 36:399–404

Dunsmuir WD, Holmes SA (1996) The aetiology and management of erectile, ejaculatory, and fertility problems in men with diabetes mellitus. Diabetic Med 13:700–708

Farthing MJR, Dawson AM (1983) Impaired semen quality in Crohn's disease – drugs, ill health, or undernutrition? Scand J Gastroenterol 18:57–60

Fenwick PB, Toone BK, Wheeler MJ, Nanjee MN, Grant R, Brown D (1985) Sexual behaviour in a centre for epilepsy. Acta Neurol Scand 71:428–435

Ford HC, Cooke RR, Keightley EA, Feek CM (1992) Serum levels of free and unbound testosterone in hyperthyroidism. Clin Endocrinol (Oxf) 36:187–192

Francis RB, Kasper CK (1983) Reproduction in hemophilia. J Am Med Assoc 250:3192–3195

Gluud C, Bennett P, Dietrichson O, Johnsen SG, Ranek L, Svendsen LB, Juhl E (1981) Short-term parenteral and peroral testosterone administration in men with alcoholic cirrhosis. Scand J Gastroenterol 16:749–755

Gordon D, Beastall GH, Thomson JA, Sturrock RD (1986) Androgenic status and sexual function in males with rheumatoid arthritis and ankylosing spondylitis. Q J Med 231:671–679

Gray A, Feldman HA, McKinlay JB, Longcope C (1991) Age, disease, and changing sex hormone levels in middle-aged men: results of the Massachussetts Male Aging Study. J Clin Endocrinol Metab 73:1016–1025

Griggs RC, Pandya S, Florence JM, Brooke MH, Kingston W, Miller JP, Chutkow J, Herr BE, Moxley RT (1989) Randomized controlled trial of testosterone in myotonic dystrophy. Neurology 39:219–222

Grunnert E, Nyfors A, Hansen KB (1977) Studies on human semen in topical corticosteroid-treated and in methotrexate-treated psoriatics. Dermatologica 154:78–84

Grunstein RR, Handelsman DJ, Lawrence SJ, Blackwell C, Caterson ID, Sullivan CE (1989) Hypothalamic dysfunction in sleep apnea: reversal by nasal continuous positive airways pressure. J Clin Endocrinol Metab 68:352–358

Handelsman DJ (1985) Hypothalamic-pituitary gonadal dysfunction in chronic renal failure, dialysis, and renal transplantation. Endocr Rev 6:151–182

Handelsman DJ, Dong Q (1992) Ontogenic regression: a model of stress and reproduction. In: Sheppard K, Boublik JH, Funder JW (eds) Stress and reproduction. Raven, New York, pp 333–345

Handelsman DJ, Dong Q (1993) Hypothalamo-pituitary gonadal axis in chronic renal failure. Endocrin Metab Clin 22:145–161

Handelsman DJ, Yue DK, Turtle JR (1983) Hypogonadism and massive testicular infiltration with amyloidosis. J Urol 129:610–612

Handelsman DJ, Conway AJ, Boylan LM, Turtle JR (1984) Youngs syndrome: obstructive azoospermia and chronic sinopulmonary infection. N Engl J Med 310:3–9

Handelsman DJ, Staraj S (1985) Testicular size: the effects of aging, malnutrition and illness. J Androl 6:144–151

Handelsman DJ, Strasser S, McDonald JA, Conway AJ, McCaughan GW (1995) Hypothalamic-pituitary testicular function in end-stage non-alcoholic liver disease before and after liver transplantation. Clin Endocrinol (Oxf) 43:331–337

Hughes GS, Mathur RS, Margolius HS (1989) Sex steroid hormones are altered in essential hypertension. J Hypertens 7:181–187

Iranmanesh A, Lizzaralde G, Veldhuis JD (1991) Age and relative adiposity are specific negative determinants of the frequency and amplitude of growth hormone (GH) secretory bursts and the half-life of endogenous GH in healthy men. J Clin Endocrinol Metab 73:1081–1088

Isojarvi JI, Pakarinen AJ, Myllyla VV (1989) Effects of carbamazepine on the hypothalamic-pituitary gonadal axis in male patients with epilepsy: a prospective study. Epilepsia 30:446–452

Jaffe A, Chen Y, Kisch ES, Fischel B, Alon M, Stern N (1996) Erectile dysfunction in hypertensive subjects. Assessment of potential determinants. Hypertension 28:859–862

Jannini EA, Ulisse S, D'Armiento M (1995) Thyroid hormone and male gonadal function. Endocr Rev 16:443–59

Jin B, McCaughan G, Handelsman D (1999) Effects of liver disease and transplantation on the human prostate. J Androl 20:559–565

Kandeel FR, Swerdloff RS (1988) Role of temperature in regulation of spermatogenesis and the use of heating as a method for contraception. Fertil Steril 49:1–23

Khaw KT, Barrett-Connor E (1988) Blood pressure and endogenous testosterone in men: an inverse relationship. J Hypertens 6:329–332

Kley HK, Strohmeyer G, Kruskemper HL (1979) Effect of testosterone application on hormone concentrations of androgens and estrogens in male patients with cirrhosis of the liver. Gastroenterology 76:235–241

Kley HK, Stremmel W, Kley JB, Schlaghecke R (1992) Testosterone treatment of men with idiopathic hemochromatosis. Clin Invest 70:566–572

Knigge U, Dejgaard A, Wollesen F, Ingerslev O, Bennett P, Christiansen PM (1983) The acute and long term effect of the H2-receptor antagonists cimetidine and ranitidine on the pituitary-gonadal axis in men. Clin Endocrinol (Oxf) 18:307–318

Kreuser ED, Klingmuller D, Thiel E (1993) The role of LHRH-analogues in protecting gonadal functions during chemotherapy and irradiation. Eur Urol 23:157–164

Kumar BJ, Kurana ML, Ammini AC, Karmarkar MG, Ahuja MM (1990) Reproductive endocrine functions in men with primary hypothyroidism: effect of thyroxine replacement. Horm Res 34:215–218

La Spada AR, Wilson EM, Lubahn DB, Harding AE, Fischbeck KH (1991) Androgen receptor gene mutation in X-linked spinal and bulbar muscular atrophy. Nature 352:77–79

La Spada AR, Rollin DB, Harding AE, Warner CL, Spiegel R, Hausmanowa-Petrusewicz I, Fischbeck KH (1992) Meiotic instability and genotype-phenotype correlation of the trinucleotide repeat in X-linked spinal and bulbar muscular atrophy. Nature Genet 2:301–304

Lange D, Henning H, Schirren C (1978) Andrologische Untersuchungen bei der Immun-suppressive-therapie der chronisch-aggressiven Hepatitis. Andrologia 10:373–379

Linnet L, Hjort T, Fogh-Andersen P (1981) Association between failure to impregnate after vasovasostomy and sperm agglutinins in semen. Lancet i:117–119

Liu PY, Handelsman DJ (1998) Androgen therapy in non-gonadal disease. In: Nieschlag E, Behre HM (eds) Testosterone: action, deficiency and substitution. Springer, Berlin Heidelberg New York, pp 473–512

Luton JP, Thieblot P, Valcke JC, Mahoudeau JA, Bricaire H (1977) Reversible gonadotropin deficiency in male Cushings disease. J Clin Endocrinol Metab 45:488–495

Mastrogiacomo I, Bonanni G, Menegazzo E, Santarossa C, Pagani E, Gennarelli M, Angelini C (1996) Clinical and hormonal aspects of male hypogonadism in myotonic dystrophy. Ital J Neurol Sci 17:59–65

Matsumoto A, Sandblom RE, Schoene RB, Lee KA, Giblin EC, Pierson DJ, Bremner WJ (1985) Testosterone replacement in hypogonadal men: effects on obstructive sleep apnea, respiratory drive and sleep. Clin Endocrinol (Oxf) 22:713–721

Meistrich ML, van Beek MEAB (1990) Radiation sensitivity of the human testis. Adv Radiat Biol 14:227–268

Meschede D, Behre HM, Nieschlag E (1995) Endocrine and spermatological characteristics of 135 patients with bilateral megalotestis. Andrologia 27:207–12

Neugebauer D, Neuwinger J, Jockenhovel F, Nieschlag E (1990) '9+0' axoneme in spermatozoa and some nasal cilia of a patient with totally immotile spermatozoa associated with thickened sheath and short midpiece. Hum Reprod 5:981–986

Nicholls RD (1993) Genomic imprinting and uniparental disomy in Angelman and Prader-Willi syndromes: a review. Am J Med Genet 46:16–25

Obermayer-Straub P, Manns MP (1998) Autoimmune polyglandular syndromes. Baillieres Clin Gastroenterol 12:293–315

O'Brien IAD, Lewin IG, O'Hare JP, Corrall RJM (1982) Reversible male subfertility due to hyperthyroidism. BMJ 285:691

Patrizio P, Asch RH, Handelin B, Silber SJ (1993) Aetiology of congenital absence of the vas deferens: genetic study of three generations. Hum Reprod 8:215–220

Petitti DB (1986) Epidemiologic studies of vasectomy. In: Zatuchni GI, Goldsmith A, Spieler JM, Sciarra JJ (eds) Male contraception: advances and future prospects. Harper and Row, Philadelphia, pp 24–33

Petzke F, Heppner C, Mbulamberi D, Winkelmann W, Chrousos GP, Allolio B, Reincke M (1996) Hypogonadism in Rhodesian sleeping sickness: evidence for acute and chronic dysfunction of the hypothalamic-pituitary-gonadal axis. Fertil Steril 65:68–75

Post FA, Soule SG, Willcox PA, Levitt NS (1994) The spectrum of endocrine dysfunction in active pulmonary tuberculosis. Clin Endocrinol (Oxf) 40:367–370

Puliyel MM, Vyas GP, Mehta GS (1977) Testosterone in the management of cirrhosis of the liver – a controlled study. Aust NZ J Med 7:17–30

Raffi F, Brisseau JM, Planchon B, Remi JP, Barrier JH, Grolleau JY (1991) Endocrine function in 98 HIV-infected patients: a prospective study. AIDS 5:729–733

Rimoin DL, Schimke RN (1971) The gonads. In: Rimoin DL, Schimke RN (eds) Genetic disorders of the endocrine glands. Mosby, St. Louis

Rowley MJ, Leach DR, Warner GA, Heller CG (1974) Effect of graded doses of ionizing radiation on the human testis. Radiat Res 59:665–678

Samojlik E, Kirschner MA, Ribot S, Szmal E (1992) Changes in the hypothalamic-pituitary-gonadal axis in men after cadaver kidney transplantation and cyclosporine therapy. J Androl 13:332–336

Sandblom RE, Matsumoto AM, Scoene RB, Lee KA, Giblin EC, Bremner WJ, Pierson DJ (1983) Obstructive sleep apnea induced by testosterone administration. N Engl J Med 308:508–510

Schlatt S (1999) Prospects and problems for germ cell transplantation in the male. Int J Androl 22:13–18

Schneider BK, Pickett CK, Zwillich CW, Weil JV, McDermott MT, Santen RJ, Varano LA, White DP (1986) Influence of testosterone on breathing during sleep. J Appl Physiol 61:618–623

Schramm P, Seyfeddinpur N (1980) Spermiogrammuntersuchungen bei Patienten unter Langzeithydantoinbehandlung. Andrologia 12:97–101

Semple CG, Robertson WR, Mitchell R, Gordon D, Gray CE, Beastall GH, Reid WH (1987) Mechanisms leading to hypogonadism in men with burn injuries. BMJ 295:403–407

Spector TD, Perry LA, Tubb G, Silman AJ, Huskisson EC (1988) Low free testosterone levels in rheumatoid arthritis. Ann Rheum Dis 47:65–68

Stahl NI, Decker JL (1978) Androgenic status of males with systemic lupus erythematosus. Arthritis Rheum 21:665–668

Stillman RJ, Rosenberg MJ, Sachs BP (1986) Smoking and reproduction. Fertil Steril 46:545–566

Suzuki H, Tominaga T, Kumagai H, Saruta T (1988) Effects of first-line antihypertensive agents on sexual function and sex hormones. J Hypertens 6:S649–651

Vazquez JA, Pinies JA, Martul P, de los Rios A, Gatzambide S, Busturia MA (1990) Hypothalamo-pituitary-testicular function in 70 patients with myotonic dystrophy. J Endocrinol Invest 13:375–379

Villalta J, Ballesta JL, Nicholas JM, Martinez de Osaba MJ, Antunez E, Pimentel C (1997) Testicular function in asymptomatic chronic alcoholics: relation to ethanol intake. Alcohol Clin Exp Res 21:128–133

Villette JM et al (1990) Circadian variations in plasma levels of hypophyseal, adrenocortical and testicular hormones in men infected with human immunodeficiency virus. J Clin Endocrinol Metab 70:572–577

Viviani S, Santoro A, Ragni G, Bonfante V, Bestetti O, Bonadonna G (1985) Gonadal toxicity after combination chemotherapy for Hodgkin's disease. Comparative results of MOPP vs ABVD. Eur J Cancer Clin Oncol 21:601–605

Wang C, Tso SC, Todd D (1989) Hypogonadotropic hypogonadism in severe beta-thalassemia: effect of chelation and pulsatile gonadotropin-releasing hormone therapy. J Clin Endocrinol Metab 68:511–516

Warner CL, Griffin JE, Wilson JD, Jacobs LD, Murray KR, Fischbeck KH, Dickoff D, Griggs RC (1992) X-linked spinomuscular atrophy: a kindred with associated abnormal androgen receptor binding. Neurology 42:2181–2184

Whitehead E, Shalet SM, Blackledge G, Todd I, Crowther D, Beardwell CG (1982) The effects of Hodgkin's disease and combination chemotherapy on gonadal function in the adult male. Cancer 49:418–422

Woolf PD, Hamill RW, McDonald JV, Lee LA, Kelly M (1985) Transient hypogonadotropic hypogonadism caused by critical illness. J Clin Endocrinol Metab 60:444–450

Zelissen PM, van Hattum J, Poen H, Scholten P, Gerritse R, te Velde ER (1988) Influence of salazosulphapyridine and 5-aminosalicylic acid on seminal qualities and male sex hormones. Scand J Gastroenterol 23:1100–1104

CHAPTER 13

Environmental Influences on Male Reproductive Health **13**

M. H. BRINKWORTH · D. J. HANDELSMAN

Humans are exposed to a vast array of chemicals through a wide range of portals. Innumerable environmental, toxic hazards arising from nature have always existed but the additional exposures to man-made chemicals has increased progressively since the Industrial Revolution. Regulatory agencies, themselves the product of public demand for drug regulation following thalidomide and other catastrophes, have developed licensing guidelines for new chemicals in order to protect human populations from damaging environmental exposures, yet permitting the production and use of important new chemicals. Over the last three decades the scope and sophistication of testing requirements has increased greatly as the quantity and diversity of chemical entities to which humans may be exposed continues to increase. The earliest safety screening mainly concerned **acute toxicity**, **carcinogenesis** and **teratogenesis**, however, currently **reproductive and genetic toxicity** are being evaluated to an increasing extent. Although historically, reproductive effects have been most studied in females, it is now recognized that adverse effects on **male reproductive function** are also important.

The need to regulate human exposure to chemicals is widely accepted and regulations intended to govern acceptable exposure apply, in descending order of stringency, to medical drugs, foods and food supplements, cosmetics, veterinary drugs, agricultural products (including herbicides and pesticides), domestic and industrial chemicals. Ironically, equally hazardous medical procedures like surgery are not similarly regulated for safety and efficacy, unlike the drugs they require. Complex regulatory standards exist for all these categories of chemicals with the stringency of the testing and safety margin required varying pragmatically according to likely human exposure and risk. Unfortunately, scientific methodologies to evaluate human health risks, including those to reproduction, remain in their infancy while the task grows in scope and complexity. In principle, **human toxicology** is based on an amalgam of

- limited **observational human data**, usually retrospective epidemiological studies, and
- more abundant **experimental studies in animals and cells.**

The former lacks the rigorous control of randomized or controlled prospective studies, while the latter has uncertain applicability to humans. Neither approach is entirely satisfactory or even complementary, as species-specific variability can lead to contradictory findings. Nevertheless, these are the only tools currently available to bridge rationally the gulf between, on the one hand, the essential task of providing some assurances of safety for current and future exposures to chemicals, while on the other, allowing for the timely introduction of new agents into medicine, industry and, inevitably, into the shared environment.

> The contrast between observational data in humans and data from experimental studies exemplifies **an important distinction in toxicology,** that **between hazard and risk.**

Experiments aimed purely at determining whether an agent has **the potential to damage a biological system** are concerned with **hazard.** The concept of **risk combines hazard and biological context.** It incorporates not only the level of exposure but levels reaching the target tissue, the effects of toxifying/detoxifying metabolic systems, repair processes and any other factors modulating the final response. The ultimate objective of toxicological investigations is thus not just to identify particular compounds as hazardous but to provide the best possible assessment of the risks they pose to humans.

13.1 Potential Adverse Effects on Spermatogenesis

Spermatogenesis involves the continuous replication and complex metamorphosis of relatively undifferentiated, diploid, stem cells into highly specialized, motile, haploid cells (see Chap. 3). These haploid gametes must, furthermore, be capable of traveling through the female reproductive tract and fertilizing an ovum (see Chap. 4). This highly complex process occurring in the reproductive tract is closely governed by hypothalamic-pituitary and testicular hormones, thereby making it also susceptible to influences on endocrine organs, notably the brain. It is, therefore, not surprising that environmental agents can adversely affect germ cell development at many different stages and by different means. Indeed, this may explain why huge numbers of sperm are produced (around 2×10^8 per day [see Chap. 3] and 2×10^{12} in a lifetime), while only one is required for fertilizing an ovum, an event usually occurring less than ten times per lifetime.

Chemicals can theoretically damage spermatogenesis potentially at any stage from proliferating sper-

matogonia to mature spermatozoa. Broadly three different and not mutually exclusive toxic effects are possible: **cell death, sub-lethal cell damage** or **genetic change.**

Lethally damaged cells either die within the epithelium or are shed into the lumen of the seminiferous tubule. Those dying *in situ* may do so by

- **necrosis,** an uncontrolled lysis and non-specific spilling of cellular contents, or by
- **apoptosis,** a physiological process of programmed cell death whereby a doomed cell breaks down into smaller, apoptotic bodies that are then phagocytosed by Sertoli cells (Kerr et al. 1972).

Apoptosis is the orderly mechanism by which spermatogenic cells die within the germinal epithelium without collateral damage to adjacent Sertoli or germ cells. Recent evidence suggests that apoptosis is a major mechanism of action of testicular toxins such as methoxyacetic acid (MAA) (Brinkworth et al. 1995) or adverse physiological conditions such as gonadotropin deprivation (Tapanainen et al. 1993; Billig et al. 1995; Brinkworth et al. 1995). There is evidence that **the Fas – Fas-ligand system** may be involved in mediating some toxin-induced apoptosis in the rodent (Lee et al. 1997). According to this model, constitutive expression of Fas ligand in Sertoli cells leads to apoptosis in germ cells that are stimulated to express Fas as a result of an apoptotic signal. However, it is not yet clear whether human Sertoli cells express Fas ligand so the significance of the model is currently uncertain. Other genes that appear to have a role in male germ-cell apoptosis are **p53** (Yin et al. 1998), **Bcl-2** (Furuchi et al. 1996; Rodriguez et al. 1997), **Bcl-w** (Print et al. 1998) and **Bax** (Knudson et al. 1995).

An alternative influence of apoptosis on germ-cell toxicity is suggested by the recent finding that cyclophosphamide administration to male rats that leads to the induction of fetal abnormalities among a proportion of their offspring (Trasler et al. 1985) also reduces the level of apoptosis among their germ cells (Brinkworth and Nieschlag 2000). Thus, not only may apoptosis be a response to male reproductive toxicity but disturbances of apoptosis could also influence the vertical transmission of mutation.

Non-lethal germ cell damage will either be **repaired** or leave permanent effects on the structure or function of the mature spermatozoa, including the possibility of **transgenerational genetic effects.** It has been suggested that **chronic, low-dose exposures** can be more effective at inducing **paternally-mediated effects in the offspring** (Anderson et al. 1996) than the high, acute exposures. Effects observed are most commonly gross morphological abnormalities in the fetuses (Trasler et al. 1985) but there is evidence that certain, specific, dosing regimens can induce cancer in the offspring (Lord et al. 1998). It has been suggested that these could be the result either of a suppression of apoptosis or the induction of genomic instability (Brinkworth 2000). Clinical implications are far from clear due to the lack of evidence for similar effects in human populations.

Almost nothing is known about the **repair of non-genetic damage** in germ cells and although DNA repair occurs, little is known about the specific mechanisms involved. DNA repair capacity is believed to diminish during spermatid elongation and to be virtually non-existent in spermatozoa. This can make them more susceptible to the effects of hazards such as radiation and alkylating drugs, although some protection may be afforded by the progressive chromatin condensation that accompanies spermatid elongation.

13.2 Targets for Toxicity

Testicular function, including androgen secretion and the production of fertile spermatozoa, can be adversely affected by pre-testicular, testicular and post-testicular mechanisms.

The following mechanisms may apply not necessarily to the whole population but also to vulnerable subgroups who may have genetic polymorphisms that enhance or reduce individual or group susceptibility to toxicological processes as they have been observed in pharmacogenetics. Such systematic variation in susceptibility may result in apparent enhancement of effects in small, but vulnerable, subpopulations. Further toxicological studies of genetic polymorphisms in susceptibility to environmental agents are needed.

13.2.1 Pre-testicular Targets for Toxicity

Testicular function is regulated by the pituitary hormones FSH and LH (see Chap. 3) and toxicity that disturbs this level of control is considered to be pre-testicular. This includes **occupational exposure to sex steroids** such as estrogens, which, if absorbed sufficiently, can inhibit pituitary gonadotropin secretion resulting in sexual dysfunction, gynecomastia and hypogonadotrophic hypogonadism. Examples reported include sentinel populations such as men working in the industrial manufacture of synthetic contraceptive estrogens (Harrington et al. 1978) or handling large quantities of a non-steroidal estrogenic chemical (Finkelstein et al. 1988). More recently it has been claimed that community-wide prenatal exposure to estrogen-mimicking compounds could potentially act through such a mechanism, by inhibition of fetal gonadotropin secretion and a conse-

quent **reduction in Sertoli cell proliferation** (Sharpe and Skakkebaek 1993; Toppari et al. 1996). The opposite effect can be produced experimentally by neonatal exposure of rats to **polychlorinated biphenyls** that have the ability to reduce serum thyroxine levels. This leads to hypothyroidism and a consequent increase in **Sertoli cell numbers, testis weight** and **daily sperm production** (Cooke et al. 1996).

13.2.2 Testicular Targets for Toxicity

Direct testicular toxicity may affect any of the various cell types within the testis including Leydig, Sertoli and germ cells. In practice, the primary effects of toxic chemicals appear to act relatively specifically on individual cell types, although the complex interdependence of spermatogenesis and steroidogenesis dictates that, following the initial impact, more universal, pan-testicular effects are often observed.

Selective Leydig cell damage is well known experimentally in animals given the drug ethane dimethane sulphonate (EDS). This is an alkylating agent that selectively destroys Leydig cells by an unexplained mechanism, leading subsequently to degeneration of the most androgen-dependent germ cells, pachytene spermatocytes in rat stages VII–VIII (Bartlett et al. 1986). However, no human counterpart of this model exhibiting selective Leydig cell toxicity is known and non-human primates are insensitive to EDS.

Leydig cell adenoma is a relatively rare clinical condition that, along with Leydig cell hyperplasia, nonetheless occurs quite commonly in chronic toxicity studies undertaken in rodents for safety evaluation purposes. The discrepancy between the frequency of occurrence in test species and humans suggests that such a finding does not necessarily have relevance for humans (Clegg et al. 1997). However, if the mode of action of, and potential exposure to a toxin is considered relevant, this should be taken into account in the risk assessment procedure (Clegg et al. 1997).

Sertoli cells fulfill an enormous array of functions, playing a cardinal role in regulating and supporting spermatogenesis as well as forming the scaffolding of the seminiferous tubule and creating its unique internal milieu. Consequently, **direct toxicity to Sertoli cells** should have marked effects on sperm production and function (Boekelheide 1993). Identification of selective Sertoli cell toxicity in experimental animals is difficult and relies on observation of early vacuolation and loss of seminiferous tubular fluid production followed by loss of germ cells and reflex increases in gonadotropin secretion (Boekelheide 1993). Three classes of industrial chemical have been implicated as Sertoli cell-specific toxicants:

- **phthalates**, used as plasticizers,
- **nitroaromatic compounds**, intermediates in production of dyes and explosives; and
- **γ-diketones**, used as solvents,

Dibromoacetic acid has recently been found to be a further example of a Sertoli cell toxin (Linden et al. 1997). The molecular mechanisms of Sertoli cell toxicity from all these agents, however, remain unclear. The germ-cell loss that is always consequent upon Sertoli cell damage may be mediated by an up-regulation of FasL expression (see 13.2) in order to facilitate the elimination of germ cells that can no longer be supported (Lee et al. 1999). While experimental models of chemicals with relatively selective toxicity on Sertoli cells have been established, at present no specific, human Sertoli cell toxins are well described.

Germ cells are mostly located within the diffusion-tight blood-testis barrier, thereby achieving some protection from extrinsic chemicals. The best established evidence for **direct toxicity to human germ cells** is the exquisite sensitivity of spermatogonia to ionizing irradiation and alkylating agents. The most sensitive cells are the spermatogonia, which are the only germ cell type to develop at the base of the Sertoli cells, outside the blood-testis barrier.

Spermatogonial sub-types differ in sensitivity to cytotoxins, leading to important implications for recovery from toxicity. For example the A_0, or **non-proliferating, spermatogonia** constitute the germinal stem-cell population, **destruction** of which **leads to irreversible spermatogenic damage**. Examples of stem-cell toxins include adriamycin in the mouse (but not humans) and **MOPP** combination chemotherapy (**nitrogen mustard, vincristine, procarbazine, prednisone**) in men treated for Hodgkin disease, both of which exhibit essentially irreversible spermatogenic damage presumably due to A_0 spermatogonia ablation. In contrast, proliferating spermatogonia, though even more sensitive to such cytotoxic effects, can be replaced from stem cell reserves that are activated by the depletion of these dividing cell populations. Thus, spermatogenic damage from selective toxicity to proliferating spermatogonia (eg as with lower doses of ionizing radiation and many cytotoxic drugs) can lead to complete, but temporary, loss of spermatogenesis, although its reversal through stem-cell replenishment may take years. Furthermore, non-lethal germ cell damage may induce genetic mutations in stem cell DNA, which can lead to persistent genetic changes in sperm formed subsequently. Although such chromosome defects have been detected up to 20 years after cancer therapy in humans (Brandriff et al. 1994), present evidence indicates no excess of congenital malformations or carcinogenesis among progeny of male cancer treatment survivors (Byrne et al. 1998).

Spermatocytes and spermatogonia are the germ cell types involved in meiosis, a unique genetic process involving one round of DNA replication (spermatogonia) and two of cellular division (spermatocytes), making these cells vulnerable to certain toxins as well as to genetic mutations. 2-methoxyethanol (ME), a constituent of varnishes and paints, is the best characterized spermatocyte toxin (Creasy et al. 1985; Anderson et al. 1987), an effect manifested through its metabolite, methoxyacetic acid (MAA). At high doses, MAA causes almost complete and selective elimination of pachytene spermatocytes in rats by an apoptotic rather than necrotic process (Brinkworth et al. 1995). It has been reported that rabbits are 10-fold more sensitive than rodents (Berndtson and Foote 1997) but it is not known which is the more relevant model for the human in this respect. Occupational exposure to ME has, however, been suggested to have adverse effects on spermatogenesis in humans (Welch et al. 1988).

Diploid germ cells may be more vulnerable than their haploid equivalents to spontaneous cell death (Kerr 1992) and possibly also to apoptosis induced by testicular toxicants. In addition to outright death, round spermatids can also be lost by germinal exfoliation, a process whereby large numbers are released prematurely, although their subsequent fate is unclear. Sertoli cell toxicity can also sometimes have the same effect as the stricken Sertoli cell becomes unable to maintain its attachment to the spermatids.

Meiotic recombination involves a variety of different processes, which may result in the duplication, deletion or rearrangement of stretches of DNA along a chromosome and the exchange of genetic material between chromosomes. Whilst this is a normal process that contributes to genetic diversity among gametes, it is potentially a target for genotoxins. **Minisatellites** are stretches of DNA containing tandemly repeated sequence motifs, distributed apparently randomly throughout the genome in humans. They are believed to be particularly prone to **rearrangement** during meiosis (Dubrova et al. 1998) and have spontaneous mutation rates up to 1,000-fold greater than protein-coding sequences. Therefore, they may be suitable sentinel sequences for the determination of exposure to germ-cell mutagens and of alterations in mutation rates. The children of men exposed to radiation at Chernobyl have been found to have elevated levels of minisatellite mutations in their sperm (Dubrova et al. 1996) and similar findings exist for rodents (Fan et al. 1995). Intriguingly, however, data from the sperm of two men before and after chemotherapy show no sign of a treatment-induced increase in the germ-line minisatellite mutation rate (Armour et al. 1999), a finding that is being investigated for radiation therapy. These data accord with the lack of effect on offspring following cancer treatment referred to above and may highlight a difference between environmental and therapeutic exposures or more effective human DNA repair mechanisms.

13.2.3 Post-testicular Targets for Toxicity

In contrast to testicular toxicity, post-testicular toxic effects on sperm after leaving the rete testis appear relatively uncommon. In experimental animals for example, mature spermatozoa are more resistant to DNA strand-breaking by high-dose ionizing radiation (Rousseaux et al. 1993) than are testicular germ cells. Nonetheless, the radiomimetic drug cyclophosphamide can induce mutagenic lesions in maturing sperm that result in **pre-implantation losses** following fertilization (Hales and Robaire 1993). Most post-testicular toxicity has been discovered during the search for novel non-hormonal chemical contraceptives for men (Cooper and Yeung 1999). The neuromusculature of the epididymis can be affected by adrenolytic drugs such as guanethidine or methoxamine that lead to **stasis of sperm in the epididymis,** which may even swell and rupture as a result. Conversely, **sperm transport** through the epididymis may also be **accelerated,** resulting in ejaculates containing fewer or immature sperm. Toxins acting on the epididymal epithelium, such as gossypol, interfere with **epididymal fluid secretion.** Another target for post-testicular toxicity are sperm undergoing epididymal transport. Compounds such as α-chlorhydrin and the 6-chloro-6-deoxysugars (Tsang et al. 1981) or ornidazole have highly specific effects on rat epididymal sperm, resulting in

complete **loss of motility** and hence sterility (Oberländer et al 1994). These mechanisms may be illustrated by the clinical syndrome of epididymal necrospermia described in infertile men (Wilton et al. 1988) in which normally developed sperm appear to undergo lethal damage during epididymal transit although the toxicological basis remains unknown.

13.3 Specific Instances of Environmental or Occupational Toxicity of Possible Relevance to Humans (Table 13.1)

13.3.1 Radiation

Ionizing radiation is the best studied and among the first agents to be known to have anti-spermatogenic effects in humans. Detailed studies, including serial sperm counts and testicular biopsies following single measured doses of ionizing radiation administered to the testes of US prisoner volunteers, were conducted during the 1950's and 60's and demonstrated clear dose-dependent and reversible damage to spermatogenesis (Rowley et al. 1974). These findings (Table 13.2) were most consistent with the interpretation that direct damage to **proliferating spermatogonia** was the **most sensitive** element, leading to depression in sperm output from as little as 20 cGy and azoospermia above 75 cGy doses. Higher doses caused delay in recovery of sperm output, which was proportional to dose and beyond 400 cGy the spermatogenic damage persisted for up to 5 years and may

Table 13.1. Examples of occupational exposures and their potential adverse effects on male reproductive function. Data from sources as cited in the text and Giwercman and Bonde (1998)

Exposure	Effects on
Heat	Sperm morphology, motility, fertility
Radiation X-rays	Sperm count, minisatellite mutations. Fertility?
Heavy metals Lead	Sperm morphology, count, motility, semen volume. Fertility?

Synthetic estrogens
  Diethylstilboestrol
  Oral contraceptives
	Hormone levels, genital malformations
	Gynecomastia, libido, impotence

Glycol ethers
  2-methoxyethanol
  2-ethoxyethanol
	Sperm morphology, count
	Sperm morphology, count

Pesticides
  Dibromochloropropane
  Ethylenedibromide
	Sperm count, motility, fertility
	Sperm morphology, count, motility

Solvents Carbon disulfide	Sperm morphology, count, impotence

Table 13.2. Summary of the effects of ionizing radiation on the human testis by dose. Data from Rowley et al (1974) and Jockenhövel (1993)

Dose (cGy)	Effect	Reversibility
< 10	Little effect	–
10–50	Moderate oligozoospermia	6 months
50–75	Severe oligozoospermia	6 months
75–100	Azoospermia	6 months
200–300	Azoospermia	1–2.5 years
> 300	Azoospermia	~ 5 years or none

Table 13.3. Incidence of genetic disease in the offspring of parents surviving cancer and in sibling controls. Data from Byrne 1999

	Birth defects in the offspring of:	
	Survivors	Sibling controls
Offspring with birth defects	74	142
Total number of offspring	2,198	4,544
Percentage	3.4%	3.1%

have been irreversible, consistent with stem cell killing. Subsequently, studies of men exposed to accidental, atomic bomb-related, occupational or therapeutic irradiation confirmed these findings (Neel 1998). In contrast to somatic cells, dose fractionation enhances germinal cell killing (Meistrich and van Beek 1990).

Among germ cells that survive irradiation, chromosomal damage can be observed. This can lead to cell death, repair or to transmission of cytogenetic alterations. Effects on the quality of the sperm may also occur. Workers involved in the clean-up operation following the accident at Chernobyl were reported to show reduced sperm motility and ultrastructural defects (Bartoov et al. 1997). More controversially, environmental irradiation has also been suggested as contributing, via paternal radiation exposure, to childhood leukemia clusters around nuclear plants such as at Sellafield (UK) (Gardner et al. 1990). These claims have been criticized (Doll et al. 1994) as lacking a specific mechanism, being inconsistent with the lack of similar effects from atom bomb survivors (Kodama et al. 1996) as well as not being replicated at other nuclear plants (Kinlen et al. 1993). The most recent data, from 35,949 children with cancer in Great Britain over 38 years, indicate no causal link with paternal radiation exposure (Draper et al. 1997). The original observation thus remains unexplained though it may have been a chance event or due to infection caused by the mixing of viral infected and nonin-

fected populations, as has been proposed as the explanation for higher rates of leukemia among infants in rural British 'new towns' (Kinlen et al. 1990). Nonetheless, concerns about the hazards of chronic exposure to low doses of radiation persist and a recent study has reported a significant association between stillbirths and total radiation dose before conception among male workers at Sellafield (Parker et al. 1999).

13.3.2 Cancer Therapies

Exposures to X-radiation and cytotoxic mutagens are central to the treatment of malignancy. Collateral to their cell-killing therapeutic effects, surviving cells may theoretically accumulate genetic damage, especially in germinal stem cells, which could lead to **transmission of mutations and/or malformations**. As a form of fertility insurance in the event that fertility is not recovered in a timely fashion, patients undergoing potentially sterilizing treatments should now be routinely offered **sperm cryopreservation** before commencing therapy (see Chap. 18). It remains controversial whether semen samples obtained after the start of treatment should also be cryostored and what delay in fathering a child after treatment (if any) should be advised on genotoxicity grounds (Carson et al. 1991; Carson 1993; Meistrich 1993). At the heart of this dilemma is the **relevance of an-**

imal data to humans, a problem common in human toxicology. Whereas experimental studies in laboratory rodents suggest that irradiation and chemotherapeutic agents consistently increase the risk of genetic alterations in post-spermatogonial germ cells, no such risks have been observed among children born to men surviving oncological treatment (Byrne et al. 1998; Sankila et al. 1998) (Table 13.3). Whether this represents a lack of power to detect heritable effects in the epidemiology studies (Byrne 1999), **species-variability**, an undetected increase in early human **abortions** of abnormal fetuses, or a **difference in susceptibility** between **stem cells and proliferating spermatogonia**, remains to be clarified.

13.3.3 Dibromochloropropane

The nematocide dibromochloropropane (DBCP) was widely used for pest control in banana and other plantations during the 1970's until production workers and crop sprayers in the USA and Israel were discovered to be infertile (Whorton et al. 1977). DBCP caused testicular damage manifested by oligozoospermia and azoospermia with increased blood FSH and LH levels, the degree of damage being proportional to duration of exposure (Whorton et al. 1977). Subsequent follow-up demonstrated recovery only in some of the heavily exposed men with the remainder believed to have **irreversible damage** (Eaton et al. 1986). Although this was not the first agent identified to cause human male infertility, the effects of DBCP were so dramatic and clearly related to the industrial exposure that the incident became the classic example of occupational male reproductive toxicity.

Partly as a result of the considerable concern aroused by the widespread use of pesticides, many efforts have been made to reduce the risks of exposure to hazardous components. This includes not only stringent safety testing but also refinements in spraying techniques that have reduced exposures. A recent study of Danish workers using pesticides found that they had no influence on sperm counts (Larsen et al. 1998), indicating that, at least for those chemicals studied, their use is unlikely to have an impact on human reproductive health.

13.3.4 Metals

Numerous published reports have linked exposure to heavy metals such as lead, cadmium and mercury with male infertility; however, this data is mostly unconvincing due to technical inadequacies of the studies, especially the lack of standardized protocols, small sample sizes and inadequate control groups. The best available evidence concerns occupational exposure to **lead**, which at **high body burdens** is associated with **testicular dys-**

function (Lancranjan et al. 1975). A Chinese study of occupational lead exposure found a positive association between blood levels of > 400 µg/l lead and adverse effects on total sperm count, semen volume etc (Xuezhi et al. 1992) and similar results were found in a study of workers at a lead smelter (Alexander et al. 1996). However, the lower lead levels achieved through industrial hygiene measures as well as community measures such as elimination of lead-based paints, pipes and petrol, means that exposures to ambient levels under normal community conditions no longer appear to be sufficient to cause adverse effects on human male reproduction, as is borne out by a lack of effect on time to pregnancy (Joffe et al. 1999). Less convincing is evidence linking elevated seminal plasma cadmium levels (Chia et al. 1992) or mercury intoxication among battery workers, with defects in spermatogenesis. A detailed study of two individuals with high levels of intra-testicular cadmium found no clear correlation between the heavy metal residues in seminal plasma and fertility (Keck et al. 1995).

Welding is an occupation that has been investigated in a number of studies for adverse effects on male reproduction. It is, however, an occupation with a variety of potential risk factors, including exposure to fumes containing the metals used in the welding, to the heat generated and to electromagnetic fields. The early studies produced contradictory results but the most recent data suggest no significant influence on semen parameters, gonadotropins or testosterone (Hjollund et al. 1998a), or on time to pregnancy (Hjollund et al. 1998b). In the latter study, however, there was evidence of a possible effect on welders who also smoked.

13.3.5 Complex Organochlorine Compounds

Complex organochlorine compounds include diverse chemicals such as dioxins, **polychlorinated biphenyls** and **bifurans**. Many are widely distributed throughout the environment of all populated parts of the world and have been suspected of causing reproductive toxicity. Many are **teratogens** and can have very weak hormonal properties as **estrogens**, **anti-estrogens** or **anti-androgens**. Those with estrogenic activity have been termed **xenoestrogens** but there is also concern over the role of anti-androgens, which may have analogous effects (Kelce and Wilson 1997). There is often overlap in the activity of these chemicals with some xenoestrogens showing anti-androgenic activity (Sohoni and Sumpter 1998). The non-specific term **endocrine disruptors** has been widely used to describe chemicals with any of these activities.

Prenatal exposure to xenoestrogens has been **proposed to inhibit fetal testicular development**, thereby leading to **reduced sperm production** and impaired male fertility (Sharpe and Skakkebaek 1993). Such hormonally active compounds could, according to the hypothesis, inhibit Sertoli cell proliferation either indirectly via inhibition of pituitary FSH secretion or directly at a testicular level. They would thus reduce final Sertoli cell numbers populating the testis and, since the germ cell carrying capacity of Sertoli cells is limited, could ultimately lower the numbers of germ cells eventually supported by the seminiferous epithelium (Sharpe 1993). In addition, it has been suggested that endocrine disruptors could be responsible for an increase in the incidence of reproductive system malformations and testicular cancer (Skakkebaek et al. 1998).

Xenoestrogens have only very weak steroidal activity, however, and are unlikely to be present at **biologically effective levels** in the male fetus, which resides within the pregnant uterus, the most estrogen-rich environment at any time of human life. The hypothesis therefore has a questionable biological basis and little direct evidence has been adduced to support it. Nevertheless, it has received extensive public attention, which unfortunately can appear to transmute science speculation into public fact. A follow-up of a controlled study of men born to women who received high doses of diethylstilbestrol or placebo during pregnancy shows that *in utero* exposure to this estrogen had no effect on their fertility. Only inconsistent effects on their reproductive organs were observed, amongst which was a small increase in genital malformations (Wilcox et al. 1995).

> Since diethylstilbestrol is a very potent estrogen, the low incidence of adverse effects casts doubt on the ability of non-steroidal estrogens, anti-estrogens or anti-androgenic chemicals, that are orders of magnitude less potent than estradiol, to have any effect on the male fetus (Golden et al. 1998).

Nonetheless, it has been shown that high doses of diethylstilbestrol administered neonatally to rats can affect subsequent Sertoli cell function in the adult (Sharpe et al. 1998). It is not yet known whether this is a species-specific effect.

Enormous scientific research efforts are currently underway in Europe, America and Asia designed to test the hypothesis that xenoestrogens can have adverse effects on the male reproductive system. Exposure of adult male rats to 4-*tert*-octylphenol disturbed gonadotropin levels and spermatogenesis, though food consumption and bodyweight were also affected (Boockfor and Blake 1997). p-Nonylphenol was also associated with disturbed spermatogenesis but only at doses close to the LD_{50} and above (de Jager et al. 1999), which questions the relevance of the findings to endocrine disruption. Effects at lower doses and with more environmentally-relevant routes of exposure are much more difficult to

demonstrate experimentally, mainly because of problems with reproducibility. Thus: the finding that rats exposed to butyl benzyl phthalate during gestation through to weaning had impaired sperm production (Sharpe et al. 1995) could not be repeated (Ashby et al. 1997); an initial report of estrogenic synergism between various xenoestrogens (Arnold et al. 1996) was subsequently retracted because the data could not be replicated by others or by the authors (McLachlan 1997); increases in adult mouse prostate weight following bisphenol A exposure *in utero* (Nagel et al. 1997) could not be replicated in an experiment that was designed to mimic the original study as closely as possible (Ashby et al. 1999). The reasons for these contradictory findings are not clear but they may relate to the very small magnitude of the changes being observed (Ashby and Odum 1998) and to the high degree of species- interindividual- and tissue-specificity of endocrine-disruptor effects (Walker et al. 1999).

Added impetus was given to the area of xenoestrogen effects on the male reproductive system by the discovery of estrogen receptors in the male reproductive tract and that estrogen is necessary for its development (Eddy et al. 1996; Hess et al. 1997; see also Chap. 3 and 4). This suggested that these receptors could be targets for xenoestrogens. A recent series of experiments has shown that xenoestrogens administered neonatally have effects via estrogen receptors in the male reproductive tract of the rat (Fisher et al. 1999). The magnitude of these effects is proportional to the estrogenicity of each compound, which reinforces the conclusion that the rat model suggests that ambient environmental exposures are unlikely to have any impact on the male human reproductive system.

More recently, it has been proposed that the balance between estrogenic and androgenic factors in the uterine environment may be more important than estrogenicity alone. Greater emphasis is now being placed on investigations of compounds that antagonise the action of androgens. An example of this is the plasticizer **di(*n*-butyl)phthalate**, which does not interact with either the estrogen or the androgen receptors but does interfere with androgen-dependent development of the male reproductive system in rats (Mylchreest et al. 1999).

13.3.6 Smoking

Inhaled cigarette smoke contains many hazardous compounds, some of which (such as acrolein) are reproductive toxins. Furthermore, it can induce oxidative damage to macromolecules that is detectable in the testis. Most of the few scientifically valid studies have demonstrated some reduction in sperm output and motility among smokers, effects that may be due to biological effects of smoking but could even result from **psychological self-**

selection, ie: smokers are likely to be the type of people more heavily exposed to other hazards that could cause the adverse effects seen (Vogt et al. 1984). Smoking in men trying to conceive is not associated with decreased fecundity as measured by time to pregnancy (Bolumar et al. 1996) and is more likely to be important if there is a danger that fertility could be compromised by other factors, as has been indicated, for example, by investigations of sub-fertility among welders (Hjollund et al. 1998b).

Of concern in recent years has been the growing recognition that smoking can cause DNA damage in sperm detected as chromatin disturbances (Potts et al. 1999), sperm DNA adducts (Fraga et al. 1996) and even DNA adducts in the embryo (Zenzes et al. 1999). The ultimate fate of this damage, whether it is repaired in the embryo or fixed as mutations, is not known but clearly there is a potential risk that smoking could cause transmissible abnormalities in the offspring. More substantial studies have now shown a positive association between paternal smoking and the incidence of cancer, especially leukemia among their offspring (Ji et al. 1997; Sorahan et al. 1997a; Sorahan et al. 1997b). This has since been questioned by a further study (Brondum et al. 1999) but since these contradictory data were obtained by telephone interviews and self-reported cigarette consumption, they may not be as reliable.

13.3.7 Diet, Alcohol and Social Drugs

Many specific dietary factors have been found to have a direct influence on the male reproductive system in domestic and experimental animals (Brinkworth et al. 1992), possibly partly as a result of an inhibition of LH secretion (Dong et al. 1994). However, there is little convincing evidence that similar effects can be induced in humans. This probably reflects a resilience of human spermatogenesis to fluctuations in dietary intake except in extreme cases (Keys 1950; Baker 1998). Furthermore, in such cases numerous other physiological disorders are likely also to be present, making it difficult to ascribe the impairment of spermatogenesis solely to the dietary restriction. Of probably greater, but as yet undefined importance is possible **synergism** between **dietary deficiencies** and **environmental reproductive toxins**.

As for many life-style exposures, the influence of recreational drug use on human male reproductive function remains unclear and difficult to study in a scientifically convincing fashion. Most studies are retrospective and therefore lack stringent controls for bias among confounding variables.

Excessive alcohol intake is associated with direct testicular toxicity (Pajarinen and Karhunen 1994) in addition to indirect effects due to chronic liver disease and undernutrition among alcoholics. Whether there is a testicular equivalent of the so-called 'French Paradox', whereby moderate alcohol consumption has a beneficial effect on the incidence of coronary heart disease, is not known.

Abusers of **marijuana**, **cocaine** and **opiates** are harder to study due to the illicit nature of their drug usage, and the available studies often do not adequately control for socio-economic status, nutritional intake and concomitant drug use (eg alcohol, smoking). Nevertheless, these agents appear to have only minimal effects on spermatogenesis even though opiates including heroin, morphine and methadone all markedly suppress LH and testosterone secretion due to their central activation of **opiatergic mechanisms**, causing **inhibition of hypothalamic GnRH secretion** (Cicero et al. 1974).

13.3.8 Electromagnetic Radiation

Magnetic fields are generated by domestic as well as industrial electrical equipment and vary in frequency, intensity and waveform. The frequency of electricity transmission is 50 Hertz (Hz) in Europe and 60 Hz in North America, both of which fall into the Extremely Low Frequency (ELF) range. The intensity of the magnetic component these fields is measured in Teslas (T) and is a function of distance from, and strength of the electric current. It is known that high intensity, low-frequency magnetic fields ($>$10 mTesla at 50–60 Hz) can be damaging but normal environmental exposure to ELF's does not usually exceed 0.3 mT. Of particular concern recently, however, are portable (mobile) telephones, which can generate magnetic fields of moderate intensity but high frequency in the GHz range. Also of interest is the interaction of electromagnetic radiation exposures with other risk factors such as welding (Skotte and Hjollund 1997).

Work to assess the risk to humans of magnetic fields has largely focused on carcinogenicity but reproductive effects are also well studied. Principally, however, the emphasis has been on risks during pregnancy, which are very minor in the rat (Jensh 1997) and there are very few papers relating to effects on the male. Those studies that have been undertaken are reviewed in Lundsberg et al. (1995). The consensus of opinion is that **ELF magnetic fields** have **no effect on spermatogenesis** in rodents or on the offspring sired from treated males. Furthermore, a limited study of time to pregnancy failed to reveal convincing evidence of an effect of ELF fields (Hjollund et al. 1999). **High frequency, moderate intensity fields** of the type generated by mobile telephones, however, have been found to **affect** the proportions of **spermatogenic cells in hamsters** (Niehaus et al. 1997). The possibility that these high frequency fields could be associated with an increase in testicular cancer (amongst other disorders) has been discussed (Goldsmith 1997).

13.3.9 Heat

Heat is among the best established testis-damaging agents (Setchell 1998). Brief periods of elevated temperature in experimental animals can markedly **reduce sperm production and fertility** and adverse effects have also been noted in men occupationally or experimentally exposed to heat (reviewed in: Kandeel and Swerdloff 1988; Bonde and Giwercman 1995). Mild heating can also lead to **embryonic death** among the offspring of heat-treated rams (Mieusset et al. 1992) and cause transient growth retardation of fetuses of male mice in whom the testes have been heated (Setchell et al. 1998).

Impairment of sperm output in humans has also been demonstrated in the course of work designed to explore the possibility of using local scrotal heating as a form of contraception in men (Mieusset and Bujan 1994). However, the utility of this method has been questioned by a year-long study in which scrotal temperature was elevated by about 1°C without any apparent effect on sperm production or function (Wang et al. 1997). Occupational exposure to heat such as in the ceramics industry (Figa-Talamanca et al. 1992) and among welders (Hjollund et al. 1998a,b) has also been suggested to affect the male reproductive system adversely. Varicoceles can be associated with suboptimal spermatogenesis and elevated day-night scrotal temperatures (Lerchl et al. 1993). It remains unclear whether there is a causal relationship between scrotal temperature and reduced semen parameters. More recent work on men who drive for more than 3 hours per day has also claimed effects (Thonneau et al. 1998) but it is not clear whether, if confirmed, these are the result of heat, posture or other causes.

13.3.10 Unknown Factors

The possibility that sperm output has been changing systematically in the **general male population** has long attracted interest. In the 1970's a debate about **falling sperm counts** based on data from large numbers (1,000's) of infertile men studied at single laboratories was resolved in the negative (Nelson and Bunge 1974; MacLeod and Wang 1979). The studies were then criticized, without public furore, for reliance on populations of infertile men as representative of the general male population when the operation of various distorting factors such as selection and referral bias would have overshadowed any real effects in question (Sloan 1982).

The issue was re-ignited by a **meta-analysis** of mean sperm counts from 61 studies from various centers over the preceding 50 years (Carlsen et al. 1992). This meta-analysis of semen samples from non-infertile men produced the startling claim of an apparent 50% decrease in the mean sperm counts over that time, a claim that has generated enormous public attention and scientific scrutiny. In order to explain the data, it was proposed that increased prenatal exposure to environmental estrogens (see 13.3.10) may have resulted in a global decline in sperm counts (Sharpe and Skakkebaek 1993). This suggestion was supported by a **retrospective study** of the sperm counts of sperm donors at a single Parisian center over a 20 year period also showing a similar decrease (Auger et al. 1995). Subsequent reports from Scotland (Irvine et al. 1996) and Belgium (Van Waeleghem et al. 1996) also supported the claim but studies from Finland (Vierula et al. 1996), the USA (Fisch et al. 1996), Toulouse in France (Bujan et al. 1996) and Australia (Handelsman 1997), failed to find supporting evidence. In consequence it was proposed that there is **geographical variation** in sperm count between different populations (Fisch and Goluboff 1996). Interestingly, a study of sperm counts among **domesticated animals** also showed no evidence of a secular decline in sperm counts over more than the last 60 years (Setchell 1997). Furthermore, human infertility overall is declining (Akre et al. 1999) making any claimed increase in male infertility unlikely.

No **prospective** and little conclusive **experimental evidence** yet supports these provocative suggestions, which are highly controversial (Lerchl and Nieschlag 1996). The original meta-analysis has been largely refuted on methodological grounds including failure to adjust adequately for the skewed distribution of sperm concentrations, reliance on sub-optimal linear models and inappropriate application of meta-analysis (Brake and Krause 1992; Olsen et al. 1995). Meta-analysis, a controversial statistical technique, treats summary data from published studies as equally valid data points in a retrospective observational study. It was originally designed to aggregate quantitatively the overall effect sizes from many small controlled studies by using the same method to measure the same variable in equally well-defined populations. Where these criteria are not met, meta-analysis may be seriously flawed by biases that are impossible to predict or correct (Egger et al. 1998). By these standards the Carlsen meta-analysis is clearly invalid. The 61 studies had little in common apart from control groups of non-infertile men such as sperm donors, and men who were recently fertile, once fertile, or of undefined fertility. The comparability of selection/rejection criteria between studies could not be fully evaluated. Furthermore, during the period from which the 61 studies were drawn, the accepted standards for what constituted the minimum "normal" or "fertile" sperm concentration had fallen progressively from 60 to 40 then 20×10^6 sperm/ml. This progressive fall alone could have produced the apparent secular trend in sperm concentrations by more liberal selection/rejection criteria for the control groups (Brake and Krause 1992). In addition, the **decrease in semen volume** in the Carlsen study suggests that the mean **sexual abstinence intervals** of participants – the most important known determinant of sperm output – also decreased during the period under observation. Alleged geographical differences in sperm counts (see above), if real, may also contribute a confounding factor in the meta-analysis (Fisch and Goluboff 1996; Paulsen et al. 1996). Discrepancies between studies conducted in different cities can be considered genuine geographical differences only if the participants in each study are representative of that city. Since participation bias makes that highly unlikely in any single center, such discrepancies between studies can only lead to discussion of differences in recruitment between studies and not to valid inferences based on geography. Finally, more appropriate statistical models of the same data actually indicate an increase in sperm counts over the last 20 years (Brake and Krause 1992; Olsen et al. 1995). For these reasons, no sound conclusions can be drawn from the Carlsen meta-analysis; indeed it constitutes an excellent example of the misuse of meta-analysis. The Parisian study (Auger et al. 1995) also does not overcome the defects of its retrospective uncontrolled design. The **self-selected** source population of married, fertile men volunteering to become sperm donors is not representative of the general male population and this selection bias is likely to have changed during the study period. The results of Auger et al. are therefore more likely to reflect changes in selection of the population rather than changes in the underlying population.

13.4 Design and Interpretation of Toxicological Studies

13.4.1 Design of Non-human Studies

The ultimate value of non-human studies is judged by their contribution to the understanding of human toxicology. This rests on the balance between the strengths of experimental toxicology – such as the ability to make carefully controlled, reproducible observations on any relevant physiological variables, and its deficiencies – including the uncertain validity of extrapolation from a test system to humans. **Randomization** is essential to ensure **balance** between **known** as well as **unknown covariables in the control and treatment groups**. Precision, reproducibility and replication are all additional key features of the optimal experimental design expected in such studies. **Interpretation must consider** carefully the possibility of **species differences in** relevant factors such as **route of administration, distribution, metabolism, excretion and mode of action** of the chemical under consideration.

13.4.2 Design of Human Studies

Human toxicological studies usually yield retrospective epidemiological or clinical data relating to uncontrolled exposures so that controlling for covariables may be difficult or impossible. A major **source of bias** in human studies, particularly those requiring collection of semen samples, is the **participation rate**. Although the social acceptability of providing semen samples may have increased in recent years, most men are unwilling to participate unless they are concurrently concerned about their fertility. This inevitably means that **participants** in such studies **are self-selected** and introduce an ineradicable bias for which it is impossible to adjust. Typical end-points measured in human studies are derived from a medical history, a physical examination and samples of blood and semen. These will yield information on testicular volume, semen variables (sperm count, motility, morphology, seminal volume, other special tests of sperm function) and blood FSH concentration. Serial observations are particularly useful in adjusting for the between-subject variability in many of these parameters. Normal-range values can provide some indication of whether an individual may have been intoxicated, especially if serial observations are not available.

13.4.3 Regulatory Testing for Reproductive Toxicity

Regulatory Reproductive Research Strategies

In regulatory terms, chemicals are regarded as **food chemicals, pharmaceuticals** or **compounds for environmental use.** The first category contains food additives and packaging components that come into contact with foodstuffs. The second covers drugs and compounds used in human and veterinary medicine, while the third includes any chemical whose use causes it to be released into the environment. This enormous range of chemicals and uses handled by independent regulatory agencies has further diversified testing requirements according to the proposed use of the compound and the country in which the application is made. The need to unify the safety-testing demands for chemical entities intended for international usage has resulted in agreement on **common strategies for drug toxicity testing** between the European Community, the United States and Japan. Through the mutual establishment of the International Committee on Harmonization of Technical Requirements for Registration of Pharmaceuticals for Human Use, recommendations for assessment of reproductive toxicity have now been presented and adopted by the regulatory authorities in each domain. Based on the '3 segment' design first introduced by the US Food and Drug Administration (FDA) in 1966 (see Sullivan 1988), they involve a **fertility study in male and female rats, a pre and postnatal study in pregnant female rats and a teratology study** in the rat and one other mammalian species. Only the first can identify direct effects on male reproduction, although any preliminary studies performed to set dose levels should obtain data on testicular histology, sperm motility and viability. If good data are available from such studies, seminology data are not required from the fertility study. Remarkably, these requirements represent the first time that specific testing of male reproductive effects of new chemical entities has been requested.

Food chemical and environmental chemical regulation is overseen by the FDA and the Environmental Protection Agency respectively, in the USA, by the Organization for Economic Cooperation and Development in Europe and by the Japanese Ministry for Agriculture, Fisheries and Food in Japan. All these agencies require essentially the same testing for these chemicals, which involves

- a **teratology study in two species,**
- a **one-generation toxicity study** and
- a **two-generation toxicity study.**

Testicular pathology and **seminology data** are now required from all generations.

Directive 93/21/EEC of the European Union (an addition to the Council Directive on Classification, Packaging and Labelling of Dangerous Substances, 67/548/EEC) divides reproductive toxins into three categories. These indicate a risk (labeled "R60" or "R61") or possible risk (R62, R63) to fertility or to the unborn child respectively, or a risk to breast-fed babies (R64). This labeling is designed to reflect the existing state of scientific knowledge regarding the reproductive safety of any compound to which humans may be exposed in Europe.

Experimental Methods in Male Reproductive Research

Regulatory male reproductive toxicology is increasingly adopting techniques used in basic research (reviewed in Chapin and Heindel 1993). In addition to the basic techniques already in wide use, these include

- detailed **histological evaluation of the germinal epithelium,**
- recognizing the characteristic associations and stages (Hess 1990);
- **flow cytometry,** which quantitates both total sperm numbers as well as the proportions of haploid, diploid and tetraploid cells in the testis;
- **vital dye staining** to determine the numbers of cells with intact membranes as an estimate of viability;
- and **computerized techniques for objective assessment of sperm motion** (Seed et al. 1996).

A variety of *in vivo* genotoxicity assays have also been developed to detect potentially transmissible genetic mutations in germ cell DNA. These include tests for **dominant lethal mutations, specific-locus mutations, dominant skeletal mutations, heritable translocations** and **aneuploidy.** Other research techniques such as stereological quantitation of germ cell numbers and genetic evaluation of germinal epithelium are yet to be widely adopted.

> Critically, however, no single test provides an overall prediction of toxicity to the male reproductive system.

13.4.4 Criteria for the Evaluation of Human Toxicology Data

Regulatory decisions concerning human safety involve difficult evaluations of human risk. This inevitably involves an amalgam of human data, which is usually retrospective, observational and uncontrolled, with designed and controlled laboratory experimentation on animals, cells and *in vitro* systems. The former lacks scientific rigor in that confounding variables may remain unidentified and unaccounted for, while the latter lacks reliable extrapolation to humans. With many new chemical entities, relevant human data may be totally lacking, making complete reliance on laboratory evaluation necessary. In other situations human sentinel populations such as those receiving medicinal drugs or those occupationally exposed to non-medicinal chemicals (eg manufacturers, applicators) may provide crucial, albeit limited, information.

Controlled experimentation of chemical effects in healthy humans is severely limited, largely being restricted to medically-used drugs with minimized toxicity. Otherwise, the best opportunity for scientifically valid studies of chemical effects on human reproduction is in occupational health where exposure to various specified chemicals can be measured and unexposed control groups can be studied concurrently. Interpretation of such studies are, however, fraught with difficulties due to **systematic biases** arising from **non-randomization, entry bias** (the reproductive analogy of the "healthy worker effect") and **low and selective participation rates,** especially among control groups. The requirement for semen analysis is a major and almost insurmountable stumbling block for the validity of such human field studies. At present it remains highly characteristic of male employees to participate in studies requiring semen analyses only if they have prior concerns about their own fertility and/or toxic exposures. Participation rates in control groups in industrial settings is typically as low as 10–20%, leaving great scope for intractable biases.

13.5 Future Perspectives

13.5.1 Experimental Studies

Non-human studies

The suggestion that intra-uterine exposure to hormonally active chemicals can affect future reproductive potential is a hypothesis that requires further testing in experimental animals. A variety of studies have reported that both potent and relatively weak xenoestrogens can affect the reproductive system in male rodents following pre-/neo-natal exposure just as a number have reported negative effects. Of critical importance for future work will be the reproducibility of effects that can be induced and whether the dose levels at which they occur are in any way comparable to likely human exposure. At the same time, it will be essential to establish the relevance to humans of the animal model used. This latter point is of great general significance because of the inevitable reliance on cross-species comparisons in experimental toxicology. The wider search for better predictors of human reproductive toxicity is acquiring greater urgency as public attention is increasingly focused on real or alleged instances of adverse environmental influences on reproduction. In this respect, studies using chronic, low-dose regimens that mimic actual human exposures more closely than conventional acute dosing need to be developed and validated further.

Recent progress towards the understanding of how heritable mutations can be induced in the male germline means that progress can now be made towards establishing with greater certainty whether specific agents can have such effects. When likely mechanisms have been demonstrated experimentally, appropriate testing strategies can be developed for the evaluation of suspect or novel chemicals.

Human Studies

An increasing awareness that many chemicals can adversely affect male reproductive function is an important starting point for future development in human reproductive toxicology. In future, more **systematic collections of reproductive information** from **exposed** and **unexposed workers** as well as more public availability of **pre-registration testing of new drugs** would greatly facilitate early and sensitive detection of previously unrecognized hazards to male reproduction. This might reduce the proportion of infertile men in whom the diagnosis of male infertility remains unexplained.

Analysis of semen samples for both clinical and research purposes is standardized by universal adoption of the WHO *Laboratory Handbook for the Examination of Human Semen and Sperm-Cervical Mucus Interaction*, which is in its 4th edition (1999). Inter- and intra-laboratory variability in semen evaluation is increasingly being reduced by **quality control programs for semen analysis**. The establishment of **normal ranges**, however, remains a difficult task. Data collected from any population, whether on numbers of children or sperm counts, may be difficult to interpret unless an appropriate control group can be identified.

The collection of sperm data from 'at risk' populations is fraught with practical difficulties including low and biased participation rates according to perceived risk, as well as deterministic interpretations of sporadic clusters of cases. The limited acceptability of semen collections makes it desirable that different monitoring systems less reliant on sexual function should be available. An effective alternative is the **Time-To-Pregnancy** (TTP) **questionnaire-based data collection system** developed by Joffe et al. (1993), which supersedes the previous **standardized fertility ratio** described by Levine et al. (1980). The TTP methodology allows quantitative estimation of fertility performance of groups of men as a means of monitoring fertility in occupational or other settings. Thus, the routine collection of reproductive data in the workplace, whether from questionnaire or semen samples, would greatly improve the possibility for early warning of potential fertility problems.

13.5.2 Clinical Implications

Historical Perspective

It is a curious paradox of modern life that at a time when life expectancy is longer than ever in human history, public clamor about the damaging effects of environmental chemicals and radiation on human health is ever increasing. Ironically, these preoccupations originate within affluent Western economies rather than among developing countries where life expectancy has yet to catch up with Western standards; such concerns were unheard of in post-industrial European countries while life expectancy was much shorter than it is now. Together with the flourishing fad diet and artificial exercise industries, these constitute the remarkably popular modern hobby of health consciousness in wealthy countries. This narcissistic luxury reflects the modern version of the "conspicuous consumption" that Thorstein Veblen (1857–1929) identified as emblematic of the growing affluence of the emergent mercantile middle class a century ago in the USA ("Theory of the Leisure Classes" 1899). Like other fashions, health consciousness has only a casual relationship with rationality, consisting at its most extreme, of largely irrational phobias and passions superficially disguised by a layer of scientific patois and eagerly captured by endlessly inventive and avaricious marketers. Often ignited by crusading journalists or ecologists with a commercial interest in sensation, such histrionic 'revelations' are fueled among the public by ignorance, superstition and fear of technological progress.

Coinciding with the rise of the health consciousness fashion during the prosperity of the latter half of the 20th century, several public health crises, notably Thalidomide®-induced teratogenesis, created political pressure that propelled the inception of increasingly stringent regulations regarding medical, occupational, environmental, domestic and recreational exposures to chemicals, radiation and devices. Unfortunately, precipitate political action that outstrips genuine scientific knowledge often results in poor science policy as, in an unfortunate analogy to Gresham's law of monetary flows, bad science drives out the good (Thomas Gresham, 1519–1579). One consequence of this has been the conducting of regulatory testing with little consideration of what actually constitutes a 'safe' compound. As proving a negative is impossible, defining safety is an unachievable goal unless carefully qualified and delineated. If not, like the drunk's use of a lampost, science becomes relegated to being used for support rather than illumination. Another problem is that the long-term predictions of newer tests developed from fundamental research cannot be based on empirical data but rest largely on plausible supposition.

At present, licensing authorities require a negative data set from a limited battery of assays for registration of a new compound for human use. This necessarily ignores the possibility that a **potentially hazardous compound may present no risk at likely human exposure levels** and that certain **ostensibly benign compounds** could have **unpredicted effects**, for example, by acting in concert with other chemicals. Currently, then, there is an acute need for consensus as to what should be the true level of concern over potential reproductive toxins.

Clinical Practice

In routine clinical practice **the possibility of environmental and toxic factors in causing infertility and other andrological disorders should always be considered carefully**. The accurate identification of such influences is largely dependent upon an **index of suspicion** together with confirmation by a careful **history of occupational**, domestic, recreational and other potential **environmental exposures**. Laboratory confirmation of specific forms of intoxication may occasionally be helpful but is rarely possible. Although measurement of suspected toxins in body fluids (eg blood, seminal plasma) may be possible, its significance needs to be established by properly controlled clinical studies. Without these, interpretation can be impossible. A careful and thorough occu-

pational history remains an essential part of proper evaluation of men for infertility or other andrological disorders. Specific attention should be paid to the type of work routinely performed, and compliance with and results of health monitoring, if applicable. In addition, domestic exposures from gardening (pesticide exposure), holidays (visiting farms or zoos) and hobbies should be considered. In addition to its value for counseling patients, such categorization of life-styles of patients may become useful for retrospective studies. In the case of patients who believe they have been intoxicated by various environmental agents, a full evaluation of reproductive function is usually necessary to dispel any concerns or identify the extent of damage.

13.6 References

Akre O, Cnattingius S, Bergstrom R, Kvist U (1999) Human fertility does not decline: evidence from Sweden. Fertil Steril 71:1066–1069

Alexander BH, Checkoway H, van Netten C, Muller CH, Ewers TG, Kaufman JD, Mueller BA, Vaughan TL, Faustman EM (1996) Semen quality of men employed at a lead smelter. Occup Environ Med 53:411–416

Anderson D, Brinkworth MH, Jenkinson PC, Clode SA, Creasy DM, Gangolli SD (1987) Effect of ethylene glycol monomethyl ether on spermatogenesis, dominant lethality, and F1 abnormalities in the rat and the mouse after treatment of F0 males. Teratog Carcinog Mutagen 7:141–158

Anderson D, Edwards AJ, Brinkworth MH, Hughes JA (1996) Male-mediated F1 effects in mice exposed to 1,3-butadiene. Toxicology 113:120–127

Armour JAL, Brinkworth MH, Kamischke A (1999) A direct analysis by small-pool PCR of MS205 minisatellite mutation rates in sperm after mutagenic therapies. Mutat Res 15:73–80

Arnold SF, Klotz DM, Collins BM, Vonier PM, Guillette LJ Jr, McLachlan JA (1996) Synergistic activation of estrogen receptor with combinations of environmental chemicals. Science 272:1489–1492

Ashby J, Odum J (1998) The importance of protocol design and data reporting to research on endocrine disruption. Environ Health Perspect 106:A315–316; discussion A316–317

Ashby J, Tinwell H, Haseman J (1999) Lack of effects for low dose levels of bisphenol A (BPA) and diethylstilbestrol (DES) on the prostate gland of CF1 mice exposed in utero. Regul Toxicol Pharmacol 30:156–166

Ashby J, Tinwell H, Lefevre PA, Odum J, Paton D, Millward SW, Tittensor S, Brooks AN (1997) Normal sexual development of rats exposed to butyl benzyl phthalate from conception to weaning. Regul Toxicol Pharmacol 26:102–118

Auger J, Kunstmann JM, Czyglik F, Jouannet P (1995) Decline in semen quality among fertile men in Paris during the past 20 years. N Engl J Med 332:281–285

Baker HW (1998) Reproductive effects of nontesticular illness. Endocrinol Metab Clin North Am 27:831–850

Bartlett JM, Kerr JB, Sharpe RM (1986) The effect of selective destruction and regeneration of rat Leydig cells on the intratesticular distribution of testosterone and morphology of the seminiferous epithelium. J Androl 7:240–253

Bartoov B, Zabludovsky N, Eltes F, Smirnov VV, Grischenko VI, Fischbein A (1997) Semen quality of workers exposed to ionizing radiation in decontamination work after the Chernobyl nuclear reactor accident. Int J Occup Environ Health 3:198–203

Berndtson WE, Foote RH (1997) Disruption of spermatogenesis in rabbits consuming ethylene glycol monomethyl ether. Reprod Toxicol 11:29–36

Billig H, Furuta I, Rivier C, Tapanainen J, Parvinen M, Hsueh AJ (1995) Apoptosis in testis germ cells: developmental changes in gonadotropin dependence and localization to selective tubule stages. Endocrinology 136:5–12

Boekelheide K (1993) Sertoli cell toxicants. In: Russell LD, Griswold MD (eds) The Sertoli Cell. Cache River Press, Clearwater, pp 551–575

Bolumar F, Olsen J, Boldsen J (1996) Smoking reduces fecundity: a European multicenter study on infertility and subfecundity. The European Study Group on Infertility and Subfecundity. Am J Epidemiol 143:578–587

Boockfor FR, Blake CA (1997) Chronic administration of 4-tert-octylphenol to adult male rats causes shrinkage of the testes and male accessory sex organs, disrupts spermatogenesis, and increases the incidence of sperm deformities. Biol Reprod 57:267–277

Bonde JP, Giwercman A (1995) Occupational hazards to male fecundity. Reprod Med Rev 4:59–73

Brake A, Krause W (1992) Decreasing quality of semen. Br Med J 305:1498

Brandriff BF, Meistrich ML, Gordon LA, Carrano AV, Liang JC (1994) Chromosomal damage in sperm of patients surviving Hodgkin's disease following MOPP (nitrogen mustard, vincristine, procarbazine, and prednisone) therapy with and without radiotherapy. Hum Genet 93:295–299

Brinkworth MH (2000) Paternal transmission of genetic damage: findings in animals and humans. Int J Androl 23:123–135

Brinkworth MH, Nieschlag E (2000) Association of cyclophosphamide-induced male-mediated, foetal abnormalities with reduced paternal germ-cell apoptosis. Mutat Res 447:149–154

Brinkworth MH, Anderson D, McLean AM (1992) Effects of dietary imbalances on spermatogenesis in CD-1 mice and CD rats. Food Chem Toxicol 30:29–35

Brinkworth MH, Weinbauer GF, Schlatt S, Nieschlag E (1995) Identification of male germ cells undergoing apoptosis in adult rats. J Reprod Fertil 105:25–33

Brondum J, Shu XO, Steinbuch M, Severson RK, Potter JD, Robison LL (1999) Parental cigarette smoking and the risk of acute leukemia in children. Cancer 85:1380–1388

Byrne J (1999) Long-term genetic and reproductive effects of ionizing radiation and chemotherapeutic agents on cancer patients and their offspring. Teratology 59:210–215

Byrne J, Rasmussen SA, Steinhorn SC, Connelly RR, Myers MH, Lynch CF, Flannery J, Austin DF, Holmes FF, Holmes GE, Strong LC, Mulvihill JJ (1998) Genetic disease in offspring of long-term survivors of childhood and adolescent cancer. Am J Hum Genet 62:45–52

Bujan L, Mansat A, Pontonnier F, Mieusset R (1996) Time series analysis of sperm concentration in fertile men in Toulouse, France between 1977 and 1992. Br Med J 312:471–472

Carlsen E, Giwercman A, Keiding N, Skakkebaek NE (1992) Evidence for decreasing quality of semen during past 50 years. Br Med J 305:609–613

Carson SA (1993) Mutagenic sensitivity of human post-spermatogonial cells. Hum Reprod 8:982

Carson SA, Gentry WL, Smith AL, Buster JE (1991) Feasibility of semen collection and cryopreservation during chemotherapy. Hum Reprod 6:992–994

Chapin RE, Heindel JJ (eds) (1993) Male reproductive toxicology. Methods in toxicology, volume 3, part A: male reproductive toxicology. Academic, San Diego

Chia SE, Ong CN, Lee ST, Tsakok FH (1992) Blood concentrations of lead, cadmium, mercury, zinc, and copper and human semen parameters. Arch Androl 29:177–183

Cicero TJ, Meyer ER, Bell RD, Wiest WG (1974) Effects of morphine on the secondary sex organs and plasma testosterone levels of rats. Res Commun Chem Pathol Pharmacol 7:17–24

Clegg ED, Cook JC, Chapin RE, Foster PM, Daston GP (1997) Leydig cell hyperplasia and adenoma formation: mechanisms and relevance to humans. Reprod Toxicol 11:107–121

Cooke PS, Zhao YD, Hansen LG (1996) Neonatal polychlorinated biphenyl treatment increases adult testis size and sperm production in the rat. Toxicol Appl Pharmacol 136:112–117

Cooper TG, Yeung CH (1999) Recent biochemical approaches to post-testicular, epididymal contraception. Hum Reprod Update 5:141–152

Creasy DM, Flynn JC, Gray TJ, Butler WH (1985) A quantitative study of stage-specific spermatocyte damage following administration of ethylene glycol monomethyl ether in the rat. Exp Mol Pathol 43:321–336

de Jager C, Bornman MS, van der Horst G (1999) The effect of p-nonylphenol, an environmental toxicant with oestrogenic properties, on fertility potential in adult male rats. Andrologia 31:99–106

Doll R, Evans HJ, Darby SC (1994) Paternal exposure not to blame. Nature 367:678–680

Dong Q, Rintala H, Handelsman DJ (1994) Androgen receptor function during undernutrition. J Neuroendocrinol 6:397–402

Draper GJ, Little MP, Sorahan T, Kinlen LJ, Bunch KJ, Conquest AJ, Kendall GM, Kneale GW, Lancashire RJ, Muirhead CR, O'Connor CM, Vincent TJ (1997) Cancer in the offspring of radiation workers: a record linkage study. Br Med J 315:1181–1188

Dubrova YE, Nesterov VN, Krouchinsky NG, Ostapenko VA, Neumann R, Neil DL, Jeffreys AJ (1996) Human minisatellite mutation rate after the Chernobyl accident. Nature 380:683–686

Dubrova YE, Plumb M, Brown J, Jeffreys AJ (1998) Radiation-induced germline instability at minisatellite loci. Int J Radiat Biol 74:689–696

Eaton M, Schenker M, Whorton MD, Samuels S, Perkins C, Overstreet J (1986) Seven-year follow-up of workers exposed to 1,2-dibromo-3-chloropropane. J Occup Med 28:1145–1150

Eddy EM, Washburn TF, Bunch DO, Goulding EH, Gladen BC, Lubahn DB, Korach KS (1996) Targeted disruption of the estrogen receptor gene in male mice causes alteration of spermatogenesis and infertility. Endocrinology 137:4796–4805

Egger M, Schneider M, Davey Smith G (1998) Spurious precision? Meta-analysis of observational studies. Br Med J 316:140–144

Fan YJ, Wang Z, Sadamoto S, Ninomiya Y, Kotomura N, Kamiya K, Dohi K, Kominami R, Niwa O (1995) Dose-response of a radiation induction of a germline mutation at a hypervariable mouse minisatellite locus. Int J Radiat Biol 68:177–183

Figa-Talamanca I, Dell'Orco V, Pupi A, Dondero F, Gandini L, Lenzi A, Lombardo F, Scavalli P, Mancini G (1992) Fertility and semen quality of workers exposed to high temperatures in the ceramics industry. Reprod Toxicol 6:517–523

Finkelstein JS, McCully WF, MacLaughlin DT, Godine JE, Crowley WF Jr (1988) The mortician's mystery. Gynecomastia and reversible hypogonadotropic hypogonadism in an embalmer. N Engl J Med 318:961–965

Fisch H, Goluboff ET (1996) Geographic variations in sperm counts: a potential cause of bias in studies of semen quality. Fertil Steril 65:1044–1046

Fisch H, Goluboff ET, Olson JH, Feldshuh J, Broder SJ, Barad DH (1996) Semen analyses in 1,283 men from the United States over a 25-year period: no decline in quality. Fertil Steril 65:1009–1014

Fisher JS, Turner KJ, Brown D, Sharpe RM (1999) Effect of neonatal exposure to estrogenic compounds on development of the excurrent ducts of the rat testis through puberty to adulthood. Environ Health Perspect 107:397–405

Fraga CG, Motchnik PA, Wyrobek AJ, Rempel DM, Ames BN (1996) Smoking and low antioxidant levels increase oxidative damage to sperm DNA. Mutat Res 351:199–203

Furuchi T, Masuko K, Nishimune Y, Obinata M, Matsui Y (1996) Inhibition of testicular germ cell apoptosis and differentiation in mice misexpressing Bcl-2 in spermatogonia. Development 122:1703–1709

Gardner MJ, Snee MP, Hall AJ, Powell CA, Downes S, Terrell JD (1990) Results of case-control study of leukaemia and lymphoma among young people near Sellafield nuclear plant in West Cumbria. Br Med J 300:423–429

Giwercman A, Bonde JP (1998) Declining male fertility and environmental factors. Endocrinol Metab Clin North Am 27:807–830, viii

Golden RJ, Noller KL, Titus-Ernstoff L, Kaufman RH, Mittendorf R, Stillman R, Reese EA (1998) Environmental endocrine modulators and human health: an assessment of the biological evidence. Crit Rev Toxicol 28:109–227

Goldsmith JR (1997) Epidemiologic evidence relevant to radar (microwave) effects. Environ Health Perspect 105 [Suppl 6]:1579–1587

Hales BF, Robaire B (1993) Paternally mediated effects on progeny outcome. In: Whitcomb RW, Zirkin BR (eds) Understanding male fertility: basic and clinical approaches. Raven, New York, pp 307–320

Handelsman DJ (1997) Sperm output of healthy men in Australia: magnitude of bias due to self-selected volunteers. Hum Reprod 12:2701–2705

Harrington JM, Stein GF, Rivera RO, de Morales AV (1978) The occupational hazards of formulating oral contraceptives – a survey of plant employees. Arch Environ Health 33:12–15

Hess RA (1990) Quantitative and qualitative characteristics of the stages and transitions in the cycle of the rat seminiferous epithelium: light microscopic observations of perfusion-fixed and plastic-embedded testes. Biol Reprod 43:525–542

Hess RA, Bunick D, Lee KH, Bahr J, Taylor JA, Korach KS, Lubahn DB (1997) A role for oestrogens in the male reproductive system. Nature 390:509–512

Hjollund NH, Bonde JP, Jensen TK, Ernst E, Henriksen TB, Kolstad HA, Giwercman A, Skakkebaek NE, Olsen J (1998a) Semen quality and sex hormones with reference to metal welding. Reprod Toxicol 12:91–95

Hjollund NH, Bonde JP, Jensen TK, Henriksen TB, Kolstad HA, Ernst E, Giwercman A, Pritzl G, Skakkebaek NE, Olsen J (1998b) A follow-up study of male exposure to welding and time to pregnancy. Reprod Toxicol 12:29–37

Hjollund NH, Skotte JH, Kolstad HA, Bonde JP (1999) Extremely low frequency magnetic fields and fertility: a follow up study of couples planning first pregnancies. The Danish First Pregnancy Planner Study Team. Occup Environ Med 56:253–255

Irvine S, Cawood E, Richardson D, MacDonald E, Aitken J (1996) Evidence of deteriorating semen quality in the United Kingdom: birth cohort study in 577 men in Scotland over 11 years. Br Med J 312:467–471

Jensh RP (1997) Behavioral teratologic studies using microwave radiation: is there an increased risk from exposure to cellular phones and microwave ovens? Reprod Toxicol 11:601–611

Ji BT, Shu XO, Linet MS, Zheng W, Wacholder S, Gao YT, Ying DM, Jin F (1997) Paternal cigarette smoking and the risk of childhood cancer among offspring of nonsmoking mothers. J Natl Cancer Inst 89:238–244

Jockenhövel F (1993) Hypogonadism and infertility as sequelae of general diseases and toxins. Internist (Berl) 34:741–755

Joffe M, Villard L, Li Z, Plowman R, Vessey M (1993) Long-term recall of time-to-pregnancy. Fertil Steril 60:99–104

Joffe M, Bisanti L, Apostoli P, Shah N, Kiss P, Dale A, Roeleveld N, Lindbohm ML, Sallmen M, Bonde JP (1999) Time to pregnancy and occupational lead exposure. Asclepios. Scand J Work Environ Health 25:64–65

Kandeel FR, Swerdloff RS (1988) Role of temperature in regulation of spermatogenesis and the use of heating as a method for contraception. Fertil Steril 49:1–23

Keck C, Bramkamp G, Behre HM, Muller C, Jockenhovel F, Nieschlag E (1995) Lack of correlation between cadmium in seminal plasma and fertility status of nonexposed individuals and two cadmium-exposed patients. Reprod Toxicol 9:35–40

Kelce WR, Wilson EM (1997) Environmental antiandrogens: developmental effects, molecular mechanisms, and clinical implications. J Mol Med 75:198–207

Kerr JB (1992) Spontaneous degeneration of germ cells in normal rat testis: assessment of cell types and frequency during the spermatogenic cycle. J Reprod Fertil 95:825–830

Kerr JF, Wyllie AH, Currie AR (1972) Apoptosis: a basic biological phenomenon with wide-ranging implications in tissue kinetics. Br J Cancer 26:239–257

Keys A. (ed) (1950) The biology of human starvation. University of Minnesota Press, Minneapolis

Kinlen LJ, Clarke K, Hudson C (1990) Evidence from population mixing in British New Towns 1946–85 of an infective basis for childhood leukaemia. Lancet 336:577–582

Kinlen LJ, Clarke K, Balkwill A (1993) Paternal preconceptional radiation exposure in the nuclear industry and leukaemia and non-Hodgkin's lymphoma in young people in Scotland. Br Med J 306:1153–1158

Knudson CM, Tung KS, Tourtellotte WG, Brown GA, Korsmeyer SJ (1995) Bax-deficient mice with lymphoid hyperplasia and male germ cell death. Science 270:96–99

Kodama K, Mabuchi K, Shigematsu I (1996) A long-term cohort study of the atomic-bomb survivors. J Epidemiol 6:S95–105

Lancranjan I, Popescu HI, Gravenescu O, Klepsch I, Serbanescu M (1975) Reproductive ability of workmen occupationally exposed to lead. Arch Environ Health 30:396–401

Larsen SB, Giwercman A, Spano M, Bonde JP (1998) A longitudinal study of semen quality in pesticide spraying Danish farmers. The ASCLEPIOS Study Group. Reprod Toxicol 12:581–589

Lee J, Richburg JH, Younkin SC, Boekelheide K (1997) The Fas system is a key regulator of germ cell apoptosis in the testis. Endocrinology 138:2081–2088

Lee J, Richburg JH, Shipp EB, Meistrich ML, Boekelheide K (1999) The Fas system, a regulator of testicular germ cell apoptosis, is differentially up-regulated in Sertoli cell versus germ cell injury of the testis. Endocrinology 140:852–858

Lerchl A, Nieschlag E (1996) Decreasing sperm counts? A critical (re)view. Exp Clin Endocrinol Diabetes 104:301–307

Lerchl A, Keck C, Spiteri-Grech J, Nieschlag E (1993) Diurnal variations in scrotal temperature of normal men and patients with varicocele before and after treatment. Int J Androl 16:195–200

Levine RJ, Symons MJ, Balogh SA, Arndt DM, Kaswandik NT, Gentile JW (1980) A method for monitoring the fertility of workers. 1. Method and pilot studies. J Occup Med 22:781–791

Linder RE, Klinefelter GR, Strader LF, Veeramachaneni DN, Roberts NL, Suarez JD (1997) Histopathologic changes in the testes of rats exposed to dibromoacetic acid. Reprod Toxicol 11:47–56

Lord BI, Woolford LB, Wang L, Stones VA, McDonald D, Lorimore SA, Papworth D, Wright EG, Scott D (1998) Tumour induction by methyl-nitroso-urea following preconceptional paternal contamination with plutonium-239. Br J Cancer 78:301–311

Lundsberg LS, Bracken MB, Belanger K (1995) Occupationally related magnetic field exposure and male subfertility. Fertil Steril 63:384–391

MacLeod J, Wang Y (1979) Male fertility potential in terms of semen quality: a review of the past, a study of the present. Fertil Steril 31:103–116

McLachlan JA (1997) Synergistic effect of environmental estrogens: report withdrawn. Science 277:462–463

Meistrich ML (1993) Potential genetic risks of using semen collected during chemotherapy. Hum Reprod 8:8–10

Meistrich ML, van Beek MEAB (1990) Radiation sensitivity of the human testis. Adv Radiat Biol 14:227–268

Mieusset R, Bujan L (1994) The potential of mild testicular heating as a safe, effective and reversible contraceptive method for men. Int J Androl 17:186–191

Mieusset R, Quintana Casares P, Sanchez Partida LG, Sowerbutts SF, Zupp JL, Setchell BP (1992) Effects of heating the testes and epididymides of rams by scrotal insulation on fertility and embryonic mortality in ewes inseminated with frozen semen. J Reprod Fertil 94:337–343

Mylchreest E, Sar M, Cattley RC, Foster PM (1999) Disruption of androgen-regulated male reproductive development by di(n-butyl) phthalate during late gestation in rats is different from flutamide. Toxicol Appl Pharmacol 156:81–95

Nagel SC, vom Saal FS, Thayer KA, Dhar MG, Boechler M, Welshons WV (1997) Relative binding affinity-serum modified access (RBA-SMA) assay predicts the relative in vivo bioactivity of the xenoestrogens bisphenol A and octylphenol. Environ Health Perspect 105:70–76

Neel JV (1998) Reappraisal of studies concerning the genetic effects of the radiation of humans, mice, and Drosophila. Environ Mol Mutagen 31:4–10

Nelson CM, Bunge RG (1974) Semen analysis: evidence for changing parameters of male fertility potential. Fertil Steril 25:503–507

Niehaus M, Bruggemeyer H, Behre HM, Lerchl A (1997) Growth retardation, testicular stimulation, and increased melatonin synthesis by weak magnetic fields (50 Hz) in Djungarian hamsters, *Phodopus sungorus*. Biochem Biophys Res Commun 234:707–711

Oberländer G, Yeung CH, Cooper TG (1994) Induction of reversible infertility in male rats by oral ornidazole and its effects on sperm motility and epididymal secretions. J Reprod Fertil 100:551–559

Olsen GW, Bodner KM, Ramlow JM, Ross CE, Lipshultz LI (1995) Have sperm counts been reduced 50 percent in 50 years? A statistical model revisited. Fertil Steril 63:887–893

Pajarinen JT, Karhunen PJ (1994) Spermatogenic arrest and 'Sertoli cell-only' syndrome – common alcohol-induced disorders of the human testis. Int J Androl 17:292–299

Parker L, Pearce MS, Dickinson HO, Aitkin M, Craft AW (1999) Stillbirths among offspring of male radiation workers at Sellafield nuclear reprocessing plant. Lancet 354:1407–1414

Paulsen CA, Berman, NG, Wang C (1996) Data from men in greater Seattle area reveals no downward trend in semen quality: further evidence that deterioration of semen quality is not geographically uniform. Fertil Steril 65:1015–1020

Potts RJ, Newbury CJ, Smith G, Notarianni LJ, Jefferies TM (1999) Sperm chromatin damage associated with male smoking. Mutat Res 423:103–111

Print CG, Loveland KL, Gibson L, Meehan T, Stylianou A, Wreford N, de Kretser D, Metcalf D, Kontgen F, Adams JM, Cory S (1998) Apoptosis regulator bcl-w is essential for spermatogenesis but appears otherwise redundant. Proc Natl Acad Sci USA 95:12424–12431

Rodriguez I, Ody C, Araki K, Garcia I, Vassalli P (1997) An early and massive wave of germinal cell apoptosis is required for the development of functional spermatogenesis. EMBO J 16:2262–2270

Rousseaux S, Sele B, Cozzi J, Chevret E (1993) Immediate rearrangements of human sperm chromosomes following invivo irradiation. Hum Reprod 8:903–907

Rowley MJ, Leach DR, Warner GA, Heller CG (1974) Effect of graded doses of ionizing radiation on the human testis. Radiat Res 59:665–678

Sankila R, Olsen JH, Anderson H, Garwicz S, Glattre E, Hertz H, Langmark F, Lanning M, Moller T, Tulinius H (1998) Risk of cancer among offspring of childhood-cancer survivors. Association of the Nordic Cancer Registries and the Nordic Society of Paediatric Haematology and Oncology. N Engl J Med 338:1339–1344

Seed J, Chapin RE, Clegg ED, Dostal LA, Foote RH, Hurtt ME, Klinefelter GR, Makris SL, Perreault SD, Schrader S, Seyler D, Sprando R, Treinen KA, Veeramachaneni DN, Wise LD (1996) Methods for assessing sperm motility, morphology, and counts in the rat, rabbit, and dog: a consensus report. ILSI Risk Science Institute Expert Working Group on Sperm Evaluation. Reprod Toxicol 10:237–244

Setchell BP (1997) Sperm counts in semen of farm animals 1932–1995. Int J Androl 20:209–214

Setchell BP (1998) The Parkes Lecture. Heat and the testis. J Reprod Fertil 114:179–194

Setchell BP, Ekpe G, Zupp JL, Surani MA (1998) Transient retardation in embryo growth in normal female mice made pregnant by males whose testes had been heated. Hum Reprod 13:342–347

Sharpe RM (1993) Declining sperm counts in men – is there an endocrine cause? J Endocrinol 136:357–360

Sharpe RM, Skakkebaek NE (1993) Are oestrogens involved in falling sperm counts and disorders of the male reproductive tract? Lancet 341:1392–1395

Sharpe RM, Fisher JS, Millar MM, Jobling S, Sumpter JP (1995) Gestational and lactational exposure of rats to xenoestrogens results in reduced testicular size and sperm production. Environ Health Perspect 103:1136–1143

Sharpe RM, Atanassova N, McKinnell C, Parte P, Turner KJ, Fisher JS, Kerr JB, Groome NP, Macpherson S, Millar MR, Saunders PT (1998) Abnormalities in functional development of the Sertoli cells in rats treated neonatally with diethylstilbestrol: a possible role for estrogens in Sertoli cell development. Biol Reprod 59:1084–1094

Skakkebaek NE, Rajpert-De Meyts E, Jorgensen N, Carlsen E, Petersen PM, Giwercman A, Andersson AG, Jensen TK, Andersson AM, Muller J (1998) Germ cell cancer and disorders of spermatogenesis: an environmental connection? Apmis 106:3–11

Skotte JH, Hjollund HI (1997) Exposure of welders and other metal workers to ELF magnetic fields. Bioelectromagnetics 18:470–477

Sloan DG (1982) Male fertility potential. Fertil Steril 37:126

Sohoni P, Sumpter JP (1998) Several environmental oestrogens are also anti-androgens. J Endocrinol 158:327–339

Sorahan T, Lancashire RJ, Hultén MA, Peck I, Stewart AM (1997a) Childhood cancer and parental use of tobacco: deaths from 1953 to 1955. Br J Cancer 75:134–138

Sorahan T, Prior P, Lancashire RJ, Faux SP, Hultén MA, Peck IM, Stewart AM (1997b) Childhood cancer and parental use of tobacco: deaths from 1971 to 1976. Br J Cancer 76:1525–1531

Sullivan FM (1988) Reproductive toxicity tests: retrospect and prospect. Hum Toxicol 7:423–427

Tapanainen JS, Tilly JL, Vihko KK, Hsueh AJ (1993) Hormonal control of apoptotic cell death in the testis: gonadotropins and androgens as testicular cell survival factors. Mol Endocrinol 7:643–650

Thonneau P, Bujan L, Multigner L, Mieusset R (1998) Occupational heat exposure and male fertility: a review. Hum Reprod 13:2122–2125

Toppari J, Larsen JC, Christiansen P, Giwercman A, Grandjean P, Guillette LJ Jr, Jegou B, Jensen TK, Jouannet P, Keiding N, Leffers H, McLachlan JA, Meyer O, Muller J, Rajpert-De Meyts E, Scheike T, Sharpe R, Sumpter J, Skakkebaek NE (1996) Male reproductive health and environmental xenoestrogens. Environ Health Perspect 104 [Suppl 4]:741–803

Trasler JM, Hales BF, Robaire B (1985) Paternal cyclophosphamide treatment of rats causes fetal loss and malformations without affecting male fertility. Nature 316:144–146

Tsang AY, Lee WM, Wong PY (1981) Effects of antifertility drugs on epididymal protein secretion, acquisition of sperm surface proteins and fertility in male rats. Int J Androl 4:703–712

Van Waeleghem K, De Clercq N, Vermeulen L, Schoonjans F, Comhaire F (1996) Deterioration of sperm quality in young healthy Belgian men. Hum Reprod 11:325–329

Vierula M, Niemi M, Keiski A, Saaranen M, Saarikoski S, Suominen J (1996) High and unchanged sperm counts of Finnish men. Int J Androl 19:11–17

Vogt HJ, Heller WD, Obe G (1984) Spermatogenesis in smokers and non-smokers: an andrological and genetic study. In: Obe G (ed) Mutation in man. Springer, Berlin Heidelberg New York, pp 247–291

Walker C, Ahmed SA, Brown T, Ho SM, Hodges L, Lucier G, Russo J, Weigel N, Weise T, Vandenbergh J (1999) Species, interindividual, and tissue specificity in endocrine signaling. Environ Health Perspect 107:619–624

Wang C, McDonald V, Leung A, Superlano L, Berman N, Hull L, Swerdloff RS (1997) Effect of increased scrotal temperature on sperm production in normal men. Fertil Steril 68:334–339

Welch LS, Schrader SM, Turner TW, Cullen MR (1988) Effects of exposure to ethylene glycol ethers on shipyard painters: II. Male reproduction. Am J Ind Med 14:509–526

Whorton D, Krauss RM, Marshall S, Milby TH (1977) Infertility in male pesticide workers. Lancet 2:1259–1261

Wilcox AJ, Baird DD, Weinberg CR, Hornsby PP, Herbst AL (1995) Fertility in men exposed prenatally to diethylstilbestrol. N Engl J Med 332:1411–1416

Wilton LJ, Temple-Smith PD, Baker HW, de Kretser DM (1988) Human infertility caused by degeneration and death of sperm in the epididymis. Fertil Steril 49:1052–1058

World Health Organization (1999) WHO Laboratory Handbook for the Examination of Human Semen and Sperm-Cervical Mucus Interaction. Cambridge University Press, Cambridge

Xuezhi J, Youxin L, Yilan W (1992) Studies of lead exposure on reproductive system: a review of work in China. Biomed Environ Sci 5:266–275

Yin Y, Stahl BC, DeWolf WC, Morgentaler A (1998) p53-mediated germ cell quality control in spermatogenesis. Dev Biol 204:165–171

Zenzes MT, Puy LA, Bielecki R, Reed TE (1999) Detection of benzo[a]pyrene diol epoxide-DNA adducts in embryos from smoking couples: evidence for transmission by spermatozoa. Mol Hum Reprod 5:125–131

CHAPTER 14

Gynecology Relevant to Andrology

14

U. A. KNUTH · H. P. G. SCHNEIDER · H. M. BEHRE

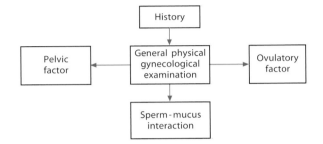

Fig. 14.1. Main diagnostic areas of female infertility work-up

The care and the successful treatment of the infertile couple requires a multidisciplinary approach which supports and counsels the couple as an entity. The flowchart in Fig. 14.1 enables the non-gynecologist to appreciate the main diagnostic and therapeutic steps necessary for the evaluation and treatment of female factors of a couple's infertility.

14.1 Medical History and Somatic Factors

14.1.1 Age

The decline in female fecundity with advancing age is well known; donor insemination studies which allow for a constant male factor show a decrease in female fertility with increasing female age. Fig. 14.2 shows exemplary studies (Schwartz and Mayaux 1982; Yeh and Seibel 1987). IVF/ICSI cycles reported in the German IVF Register (1998) and evaluated prospectively showed a pregnancy rate per transfer of 25.8% for the 30–34 year-old group (n = 8383); this dropped to 20.4% in the following group of 35–39 year-olds (n = 5517) and fell further to 11.7% in patients (n = 1568) even older. Declining female fertility is ascribed to an age-dependent decrease in ovarian function. An increase in FSH levels parallel to female age begins at the age of 25 (Ebbiary et al. 1994).

The FSH level, in addition to inhibin B in the early follicular phase, combined with estradiol and progesterone, is the most important parameter for diagnosing de-

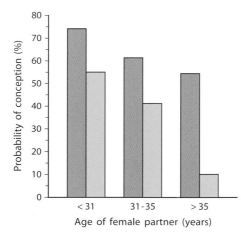

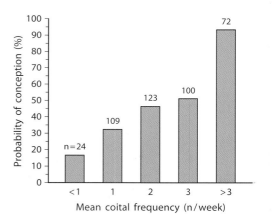

Fig. 14.2. Relationship between probability of conception and female age according to two independent studies. *Red columns*: redrawn from Federation CECOS, Schwartz and Mayaux (1982) reprinted with permission (New England Journal of Medicine 1982, 306:404–406). *Pink columns*: redrawn from Yeh and Seibel (1987), reprinted with permission from the American College of Obstetricians and Gynecoligists (Obstetrics and Gynecology 1987, 70:313–316)

Fig. 14.4. Rate of conception depending on coital frequency per week in couples who achieved a pregnancy within 6 months of unprotected intercourse. Adapted from MacLeod J, Gold RZ. The male factor in fertility and infertility: IV. Semen quality and certain other factors in relation to ease of conception. (Fertil Steril 1953, 4:10–33. Reproduced with permission of the publisher, the American Society for Reproductive Medicine [formerly The American Fertility Society])

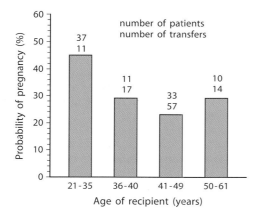

Fig. 14.3. Pregnancy rates after transfer of donated oocytes depending on recipient's age. Adapted from Flamigni et al. (1993) with permission of the publisher (Human Reproduction 1993, 8:2088–2092)

clining ovarian function (Gülekli et al. 1999; Corson et al. 1999). Conversely, assisted reproduction studies of couples in which older women receive oocytes from younger donors show normal fertility rates (Fig. 14.3). However, even here fertility rates decline after the age of 35 years.

The older woman undeniably bears an increased risk of pathological alterations of her reproductive organs. Moreover, a subgroup of patients with decreased fertility evolves among those who do not conceive despite

years of unprotected intercourse. In these cases age is only an apparent factor for the decline in fertility. A retrospective study by structured interview after delivery showed that no change occurs in the latency rates until conception in normal fertile women between the ages of 26 and 35 years (Knuth and Mühlenstedt 1991).

14.1.2 Coital Frequency

The decline in fecundity with advancing age is seen by some authors to result solely from a decrease in coital frequency per cycle (James 1979). Other studies have shown that this factor must be assessed before forming a prognosis in the treatment of the infertile couple (Fig. 14.4).

Increased coital frequency augments the probability of fertile sperm reaching the Fallopian tubes at the optimal time. One could thus deduce that low coital frequency, perhaps only at the time of ovulation, could result in acceptable rate of conception. Such a recommendation is, however, often counterproductive. Recommendations to have intercourse on certain days or even at a certain time of day cause considerable stress, often preventing couples from having normal intercourse with intravaginal ejaculation (Agarwal and Haney 1994). The experienced physician will only suggest timed intercourse before and during the "fertile days". Recommendations as to the frequency or time of day for intercourse should be withheld. Natural conception studies have shown that a single act of intercourse timed between 6 days before and 3 days after ovulation results in pregnancy (France et al. 1992). Reevaluation of earlier publications shows that the highest rates of spontaneous conceptions occur when coitus takes place on the day prior to ovulation (Dunson et al. 1999).

14.1.3 Length of Childlessness

The duration of barrenness is directly related to the probability of conceiving and represents an important prognostic parameter. A clinical study of 969 Dutch couples (Eimers et al. 1994) showed an 11% decline in the fertility rates with the numbers of years of unprotected intercourse. A woman who has spent seven years unintentionally childless thus has only a 50% chance of becoming pregnant compared to a woman with one year of infertility. If, however, she had an earlier pregnancy, the factor increases chances for probable conception by 74% compared with a population with primary infertility.

14.1.4 Risk of Infection

The probability that the couple's infertility is due to a tubal factor rises with the number of sexual partners in the past and is also correlated with age at first intercourse.

14.1.5 Psychological Factors

Female sexual interest seems to be correlated with the menstrual phase. Increased libido in the follicular phase results in a natural rise in coital frequency during the fertile phase (Dennerstein et al. 1994). Infertility therapy can, however, deeply disturb the couple's sexuality, interrupting physiological events and resulting in functional infertility. During infertility therapy inherent sexual dysfunction is often magnified. It can be symptomatically divided into three groups: loss of libido, orgasmic dysfunction, and inability for intravaginal intercourse (Herms 1989).

Libido Dysfunction and Orgasmic Disturbances

The primary absence of sexual desire (**alibidinia**) is extremely rare. The decrease or loss of libido is usually a secondary change. Psychological causes, such as deep-rooted fear or depression, can result in aversion reactions, in a loss of sexual interest, or even in sexual deviations. The group of organic causes includes chronic dyspareunia, endocrinological imbalance and debilitating disease. Psychotropic drugs such as antihypertensives, tranquilizers or sedatives can alter the patient's libido. Even the constant availability of a sexual partner can re-

sult in apathy, a loss of sexual interest and even in sexual aversion. This, of course, results in reduced coital frequency and thus reduced fertility. Factors which cause a change in libido can also influence orgasmic capability.

Dyspareunia

In contrast to inhibited sexual desire and orgasmic dysfunction, which are usually psychological disturbances, the main factor for dyspareunia is physical discomfort. Painful intercourse, called **algopareunia**, can have organic as well as psychological origins, which may occur sequentially. Timed intercourse recommended during an infertility treatment program can itself be a major factor in initiating this symptom.

In some patients, **vaginismus**, an involuntary painful spasm of the pelvic floor, inhibits intercourse. This is often combined with a defensive reaction of the entire body in the form of lordosis and adduction of the lower extremities. This reaction is always psychological in nature, and is often combined with sexual fear or a traumatic sexual experience in the past. The care of the patient must be in the form of psychotherapy, and never of surgical nature.

14.1.6 Hormones and Female Sexuality

The influence of hormonal factors on female sexuality is not as clear as it is for male sexuality. **Estrogens** are necessary for normal vaginal reaction during sexual arousal, but their influence on sexual desire and female orgasm is not as distinct. An important role in female libido is ascribed to testosterone. In women with androgen deficiency loss of libido is the dominant clinical symptom (Davis 1999a). This loss can be effectively compensated by appropriate substitution of androgens or androgen precursors such as dehydroepiandrosterone (Arlt et al. 1999; Davis 1999b). However, the role of hormones in female sexuality is either strongly modified by **psychosocial factors** or results in a much more individualized reaction when compared to that of males (Bancroft 1993).

14.1.7 Stress

During the treatment of infertility stress is often mentioned as one of the possible causes of failed conception. However, there is no clear definition of this entity which could be used for a reproducible experimental study. Stress implies a pooling of many negative factors which influence well-being, such as exhaustion stemming from rest or sleep deficiency, tension and inability to find relief from real or imagined pressure. An investigation of

420 Danish couples seeking infertility treatment for the first time showed a reduction in the probability of conception from 16.5% to 12.8% in couples with a high stress score, i.e. >80th percentile on the General Health Questionnaire (Hjollund et al. 1999). Over and beyond such systematic studies, often anecdotal and casuistic evidence is offered to support the thesis that stress factors decrease female fertility. One example often cited is the supposedly increased pregnancy rate after adoption. A systematic study, however, shows that the conception rate of 4.3% post adoption is equal to that of couples who do not adopt (Banks 1961). That acutely stressful situations need not be an obstacle to pregnancy can be inferred from high pregnancy rates (5%) following rape (Holmes et al. 1996). Menstrual cycle changes which are caused by stress are, however, well documented and are discussed in section 14.2.4.

Immunological Modulation and Stress

Recently reciprocal relationships between stress and immunological events have been increasingly noted. Especially in the female there seem to be powerful mechanisms in which immunological factors stimulate stress factors and result in decreased fertility.

An increased secretion of corticotropin-releasing hormone (CRH), with the resulting stimulation of ACTH, causes a rise of glucocorticoid secretion. This modulates precursors of prostaglandin synthesis, platelet activating factor, serotonin, cytokinins, interleukin-1 and -6 and tumor necrosis factor (TNF). CRH is a part of the proopiomelanocortin system, and thus regulates the secretion of α-MSH and β-endorphin, which, in combination with met-encephalin, directly influences the function and activity of the immunocytes. It can be concluded that a stress situation can negatively influence implantation via autoimmune factors. This complex interaction promises to become a major area of female infertility research in the future (Negro-Vilar 1993; Chrousos 1995).

14.1.8 Environmental Factors

So-called **"environmental factors"** are often cited while searching for a cause for infertility. It is, however, almost never possible to make a clear statement pertaining to particular environmental factors on female infertility and their influence on an individual couple's infertility.

Definitions

Several years ago the WHO initiated a study of environmental factors relevant to fertility (Baranski 1993). To measure the influence of potentially harmful substances, a measurable parameter is required. An often cited parameter is the infertility rate. Using this parameter, the rate of infertility in a group of normal patients is compared to the infertility rate in a group of patients who are under the influence of a certain external environmental factor. Methodical problems arise whenever infertility is to be characterized, as the definition may be subject to varying preconditions:

- Failure to conceive after one year of unprotected intercourse.
- Failure to achieve a clinically discernable pregnancy after one year of unprotected intercourse.
- Failure to deliver a viable baby after one year of unprotected intercourse.

These three different definitions already demonstrate that methods of confirming a pregnancy alone may influence the parameter "infertility rate" as well as results.

Since the organism is never exposed exclusively to one potentially noxious environmental factor, the influence of possible cofactors such as nicotine, alcohol, caffeine and other substance abuse must be considered in first instance. Certain behavioral patterns are also correlated with other socio-economic factors, which again influence the fertility rate.

Epidemiology

Although extensive lists exist of environmental factors possibly influencing female fertility (Baranski 1993), they are usually of little use for practical counselling of the individual infertile couple, since even the best epidemiological studies only show a slightly elevated risk for a population exposed to a potential environmental hazard as a whole. Infertility rates in women rise when they are continually exposed to toxins such as anesthetics, asbestos, textile dyes and dry cleaning agents. The risk for infertility is increased by a factor of 2.4 in women exposed to a high level of noise (Rachootin and Olsen 1983). Even specialized databases fail to provide useful data on toxic influences on human reproductive functions (Scialli 1994). The fact that less than 1% of over 60,000 chemical substances included in lists of toxic materials has been investigated, illustrates the magnitude of the problem.

Even well-controlled studies fail to give a precise picture of the influence of certain factors on fertility. A study of dental assistants who were exposed to mercury vapor showed, for example, that the fertility of women who assisted in more than 30 fillings per week only reached 63% of the fertility of those women not exposed to mercury vapor. However, the fertility rate of those women with a low exposure to mercury vapor was better than that of the non-exposed controls (Rowland et al. 1994).

Nicotine

Compared to poorly definable environmental factors, the exposure to nicotine plays a practical role which can usually be eliminated. Although the effect of nicotine on fertility is not consistently described in the literature, a large British study clearly demonstrates a negative effect of nicotine on fertility. Female nicotine consumption resulted in a 12% rise in the conceptive latency in 11,407 persons born in 1958 and followed in Great Britain. Male smoking did not cause a negative effect on fertility after data was corrected for socio-economical factors (Joffe and Li 1994). A prospective Danish study of 430 couples showed a reduced rate of fecundity (=0.53) in women who smoked, compared with non-smokers (95% confidence interval 0.31–0.91). An important factor was whether the mothers of the women investigated had smoked during pregnancy (Jensen et al. 1998). It is also known the IVF results are poorer in women who smoke, and that ovarian function also declines earlier in this population. One of the first steps in patient education and counselling during infertility treatment should thus be to abandon nicotine consumption.

X rays and Radioactivity

Although the negative effects of smoking on female fertility have been proven, most of the affected woman do not find it necessary to change their behavior. In contrast to this, the influence of X rays and radioactivity on fertility is usually overestimated by the general population.

Epidemiological studies and detailed analysis of radioactive exposure of females before conception show no clear effects (Committee on the Biological Effect of Ionizing Radiation 1990). A study of 627 women with thyroid carcinoma who were treated with radioactive iodine (^{131}I) showed no significant difference in the fertility rate when compared to controls (Dottorini et al. 1995). The ovarian radioactive dose in such a therapy was determined to be 1.14 ± 0.34 Gy (mean$\pm$SEM) (Izembart 1992). In this study 12 of 50 patients developed amenorrhoea and 38 showed no change in ovarian function. The effect of age on onset of menopause was, however, not clearly delineated in the study. Total body radiation because of neoplastic disease during childhood results in definitively higher total body doses. These cover a range between 20 and 30 Gy. Women who have survived this form of treatment and have continuing ovarian function often deliver low birth weight infants. This is explained by hypoplasia of uterine tissue and im-

paired vascularization (Critchey et al. 1992). Research data show a variable influence of radiation on female fertility. It cannot be deduced that a pregnancy will not be achievable in these patients. An ovarian dose of 4 Gy can cause sterility in about 30% of young women and in 100% of women over the age of 40 years (Ogilvy-Stuart and Shalet 1993). These results are underlined by data obtained from patients treated with chemotherapy and radiation in Hodgkin disease (Bokemeyer et al. 1994).

Electromagnetic Fields

In contrast to the low number of patients who have been exposed to radioactive materials or X rays, almost every patient seen for infertility counselling has been or is exposed to weak electromagnetic fields. Some consider so-called "electro-smog" as the causal factor for infertility. This has not been proven for the average patient. Even in extreme situations, such as the personnel of nuclear magnetic resonance imaging departments, no change in fertility rates was apparent (Kanal et al. 1993). The harmlessness of **ultrasonography** for the fetus will be discussed later.

14.1.9 Pertinent Medical History

Physiology of Pregnancy

An assessment of the medical history for female and male factors affecting infertility is important in infertility counselling since often causal therapeutical options become possible. Notwithstanding, consideration of diseases which may worsen during pregnancy is also necessary, so that the couple may be counselled to forego further therapy.

Such changes in pregnancy may be caused by adaptations in the cardiovascular system as well as by immunological events. Renal circulation increases 50% in early pregnancy. The circulating blood volume expands during pregnancy by between 27 and 64%. Cardiac output grows from 4.5 to 5.5 l/min and the pulse rate also rises from 70 to about 85 beat/min at the end of pregnancy. There are no major changes in the respiratory system.

The ureters dilate during pregnancy and may also become compressed. This results in a higher infection rate and/or hydronephrosis. The motility of the gastrointestinal tract decreases. Liver function is usually not altered. Thyroidal activity is stimulated with a rise in protein-bound iodine levels. Carbohydrate metabolism usually remains constant, although a slight glucosuria is common as a result of a lower renal threshold for glucose.

Pertinent Medical Disorders

Pulmonary disease. Pulmonary tuberculosis will not worsen during pregnancy. Pregnancy has a favorable influence on the course of uncomplicated sarcoidosis with a possible decrease of pulmonary hilus lymphomas. The course of asthma is also usually not altered during pregnancy.

Cardiovascular system. Manifest cardiovascular disease may deteriorate owing to the physiological changes that occur in the cardiovascular system during pregnancy. A patient with cardiac disease should thus consult a cardiologist before beginning infertility therapy. Today pregnancy is even possible following heart transplant (Morini et al. 1998).

Gastrointestinal disease. Inflammatory bowel disease usually has no effect on fertility. In severe Crohn's disease or ulcerative colitis one should, however, wait for a less active or inactive phase to plan pregnancy, if possible.

Viral hepatitis is a much more significant factor in infertility therapy. In areas endemic to hepatitis A, women usually become immune to hepatitis A before reaching reproductive age. Children of mothers who develop acute hepatitis A during pregnancy show no effects of the disease. Thus hepatitis A is not a true problem in infertility therapy.

The situation with hepatitis B infection is more serious. Prenatal care studies in Germany show a positive hepatitis B antigen in 0.73 to 1.73 % of all women examined (Joosten and Stürner 1980). Intrauterine transmission of this infection to the fetus is, however, rare. More than 90 % of infected children probably result from direct contact of the newborn with infectious maternal blood during vaginal delivery (review article by Heckers and Lasch 1986).

The relatively low risk of an intrauterine hepatitis B infection was demonstrated during an unfortunate situation in which 22 women were contaminated with hepatitis B in an IVF programme. All women suffered from acute hepatitis B during the first trimester. Hepatitis B-DNA could not, however, be isolated in the serum or in the lymphocytes of the 22 exposed children (Quint et al. 1994).

The importance of hepatitis C is more imminent than that of hepatitis B, since passive immunization does not seem to be a possibility in this infection. In northern Europe investigations in blood donors revealed a rate of disease between 0.01 % and 0.05 %.

The infection persists in about 80 % of all cases and leads to chronic persistent or chronic active hepatitis, with 20–30 % developing into cirrhosis. Passive immunization is not currently available and treatment with interferon has yielded only few data.

Intrauterine transmission of acute hepatitis C has been clearly demonstrated. Follow-up of 403 women post-delivery with hepatitis C virus antibodies and their offspring revealed infection in 13 of 403 neonates (3.2 %). This applied only to infants whose mothers were virus-RNA positive. As six infants were virus RNA-positive immediately after birth, an intrauterine infection must be assumed (Resti et al. 1998). If patient history reports hepatitis C, or if a finding of such arises during a routine diagnostic step in infertility therapy, counselling must include the risk for the fetus. The potential of interferon therapy has yet to be clarified in these particular cases.

The risk of hepatitis C transmission to spouses of carriers is not clear (Van der Poel et al. 1994).

A patient with chronic hepatitis need not expect a progression of the disease during pregnancy. In patients with chronic aggressive hepatitis, however, only the autoimmune form is not influenced by pregnancy. The prognosis in chronic aggressive hepatitis B is reduced. Experts are not, however, able to make general recommendations for this situation. In the case of esophageal varicosis due to liver cirrhosis, experts recommend prophylactic sclerosis prior to planned pregnancy.

In contrast to the various forms of hepatitis, ulcerative disease is not a problem either before or during pregnancy. An initial attack rarely occurs during pregnancy. Cholecystitis is described more frequently than peptic ulcer disease. One of 1300 cholecystectomies are performed during pregnancy. There is, however, no special need for counselling concerning this subject during infertility therapy.

HIV. In contrast to hepatitis, HIV-positive women seeking pregnancy represent only a small group in Germany. When the mother is seropositive, the probability of an intrauterine infection is about 20 % if a caesarean section is done and when the mother does not nurse. If the mother is treated (e. g. with azidothymide) during pregnancy, the risk of infant infection can be reduced to approximately 3 %. Independent of possible infant infection, HIV represents a fourfold higher risk of abortion and stillborn offspring (Brocklehurst and French 1998). The same authors documented an additional albeit weak effect of pregnancy on the further development of HIV disease (French and Brocklehurst 1998). In view of this situation, pregnancy in HIV-positive women can hardly be advocated or supported therapeutically.

Urinary tract. Pre-existing diseases of the urinary tract can cause severe complications in pregnancy. In particular cases patients should be counselled against further infertility therapy. During acute renal disease such as pyelonephritis or glomerulonephritis, pregnancy should be avoided. Treated tuberculosis of the urinary tract with negative controls is no argument against a pregnancy. A patient history of kidney stones or a surgically corrected congenital hydronephrosis do not present a contraindication for pregnancy. Progressive **polycystic degeneration of the kidneys** with restricted glomerular and tubular function have a poor prognosis in pregnancy, and thus also in infertility therapy. **Chronic glomerulonephritis** and **diabetic glomerulonephritis** are a high risk for the development of eclampsia and intrauterine fetal demise. During counselling of patients with a nephrotic syndrome one should more or less advise against further infertility therapy. After **renal transplantation**, however, patients may consider a pregnancy in consultation with a specialist 2–3 years after surgery (Kremling 1986).

Neoplasias. Malignant gynecological diseases such as **breast cancer**, **cervical cancer** and **ovarian cancer** differ as to the effects of a pregnancy on the course of the disease (Börner 1986). In summary, a pregnancy following breast cancer will not stimulate further disease or worsen the prognosis. Patients with a history of **carcinoma in situ of the uterine cervix** should allow a period of 6–12 months to pass during which cytological controls are negative before attempting therapy for infertility. Patients with **malignant ovarian tumors**, who were treated with a conservative unilateral salpingoovarectomy should be counselled to undertake contraceptive methods for a period of two years, since most recurrences appear during this period.

It is not possible to cover all of the diseases which may be influenced by pregnancy in this chapter. Most of the other diseases are quite rare, so that even gynecological obstetrical textbooks do not suffice in counselling an individual patient. A literature search will provide helpful and up-to-date information.

14.2 Ovarian Cycle and Ovulation

14.2.1 Follicles

The mainstay of female reproductive physiology is the maturation of the oocyte in conjunction with the menstrual cycle. The evaluation of the maturing ovarian follicle, of ovulation and of the luteal phase is therefore a central point in the workup of infertility patients.

Early Oocyte Development

The maturation of oocytes is a long process which begins during fetal development. Oocyte maturation is completed, however, only during fertilization, which often takes place up to more than 30 years after the beginning of oocyte development. During fetal life 6–7 million germ cells develop in the second trimester. By the time of birth, many of the germ cells have undergone atresia, and the newborn female has about two million ova. At this time, the **primary oocytes** have undergone the first part of the first meiotic division and have reached the first stage of arrest. This phase of arrest lasts until puberty, when ovulation of the oocytes begins.

Meiosis

Meiosis only continues when ovulation has taken place. One half of the paired chromosomes are expelled in the **first polar body**. The oocyte is now haploid. This phase is called the **metaphase II** and the oocyte is a **secondary oocyte**. This is the situation at the time of ovulation. If the oocyte is not fertilized, it remains in this stage. If fertilization occurs, one half of the chromatin is again expelled in form of the **second polar body**. Female meiosis, thus, in contrast to spermatogenesis, begins in the early fetal period and ends at the point of fertilization in the adult female.

Follicle Development

The development of the surrounding follicle occurs in parallel with ovarian oocyte development. During the eighth week of pregnancy the primary oocytes are surrounded by a single layer of spindle-shaped cells. These are **precursors of the later granulosa and theca cells**. The oocyte and the granulosa cells are surrounded by a basal membrane which separates the **primordial follicle** from the stroma. The follicle with layered granulosa cells is called a **secondary follicle**. In the seventh month of pregnancy an **antrum** can develop in the granulosa cell layer; the follicle is then called a **tertiary** or a **Graafian follicle**.

Regulatory Mechanisms

The granulosa cells begin to express **FSH receptors** during the fifth to sixth month of pregnancy. The number of receptors per cell remains constant; the absolute number of FSH receptors per follicle, however, rises with the increasing number of granulosa cells. During further development, receptors for estradiol, progesterone, testosterone and glucocorticoids can be detected. For the further development of the follicle FSH is required. This is supported by the influence of the estrogens. Thus a **positive feedback** exists in which even minimal FSH concentrations in the follicular fluid are answered by a positive feedback. It is of note that FSH is only detectable in the follicular fluid if the ratio of estrogens to androgens is dominated by estrogens and the quotient is above 1. If androgens increase, FSH is not detectable.

In addition to estradiol and FSH, other factors influence the mitotic division of the granulosa cells. Aromatase and LH receptors are induced depending on the FSH concentration and the time phase. The aromatases convert androgens into estrogens. The development of LH receptors in the **dominating follicle** prepares it for the midcyclic LH surge and thus for ovulation. Additionally, the LH receptors are necessary for the production of progesterone which occurs later in the corpus luteum. During follicle development, estradiol seems to act synergistically with FSH to facilitate the development of FSH receptors. Later in the cycle estradiol stimulates LH receptor density and the activity of the LH receptors. When estrogen synthesis is blocked, none of the Graafian follicles will grow in diameter over 2.2 mm. If FSH stimulation is blocked during follicle development, FSH and LH receptor numbers decline, and granulosa cells die.

Follicle Selection. Knowledge of follicular development is important for understanding impaired follicular maturation. The preovulatory rise in estradiol initiates a negative feedback, and thus a suppression of pituitary FSH secretion. Since the pre-ovulatory follicle has a higher receptor density than the other smaller follicles, further maturation is possible, whereas the smaller follicles must degenerate to **atretic** follicles. The effect of FSH can be modulated by prolactin and sexual steroids. Estrogen, insulin and other somatotropic factors can influence the aromatase activity and the development of LH receptors. The stimulation of aromatase, LH receptors and prolactin receptors by FSH seems to be restricted to the membranes of the granulosa cells. Thus a very complicated system of endocrine and paracrine regulatory mechanisms exist in which there are a multitude of steps during which the maturation of follicles can be disturbed.

Two-cell-theory. Further LH receptors develop in the cells of the **theca interna** of the Graafian follicle. The theca interna consists of mesenchymal cells surrounding the entire follicle. Under the influence of LH, the theca interna cells change into epithelial cells which are able to produce androgens, of which the most important is **androstenedione**. This androgen is the main precursor for follicular estradiol production and a significant factor for further follicle development. An excessive production of androgens, which exceeds the capacity of the aromatase to synthesize estrogens, causes a decline in the estrogen/androgen quotient and thus follicular atresia as already described. In an androgen-rich environment, the direction of conversion of androstenedione is changed even further from estrogen formation into additional androgen production. An optimal follicle can only develop if androgen production in the theca cells is followed by estrogen production from these androgens in the granulosa cells. This mechanism is called the **two-cell-theory** of follicular estrogen production. Like granulosa cells, the theca cells can also be influenced by other hormones. The regulation of the hypothalamic pituitary ovarian axis and the target organs is simplified in Fig. 14.5.

Paracrine regulation of ovarial function. In the light of recent investigations, the classic model of ovarian regulation appears inadequate. Follicle selection, growth, maturation and ovulation seem to be regulated by complex intraovarian mechanisms in conjunction with gonadotropins and sex steroids. These local factors presumably have both paracrine and autocrine effects. In the paracrine system, locally secreted messenger substances influence neighboring target cells of the same organ, whereas autocrine regulation influences secretory cells within the organ via surface receptors.

The list of autocrine/paracrine factors is growing rapidly. Current research is concentrated on the **IGF (insulin-like growth factor) system**. Beside the liver, the ovary is the main source of insulin-like growth factor I (IGF I). **IGF I** and **IGF II** are produced by the granulosa cell. IGF I increases the effect of LH and FSH and seems to be important in the coordination between theca and granulosa cell functions. FSH and LH increase the number of receptors on the granulosa cell and this reaction is additionally intensified by estrogens. In the theca cell, IGF I stimulates and increases steroid formation. On the whole, IGF I is important for the formation and increase of FSH and LH receptors, for steroidogenesis, for secretion of inhibin and oocyte maturation.

Along with IGF I receptors, the granulosa cell has receptors for **insulin**, which binds directly to IGF receptors. This cross-reactivity is important for many pathophysiologic events in the ovary, as insulin causes a modulation of ovarian function. The regulatory cascade is complicated by the fact that IGF molecules are bound and neutralized by IGF-binding proteins. Thus the concentration of IGF-binding proteins directly affects cell regulation. In addition, the **TGF (transforming growth factor) β gene** family is important. This term comprises substances such as **activin**, **inhibin** and "**growth and differentiation factor 9**" which modulates both stimulatory and inhibiting effects of gonadotropins. "Growth and differentiation factor 9" seems to be an oocyte-specific growth factor which is important for development beyond the primordial follicle. Additionally, an intraovarian **interleukin-1 system** seems to regulate periovulatory events reciprocally with LH (Udoff and Adashi 1999).

Beside growth processes which are connected with an increase of cell numbers in follicle maturation and ovulation, the elimination of supernumerary cells in the ovary is a decisive factor in normal ovarian function. This programmed cell death (apoptosis) is becoming a major research interest (Chun and Hsueh 1999).

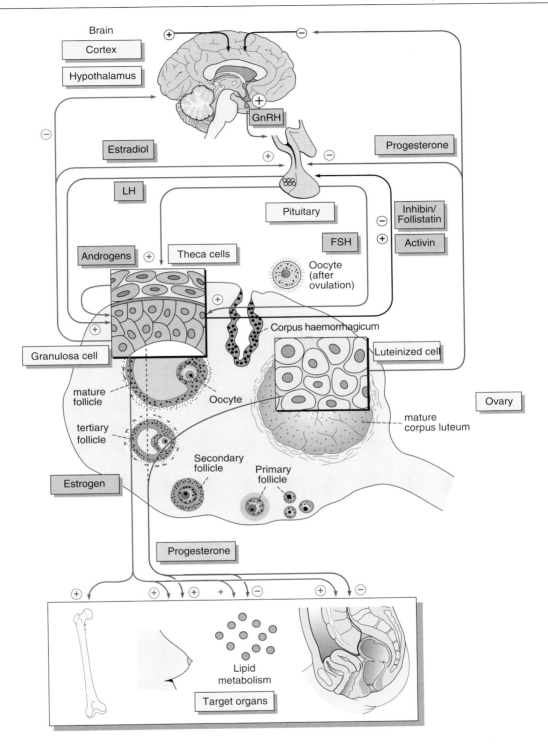

Fig. 14.5. Feed-back mechanism of hypothalamo-pituitary-go-nadal axis and interdependence of hormone production in the structures of theca and granulosa cell layers. The schematic drawing of the ovary shows the cyclic changes of the growing follicle. (From Nieschlag et al. 1999)

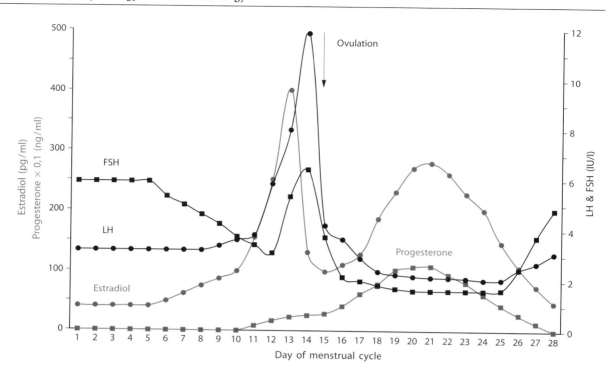

Fig. 14.6. Serum hormone concentrations during the menstrual cycle

Clinically, most of the paracrine parameters which have been discussed cannot be quantified. To evaluate normal or pathological development of follicle maturation, one still has to rely on classical measurement of sexual steroids and gonadotropins. Fig. 14.6 shows the course of the serum hormone concentrations used in routine clinical diagnosis.

14.2.2 Menstrual Cycle

Hormone Variations

The normal menstrual cycle can be divided into two phases: the follicular phase and the luteal phase. The first day of menstruation represents the first day of the cycle. The **follicular phase** lasts from the first day of menstruation until the pre-ovulatory LH surge. **Ovulation** occurs about 36–38 hours after the LH surge. As discussed above, estradiol concentrations rise during follicular development and cause a reduction in FSH during the second half of the follicular phase. Conversely, the rise of estradiol has a positive feedback effect on the production of LH, and thus causes the mid-cyclic LH surge. In clinical practice, one can expect normal peri-ovulatory mono-follicular development with an estradiol concen-

tration of 250 pg/ml in the serum. If during **ovulation** the ovum is extruded from the Graafian follicle, the remaining follicle develops into the **corpus luteum**, which produces progesterone, estradiol, and 17α-hydroxyprogesterone. The production of these hormones is stimulated by LH and choriogonadotropin. Progesterone secretion, combined with estradiol release, causes a negative feedback on gonadotropin secretion, so that serum levels gradually decrease at the end of the luteal phase.

LH is secreted in **pulses**; the interval between peaks during the follicular phase ranges from 60 to 90 minutes. The amplitude and the frequency rise continually as mid cycle is reached. After ovulation, a lower frequency of 100 to 300 minutes is attained. The amplitude, however, rises in the luteal phase. The pulsatile secretion of LH is caused by the pulsatile secretion of GnRH. This discontinual release is very important for infertility therapy (see below).

Luteal phase. Progesterone secretion after ovulation has a central thermogenic effect on the hypothalamus. Therefore, graphic representation of measurement of basal temperature (basal body temperature chart) can provide a first impression of cycle quality. A rise in morning temperature usually occurs when progesterone levels exceed 3 ng/ml. This level is, however, not representative for normal luteal function, so that even a basal temperature curve with a normal hyperthermic phase must not necessarily have an underlying normal follicular development with a normal luteal phase. On the

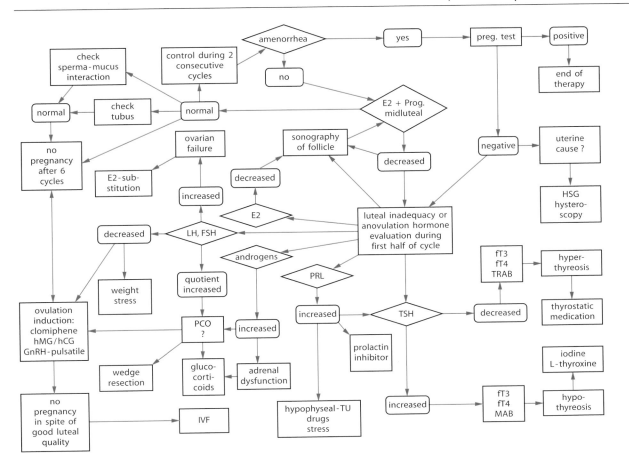

Fig. 14.7. Flow chart for the systematic diagnosis of impaired follicular growth. Only main areas are shown to facilitate readability. For more details see text

other hand, some women do not show a rise in basal temperature after producing the thermogenic pregnen-3α-ol-20-one so that the absence of a hyperthermic phase must not necessarily imply anovulation. The basal body temperature chart (BBT chart) is thus no longer such a central diagnostic tool as it was when **follicular development** and **ovulation** could not be followed **sonographically.**

> One must be especially careful not to use the BBT chart to set the time for insemination or timed intercourse, since the progesterone level described occurs 1–2 days after ovulation. The basal temperature curve should be used only in order to show variations of cycle quality and/or to time diagnostic procedures.

The second cyclic phase, the luteal phase, is relatively constant, and lasts 13–14 days in most women. The first half of the menstrual cycle can, however, vary greatly so that a menstrual cycle length between 21 and 35 days can be seen as normal, if the luteal phase remains constant.

Ovulation. The midpoint of the menstrual cycle is, naturally, ovulation, which must be recorded during the evaluation of the menstrual cycle (see Fig. 14.7). Next to ovulation, cyclic changes in the uterine cervix and the endometrium occur. The changes in cervical mucus are of eminent importance in the evaluation of the sperm-mucus-interaction (see Fig. 14.8).

Changes in the Uterine Cervix and in Cervical Mucus Production

The cervical os is the entrance to the uterine cavity and consists of a system of folds and gaps called cervical crypts or endocervical glands. These endocervical glands have a secretory epithelium combined with ciliated epithelium in a ratio of 10:1. The secretory cells produce the cervical mucus and lie mainly in the upper part

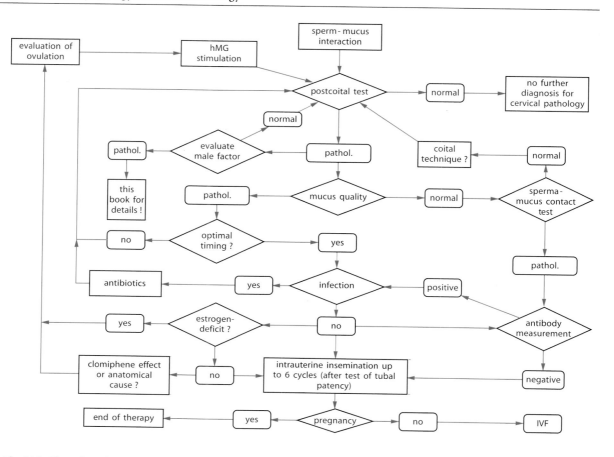

Fig. 14.8. Flow chart for the systematic evaluation of sperm-mucus-interaction. Only main areas are shown to facilitate readability. For more details see text.

of the cervix, close to the uterus. The secretory activity of the cervical epithelium undergoes cyclic changes, and thus can give easily obtainable information on the stage of the menstrual cycle. Important information is yielded by the **amount of mucus**, the **width of the external cervical os**, the **Spinnbarkeit** of the mucus, and the **fern-like pattern** which develops when drying. The amount of estrogen necessary to stimulate cervical mucus secretion varies in individual patients, and can vary from cycle to cycle. Cervical secretion is influenced by cervical infection, or after surgical procedures on the cervix. In some patients, cervical mucus production can be seen several days prior to ovulation; in other cases optimal cervix secretion occurs only a few hours before the LH surge. This must be taken into account when examining sperm-mucus-interaction. The development of the cervical factor can be judged using the **cervical index** of **Insler**. The technique of cervical mucus diagnosis is described in WHO 1999.

The uterine cervix and the cervical mucus are important for the ascent of the sperm, since they protect the

sperm from the acidic vaginal environment. The uterine cervix provides an energy-rich substrate for the spermatozoa, facilitates the transport of the sperm from the vagina into the uterine cavity, provides a reservoir for the sperm in the cervical crypts, and also acts as a filter which separates normally formed sperm from those that are malformed. (For a review on the cervix see Insler and Bettendorf 1977.)

Endometrium

The cyclic changes of the endometrium, like the changes of the cervical factor, reflect cyclic ovarian function and are of eminent importance for the nidation of the fertilized oocyte. The endometrium becomes thicker during the follicular phase. Uterine glands are drawn out so that they become lengthened. This proliferation has given the first half of the menstrual cycle its name. After ovulation is complete, vascularization of the endometrium is increased. Edema develops, the glands of the endometrium become convoluted and begin to secrete a clear fluid. Consequently, this phase of the cycle is the so-called secretory or luteal phase.

If pregnancy does not occur, the corpus luteum regresses; hormonal stimulation of the endometrium decreases and it becomes thinner. This adds to the curling of the arteries and focal necrosis occurs with local hemorrhage, which finally confluates and causes the menstrual flow. The cause of vascular necrosis is not known. Since the endometrium and the menstrual blood contain high concentrations of prostaglandins, and the infusion of prostaglandin PGF2α-causes necrosis of the endometrium, it seems possible that the prostaglandin release causes contraction of the blood vessels.

Seventy-five percent of menstrual blood is of arterial origin. It contains necrotic endometrial cells, prostaglandins, and a relatively high proportion of fibrinolysin. This is why usually no coagulation of the menstrual blood occurs. **Menstrual blood flow** usually lasts 3–5 days. A flow of 1–8 days can still be considered normal, unless a sudden change in the regular blood flow of a patient occurs. The average woman loses around 30 ml blood per cycle. This varies between slight smearing and up to a blood loss of 80 ml. If more than 80 ml is lost, a pathological cause must be considered. After menstruation the endometrium once again develops from the remaining cells of the basal layer.

Vaginal Epithelium

The vaginal epithelium undergoes cyclic changes under the influence of estrogen secretion as does the endometrium (for a review see Schnell 1973). Although alterations in the vaginal epithelium can indicate cycle phases, these are subject to great variation, so that no clearcut cyclic diagnosis can be obtained through cytological analysis of the vaginal epithelium.

tion and follicle maturation, ultrasound provides the possibility of following the **maturation of the follicle** and of ascertaining **ovulation**. Sonography thus constitutes a major component in the evaluation of the female factor in infertility, and is an indispensible tool.

Transabdominal sonography formerly used has been replaced by vaginal investigation. One major advantage is that the patient does not need to have a full bladder in order to provide an "acoustic window" through which the uterus and ovaries can be visualized. The vaginal probe lies in close approximation to pelvic structures so that a higher frequency can be used, leading to better resolution. In addition to classic sonography, measuring blood flow by doppler sonography provides further information. Tissue damage due to energy produced by the ultrasound waves has never been shown during clinical use of this diagnostic tool. The negative effects which have been described in animal experiments require a higher output level than is used in clinical sonography.

The sonographic picture of an ovary is a rotational ellipsoid with a volume below 6 ml. Pathological changes can be seen quite readily. An important pathological picture is that of the **polycystic ovary (PCO)**, the pathophysiology of which will be discussed later. Typically, small follicles under 1 cm arranged like a string of pearls along with an ovary larger than normal with increased stroma are seen (Fig. 14.9). In addition to PCO syndrome, **endometriosis** and other **cystic changes** of the ovary can at times also be identified by ultrasound. Changes in the Fallopian tube such as a **sactosalpinx**, in which peripheral closure of the tube causes tubal dilation by intratubal fluids, can often be diagnosed sonographically. If a sactosalpinx can be identified sonographically, women seeking pregnancy can benefit from

14.2.3 Diagnostic Evaluation of the Cycle

Essentially, evaluation of the female cycle requires the identification of optimal follicle maturation with ovulation, the development of a corpus luteum of good quality, as well as the physiological cyclic development of the endometrium which is necessary for nidation of a fertilized oocyte. It is important to remember that all the tests used in the evaluation of the cycle are indirect tests which have their limits.

Ultrasound

Although the basal body temperature chart, and the measurement of hormone concentrations in serum, urine, and saliva give indirect information about ovula-

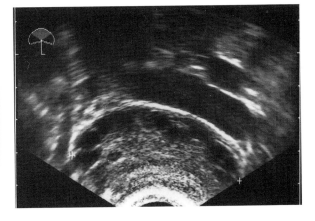

Fig. 14.9. Sonographic picture of polycystic ovary

salpinectomy prior to IVF therapy (Strandell et al. 1999). The most important aspect of sonography in infertility therapy is, however, the evaluation of follicle growth in the normal and the stimulated cycle. Additionally, the endometrium can be evaluated and invasive procedures can be avoided.

Endometrial Evaluation. Ultrasonographically, the endometrium presents as a relatively thin and homogenous echo during the proliferative phase. During the late proliferative phase the thickness increases and measures about 5 mm in the anterior-posterior diameter. Edema of the stroma often causes an echo-dense edge of the uterine cavity, so that prior to ovulation often a multi-layered picture of the endometrium is seen. In the luteal phase the thickness of the endometrium lies between 7 and 9 mm.

Evaluation of the Ovaries. In optimal cases, ultrasound resolution identifies ovarian structures up to 2 mm. As early as day 5 of the cycle, the dominant follicle is selected from the other primordial follicles. Between the eighth and the twelfth day it has reached a diameter of 14 mm. During the last 4–5 days prior to ovulation, the diameter of the dominant follicle increases between 2 and 3 mm per day. The follicle thus reaches a diameter of 16–28 mm. The variable size does not allow the prediction of the time of ovulation on the basis of ultrasound alone, so that ultrasound diagnosis should always be combined with determination of estradiol and LH levels during the pre-ovulatory phase (Queenan et al. 1980). The prediction of the LH surge on the basis of ultrasound is quite inaccurate, is equal to that of predicting the surge on the basis of the day of the cycle (Buttery et al. 1983). Transvaginal ultrasonography in combination with the endocrinological methods can, however, double the fertility rate during insemination procedures.

After the LH surge, theca tissue becomes increasingly vascularized and the granulosa layer separates from the theca cells. This process can be visualized sonographically approximately 24 hours prior to begin of ovulation and is usually accompanied by a discrete rise of plasma progesterone levels. Additionally, the cumulus oophoros can be seen sonographically in about one fifth of all follicles larger than 18 mm. If the vascular supply of the follicle, which can be ascertained by color Doppler sonography, is also taken into consideration, the quality of the egg cell can be evaluated even better and conception rates can be improved (Bhal et al. 1999).

About 25 % of patients show ultrasonographically demonstrable fluid in the culdesac after ovulation. The transition from follicle to corpus luteum is seen by an indentation of the capsule and an increase of intrafollicular echo-density. Sometimes, however, the corpus luteum is a rather solid structure which cannot readily be identified by ultrasound.

LUF Syndrome. Impaired ovulation, which is usually caused by problems of follicular maturation, is often a cause of infertility. This is frequently diagnosed by ultrasound examination, since other objective tests are often normal. A typical clinical picture is that of the syndrome of **luteinization of the unruptured follicle** (LUF syndrome) which was first discussed in 1967 (Kase et al. 1967). In this clinical entity, the hormone profiles are in a normal range and yet a rupture of the follicle does not occur. About 5 % of all normal cycles are said to occur in this form. However, the significance for infertility is not yet proven since this syndrome is not one of continuous anovulation. Ultrasound examination can lead to diagnosis when 36 hours after the LH surge the cystic follicle remains unchanged and no shrinkage can be shown.

A menstrual cycle can be anovulatory even if menstruation occurs at the proper time. In anovulatory cycles, however, usually low progesterone levels are found in the luteal phase. The rise in estradiol levels in the luteal cycle is also reduced, so that the measurement of progesterone and estradiol in the second half of the menstrual cycle gives important information pertaining to ovulation. An exception is, of course, the above-mentioned LUF syndrome.

In addition to the diagnostic evaluation of follicle growth and corpus luteum development, ultrasound can be used in the luteal phase to determine the quality of the endometrium. Deichert et al. (1986) compared the endometrial thickness with hormonal parameters, and concluded that endometrial thickness below 10 mm is an indication for hormonal stimulation or substitution in order to optimize implantation of the blastocyte. In a prospective cohort study comprising 1186 women seeking treatment for infertility, no correlation between thickness of the endometrium and pregnancy rate following IVF or ICSI could be found. Conversely, the pregnancy rate was found to be significantly lower in women with a thin endometrium undergoing intrauterine insemination (De Geyter et al. 2000).

Endometrial Biopsy

Most gynecologists consider the histological examination of an endometrial biopsy the primary method for judging luteal quality. Classically, the examination is carried out just before onset of the menstrual flow. Ideally an endometrial strip is obtained through outpatient curettage on day 27 or 28, or, in a longer menstrual cycle, 1–2 days before the beginning of menstrual flow. The endometrial strip should enclose all layers of the endometrium up to the myometrium, so that the functional and basal layer may be examined. For evaluation of the endometrial biopsy, the date of the next menstrual period must be known. This date is set equal to day 28. If the biopsy is obtained two days earlier, then the endometrium should show the histological picture of the 26th cyclic day. If the histological picture deviates by more than two days, luteal insufficiency is diagnosed. Although this is a standard method, in some patients serial endometrial biopsies at different times in the menstrual cycle show a pathological development in the early luteal phase which becomes normal shortly before the beginning of menstrual flow. This indicates that an endometrial biopsy obtained at an earlier time during the luteal cycle may be of diagnostic importance, since the structure of the endometrium on day 20–24 of the cycle is important for the blastocyte. Of major importance is the synchronous development of the endometrial glands and stroma (see Blasco 1994).

Progesterone Levels and Evaluation of Luteal Quality

The endometrial biopsy is the standard method for evaluation of luteal quality in clinical research. This diagnostic test is, however, not usually used in the clinical setting because of its invasive character. Instead, the **measurement of progesterone and estradiol** in the luteal phase is usually applied. Since progesterone secretion is pulsatile, this method is often criticized as having a high discrepancy rate. However, a single midluteal progesterone serum level below 10 ng/ml (31.8 nmol/l) or the sum of three progesterone levels below 30 ng/ml (95.4 nmol/l) are better correlated with the integrated progesterone concentration in the luteal phase than the basal body temperature chart, the length of luteal phase, or the pre-ovulatory diameter of the follicle. According to some data, **serum progesterone levels predict the quality of the luteal phase even better than the endometrial biopsy** (Jordan et al. 1994).

Progesterone is the primary hormone of the corpus luteum and of eminent importance for nidation and the maintenance of early pregnancy. A lutectomy in the sev-enth week of pregnancy causes miscarriage (Csapo et al. 1973). The removal of the corpus luteum during the ninth week of pregnancy, however, causes only a transitory drop in progesterone serum levels and pregnancy continues to develop. If an early decrease of progesterone concentration in the seventh week of pregnancy is compensated by substitution of this hormone, pregnancy continues to develop.

Pregnancies in women with ovarian insufficiency who become pregnant after oocyte donation can be supported by progesterone substitution during the first weeks of pregnancy. Serum levels of 20 ng/ml are sufficient. This serum level is obtained by giving 50 mg progesterone daily. Physiologically, the daily production of progesterone in the luteal phase is about 25 mg. A midluteal progesterone concentration under 3.1 ng/ml in a natural cycle signals anovulation. The median progesterone levels in conceptive cycles are around 17.8 ng/ml, although in extreme cases single conceptions also occur at lower levels around 3.8 ng/ml. In clinical practice, a midluteal progesterone level eight days post-ovulation greater than 10 ng/ml demonstrates sufficient luteal function (review in Wathen et al. 1984).

The daily fluctuations of progesterone serum levels (shown in Fig. 14.10) lead one to expect that statistically about a third of all progesterone measurements will lie below 10 ng/ml, even though a normal luteal phase is present. The measurement of progesterone in combination with estradiol is, however, a clinically relevant diagnostic tool which gives a first impression of follicular maturation when estradiol and progesterone are deter-

Fig. 14.10. Fluctuations in serum progesterone concentrations during a 24-hour period. Adapted from McNeely MJ, Soules MR. The diagnosis of luteal phase deficiency: a critical review. (Fertil Steril 1988, 50:1–15. Reproduced with permission of the publisher, the American Society for Reproductive Medicine [formerly The American Fertility Society])

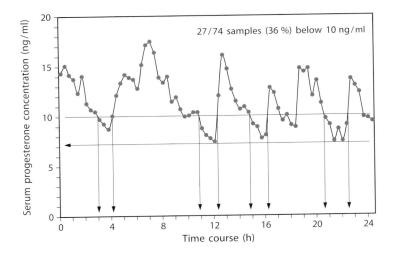

27/74 samples (36 %) below 10 ng/ml

mined on the eighth post-ovulatory day. Within the above-mentioned limits, it is then possible to establish whether ovulation has occurred. Several menstrual cycles must be monitored to show whether the patient has a continual restriction of her luteal quality or not. In such a case, the cause of impaired follicle maturation must be obtained before deciding on further therapy.

14.2.4 Impairment of Follicle Maturation

> The extreme form of impaired follicle maturation is that of anovulation with amenorrhea, although these cases are far less common than those in which the menstrual cycle remains unimpaired (Fig. 14.11).

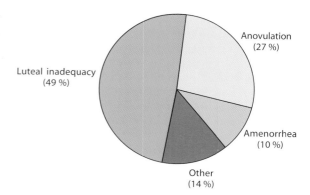

Fig. 14.11. Relative proportion of impaired follicular growth among patients of an infertility clinic according to severity of disturbance. (Adapted from Bohnet 1985)

Amenorrhea

Amenorrhea is a symptom that occurs in a large group of disorders, resulting in the absence of menstruation. Amenorrhea can be a result of dysfunctional endometrium with normal hormone levels or it can be due to disturbance of the hypothalamo-pituitary-gonadal axis with a normal endometrial reaction following exogenous hormone substitution. For scientific purposes, amenorrhea can be classified according to WHO criteria (Fig. 14.12).

Amenorrhea can be either primary or secondary. This classification says nothing about the cause of amenorrhea, since the same disorder can result in either primary or secondary amenorrhea. **Primary amenorrhea** is defined as the absence of menses by age 16. This is clinically important, since in 35–40 % of the patients primary amenorrhea is a result of **primary ovarian insufficiency** or urogenital dysgenesis. **Secondary amenorrhea** is the absence of menstruation for at least 4 months in a woman who had had at least one spontaneous menstrual cycle in her history.

Primary Amenorrhea. Patients with primary amenorrhea do not often present in infertility practice, since most of the causes are of genetic origin and have been diagnosed in puberty or in early adulthood. The primary cause of primary amenorrhea is **Turner syndrome** with the classical karyotype X0. In extremely rare cases, patients with Turner syndrome do have a menstrual period and later develop secondary amenorrhea as a result of premature ovarian insufficiency.

The second most common cause of primary amenorrhea is Muellerian duct dysgenesis, which is characterized by the congenital failure of the Fallopian tubes, the uterus and/or the vagina to develop. An example is **Ro-**kitansky-Küster-Hauser syndrome**, which is a clinical entity with vaginal aplasia, a rudimentary uterus and normal Fallopian tubes. In Muellerian duct dysgenesis, ovarial function is intact, so that the gonadotropins and sexual steroids show normal levels. Diagnosis is obtained after clarification of the anatomy through a gynecological examination, imaging diagnostics, hysteroscopy, and possibly diagnostic laparoscopy.

Patients who are underweight in relation to height can present with primary amenorrhea. The importance of body weight for normal development of the hypothalamic pituitary ovarian axis is seen in the hypothesis of critical body weight, which postulates that a particular body weight must be obtained in relation to height before menstruation can begin (for review see Knuth et al. 1977). In addition to these common causes of primary amenorrhea, a number of congenital and exogenic defects can disrupt the hypothalamic pituitary axis, which results in a defect in hormonal regulation analogous to that which has been described in men.

Secondary Amenorrhea. Secondary amenorrhea plays a much more important role in infertility practice than primary amenorrhea described above.

> A major cause of secondary amenorrhea is pregnancy. This fact has to be considered in every patient presenting with this symptom.

Even if a patient has been diagnosed with another cause of amenorrhea, it must be remembered that pregnancy can develop out of an amenorrheic phase, and that menstruation need not have occurred. This is often seen in the effective therapy of hyperprolactinemic amenorrhea.

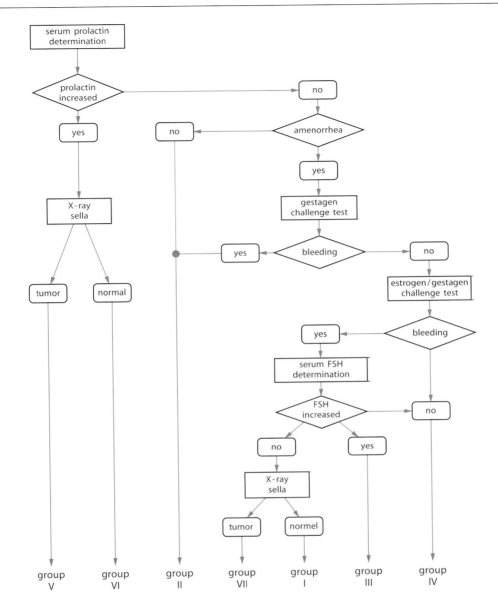

Fig. 14.12. Classification of impaired ovarian function according to WHO guidelines

A rare cause of amenorrhea are **intrauterine synechia** which can cause **Asherman's syndrome**, in which a destruction of the endometrium has occurred with a resulting internal adhesion of the uterine cavity. This is usually caused by a complicated dilatation and curettage such as in infected abortion, or extremely vigourous curettage, but the syndrome can also occur after unspecific or tuberculous endometriosis. Patient history is important for diagnosis. A suspicion of Asherman's syndrome can be strengthened by normal estradiol and progesterone levels in the luteal phase, or through con-

tinuing amenorrhea after hormonal stimulation. Diagnosis is obtained through hysteroscopy or, with limitations, by hysterosalpingography. Therapeutically, adhesiolysis of the uterine cavity must be followed by sequential estrogen and progesterone substitution in the form of a pseudo-pregnancy. Simultaneously, an IUD can be used in order to deter the development of new adhesions while the endometrium regenerates.

If Asherman syndrome and a hysterectomy can be ruled out, the cause of secondary amenorrhea in the remaining cases which present in infertility practice can be divided into those with hypothalamic and pituitary defects, and those with ovarian failure.

Hypothalamic amenorrhea is a diagnosis of exclusion and represents a functional defect of the secretion of gonadotropins caused by rapid weight loss, rapid weight gain, systemic diseases, extreme physical activity and/or extreme stress situations (see Sect. 14.1.7). Hypothalamic amenorrhea is the extreme case of impaired follicle maturation, in which luteal insufficiency or anovulation with normal menstruation occur because of the above-named causes prior to the development of secondary amenorrhea.

Hyperprolactinemia is often a cause of absent menstruation. Here again amenorrhea is the extreme endpoint of hyperprolactinemia; luteal insufficiencies and anovulation with normal menstruation are seen much more commonly. In hyperprolactinemia one must think of a **pituitary adenoma** or **hypothyroidism** as causative factors.

An important cause of impaired follicular maturation, and thus of amenorrhea, is the **polycystic ovarian syndrome** (PCO syndrome). Primarily one thinks of an obese patient with hyperandrogenic symptoms and the typical picture in ultrasound diagnosis described above. The so-called PCO-syndrome or Stein-Leventhal-syndrome is, however, only an endpoint of a group of various different pathological disturbances and represents a disruption of the cyclic ovarian function with elevated androgen/estradiol levels and an unbalanced LH/FSH ratio.

In addition to these three common causes of secondary amenorrhea and impaired follicle maturation, rare causes of hypothalamic tumors and cysts, and infiltrative diseases of the hypothalamus or the pituitary gland such as tuberculosis, sarcoidosis or histiocytosis X exist. These are, however, rarities even in specialized centers.

In contrast to dysfunction of the hypothalamo-pituitary axis, which can be readily treated, the common diagnosis of primary ovarian failure is usually the endpoint of infertility workup in countries where oocyte donation is prohibited by law, since atresia of the primordial follicles results in an absolute loss of oocytes. Premature ovarian failure is characterized by the loss of ovarian function before the age of 35 years. This can be a result of chemotherapy or radiation therapy or also may have an immunological cause.

Hyperprolactinemia

The existing relationship between disturbed reproductive function and lactation has long been known. Designation names are found in the older literature such as the Chiari-Frommel syndrome (postpartal amenorrhea with persisting lactation); Argonz-Ahumada-Castillo syndrome (galactorrhea and reduced urinary estrogen concentrations) and Albright-Forbes syndrome (amenorrhea, reduced urinary FSH concentrations and galactorrhea). After 1972, when it first became possible to

measure human prolactin, all of these syndromes were found to have a common denominator, namely that of hyperprolactinemia.

In contrast to the other hormones of the pituitary gland, prolactin is mainly regulated through a hypothalamic inhibitory factor. The main inhibitor is dopamine. In rat experiments 70 % of prolactin secretion can be inhibited through a dopamine infusion, if the endogenic dopamine synthesis has been blocked beforehand. γ-aminobutyric acid (GABA) is another inhibitory factor which, however, is weaker in its effect than dopamine.

A number of stimulating substances have also been found which are important for the short-term secretion of prolactin. These substances include thyrotropin-releasing hormone (TRH), vasoactive intestinal peptide (VIP) and angiotensin. Serotonin precursors cause a significant rise in prolactin concentrations. Consequently, the blockade of serotonin inhibits prolactin secretion. Endogenous opioids increase prolactin secretion by inhibiting dopamine synthesis and reducing dopamine secretion. Histamine and substance P both stimulate prolactin secretion, although the exact regulatory mechanisms are not yet known.

The differentiated regulation of prolactin secretion explains the various causes of hyperprolactinemia. A slight rise in serum prolactin concentration can be a symptom of central neurogenic dysregulation, such as the stress reaction, in the form of a functional dysregulation. Hyperprolactinemia can be due to the ingestion of a variety of drugs. **Primary hypothyroidism** can also be the cause of increased prolactin. Even hormonally inactive tumors close to the pituitary gland can cause hyperprolactinemia through changes in portal circulation. Very high prolactin concentrations are usually, however, caused by prolactin secreting tumors (**prolactinoma**).

About one third of all patients with secondary amenorrhea have a **pituitary adenoma**. In patients with simultaneously occurring galactorrhea, 50 % of those women exhibit an abnormal cone view of the sella turcica. The infertility in these patients is related more closely to hyperprolactinemia than to tumor size except, of course, in extreme cases.

A prolactinoma causes a rise in hypothalamic dopamine concentration, which in turn causes a negative feedback on GnRH secretion. This causes a decrease of gonadotropin secretion, which then results in anovulation. Therapeutically, one must thus either remove the adenoma or lower the prolactin concentration by giving a specific inhibitor.

Since not all cases of hyperprolactinemia develop the typical symptoms, a check of the prolactin serum concentration belongs to the routine diagnostic workup of female factor infertility.

A blood sample is best taken during basal conditions in the early morning hours. Since this is usually not obtainable in clinical routine, one must consider the circadian rhythm and subjective situation during which the blood sample was drawn when evaluating the serum level obtained. If hyperprolactinemia is diagnosed, then the level needs to be checked in a second sample. Prolactin serum levels show great fluctuations which can be caused by a variety of physiological stimuli such as nutrition and sleep behavior, stress, and physical activity. The intake of prolactin-stimulating drugs must also be considered.

Before beginning treatment of a slight to medium hyperprolactinemia (lower than 50 ng/ml) with a prolactin inhibiting drug the TSH level (less than 3 μU/l) should be obtained from the same blood sample in order to rule out thyroid dysfunction. In this case, treatment of the thyroid may be pertinant. If the prolactin concentrations exceed 50 ng/ml without known physiological stimuli, one should perform a radiological check up of the sella turcica.

The probability of a pituitary adenoma is about 1:5 when prolactin serum concentrations are above 50 ng/ml. The probability rises to 1:2 if serum concentrations exceed 100 ng/ml. In cases with even higher prolactin concentrations, almost all patients have a microadenoma. When levels rise above 1000 ng/ml a macroprolactinoma is very probable.

Pituitary Adenoma. **Prolactin-secreting adenomas** are the most frequent tumor of the pituitary gland. About 50 % of all pituitary adenomas which are found in male and female autopsies fall into this group. 9–27 % of autopsied humans have a prolactinoma, with the highest incidence occurring in the sixth decade of life. There is no difference in incidence between male and female patients, although clinical symptoms are seen much more commonly in women. Hyperprolactinemia can be diagnosed five times more commonly in women than in men.

The radiological work-up has changed in the past few years. The cone view of the sella turrica can only diagnose adenomas greater than 10 mm in size. A **CT scan** of the sella in combination with radiological constrast dye allows the detection of lesions about 2 mm in size. The **MRI scan** is superior to a CT scan for identifying microadenomas, and is the best diagnostic test to rule out an adenoma. An ophthalmological checkup is only necessary when the adenoma is greater than 10 mm in diameter.

Empty-sella Syndrome. A radiologically abnormal sella can be seen in the **empty-sella syndrome.** In this case, the diaphragma sellae is congenitally malformed. This defect causes an expansion of the subarachnoidal space into the pituitary fossa, which results in a bilateral displacement of the pituitary gland causing the sella to appear empty. This syndrome is not rare. It is seen in 5 % of all autopsies, 85 % of which are female. The empty sella syndrome is usually a benign syndrome, whereas radiologically sometimes the misdiagnosis of a tumor occurs. In these cases surgical intervention must be prohibited. After the diagnosis has been made, an annual check of prolactin concentrations should be performed. If a hyperprolactinemia is found, treatment with a prolactin inhibitor may be started (for review see Speroff et al. 1994).

In the recent past, a direct inhibitory effect of elevated prolactin levels on follicular maturation has been suspected. Follicular atresia, anovulation, insufficient development of the corpus luteum, and a premature luteolysis were presumably caused solely by the pathologically elevated prolactin concentrations. These mechanisms have been established in the rat model, but it is not yet clear if the same apply in humans.

Lately an increasing number of experts are believing that the findings described above are caused by hypothalamic changes. Peripherally measured hyperprolactinemia appears to be secondary to a central nervous dysregulation caused primarily by an alteration in the pulsatile GnRH pattern. The changes in the GnRH pattern deter normal gonadotropin secretion, and thus follicular maturation. Richardson et al. (1985) showed that rhesus monkeys with hypothalamic lesions treated with exogenic pulsatile GnRH showed normal postovulatory plasma progesterone concentrations independent of the prolactin serum level. A correlation between progesterone and prolactin levels in a group of women with luteal insufficiency could not be shown when compared with normal control groups (for review see Soules 1993).

Even if it is not entirely clear whether there is a direct effect of elevated serum prolactin concentrations on follicular maturation, or if the origin lies in an alteration of gonadotropin secretion, hyperprolactinemia is undoubtedly a cause for female infertility and should thus be treated.

Surgical and Radiological Treatment of Hyperprolactinemia. In the past, before dopamine agonists were available for the treatment of hyperprolactinemia, patients with pituitary adenomas and other similar tumors were operated or received radiation therapy. Data on these patients show that transphenoidal neurosurgery resulted in ovulatory menstrual cycles in 80 % of patients with microadenomas, but only in 40 % of those with macroadenomas. In 30 % of the patients with microadenomas, however, a tumor reappeared. The recurrence rate of macroadenomas was around 90 %. Severe side-effects such as panhypopituitarism and liquorfistula occur and restrict the indication for neurosurgical treatment.

The results of radiation are inferior to those of surgery, so that this form of therapy should only be used for postoperative treatment of larger tumors which show new growth, and do not respond to pharmacological treatment.

In the past, it was feared that a treated pituitary adenoma could expand during pregnancy. This is extremely uncommon in microadenomas where even breast feeding may be allowed without having to fear the stimulation of a pituitary adenoma. The risk of pituitary adenoma growth during pregnancy rises, of course, with the size of the adenoma. In the case of a microadenoma a monthly ophthalmological checkup plus measurement of prolactin serum concentrations have been recommended. Lately, advice has become more lenient, and these checkups are recommended only in the case of headache or visual disturbances.

Since neurosurgery during pregnancy is, as in the past, only performed when acute symptoms occur, these new lenient recommendations seem consistent. Traditional monitoring can, however, be reassuring both to the patient and the physician.

Pharmacological Treatment. The development of synthetic prolactin inhibitors represented an important step in the treatment of hyperprolactinemia. The introduction of bromocriptine in the 1970s allowed the direct treatment of hyperprolactinemic amenorrhea and infertility for the first time.

- **Bromocriptine** is a lysergic acid derivative with dopamine agonistic activity, which inhibits prolactin secretion by binding at the dopamine receptor. Depending on the prolactin concentrations, a dose of 1.25 to 2.5 mg in the evening may be enough to normalize the prolactin level. In patients with pituitary adenomas, 10 mg or more daily may be needed. Although this form of treatment is very effective, adverse reactions may cause poor compliance. Headaches and nausea often occur during the beginning of treatment. Dizziness is caused by orthostatic hypotension, since noradrenergic neural transmitters are interfered with. These effects can be minimized by slowly increasing the dosage. Treatment should always begin with half a tablet taken in the evening. The dosage may be increased every three days by 1.25 mg until the final dosage is reached. Vaginal application of uncoated tablets of bromocriptine can markedly reduce side-effects of the drug (Ginsburg et al. 1992). Since this form of application results in a higher rate of resorption and eliminates the first-pass effect of the liver, a lower daily dosage can achieve the same effects. This is often clinically employed. Research data show that about 80 % of patients with hyperprolactinemic amenorrhea regularly menstruate as a result of treatment with bromocriptine. In 50–75 % of patients with pituitary adenoma, treatment with dopamine agonists has significant influ-

ence on tumor size. Neoplasias were no longer detectable in 25–30 % of these cases receiving long-term treatment. In view of this aspect, pharmacological treatment of a pituitary adenoma should be the method of choice. Transphenoidal neurosurgery should only be considered if bromocriptine therapy does not reduce tumor size. This is also relevant in cases where prolactin levels return to normal. In this case, evidence points to a non-functional tumor which causes hyperprolactinemia merely by disrupting the dopamine supply in the pituitary stalk.

If pregnancy occurs, bromocriptine treatment is usually discontinued. Three large-scale studies have shown that even with continuation of therapy, no negative consequences for the fetus have to be feared (Holmgren et al. 1986).

- A number of new prolactin inhibitors are now available. **Lisuride** has a higher activity, a longer half-life and is better tolerated by some patients, so patients unable to continue bromocriptine therapy can switch to lisuride.
- **Metagoline** is an antiserotoninergic substance which acts via a non-dopaminergic mechanism, and can be tried as an alternative product (Bohnet et al. 1986).
- A new substance is **Cabergoline**, a prolactin inhibitor, which only needs to be taken 1–2 times per week, and which seemed to be better tolerated than bromocriptine in first clinical trials.

Hyperprolactinemia which is caused by thyroidal dysfunction should be treated through adequate treatment of the thyroid gland.

Polycystic Ovarian Disease

The different entities which are combined under the term polycystic ovarian disease are, next to hyperprolactinemia, the most important cause of anovulatory infertility. The clinical picture varies from the physiologically normal patient with an anovulatory menstrual cycle to the adipose, hirsute and oligoamenorrhic patient who was first described by Stein and Leventhal.

Typical ovarian alterations, which may not be present, were originally responsible for the designation. These characteristics are bilaterally enlarged ovaries with a smooth pearl-white capsule which are 2.8 times larger in size than the normal ovary. The number of primordial follicles remains the same, but the number of maturing and atretic follicles is doubled, so that each ovary has 20–100 cystic follicles which can be seen through the capsule. The tunica is about 50 % thicker than that of a normal ovary. The hilus cells quadruple in volume, and the cortical and subcortical stroma is enlarged.

In the past these typical ovarian alterations were assumed to cause PCOS; the underlying pathophysiological mechanism was misunderstood . In fact, the anatomical situation results from a hormonal dysregulation perpetuated and aggravated in a vicious circle. These changes can be caused by hypothalamic, hypophyseal, ovarian and/or adrenal dysfunction which are all often combined with oligo- or amenorrhea, hirsutism, and infertility. The characteristic polycystic ovary is seen when no ovulation occurs during a longer period of time. "Polycystic ovarian disease" thus is not a diagnosis, but a prototypical form of chronic hyperandronemic anovulation. Recent studies show that little-known disturbances of androgen secretion and dysfunctional regulation of steroid biosynthesis are at fault. The typical ovarian morphology described above is frequent, but in no way adequate for diagnosis. Many women with no hormonal dysfunction have more than eight subcapsular follicular cysts of less than 10 mm. Epidemiological studies show that about 25 % of all premenopausal women demonstrate typical signs for polycystic ovarian disease in ultrasound examination. Even women who take oral contraceptives can show the typical ultrasound picture in 14 % of all cases (Clayton et al. 1992). The prevalence of disturbances associated with anovulation is only between 5 % and 10 %.

Increased androgen production plays an important role in the pathogenesis of PCOS. Steroid biosynthesis in the ovary and in the female adrenal cortex follows the same mechanisms as described for the male in Chap. 3. Ovarian androstenedione is the basis for both testosterone and estrogens. Unlike in the male, LH and ACTH do not control androgen production by a specific inhibitory feedback mechanism, as androgens are only byproducts of estrogens and cortisone synthesis. Rather, intraovarian control of androgen production plays a critical role. In the ovary androgens represent a "necessary evil" (Rosenfield 1999). On the one hand, they are necessary for estrogen production and accelerate growth of smaller follicles; on the other hand, when overabundant they prevent selection of the leading follicle and cause atresia. Steroidal secretory patterns of PCOS patients suggest a generalized dysregulation of androgen production, particularly affecting the level of 17-hydroxylase and 17,20 lyase activity. This dysregulation can manifest itself solely as ovarian hyperandrogenemia, but may also lead to functional hyperandrogenemia of the adrenal cortex. A combination of the two is not rare. Inherently a PCOS can derive from pathological androgen production of the adrenal cortex.

Absence of the correct rhythmic pattern of gonadotropin and sexual steroid secretion causes persistent anovulation. Serum levels of testosterone, androstenedione, dehydroepiandrosterone sulphate, 17-hydroxyprogesterone and estrone are thus elevated. The elevated production of estrogens is not due to direct ovarian secretion. The daily production of estradiol in women with polycystic ovarian disease is equal to that of normal women in the early follicular phase. The elevated serum estrogen concentration is rather due to peripheral aromatization of androstenedione to estrone in adipose tissue.

Typically, the **LH to FSH ratio** is greater than 3 in polycystic ovarian disease. 20–40 % of all patients with polycystic ovaries, however, do not have this typical change in the LH to FSH ratio. Analysis of the LH pulse pattern in PCO-patients shows a frequency identical to that of normal controls. The individual pulse amplitude, however, is elevated (12.2 ± 2.7 mU/ml) when compared to normal controls in early or midfollicular phase (6.2 ± 0.8 mU/ml) (Kazer et al. 1987). This seems to be a result of a change in GnRH pulse frequency.

An increase in the GnRH pulse amplitude with constant pulse frequency reduces peripheral FSH concentrations in the presence of normal LH patterns. This causes the typical reversal in the LH/FSH ratio. Research data thus demonstrate that the change in gonadotropin secretion often associated with polycystic ovarian disease is due to a malfunction in the frequency and amplitude modulation of GnRH production. A primary disturbance of LH secretion does not, however, seem to be the origin of PCOS.

Endogenous opiates influence hypothalamic GnRH secretion. It has been shown that endorphin metabolism can be modulated in polycystic ovarian disease when compared to controls. β-endorphin and adrenocorticotrope hormone (ACTH) stem from the same precursor called proopiomelanocortin (POMC). It is known that β-endorphin levels are elevated in situations in which ACTH production is increased. The concentrations of ACTH and cortisol are normal in PCO patients, but this does not rule out a higher rate of metabolism of these substances. Since β-endorphin levels are elevated in stress situations, and patients with PCO show a higher rate of psychological stress reactions, it is possible that this may be one central factor in the impairment of normal regulatory mechanisms.

The influence of hyperprolactinemia in central hormone regulation was discussed above, and explains the high association of hyperprolactinemia with polycystic ovarian disease.

Elevated testosterone concentrations reduce the measurable free sex hormone binding globulin (SHBG), so that anovulatory women with polycystic ovaries usually have a 50 % reduced level of SHBG due to secondary hyperandrogenemia. Reduced SHBG concentration elevates the concentration of free estrogen, which again is positively correlated with a rise in the LH/FSH ratio. The elevated free estradiol concentration, and the peripheral metabolism of androstenedione to estrogen reduce the FSH level. A residual activity of FSH, however, remains so that continued stimulation of the ovaries with ensuing follicle production occurs. The hypothalamic pituitary axis is fully intact, and is even the basis for further development of polycystic ovarian disease.

Follicular maturation in PCOS does not, however, end in ovulation. The maturation of the smaller follicles extends over several months so that typically 2–6 mm large follicle cysts are produced, which in turn give this disease its name. Since the follicles are enclosed in a hyperplastic theca layer, the follicular stroma is enlarged and constantly produces steroids under continued gonadotropin stimulation. This closes the vicious circle so that the disease is perpetuated. After the follicles die off and the layer of granulosa cells disintegrates, the thecal portion remains so that the production of androstenedione and testosterone increases, according to the two-cell theory outlined above. The increased testosterone levels further reduce SHBG with a consequent rise of free estrogens. Simultaneously the free testosterone fraction increases, with the resulting effect on androgen-dependent tissue.

Insulin Resistance. About 40 % of patients with polycystic ovarian disease show increased **insulin resistance**. Although obesity and age increase the probability of insulin resistance, even non-obese women and young women with PCOS may show glucose intolerance. The infusion of glucose causes an excess secretion of insulin. It is estimated that about 10 % of all cases of glucose intolerance are caused by PCOS-induced insulin resistance. 15 % of all later diabetes type II cases show a PCOS in their history.

Although androgens can induce a slight insulin resistance, the concentrations found in PCOS are not sufficient to explain disturbances of insulin metabolism. If androgen production is inhibited, insulin sensitivity fails to normalize. Conversely, insulin resistance increases only negligibly when androgens are given, as in female-to-male trans-sexuals. Independent of the mechanism of elevated circulating insulin levels, binding of insulin to the **IGF-I receptors** in the theca cells occurs. This increases thecal androgen production by LH stimulation. The elevated circulating insulin levels thus increase androgen production in insulin resistance. Simultaneously, elevated insulin levels inhibit hepatic SHBG production and the production of IGF binding protein-I. Although there are indications that hyperandrogenemia can cause hyperinsulinemia, most experimental data suggest that disturbed insulin metabolism precedes irregular androgen metabolism (Dunaif 1999).

Obesity. Since increased body weight and abdominal adipose tissue causes hyperinsulinemia and reduced glucose tolerance, one may deduce that obesity is the major factor in polycystic ovarian disease. The typical distribution of female adipose tissue distribution in the hip area does not play such a major role. An objective method to determine the distribution of adipose tissue is the measurement of the ratio of waist-to-hip circumference. If the ratio is larger than 0.85, an android distribution of adipose tissue is probable, and hyperinsulinism should be suspected. If the ratio is below 0.75, a gynoid distribution is probable, which in turn is only rarely combined with changes in insulin metabolism.

Diagnosis. Endocrinological investigation plays the major role in excluding the possibility of a PCOS and is mandatory even if the patient shows no physiological stigmata but is anovulatory. The typical ultrasound picture is not sufficient for diagnosis, as was formerly believed (see Fig. 14.9). Determining testosterone, androstenedione, DHEAS, estradiol, LH, FSH and prolactin levels in the first half of the cycle may be helpful in deciding on a form of individual treatment. Cortisol and 17-OH-progesterone levels supplement the basic workup when adrenal involvement is suspected.

Treatment. Since polycystic ovarian disease usually encompasses elevated androgen levels, a chronic elevation of estrogen levels, and an inverse LH/FSH ratio, treatment must intervene in this vicious circle in order to allow ovulation to occur. Methods of treatment are as follows:

1) Anti-estrogens (e. g. clomiphene),
2) glucocorticoids (dexamethasone 0.25–0.5),
3) pulsatile GnRH treatment via a cyclic pump,
4) hMG-stimulation,
5) surgical reduction of ovarian stroma,
6) oral anti-diabetic medication.

Treatment forms 1–3 still allow feedback and regulatory mechanisms of follicular maturation to occur. In contrast, the treatment with hMG or hCG directly acts at the ovarian level and thus carries a higher risk of hyperstimulation. Surgical reduction of androgen producing ovarian stroma should only be tried when other forms of treatment have failed (review in Gibson 1995).

Research data show that 63 % to 95 % of the infertile women with polycystic ovarian disease ovulate after chlomiphene treatment. Chlomiphene is a weak anti-estrogen and causes a rise in gonadotropin levels. Treatment usually begins with 50 mg daily for five days, beginning between the third and seventh day of the menstrual cycle. 27–50 % of the women ovulate with this low dosage. In some cases, an increase up to 150 mg daily should be considered, in which a further 26 % to 29 % ovulate. If this dosage does not result in ovulation, one may additionally prescribe dexamethasone (0.25 to 0.5 mg daily), depending on the DHEA-sulphate serum concentration. If follicular maturation is seen in ultrasound and is shown by serum hormone concentrations and no ovulation occurs, ovulation can be induced by 5,000 to 10,000 IU hCG i.m. If one considers that normally only 50 % of all couples achieve pregnancy within three months, and that 80 % require one year for conception to occur, treatment should be continued for at least six months or cycles if ultrasound and hormone levels show an adequate luteal phase. This therapy allows for an up to 90 % success rate for chlomiphene treatment, if other cofactors for infertility have been ruled out.

hMG and FSH. If treatment with clomiphene does not result in ovulation or conception, the next step is treatment with gonadotropins. Patients with hyperandrogenemia have a poorer success rate than those with pure hypothalamic amenorrhea. Since patients with polycystic ovarian disease are very sensitive to hMG stimulation, this treatment form walks a fine line between the induction of ovulation and hyperstimulation with the risk of multiple pregnancy. After the introduction of purified FSH it was hoped that the LH/FSH ratio could be corrected in order to achieve a better form of treatment. The clinical results to date do not, however, clearly show better results in the treatment with purified FSH (Baird and Howles 1994). One advantage of the new FSH products is that of possible subcutaneous injection. Uncontrolled studies show a higher conception rate and a lower rate of hyperstimulation.

GnRH Down-regulation. Treatment with pure hMG and hCG stimulation often results in a **premature LH peak** with luteinization of the follicle. Some authors believe that this premature LH peak is the major cause for later miscarriage, which is often found in polycystic ovarian disease. Clinical data, however, are not clear, so that down-regulation is not necessarily recommended in a treatment of polycystic ovarian disease with hMG and hCG.

Pulsatile GnRH Treatment. Large-scale studies in the 1980s showed that this form of treatment resulted in a relatively high pregnancy rate without the high risk of hyperstimulation. In patients resistant to chlomiphene citrate, treatment with pulsatile GnRH resulted in a conception rate of 26 % per cycle. The conception rate could be elevated to 38 % with simultaneous down-regulation followed by pulsatile GnRH treatment. The miscarriage rate of 38 % was, however, also elevated (for review see Filicori 1994).

Ovarian Wedge Resection. If the above-mentioned forms of treatment do not result in pregnancy, ovarian wedge resection may be considered in order to reduce androgen production in the ovarian stroma. Up to 90 % of such patients show normal ovulatory cycles after surgery. About one third of the successfully operated women, however, develop oligoamenorrhoea within the following year (Buttram and Vaquero 1975). The concep-

tion rate is reduced to 1.8 % per cycle, which may be due to adnexial adhesions after such an operation (Adashi et al. 1981). Microsurgical and endoscopic techniques seem to avoid adhesion formation by replacing wedge resection by thermocauterization, laser vaporisation and electrocoagulation. A study of 106 patients with electrocoagulation showed a pregnancy rate of 70 % (Naether et al. 1994).

Oral Antidiabetic Medication. Studies were carried out with metformine and troglitazone to reduce insulin resistance. Androgen levels did indeed improve and ovulatory cycles were achieved. At the present time this treatment must be considered experimental, especially in view of the fact that troglitazone has been withdrawn from the American market (Dunaif et al. 1996; Nestler et al. 1998).

Reduced Body Weight and Follicular Maturation. Independent of the treatment modalities mentioned above, treatment of obese patients should be based on weight reduction.

Whereas the elevated body weight in many patients with polycystic ovarian disease propagates or even induces hormonal dysregulation, underweight patients also have a major risk factor for impaired follicular maturation and amenorrhea. A major proportion of the patients with hypothalamic amenorrhea fall into this group. This clinical entity is characterized by an inadequate pulsatile GnRH secretion. Diagnosis is one of exclusion in which other pituitarian disorders must be ruled out. In addition to evident low body weight, a particularly stressful situation such as flight and displacement can induce hypothalamic dysregulation. Such patients show extremely low or non-measurable gonadotropin levels. Prolactin levels lie in the normal range, and the cone view of the sella shows no pathological changes. A progesterone challenge test with a transformation dose (such as G-Farlutal 5 mg b.i.d. for 10 days) does not result in bleeding, and thus demonstrates the absence of estrogen stimulus on the endometrium.

The most extreme form of low body weight amenorrhea is that of **anorexia nervosa.** The pure form of anorexia is extremely rare in the infertility clinic, but minor forms may be seen more often in infertility patients.

In contrast to anorexia nervosa, which may have concurring central nervous dysregulation, **simple weight loss** may be a cause of impaired follicular maturation, and may be readily overlooked. The endocrine imbalance, however, is comparable to that of anorexia. Hormone studies show low FSH and LH concentrations, elevated cortisol levels, normal prolactin, TSH and L-thyroxine levels with low normal fT_3 and elevated reverse-T_3 levels. Extreme weight loss causes the loss of sleep-associated episodic LH secretion, showing a pattern usually found in early puberty. Weight gain within

15 % of ideal body weight may result in an improvement of the symptoms.

In addition to low body weight, **physical activity** may cause cyclic dysregulation. Many studies have shown menstrual dysregulation in athletes, especially in long-distance runners and ballet dancers. The percentage of amenorrhea is proportional to the weekly distance run, and inversely proportional to body weight. Decreasing body weight results in a higher incidence of anovulatory cycles and a reduction in the quality of the luteal phase. The theoretic mechanism for impaired GnRH secretion is a change in estrogen metabolism, in which estradiol is converted to catechol estrogens which seem to have anti-estrogenic properties.

Increased physical activity such as in running often results in a "**runners' high**", which is thought to be the result of an increase in endogenous opiates. These endogenous opiates may cause an elevation of corticotropin releasing hormone concentrations, which in turn reduce gonadotropin production. Hypothalamic GnRH production seems to be suppressed. In 49 of 66 patients with hypothalamic dysregulation of follicular maturation, treatment with 25 to 125 mg **Naltrexon** daily resulted in a normal menstrual cycle. The pregnancy rate was almost equal to that of normal controls (Wildt et al. 1993). Alternatively, pulsatile GnRH treatment or hMG and hCG stimulation may be considered, but here again there is a risk of multiple pregnancy. First, however, body weight should be normalized.

Primary Ovarian Failure

In patients with secondary amenorrhea primary ovarian failure must be ruled out. This can be done during the initial examination in which FSH and estradiol levels are measured. If a patient with a history of oligo-amenorrhea has elevated FSH levels and reduced estradiol concentrations, the diagnosis of primary ovarian failure can be formed. The FSH levels should lie at least two standard deviations above the mean in the follicular phase, and should be confirmed by a second sample.

1 % of all women have **precocious menopause** with ovarian failure beginning before the age of 35 years. The causes are usually unknown. Sometimes a chromosomal origin may be identified; other causes include autoimmune diseases, viral infections, previous chemotherapy and/or radiation therapy.

Turner syndrome with the loss of one X chromosome is one of the most common human chromosome defects, and is seen in one of 2500 live births. Typically, these patients show short stature and streak gonads. Ovarian dysfunction, however, shows extreme variations. An ultrasound study of 104 young Turner patients showed visually demonstrable ovaries in one third of the patients (Masserano et al. 1989).

Many of these women had an incomplete deletion of the X chromosome. This explains case reports of pregnancy and live births before premature ovarian failure begins in women with X0 syndrome and partial X deletions.

Various other genetic abnormalities are associated with hypergonadotropic hypogonadism. They are, however, so rare in a normal infertility clinic that a routine genetic diagnostic check does not seem warranted.

In addition to chromosomal diseases some genetic diseases, such as galactosemia, may cause premature ovarian failure.

Chemotherapy with antimetabolites and radiation therapy may impair ovarian function, and should be identifiable in the patient's history.

It is not clear if other exogenous toxins may play a role in premature ovarian failure. Analogous to orchitis in men, it is assumed that oophoritis may occur after mumps. There are, however, only a few case reports which do not allow a clear statement on this issue.

Autoimmune Diseases. There is some evidence that autoimmune antibodies may cause premature ovarian failure. Typical autoimmune diseases such as Hashimoto thyroiditis, Basedow disease, Addison disease, hyperthyroidism, juvenile diabetes, pernicious anemia, alopecia areata, vitiligo, and myasthenia gravis are associated with ovarian failure. Patients often have several autoimmune diseases simultaneously, which is known as the "polyglandular failure syndrome". The most common association is that of thyroidal disease and Addison's disease.

Circulating autoantibodies against ovarian stroma can be found in the serum of patients with primary ovarian failure. It is, however, not clear whether the antibodies are primary or secondary in nature. This is also true for cellular autoimmune disease in which lymphocyte infiltration of the ovaries can be found.

The fourth argument for an immunological cause for premature ovarian failure is the statistically significant correlation between human leucocyte antigens (HLA) with some autoimmune diseases (for review see Bakimer et al. 1984).

In addition to the above-mentioned causes for hypergonadotropic hypogonadism, there are rare cases with defective FSH hormone receptors, and others with biologically inactive gonadotropins. These are, however, not relevant in clinical routine (see review by Taylor et al. 1993).

Treatment. After diagnosing premature ovarian failure, substitution with an estrogen and progesterone combination should be recommended. In rare cases, patients show remission and possibly may conceive (Shangold et al. 1977). A causal therapy is, however, not possible in patients with hypergonadotropic hypogonadism. Oocyte and embryo donation are legally prohibited in Germany. In the USA success rates between 22% and 50% are achieved with these procedures.

Estrogen replacement therapy should also be recommended in **natural menopause** to minimize the risks for osteoporosis and cardiovascular disease. The lowest recommended doses are 2 mg estradiol or 2 mg estradiol valerate or 0.625 mg conjugated estrogen daily. The transdermal application of 0.05 mg estradiol optimizes pharmacokinetics and avoids the first-pass effect of the liver. Patients who have not undergone a hysterectomy must additionally take a progestin in order to counter the risk of endometrial carcinoma. Progestins may be given sequentially in a dosage of 0.35 mg norethisterone, 5 mg medroxyprogesterone acetate or 10 mg dydrogesterone daily for 10–14 days. Progestins may also be given continuously in the form of norethisterone acetate 1 mg daily; in this form of treatment amenorrhea usually follows after 2–6 cycles.

14.3 Infertility due to Disturbances of Gamete Migration

After checking ovulatory function in female infertility, one must consider a disturbance in the passage of the oocyte and the sperm (see Fig. 14.13 for an overview). Possible alterations exist in the vagina, the cervix, the uterus and the Fallopian tubes, as well as the pelviperitoneum.

14.3.1 Vagina and Cervix

Anatomical variations of the vagina, such as transverse and longitudinal septae, or even vaginal aplasia, are obvious. Changes in the vaginal environment may be another cause for infertility. The production of lactic acid through glycogenolysis gives the vagina a pH of 4–4.5, and thus represents a hostile environment for sperm. Physiological cervical mucus production at the time of ovulation creates the first prerequisite for passage of sperm into the genital tract.

Vaginal infections with increased discharge, a change in pH, and leukocyte transudation are detrimental to the motility and the ascent of sperm. The first clinical examination of the patient should thus include a wet mount of a vaginal smear in order to exclude the presence of pathogenic bacteria and leukocytes. A vaginal infection must also be ruled out if a pathological postcoital test

Fig. 14.13. Flow chart for the systematic evaluation of the uterine tubal passage. Only main areas are shown to facilitate readability. For more details see text

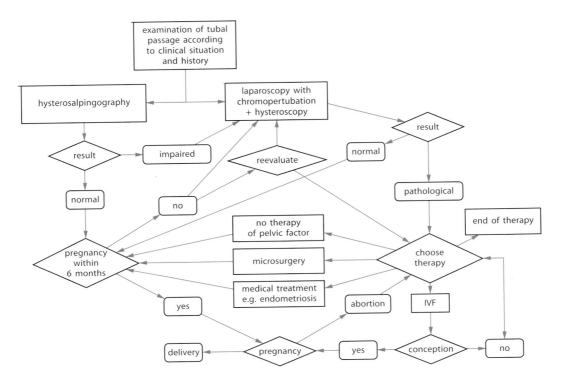

has been diagnosed due to poor mucus despite good estrogenization. Bacterial, viral, and yeast infections, as well as trichomoniasis should be considered. The most common pathogens are gardnerella vaginalis, neisseria gonorrhoea, chlamydia, mycoplasma and ureaplasma. Viral infections may be due to herpes and cytomegaly infections. Candida albicans is the most common yeast infection.

All forms of vaginitis may include cervicitis, causing a change in cervical mucus pH, and may represent a cause of infertility. Treatment can be local or systemic depending on the pathogen isolated. Post-infectious changes in the cervix can result in a stenosis or in damage to the cervical crypts with poor mucus production. Cervical smears in infertile couples have shown a mycoplasma infection in 12%, and pathogenic aerobic bacteria in 31% of the patients examined (Eggert-Kruse et al. 1992). Cervical operations such as electrocoagulation, cryotherapy, laser vaporization, or conization may be an indication for intrauterine insemination, if cervical passage of sperm is not possible.

14.3.2 Anomalies of the Female Genital Tract

The embryonic origin of the urogenital system is complex and explains many of the congenital anomalies found. A disruption in one of the many fusion steps can result in either a partial or complete agenesis of particular ducts. Congenital anomalies often include the urinary system.

Uterus

The unilateral agenesis or aplasia of the Muellerian duct results in a uterus unicornis. 0.1–3% of all women have varying uterine anomalies due to disturbed Muellerian fusion. These vary from a uterus subseptus unicollis up to the double uterus, cervix and vagina. Surgical treatment should only be recommended after considering all other possible causes for infertility, since the coexistence of infertility and, for example, a septate uterus, must not be causal.

Acquired uterine anomalies include fibroids and adhesions. Uterine leiomyomata are found in 20–25% of all women of reproductive age. They are usually asymptomatic. These fibroids may be subserous or, more importantly, intramural, submucosal, and/or pedunculated, which may be causal for infertility. A review of 27 studies from 1982–1996 reported on pregnancy rates after myectomy. Nine studies were prospective (Vercellini et al. 1998); their combined pregnancy rates were 57% (95% confidence interval 48–65%). The median interval from surgery to pregnancy varied between 8 and 20 months. Unfortunately no study compared results from surgery with non-intervention (simple waiting), so that

any improvement in probability of conception following myectomy cannot be definitely ascertained.

Fallopian Tubes

Congenital defects of the Fallopian tubes are very rare, especially if the remaining organs are normal. In rare cases, one-sided aplasia of the ovary and uterine anomaly may be combined with a one-sided aplasia of the Fallopian tube. The cause for the rare case of missing parts of the Fallopian tube is not known.

The Fallopian tube can be morphologically divided into four segments:

- The **interstitial segment** is the part of the Fallopian tube which passes through the uterine wall and is surrounded by myometrium. The endosalpinx consists of secretory and ciliated cells which form longitudinal folds in the form of a star. The diameter is about 400 µm.
- The **isthmic portion** of the tube consists of the proximal third of the Fallopian tube. The endosalpinx here has more secretory cells than ciliated cells.
- The **ampulla** consists of the other two thirds of the lateral Fallopian tube. The cilia beat towards the uterus and are important for the transport of the oocyte and embryo. Surgical procedures on the isthmic portion of the Fallopian tubes still allow for pregnancy rates of about 80%. A resection of the ampulla, however, results in a clearly lower pregnancy rate. The major portion of ectopic pregnancies are found in the ampulla, since fertilization and early embryogenic development occur in this segment of the tube.
- The **infundibulum** is fringed by the fimbriae, which have close contact with the ovary. The ostium accepts the oocyte during ovulation by means of a mechanism yet unknown. Pathological changes due to infectious diseases, adhesions or operations result in a high infertility rate, and are difficult to treat by surgery.

14.3.3 Physiology of Tubal Function

Tubal motility, secretion, and ciliary activity are the prerequisites for the complex process of sperm transport, capacitation, oocyte retrieval, fertilization, zygote development, and the transport of the oocytes and of the zygote (also see Chap. 4). The Fallopian tube shows a continuous and complex pattern of spontaneous contractions. The relationship between the contractions and gamete transport is yet unclear. In contrast to the gastrointestinal tract, no regular peristaltic movements occur over a greater distance. Individual segments simultaneously contract in opposing directions and short distances. Oocyte transport is thus discontinuous with movement towards and away from the uterus. Since the movement is primarily towards the uterus, the oocyte finally ends up at the endometrium of the uterine cavity.

The significance of tubal contractility for sperm transport is not yet clear. One would assume that tubal passage is the result of sperm motility. After insemination, however, sperm can be found 5 min. later in the peritoneal cavity, so that tubal contraction must play a major role in the primary transport of sperm. A further assumption is that contractions of the uterus and the tubes during sexual intercourse play a role in rapid sperm transport. Sperm reaching the Fallopian tube in this manner, however, do not seem to be important for fertilization.

Tubal ciliary movement is directed towards the uterus, so that the transport of sperm in the other direction must be due to other mechanisms. The secretory activity of the Fallopian tube may play a role in spermal transport. Tubal secretion is greatest at time of ovulation, and these viscous glycoproteins seem to attenuate ciliary movement in such a manner so that the sperm are able to pass the Fallopian tube on their own, as they do in the mid-cyclic cervical mucus. After mucus secretion decreases, ciliary movement towards the uterus is reactivated so that the fertilized oocytes can be transported in the correct direction.

Tubal mucus production is estrogen-stimulated and inhibited by progestins. A number of proteins found in the tubal secretion, which cannot be found in serum, seem to be of importance for reproductive function.

In contrast to the testis, female gametes are transported through an open system. After leaving the ovarian surface, the oocyte must pass through the peritoneal cavity in order to reach the Fallopian tube. Microscopy studies in humans have shown that at the time of ovulation the fimbriae and the ostium of the tube are directly in contact with the ovary. This is due to contractions of the Fallopian tube, the mesosalpinx, and the fimbriae. Interestingly, pregnancy is possible with only one ovary and a contralateral Fallopian tube.

Surgical salpingostomy in a case of a fimbrial adhesion results in only a low pregnancy rate, which shows the importance of this pick-up mechanism.

Only a very small portion of the large number of sperm deposited intravaginally during intercourse reach the Fallopian tube (see Fig. 14.14). Only optimally formed and motile sperm are able to pass the filtration and selection mechanisms of the female tract in order to reach the ampulla and thus the location of fertilization.

Fertilization probably occurs in the distal ampulla. The sperm seem to survive 24 to 48 hours in the female genital tract, with some reports of survival up to 96 hours. The oocyte can however, only be fertilized for 24 hours. The fertilized oocyte begins division in the Fallopian tube. The human zygote has no nourishment reser-

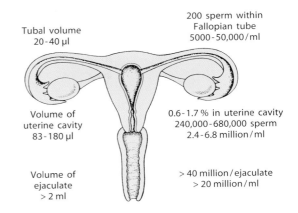

Fig. 14.14. Volume of different compartments of the female genital tract and resulting concentrations of sperm after vaginal ejaculation

voir nor constant cell contact during transport. The developing zygote must thus be maintained by the tubal secretions until it is implanted in the uterine cavity after about one week.

14.3.4 Diseases of the Fallopian Tubes

The complex processes of tubal passage show that disturbances in this area can cause infertility. Congenital anomalies are not as important as those that are acquired, such as adhesions caused by endometriosis or infections. Chlamydia infection is of primary importance.

Salpingitis

Nineteen percent of all women with salpingitis demonstrate an infection with chlamydia (Hoyme et al. 1988). Four percent of patients who underwent laparoscopy owing to tubal infertility showed culture-positive chlamydia. Since many pelvic infections have no or only unspecific symptoms, tubal passage should be checked in all patients who do not achieve pregnancy after 6 months, despite good luteal functions.

Especially in couples with clearly reduced male parameters, one should always consider further invasive diagnostic measures in the female patient.

The probability of tubal infertility in couples with secondary sterility rises by a factor of 7.5 with a history of venereal disease. A patient with appendectomy has a risk of 4.7 for tubal factor infertility when compared to controls. A history of a previous extrauterine pregnancy increases the risk 21fold, and a history of prior pelvic inflammatory disease increases the risk by a factor of 32 (Thonneau et al. 1993).

A tubal occlusion in the fimbrial part can cause a sausage-like swelling of the tube with reduction of wall structure. A meta-analysis of 14 single studies comprising over 5000 women showed that a sactosalpinx has negative consequences for conception (Camus et al. 1999). When IVF was carried out in patients with sactosalpinx, the pregnancy rate dropped by almost half compared to simple tubal obstruction close to the uterus (implantation 8.5% vs. 13.7%; birth rate 13.4% vs. 23.4%). From this it is concluded that the probability of pregnancy is reduced in cases of one-sided sactosalpinx and contralateral tubal patency. A prospective, randomized multicenter study demonstrated that IVF in patients whose sactosalpinx had been laparoscopically corrected before therapy had a significantly higher birthrate than non-operated controls (Strandell et al. 1999). This effect is markedly higher in women with sactosalpinx on both sides.

14.3.5 Diagnostic Tests of the Uterine Cavity and Tubal Patency

The available tests for tubal patency are:
- insufflation of Fallopian tube with CO_2,
- hysterosalpingography,
- chromoperturbation and diagnostic laparoscopy.

Tubal Insufflation

This method was first described in the 1920s and is unreliable. No clear information can be obtained whether the tubal obstruction lies on one or on both sides. Direct comparison with laparoscopy shows great discrepancy of the results. This method should not even be used as a screening procedure.

Hysterosalpingography

Hysterosalpingography (HSG) is a much more important procedure. It can be performed on an outpatient basis after giving an analgesic such as indomethacin 1–2 hours prior. The examination of the tubes is performed via a fluoroscope. In rare cases, tubal spasm may lead to misdiagnosis of a tubal occlusion. Spasmolytic drugs such as 1–2 ml butylscopolaminebromide i.v. should be tried.

The ovarian radiation dose varies between 1.7 mGy for a 100 mm fluoroscopic film and 2.8 mCy for a 24×30 cm spot film. This procedure is usually timed 2–5 days after menstrual bleeding in order to minimize the disturbance of a possible early pregnancy.

The risk of this radiographic diagnostic procedure is that of infection which has a probability of 1%. Identification of patients at risk has been tried through blood sampling of leukocytes, c-reactive protein, and sedimentation rates. Our own studies, however, have shown that this has a poor specificity and sensitivity (Knuth et al. 1982).

Some authors recommend prophylactic antibiotics such as 200 mg doxycycline two days before the procedure followed by five days of 100 mg. There are no uniform recommendations, and we do not use prophylactic antibiotic treatment.

During hysterosalpingography the uterine cavity is easily delineable and septae, polyps and submucosal fibroids are readily seen. In order to evaluate the significance of this diagnostic procedure, consequent pregnancy rates must be correlated to previous results. A normal hysterosalpingography was followed by pregnancy in 46% of cases with donor insemination. A uterine anomaly or defect with bilateral tubal patency resulted in a pregnancy rate of 34%. Normal uterine anatomy with unilateral tubal occlusion resulted in a pregnancy rate of 40% after donor insemination (Stovall et al. 1992).

The relatively high rate of conception despite pathological hysterosalpingography examination is probably due to optimal male factors during donor insemination. This must be considered if the male factor in the infertile couple is also impaired.

When comparing hysterosalpingography with laparoscopy and chromoperturbation a larger discrepancy is found. The predictions from HSG thus do not seem to be optimal. A positive correlation of the data is found in 62% of 104 patients examined (Adelusi et al. 1995). If the results of hysterosalpingography are normal, in 96% of the cases laparoscopy and chromoperturbation are also normal. If the HSG results are unclear and lesions are expected, laparoscopy is only correlated in 63% of cases. Suspicious lesions in the Fallopian tubes are only correlated in 54%, so that Opsahl et al. (1993) deduced that women with a normal HSG who do not conceive must undergo diagnostic laparoscopy. The interpretation of HSG can be optimized through a special catheter system which perfuses each Fallopian tube individually. In this procedure, it is possible to measure the pressure necessary to achieve patency in each individual tube. Normal tubes require a pressure of 429±376 mmHg, pathological tubes require a pressure of 957±445 mmHg (Gleicher et al. 1992). A similar procedure can be performed less invasively by duplex sonography (Allahbadia 1992). Newly developed sonographic contrast substances allow the HSG to be performed entirely by ultrasound (Degenhardt et al. 1995). This new technique may provide a simple screening procedure in the infertility clinic, although one must consider its limits in the evaluation of tubal patency.

If an HSG is performed in the classical manner an oil suspension contrast medium should be used since this results in a higher pregnancy rates compared to cases in which a hydrophilic agent is used (Watson et al. 1994). A small risk of granuloma formation following oily media must, however, be considered.

In conclusion, sono-hysterosalpingography can be recommended as a screening procedure for tubal patency in women with an uneventful prior history, negative chlamydia tests, and period of non-conception less than one year. If these requirements are not fulfilled, laparoscopy and chromoperturbation should be performed.

Hysteroscopy and Laparoscopy

The standard method for the diagnosis of pelvic conditions and tubal patency is laparoscopy combined with chromoperturbation and hysteroscopy. In contrast to hysterosalpingography, endometriosis adhesions, Fallopian tubal thinning, and ovarian alterations can be optimally diagnosed by an experienced surgeon.

Hysteroscopy. This procedure can be performed without general anesthesia if no consequent laparoscopy is planned. A rigid or flexible endoscope is passed through the cervical os into the uterine cavity which, since it is usually collapsed, must be distended by a medium. High molecular dextrin, CO_2 or 5% dextrose in water may be used. A separate instrument channel may be used, through which forceps, electrocautery or laser devices can be passed.

Laparoscopy. Laparoscopy is usually performed under general anesthesia with intubation. After subumbilical incision and insufflation of the peritoneal cavity with CO_2, the laparoscopic trocar and the laparoscope are introduced. The risks of this procedure are that of gastrointestinal or great vessel perforation. This occurs in about 0.1% of all examinations. After 1 or 2 additional incisions are made for the introduction further instruments, dye can be injected through the intrauterine cannula. Direct observation attests to tubal patency if dye spills from the ostium.

Since intraabdominal adhesions can be associated with intratubal pathology without clear disturbance of tubal patency, new diagnostic measures have been implemented. Falloscopy is performed with extremely fine endoscopes through which the internal Fallopian tube can be inspected during hysteroscopy or laparoscopy. These endoscopes have a special optical system in order to prevent damage to the Fallopian mucosa (Venezia et al. 1993).

14.3.6 Treatment

Depending on the pathology of the Fallopian tube either adhesiolysis, fimbrioplasty, salpingostomy or anastomosis may be considered. **Adhesiolysis** includes all microsurgical procedures which are performed to regain the mobility of the Fallopian tube and the ovary. **Fimbriolysis** is performed in order to mobilize fimbriae, peritoneal defects are carefully surtured. **Fimbrioplasty** is the reconstruction of the existing fimbriae in a partially or totally occluded oviduct. In the case of total occlusion, the ostium is opened and the serosa is everted in order to form a fimbriostium. If ampullary occlusion requires the resection of a part of the tube, a **salpingoneostomy** is performed. Anastomosis can be performed at every segment of the Fallopian tube.

Today the results of microsurgical procedures must be compared to those of IVF programmes. One must consider, however, that **microsurgery** may be a curative form of treatment for a patient, whereas **IVF** is only a temporary treatment form. Pregnancy rates after surgical salpingolysis, fimbriolysis and ovarialysis lie between 39–69%. In a summary statistic, a median pregnancy rate of 40% has been calculated after conventional techniques.

Post-inflammatory tubal diseases, which require fimbrioplasty and salpingostomy, however, have poorer results. A study at the University of Münster showed a pregnancy rate of only 25% in such patients (for overview see Schneider and Karbowski 1989). When deciding on the form of treatment, the availability of an experienced surgeon must be considered. The patient should be referred to a specialized microsurgical department, if an immediate IVF procedure is not to be recommended.

14.4 Endometriosis

Although it can be argued whether hysterosalpingography or laparoscopy is the better diagnostic test to check for tubal patency, laparoscopy is absolutely necessary in order to diagnose peritoneal endometriosis.

14.4.1 Pathogenesis and Epidemiology

Endometriosis is a disorder in which normal endometrium or endometrium-like tissue is found in locations other than the uterine cavity. These ectopic tissues may be involved in pathological as well as normal cyclic changes of the endometrium. The true cause of endometriosis, which can cause infertility, is unknown and many theories have been discussed. To date, the accepted theory is that endometriosis occurs through implantation of individual endometrial cells and endometrium fragments which are passed through the Fallopian tubes into the peritoneal cavity in retrograde fashion during menstruation. It is assumed that these cells then implant on the peritoneal surfaces and grow into endometrial lesions. After further proliferation these tissue particles grow to allow macroscopic visualization (Dmowski 1995).

Endometriosis is found in 5–10 % of all women of reproductive age. Its prevalence, however, is much higher in women with infertility problems.

14.4.2 Symptoms

The cardinal symptoms of endometriosis are pelvic pain, dysfunctional bleeding, and infertility. The pathophysiology by which endometriosis causes infertility is multifactorial. This includes mechanical factors, toxic derivatives in the peritoneal fluid, as well as immunological and hormonal disturbances.

The main cause for infertility, however, lies in the adhesions found in progressive stages of endometriosis. Peritubal and periovarian adhesions inhibit the interaction between the uterine tube and the ovary, which is important at the time of ovulation. Proximal tubal occlusion is often found. Although endometriosis is often present on the ovaries, small lesions probably do not play a role in fertility. Larger endometriosis, or endometriomas can invade stroma of the ovary, destroying normal tissue. These are called "chocolate cysts".

14.4.3 Pathophysiology

Physiologically, the ovaries and the tubes are surrounded by peritoneal fluid, the volume of which rises to about 20 ml at the time of ovulation. The regulation of peritoneal fluid volume is disturbed in women with endometriosis. Embryotoxic substances are also found in the peritoneal fluid of these women. After incubating sperm with the peritoneal fluid of endometriosis patients, one sees a reduction in motility in computerized analysis when compared to controls. Presumably, prostaglandins and macrophages inhibit sperm motility.

An increase in prostaglandin concentrations in the peritoneal fluid probably alters the contractility of the tubes, so that the transport of sperm, the oocyte and the zygote are modified. Normally, the peritoneal fluid contains 0.5–2 million leukocytes per ml, the major portion of which are macrophages. If endometriosis is found on the peritoneum, there is a proportional rise in macrophages. One cannot, however, discern whether these changes in the peritoneal fluid are the result or a cause of endometriosis.

Patients with endometriosis have an increased levels of IgM, IgG and IgA when compared to normal controls. An inverse correlation of the immunoglobulins with the severity of endometriosis is, however, found. Some authors presume that endometriosis is an autoimmune disease, but this has yet to be proven.

Diagnosis of endometriosis is possible by direct visual observation or histological examination during laparoscopy or laparotomy. One must be careful to search the entire pelvic peritoneum systematically in order to find discrete endometriotic lesions. It is not enough to just perform one quick diagnostic view through the endoscope and to let the patient go home with the diagnosis of endometriosis after visualizing a few topical brown-black lesions. Often only histological probes will show the typical endometriotic alterations.

14.4.4 Staging of Endometriosis

Once a diagnosis of endometriosis has been made, a staging classification must be performed. This is usually done with the help of the revised classification of the American Fertility Society (Table 14.1).

In Germany one often uses the endoscopic classification of endometriosis according to Semm, which is divided into four groups.

- **Group I:** normal patent tubes and endometriotic lesions of the epithelium under 5 mm in diameter.
- **Group II:** endometriotic lesions greater than 5 mm in diameter possibly involving the bladder, periovarian and peritubal adhesions, and/or a stenosis or phimosis of the uterine tubes.
- **Group III:** adenomyomata in the uterus or in the intramural part of the uterine tube, chocolate cysts, lesions in the sacrouterine ligaments or a sactosalpinx.
- **Group IV:** extragenital endometriosis.

Since laparoscopy is an invasive test, another screening method for endometriosis has been sought for in the past. The most commonly used parameter is the tumor marker Ca 12–5, which is a membrane antigen of epithelial origin which can be measured in the serum. Ca 12–5 levels are elevated in women with epithelial ovarian cancer and other neoplasias of the pelvis. Slight elevations are also found in women with endometriosis. The sensitivity and specificity of this parameter is, however, so low that women with slight endometriosis may have a normal level.

Table 14.1. Revised classification of endometriosis (American Society for Reproductive Medicine)

	Endometriosis	<1 cm	1–3 cm	>3 cm
Peritoneum	Superficial	1	2	4
	Deep	2	4	6
Right ovary	Superficial	1	2	4
	Deep	4	16	20
Left ovary	Superficial	1	2	4
	Deep	4	16	20
post. Culdesac-Obliteration	Partial: 4		Complete: 40	
	Adhesions	**<1/3**	**1/3–2/3**	**>2/3**
Right ovary	Filmy	1	2	4
	Dense	4	8	16
Left ovary	Filmy	1	2	4
	Dense	4	8	16
Right tube	Filmy	1	2	4
	Dense	4[a]	8[a]	16
Left tube	Filmy	1	2	4
	Dense	4[a]	8[a]	16

[a] If the fimbriated end of the Fallopian tube is completely closed, change the point assignment to 16.

Stage I   (Minimal) = 1–5,
Stage II   (Mild) = 6–15,
Stage III (Moderate) = 16–40,
Stage IV   (Severe) >40

14.4.5 Treatment

Since the pathophysiology of the disease has not been fully clarified, there is **no ideal treatment**. If adhesion formation with impaired tubal function, large endometriomas, or occluded Fallopian tubes can be diagnosed, the mainstay of therapy will be microsurgery, in some cases after prior drug treatment. In other cases it is not clear whether a specific treatment of endometriosis is even necessary. The form of treatment recommended must be tailored to the individual situation of the infertile couple.

Typical pharmacological treatment forms include
- progestins,
- danazol and
- GnRH analogs.

The estrogen and progestin combination, which has been used in the past to achieve pseudo-pregnancy, is only be used in rare cases (Schweppe 1995).

Danazol

Before GnRH analogs were introduced, danazol was the mainstay of treatment following its introduction in 1971. However, double-blind controlled studies never seem to have demonstrated a better effectiveness of danazol treatment compared to pure progestin therapy. In order to understand the mechanism of action, one must assume that receptors for estrogens and progestins are contained in endometriotic lesions, and that neutralization of these ligands will cause atrophy of the lesions. This is the main principle of the pharmacological treatment of endometriosis.

In premenopausal women, however, an extreme hypogonadotropic situation is not produced, even though the mid-cyclic LH and FSH peaks are suppressed. More importantly, danazol seems to interfere with the binding of the sex hormones to their receptors. Danazol mainly binds to progestin and androgen receptors, and interestingly enough, not to the estrogen receptor. Danazol displaces testosterone and estradiol from SHBG, and progesterone and cortisol from corticosteroid binding globulin. Consequently, an elevation of the free fractions of these hormones with the respective clinical symptoms, such as hyperandrogenemia, occur. Additionally, danazol reduces the hepatic synthesis of SHBG so that the serum concentrations of free androgen rises further. Danazol directly inhibits enzymes that synthesize estrogens.

Danazol is available in 200 mg tablets; the daily dosage is about 800 mg divided into four doses. No pregnancy can occur during this therapy, which is usually performed for six months. An attempt to lower the dosage alleviated adverse clinical symptoms, but did not show equivalent effects in control laparoscopy. In every case the goal of treatment should be amenorrhea. Estradiol serum levels should be below 40 pg/ml in minimal endometriosis, and below 20 pg/ml in more severe cases.

The **pregnancy rate** after danazol treatment lies between 28–72%. If endometrioma greater than 1 cm in diameter have been visualized, surgical treatment should be performed. One study showed that patients with minimal endometriosis who were treated for 6 months with danazol achieved a pregnancy rate of 37% after a 12-month control phase. The untreated control group, however, had a pregnancy rate of 57% (Seibel et al. 1982). This casts doubt on the rule that endometriosis necessitates treatment in all cases. Obtaining the entire clinical picture with optimal laparoscopic description and diagnosis of the disease is essential before deciding on a form of treatment.

Treatment of endometriosis by danazol is not curative, since even atrophic lesions may again proliferate after conclusion of treatment. Recurrence rates lie between 33% and 39%. Most pregnancies occur in the seven months following treatment. If no conception occurs during this time, one must consider a different form of treatment.

The elevation of androgen concentrations causes virilization in some patients. Side-effects of danazol treatment include weight gain, acne, hirsutism and reduced breast volume. In rare cases, a deepening of the voice occurs, which must be considered in those professions in which this is important. This side-effects seem to be irreversible.

GnRH Analogs

GnRH analogs are a good option for inducing reversible pseudo-menopause in which a hypogonadotropic and hypoestrogenic condition equivalent to **temporary castration** is achieved. The principle of this form of treatment has been discussed in another chapter of this book. The mechanism in females is similar to that in males, in which down-regulation results in the desired low estradiol concentration. The success of a treatment is directly proportional to the extent of estrogen reduction.

GnRH agonists probably do not have a direct effect on the ovaries. Successful treatment is due solely to estrogen deficiency. Evaluation of pregnancy rates after GnRH and danazol therapy shows similar results. Because of the hyperandrogenemic side-effects of danazol therapy, it is likely that GnRH treatment will be recommended.

The main **side-effect of GnRH agonist** treatment is that of profound hypoestrogenemia including flushes, vaginal dryness, reduced libido, and at times, depression. There is no influence on plasma lipoproteins. During a six-month treatment course, a reduction of bone mass can be reversible after conclusion of therapy.

Surgical Treatment

Surgical treatment is indicated in infertile patients with extreme adhesion formation, enlarged ovaries, and pain which is not ameliorated after pharmacological treatment, and in older patients for whom lengthy medical treatment seems inappropriate. Individualization of therapy is important, since, as in microsurgical treatment, the experience of the available surgeon has considerable significance for successful treatment.

IVF

In vitro fertilization may offer the only possibility for patients with extreme endometriosis, although results are poor in this patient group (Simon et al. 1994). Another study, however, showed pregnancy rates of 29% per transfer in endometriosis patients compared to 25% in controls (Dmowski et al. 1995).

14.5 Sperm Antibodies

If hormonal and clinical factors of female infertility have been ruled out, immunological causes are considered next.

The **mucosal immune system** represents the largest immunocompetent structure of the human body, and includes the majority of endogenous antibody-producing plasma cells. Antibodies which are detected in blood or lymph samples usually belong to the IgG-group, whereas antibodies found in secretions such as the cervical mucus are usually of the IgA group.

14.5.1 Pathophysioloy

Although a sexually active female is exposed to a great number of potential antigens in the form of spermatozoa, the female immune system can usually not be activated in this manner. Different factors may play a role in this mechanism (Jones 1994). For example, non-specific antibodies, which surround the spermatozoa in a protective fashion, deterring an immunological response, have been discussed (for review see Marshburn and Kutteh 1994).

14.5.2 Antibody Testing

Sperm antibody tests usually depend on sperm agglutination and sperm immobilization by serum antibodies. The measurement of serum antibodies against spermatozoa is without clinical significance, however, since the levels are not correlated with those of genital secretions. ELISA measurements give greatly varying results, depending on which antigen is used from the wide range of spermatozoal proteins. This explains why research data are so contradictory.

The best method to determine antibodies in the female seems to be the indirect immunobead test. Donor sperm are incubated with the body fluid to be examined, and then undergo multiple washings with a buffer. Antibodies against IgA, IgG, and, in some cases IgM, which are bound on small latex particles, are added and then the number of donor spermatozoa with attached immunobeads are counted (WHO 1999).

Spermatozoal antibodies are found in about 2–3% of the general population. The possibility of causing an amplified immunological response to intrauterine insemination using a high number of spermatozoa could not be confirmed in any of several studies (Marshburn and Kutteh 1994).

Sperm antibodies in the cervical mucus are inversely correlated with the number of live sperm during the postcoital test. However, a positive correlation between circulating antibodies and pregnancy rates cannot be proven (Eggert-Kruse et al. 1989). In conclusion, the significance of female antibodies has yet to be determined. Serum antibody testing is decidedly not an integral part of routine screening of the infertile couple. If a pathological postcoital test is found despite good cervical factors, the cervical secretion should be tested for antibodies. This is also true for other cases of unexplained infertility.

14.5.3 Treatment

The detection of sperm antibodies in combination with protracted involuntary childlessness only indicates subfertility, since studies have shown that these antibodies do not absolutely impede spontaneous pregnancy. Different strategies have been recommended to optimize the probability of conception.

- The use of **condoms** for several months has been recommended in the past in order to inhibit boostering of the immunological response. Higher pregnancy rates, have, however, not been achieved through this method.
- The results of **immune-suppressive treatment** with **glucocorticoids** vary. Since the significance of female antibodies is not clear, and the side-effects of this treatment can be severe, it should not be recommended.
- Similarly **intrauterine insemination** does not seem to elevate pregnancy rates significantly. Clinical studies showed that after 6 months of intrauterine insemination, pregnancy rates were equal to those of patients without sperm antibodies who also had poor postcoital tests (42.4% vs. 40.5%) (Check et al. 1994). This shows that these antibodies do not play a very large role in infertility.

It is not clear if IVF outcome is influenced by female sperm antibodies. Some studies show poorer fertilization results in these cases. In a study of 2363 patients, no differences in the pregnancy rates could be found between women with or without sperm antibodies (Check et al. 1995).

14.6 Early Pregnancy Abnormalities

14.6.1 Implantation

After fertilization occurs in the ampulla of the Fallopian tube, rapid cell division begins. Details of this development are described in Section 4.7. About six to eight days after conception, the blastocyte is implanted in the uterine cavity, and hCG production can be measured as a sign of implantation. Once pregnancy has been established, the gynecologist will calculate gestational age, necessary for monitoring pregnancy, and the estimated date of birth. Using Nägele's rule, the birth date can be determined by subtracting three months from the date of the last menstrual period while adding seven days to the first day of the last menstruation. This rule is based on a normal 28-day cycle, and if ovulation occurs prior to or later than the 14th day, the EDD must be corrected accordingly. Deviation from the accepted conventions of calculating gestational age can cause considerable mis-understandings and incorrect evaluation of early pregnancy.

14.6.2 Pregnancy Loss

Conception and implantation do not suffice to consider infertility treatment as successful since many couples will experience pregnancy loss.

If fetal weight is below 500 g at birth, abortion or miscarriage has occurred. Fetal weight over 500 g of a child born dead is considered a stillbirth. About 15% of all pregnancies end in abortion, with clinically recognizable fetal loss between the fourth and twentieth gestational week. The more accurate figure is about 50% of all pregnancies which end in abortion as many patients abort between the second and fourth gestational week before pregnancy becomes clinically evident, during the time in which early β-hCG measurements are not routinely performed.

80% of spontaneous abortions occur during the first twelve weeks of pregnancy. 70% of these abortions are due to chromosomal defects. Whereas young women at the age of 20 years have an abortion frequency of about 12%, older women at the end of their reproductive life have an abortion frequency of 26%. The probability of an abortion increases significantly when implanation is delayed (Wilcox et al. 1999). If a normal embryo can be detected by ultrasound, the probability of later abortion sinks to about 5%. If, however, there is a past history of several abortions, this rate rises by a factor of 4–5 (van Leeuwen et al. 1993).

Epidemiology

One miscarriage is, as can be seen above, not unusual, in fact one miscarriage is almost a normal experience of female reproductive life. Recurrent pregnancy loss is pathological and is defined as at least three consecutive miscarriages. Based on several clinical studies, the risk of a further miscarriage lies between 30–45% and does not, as was once presumed, rise further.

Etiologic Factors

A study of 500 patients with recurrent pregnancy loss gives indications of the frequency of varying possible factors (Clifford et al. 1994). 76% of the examined women had miscarriages before the 13th gestational week. Only 3% had a clinical abortion after this time.

- In 3.6% of all examined couples a **chromosomal defect** could be found, in which a balanced translocation was the most common diagnosis.

- 56% of the women had morphologic signs of **polycystic ovarian disease.** 12% of these women had mid-follicle LH levels greater than 10 IU/l.
- Further analysis of the LH concentrations using daily early morning urine analysis showed a **hypersecretion of LH** in 57% of the women.
- In the group of 372 women with early miscarriage, 14% had measurable anti-phospholipid antibodies.
- 9 women showed **uterine anomalies** in which 6 had uterine septae, and 3 a uterus bicornis. HLA-typing was not done in these patients.

A history of male chemotherapy or radiation therapy increases the potential for **chromosomal defects**, so that in addition to fetal anomalies, elevated miscarriage rates are also possible (Meistrich 1993).

Environmental factors and other **toxins** such as smoking, high caffeine intake, and alcohol have been discussed as etiological agents for miscarriage. Anesthetic gases und cleaning solvents have been discussed as typical hazards of the working environment. Elucidation of the causes is usually not possible in the individual case.

If chromosomal defects can be ruled out, endocrine factors must be considered. Thyroidal dysfunction, autoimmune diseases, and poorly adjusted diabetes mellitus have been associated with miscarriages, but probably do not play a major role in infertility patients.

The importance of an **insufficient luteal phase** and **polycystic ovarian disease** has been discussed. It is not clear whether support of the luteal phase by progesterone or hCG treatment can improve pregnancy rates. A significant effect of hCG-treatment in IVF cycles with GnRH analoga can be seen on luteal function. These results are, however, controversial in other clinical situations. In one of the latest clinical studies it could be shown that in patients with sufficient down-regulation by GnRH analogs, substitution with hCG or progesterone resulted in similar pregnancy rates (Soliman et al. 1994).

Uterine Anomalies. About 12–15% of all women with recurrent pregnancy loss have a uterine anomaly which can be confirmed by vaginal ultrasound examination and/or hysterosalpingography. In 1200 HSG examinations 188 congenital uterus anomalies were found (Makino et al. 1992). The miscarriage rate did not differ between those with a slight anomaly or those with more extreme variations. After surgical correction through metroplasty, 84% of the resulting pregnancies could be carried to term. In 74 women who had not yet received surgical treatment and were used as controls, 94% of the pregnancies ended in spontaneous abortion before the 12th gestational week. These data show the importance of checking for uterine anomalies in patients with recurrent pregnancy loss.

Infections. The significance of infectious diseases especially in abortions occurring after the 12th gestational week is noteworthy. Microbial samples should be checked for chlamydia, ureaplasma, toxoplasmosis and Listeria monocytogenis as well as Mycoplasma hominis.

Autoimmunity. 10%–16% of women with recurrent pregnancy loss have antiphospholipid antibodies (Plouffe et al. 1992). These antibodies block prostacycline synthesis, and result in high thromboxane activity with vasoconstriction and thrombosis. This in turn causes foetal growth retardation or fetal death, often in the form of recurrent miscarriage. Prothrombin time and partial thromboplastin time are elevated by antiphospholipid antibodies, and can be used as screening tests. If antiphospholipid antibodies are presumed to be the cause of recurrent pregnancy loss, treatment in form of low-dose aspirin in combination with heparin can begin as soon as pregnancy has been diagnosed. Treatment with glucocorticoids with dose titration until coagulation tests become normal have also been recommended.

Alloimmunity. A widely accepted theory states that the maternal immune systems develops a certain tolerance against the trophoblast owing to protective antibodies or blocking factors. These hypothetical factors possibly block the rejection of the autoallogenic embryo. The mechanism is, however, not clear. A rejection of the pregnancy is presumed to occur if the blocking factors fail to be produced. One possible explanation has been suggested by findings in HLA measurements, since couples with recurrent pregnancy loss often have compatible HLA antigens.

Based on this theory, patients with recurrent miscarriages were **immunized with partner lymphocytes.** The first results were very impressive with pregnancy rates of 70–80%. Clinical trials, however, have been very conflicting, and were not able to confirm the results of the early uncontrolled studies. This resulted in a rejection of this form of therapy (Frazer et al. 1993), which in turn was, however, contradicted by other investigators (Cowchock and Smith 1994). If there is an effect of immunization, it is very small and has a causal success in less than 5% of those treated. Since immunization treatment is not without risk, each individual case must be decided by the responsible physician.

As an alternative treatment form to active immunization some have recommended treatment with **unspecific immunoglobulins.** A larger multicenter study, however, came to the conclusion that the diagnostic and prognostic value of HLA-typing has been overestimated (Mueller-Eckhardt et al. 1994). Intravenous treatment with immunoglobulins and albumin was seen equal to that of placebo (Mueller-Eckhardt 1994).

14.7 Idiopathic (= Unexplained) Infertility

If all tests described above show normal results, and no causes for infertility can be found, this is called "idiopathic or unexplained infertility". This must be differentiated from the so-called idiopathic infertility of the male, which is characterized by an unexplained reduction of the semen quality. In 10–15% of infertile couples no clear cause can be defined (Crosignani et al. 1992). Prognosis of this condition is correlated with the couple's age and the length of infertility (see above).

In contrast to the normal monthly fecundity rate of 25%, couples with idiopathic or unexplained infertility have a conception rate of 1.5–3% per cycle. Patience and time alone will result in pregnancy in about 60% of the couples with idiopathic or unexplained infertility (Verkauf 1983). As a rule, no treatment should be performed if a diagnosis cannot be made. Empirical studies, however, have shown that methods of assisted reproduction result in higher pregnancy rates in couples with unexplained infertility. If a couple with unexplained infertility does not achieve pregnancy within three years, stimulation with hMG in combination with intrauterine insemination may be considered. If a conception is not achieved within 4–6 months, IVF may be performed. The results of this therapy may also be diagnostic in nature. If fertilization occurs and pregnancy does not follow, another trial of conservative therapy with hMG stimulation may be justified. Following this strategy, a cumulative pregnancy rate of 40% is achieved after six cycles with superovulation or after three cycles of IVF (Simon and Laufer 1993).

14.8 Prospects and Conclusion

If, despite all therapeutic efforts, delivery of a baby cannot be achieved, concluding treatment is a major step. Determining to end treatment signifies a failure for the couple as well as for the physician, and represents a psychological burden for everyone involved. In their despair, many couples may look for treatment by another physician and undergo the entire procedure a second time. Couples must be counselled so that they can plan the rest of their lives accordingly. Psychological counselling should be an integral part not only during treatment, but also at its conclusion. Further possibilities such as heterologous insemination or adoption must be discussed carefully and with empathy with the couple.

14.9 References

Adashi EY, Rock JA, Guzick D, Wentz AC, Jones GS, Jones HW Jr (1981) Fertility following bilateral ovarian wedge resection: a critical analysis of 90 consecutive cases of the polycystic ovary syndrome. Fertil Steril 36:320–325

Adelusi B, Alnuaim L, Makanjuola D, Khashoggi T, Chowdhury N, Kangave D (1995) Accuracy of hysterosalpingography and laparoscopic hydrotubation in diagnosis of tubal patency. Fertil Steril 63:1016–1020

Agarwal SK, Haney AF (1994) Does recommending timed intercourse really help the infertile couple? Obstet Gynecol 84:307–310

Allahbadia GN (1992) Fallopian tubes and ultrasonography – the Sion experience. Fertil Steril 58:901–907

Arlt W, Callies F, van Vlijmen JC, Koehler I, Reincke M, Bidlingmaier M, Huebler D, Oettel M, Ernst M, Schulte HM, Allolio B (1999) Dehydroepiandrosterone replacement in women with adrenal insufficiency. N Engl J Med 341:1013–1020

Baird DT, Howles CM (1994) Induction of ovulation with gonadotrophins: hMG versus purified FSH. In: Filicori M, Flamigni C (eds) Ovulation induction: Science and clinical advances. Elsevier, Amsterdam, pp 135–151

Bakimer R, Cohen JR, Shoenfeld Y (1994) What really happens to fecundity in autoimmune diseases? Immunol Allergy Clin North Am 14:701–723

Bancroft J (1993) Impact of environment, stress, occupational, and other hazards on sexuality and sexual behavior. Environ Health Perspect 101 [Suppl 2]:101–107

Banks AL (1961) Does adoption affect infertility? Int J Fertil 7:23–28

Baranski B (1993) Effects of the workplace on fertility and related reproductive outcomes. Environ Health Perspect 101 [Suppl 2]:81–90

Bhal PS, Pugh ND, Chui DK, Gregory L, Walker SM, Shaw RW (1999) The use of transvaginal power Doppler ultrasonography to evaluate the relationship between perifollicular vascularity and outcome in in-vitro fertilization treatment cycles. Hum Reprod 14:939–945

Blasco L (1994) Dyssynchrony in the maturation of endometrial glands and stromae. Fertil Steril 61:596–597

Boce J, Linet M (1994) Chernobyl, childhood cancer, and chromosome 21. Br Med J 309:139–140

Bohnet HG (1985) Prolactin und weibliche Sterilität. Leitfaden für die Praxis

Bohnet HG, Kato K, Wolf SA (1986) Treatment of hyperprolactinemic amenorrhea with Metergoline. Obstet Gynecol 67:249–251

Bokemeyer C, Schmoll HJ, Vanrhee J, Kuczyk M, Schuppert F, Poliwoda H (1994) Long-term gonadal toxicity after therapy for Hodgkins and non-Hodgkins lymphoma. Ann Hematol 68:105–110

Brevis AA (1993) Age and infertility in a Micronesean atoll population. Hum Biol 65:593–609

Brocklehurst P, French R (1998) The association between maternal HIV infection and perinatal outcome: a systematic review of the literature and meta-analysis. Br J Obstet Gynaecol 105:836–848

Buttery B, Trounson A, McMaster R, Wood C (1983) Evaluation of diagnostic ultrasound as a parameter of follicular development in an in vitro fertilization program. Fertil Steril 39:458–463

Buttram VC Jr, Vaquero C (1975) Post-ovarian wedge resection adhesive disease. Fertil Steril 26:874–876

Börner P (1986) Gynäkologische Erkrankungen. In: Künzel W, Wulf KK (eds) Die gestörte Schwangerschaft, Klinik der Frauenheilkunde und Geburtshilfe,vol 5. Urban and Schwarzenberg, Munich, pp 343–363

Camus E, Poncelet C, Goffinet F, Wainer B, Merlet F, Nisand I, Philippe HJ (1999) Pregnancy rates after in-vitro fertilization in cases of tubal infertility with and without hydrosalpinx: a meta-analysis of published comparative studies. Hum Reprod 14:1243–1249

Check JH, Bollendorf A, Katsoff D, Kozak J (1994) The frequency of antisperm antibodies in the cervical mucus of women with poor postcoital tests and their effect on pregnancy rates. Am J Reprod Immunol 32:38–42

Check JH, Katsoff D, Bollendorf A, Callan C (1995) The effect of sera antisperm antibodies in the female partner on in vivo and in vitro pregnancy and spontaneous abortion rates. Am J Reprod Immunol 33:131–133

Chrousos GP (1995) Seminars in medicine of the Beth Israel Hospital, Boston: the hypothalamic-pituitary-adrenal axis and immune-mediated inflammation. N Engl J Med 332:1351–1362

Chun SY, Hsueh AJW (1999) Paracrine mechanisms of ovarian follicle apoptosis. J Reprod Immunol 39:63–75

Clayton RN, Ogden V, Hodgkinson J, Worswick L, Rodin DA, Dyer S, Meade TW (1992) How common are polycystic ovaries in normal women and what is their significance for the fertility of the population. Clin Endocrinol 37:127–134

Clifford K, Rai R, Watson H, Regan L (1994) An informative protocol for the investigation of recurrent miscarriage: preliminary experience of 500 consecutive cases. Hum Reprod 9:1328–1332

Committee on the Biological Effect of Ionizing Radiations (1990) Health effects of exposure to low levels of ionizing radiation (BEIR V). National Academy Press, Washington, DC

Corson SL, Gutmann J, Batzer FR, Wallace H, Klein N, Soules MR (1999) Inhibin-B as a test of ovarian reserve for infertile women. Hum Reprod 14:2818–2821

Cowchock S, Smith JB (1994) Immunization as therapy for recurrent spontaneous abortion – a review and meta-analysis (letter). Obstet Gynecol 83:637–638

Critchley HOD, Wallace WHB, Shalet SM, Mamtora H, Higginson J, Anderson DC (1992) Abdominal irradiation in childhood – the potential for pregnancy. Br J Obstet Gynaecol 99:392–394

Crosignani PG, Collins J, Cooke ID, Diczfalusy E, Rubin B (1993) Unexplained infertility. Hum Reprod 8:977–980

Csapo AI, Pulkkinen MO, Wiest WG (1973) Effect of lutectomy and early progesterone replacement therapy in early pregnant patients. Am J Obstet Gynecol 115:759–765

Davis S (1999a) Androgen replacement in women: a commentary. J Clin Endocrinol Metab 84:1886–1891

Davis SR (1999b) The therapeutic use of androgens in women. J Steroid Biochem Mol Biol 69:177–184

Degenhardt F, Jibril S, Gohde M, Eisenhauer B, Schlößer HW (1995) Die ambulante Hystero-Kontrast-Sonographie (HKSG) als Möglichkeit zur Kontrolle der Tubendurchgängigkeit. Geburtsh Frauenheilkd 55:143–149

De Geyter C, Schmitter M, De Geyter M, Nieschlag E, Holzgreve W, Schneider HPG (2000) Prospective evaluation of the ultrasound appearance of the endometrium in a cohort of 1,186 infertile women. Fertil Steril 73:106–113

Deichert I, Hackeloer B, Daume E (1986) The sonographic and endocrinologic evaluation of the endometrium in the luteal phase. Hum Reprod 1:219–222

Dennerstein L, Gotts G, Brown JB, Morse CA, Farley TMM, Pinol A (1994) The relationship between the menstrual cycle and female sexual interest in women with premenstrual symptom complaints and volunteers. Psychoneuroendocrinology 19:293–304

Dmowski WP (1995) Behandlung der Minimal-Endometriose. Frauenarzt 36:535–557

Dmowski WP, Friberg J, Rana N, Papierniak C, Michalowska J, Elroeiy A (1995) The effect of endometriosis, its stage and activity, and of autoantibodies on in vitro fertilization and embryo transfer success rates. Fertil Steril 63:555–562

Dottorini ME, Lomuscio G, Mazzucchelli L, Vignati A, Colombo L (1995) Assessment of female fertility and carcinogenesis after iodine[131] therapy for differentiated thyroid carcinoma. J Nuclear Med 36:21–22

Dunaif A (1999) Insulin action in the polycystic ovary syndrome. Endocrinol Metab Clin North Am 28:341–359

Dunaif A, Scott D, Finegood D, Quintana B, Whitcomb R (1996) The insulin-sensitizing agent troglitazone improves metabolic and reproductive abnormalities in the polycystic ovary syndrome. J Clin Endocrinol Metab 81:3299–3306

Dunson DB, Baird DD, Wilcox AJ, Weinberg CR (1999) Day-specific probabilities of clinical pregnancy based on two studies with imperfect measures of ovulation. Hum Reprod 14:1835–1839

Ebbiary NAA, Lenton EA, Cooke ID (1994) Hypothalamic-pituitary ageing: progressive increase in FSH and LH concentrations throughout the reproductive life in regularly menstruating women. Clin Endocrinol 41:199–206

Eggert-Kruse W, Leinhos G, Gerhard I, Tilgen W, Runnebaum B (1989) Prognostic value of in vitro sperm penetration into hormonally standardized human cervical mucus. Fertil Steril 51:317–323

Eggert-Kruse W, Pohl S, Naher H, Tilgen W, Runnebaum B (1992) Microbial colonization and sperm mucus interaction – results in 1000 infertile couples. Hum Reprod 7:612–620

Eimers JM, Tevelde ER, Gerritse R, Vogelzang ET, Looman CWN, Habbema JDF (1994) The prediction of the chance to conceive in subfertile couples. Fertil Steril 61:44–52

Emperaire JC, Gauzere-Soumireu E, Audebert AJM (1982) Female fertility and donor insemination. Fertil Steril 37:90–93

Filicori M (1994) Use of GnRH and its analogs in the treatment of ovulatory disorders: an overview. In: Filicori M, Flamigni C (eds) Ovulation induction: basic science and clinical advances. Elsevier, Amsterdam, pp 239–243

Flamigni C, Borini A, Violini F, Bianchi L, Serrao L (1993) Oocyte donation – comparison between recipients from different age groups. Hum Reprod 8:2088–2092

France JT, Graham FM, Gosling L, Hair P, Knox BS (1992) Characteristics of natural conceptual cycles occurring in a prospective study of sex preselection – fertility awareness symptoms, hormone levels, sperm survival, and pregnancy outcome. Int J Fertil 37:244–255

Fraser EJ, Grimes DA, Schulz KF (1993) Immunization as therapy for recurrent spontaneous abortion – a review and meta-analysis. Obstet Gynecol 82:854–859

French R, Brocklehurst P (1998) The effect of pregnancy on survival in women infected with HIV: a systematic review of the literature and meta-analysis. Br J Obstet Gynaecol 105:827–835

Gibson M (1995) Reproductive health and polycystic ovary syndrome. Am J Med 98 [Suppl 1A]:S67–S75

Ginsburg J, Hardiman P, Thomas M (1992) Vaginal bromocriptine – clinical and biochemical effects. Gynecol Endocrinol 6:119–126

Gleicher N, Pratt D, Parrilli M, Karande V, Redding L (1992) Standardization of hysterosalpingography and selective salpingography – a valuable adjunct to simple opacification studies. Fertil Steril 58:1136–1141

Gülekli B, Bulbul Y, Onvural A, Yorukoglu K, Posaci C, Demir N, Erten O (1999) Accuracy of ovarian reserve tests. Hum Reprod 14:2822–2826

Heckers H, Lasch H-G (1986) Gastrointestinale Erkrankungen aus internistischer Sicht. In: Künzel W, Wulf K-K (eds) Die gestörte Schwangerschaft. Klinik der Frauenheilkunde und Geburtshilfe, vol 5. Urban and Schwarzenberg, Munich, pp 133–148

Herms V (1989) Funktionelle Sexualstörungen. In: Schneider HPG (ed) Sexualmedizin, Infertilität, Familienplanung. Klinik der Frauenheilkunde und Geburtshilfe, vol 2. Urban and Schwarzenberg, Munich, pp 52–58

Hjollund NHI, Jensen TK, Bonde JPE, Henriksen TB, Andersson AM, Kolstad HA, Ernst E, Giwercman A, Skakkebaek NE, Olsen J (1999) Distress and reduced fertility: a follow-up study of first-pregnancy planners. Fertil Steril 72:47–53

Holmes MM, Resnick HS, Kilpatrick DG, Best CL (1996) Rape-related pregnancy: estimates and descriptive characteristics from a national sample of women. Am J Obstet Gynecol 175:320–325

Holmgren U, Bergstrand G, Hagenfeldt K, Werner S (1986) Women with prolactinoma – effect of pregnancy and lactation on serum prolactin and on tumour growth. Acta Endocrinol 111:452–459

Hoyme UB, Baumler C, Kotani T, Seuffer A (1988) Chlamydia trachomatis – Nachweis bei entzündlichen Erkrankungen der Eileiter. Geburtsh Frauenheilkd 48:876–880

Insler V, Bettendorf G (eds) (1977) The uterine cervix in reproduction. Thieme, Stuttgart

Izembart M, Chavaudra J, Aubert B, Vallee G (1992) Retrospective evaluation of the dose received by the ovary after radioactive iodine therapy for thyroid cancer. Eur J Nucl Med 19:243–247

James WH (1979) The causes of the decline in fecundability with age. Soc Biol 26:330–334

Jensen TK, Henriksen TB, Hjollund, NHI, Scheike T, Kolstad H, Giwercman A, Ernst E, Bonde JP, Skakkebaek NE, Olsen J (1998) Adult and prenatal exposures to tobacco smoke as risk indicators of fertility among 430 Danish couples. Am J Epidemiol 148:992–997

Joffe M, Li ZM (1994) Male and female factors in fertility. Am J Epidemiol 140:921–929

Jones WR (1994) Gamete immunology. Hum Reprod 9:828–841

Joosten R, Stürner KH (1980) Hepatitis B Infektion des Neugeborenen durch seine scheinbar gesunde Mutter. Med Klin 75:223–224

Jordan J, Craig K, Clifton DK, Soules MR (1994) Luteal phase defect: the sensitivity of diagnostic methods in common clinical use. Fertil Steril 62:54–62

Kanal E, Gillen J, Evans JA, Savitz DA, Shellock FG (1993) Survey of reproductive health among female MR workers. Radiology 187:395–399

Kase N, Mroueh A, Olson L (1967) Clomid therapy for anovulatory infertility. Am J Obstet Gynecol 98:1037–1042

Kazer RR, Kessel B, Yen SSC (1987) Circulating luteinizing hormone pulse frequency in women with polycystic ovary syndrome. J Clin Endocrinol Metab 65:233–236

Knuth UA, Mühlenstedt D (1991) Kinderwunschdauer, kontrazeptives Verhalten und Rate vorausgegangener Infertilitätsbehandlungen. Geburtsh Frauenheilkd 51:678–684

Knuth UA, Hull MGR, Jacobs HS (1977) Amenorrhea and loss of weight. Br J Obstet Gynecol 84:801–807

Knuth UA, Mühlenstedt D, Schneider HPG (1982) Zur Effektivität von Kurzwellenbelastungstests, Blutkörperchensenkungsgeschwindigkeit und Leukozytenzahl bei der Diagnose der subakuten Adnexitis. Geburtsh Frauenheilkd 42:52–55

Kremling H (1986) Harnorgane und ihre Erkrankungen. In: Künzel W, Wulf KK (eds) Die gestörte Schwangerschaft, Klinik der Frauenheilkunde und Geburtshilfe, vol 5. Urban and Schwarzenberg, Munich, pp 163–184

MacLeod J, Gold RZ (1953) The male factor in fertility and infertility VI. Semen quality and certain other factors in relation to ease of conception. Fertil Steril 4:10–33

Makino T, Umeuchi M, Nakada K, Nozawa S, Iizuka R (1992) Incidence of congenital uterine anomalies in repeated reproductive wastage and prognosis for pregnancy after metroplasty. Int J Fertil 37:167–170

Marshburn PB, Kutteh WH (1994) The role of antisperm antibodies in infertility. Fertil Steril 61:799–811

Massarano AA, Adams JM, Preece MA, Brook CGD (1989) Ovarian ultrasound appearances in Turner syndrome. J Pediatr 114:569–573

McNeely MJ, Soules MR (1988) The diagnosis of luteal phase deficiency: a critical review. Fertil Steril 50:1–15

Meistrich ML (1993) Potential genetic risks of using semen collected during chemotherapy. Hum Reprod 8:8–10

Morini A, Spina V, Aleandri V, Cantonetti G, Lambiasi A, Papalia U (1998) Pregnancy after heart transplant: update and case report. Hum Reprod 13:749–757

Mueller-Eckhardt G (1994) Immunotherapy with intravenous immunoglobulin for prevention of recurrent pregnancy loss: European experience. Am J Reprod Immunol 32:281–285

Mueller-Eckhardt G, Mallmann P, Neppert J, Lattermann A, Melk A, Heine O, Pfeiffer R, Zingsem J, Domke N, Mohr-Pennert A (1994) Immunogenetic and serological investigations in nonpregnant and in pregnant women with a history of recurrent spontaneous abortions. J Reprod Immunol 27:95–109

Naether OG J, Baukloh V, Fischer R, Kowalczyk T (1994) Long-term follow-up in 206 infertility patients with polycystic ovarian syndrome after laparoscopic electrocautery of the ovarian surface. Hum Reprod 9:2342–2349

Negro-Vilar A (1993) Stress and other environmental factors affecting fertility in men and women – overview. Environ Health Perspect 101 [Suppl 2]:59–64

Nestler JE, Jakubowicz DJ, Evans WS, Pasquali R (1998) Effects of metformin on spontaneous and clomiphene-induced ovulation in the polycystic ovary syndrome. N Engl J Med 338:1876–1880

Nieschlag E, Weinbauer GF, Cooper TG, Wittkowski W (1999) Reproduktion. In: Deetjen P, Speckmann EF (eds) Physiologie, 3rd edn. Urban and Fischer, Munich, p 525

Ogilvy-Stuart AL, Shalet SM (1993) Effect of radiation on the human reproductive system. Environ Health Perspect 101 [Suppl 2]:109–116

Opsahl MS, Miller B, Klein TA (1993) The predictive value of hysterosalpingography for tubal and peritoneal infertility factors. Fertil Steril 60:444–448

Ouellet-Hellstrom R, Stewart WF (1993) Miscarriages among female physical therapists who report using radio- and microwave-frequency electromagnetic radiation. Am J Epidemiol 138:775–786

Plouffe L, White EW, Tho SP, Sweet CS, Layman LC, Whitman GF, McDonough PG (1992) Etiologic factors of recurrent abortion and subsequent reproductive performance of cou-

ples – have we made any progress in the past ten years? Am J Obstet Gynecol 167:313–321

Queenan JT, O'Brian GD, Bains LM, Simpson J, Collins WP, Campbell S (1980) Ultrasound scanning of ovaries to detect ovulation in women. Fertil Steril 34:99–105

Quint WGV, Fetter WPF, Vanos HC, Heijtink RA (1994) Absence of hepatitis-B virus (HBV) DNA in children born after exposure of their mothers to HBV during in vitro fertilization. J Clin Microbiol 32:1099–1100

Rachootin P, Olsen J (1983) The risk of infertility and delayed conception associated with exposure in the Danish workplace. J Occup Med 25:394–402

Resti M, Azzari C, Manelli AF, Moriondo M, Novembre E, deMartino M, Vierucci A (1998) Mother to child transmission of hepatitis C virus: prospective study of risk factors and timing of infection in children born to women seronegative for HIV-1. Br Med J 317:437–440

Richardson DW, Goldsmith LT, Pohl CR, Schallenberger E, Knobil E (1985) The role of prolactin in the regulation of the primate corpus luteum. J Clin Endocrinol Metab 60:501–504

Rosenfield RL (1999) Ovarian and adrenal function in polycystic ovary syndrome. Endocrinol Metab Clin North Am 28:265–293

Rowland AS, Baird DD, Weinberg CR, Shore DL, Shy CM, Wilcox AJ (1994) The effect of occupational exposure to mercury vapour on the fertility of female dental assistants. Occup Environ Med 51:28–34

Schneider HPG, Karbowski B (1989) In: Schneider HPG (ed) Sexualmedizin, Infertilität, Familienplanung, Klinik der Frauenheilkunde und Geburtshilfe, vol 2. Urban and Schwarzenberg, Munich, pp 373–384

Schnell JD (1973) Zytologie und Mikrobiologie der Vagina. Wissenschaftsverlag, Cologne

Schwartz P, Mayaux MJ (1982) Female fecundity as a function of age. N Engl J Med 306:404–406

Schweppe KH (1995) Therapieprinzipien der Endometriose. Frauenarzt 36:558–571

Scialli AR (1994) Data availability in reproductive and developmental toxicology. Obstet Gynecol 83:652–656

Seibel MM, Berger MJ, Weinstein FG, Taymor ML (1982) The effectiveness of danazol on subsequent fertility in minimal endometriosis. Fertil Steril 38:534–537

Shangold MM, Turksoy RN, Bashford RA, Hammond CB (1977) Pregnancy following the "insensitive ovary syndrome". Fertil Steril 28:1179–1181

Simon A, Laufer N (1993) Unexplained infertiliy: a reappraisal. Assist Reprod Rev 3:26–31

Simon C, Gutierrez A, Vidal A, Delossantos MJ, Tarin JJ, Remohi J, Pellicer A (1994) Outcome of patients with endometriosis in assisted reproduction: results from in-vitro fertilization and oocyte donation. Hum Reprod 9:725–729

Soliman S, Daya S, Collins J, Hughes EG (1994) The role of luteal phase support in infertility treatment: a meta-analysis of randomized trials. Fertil Steril 61:1068–1076

Soules MR (1993) Luteal dysfunction. In: Adashi EY, Leung PCK (eds) The ovary. Raven, New York, pp 607–627

Speroff L, Glass RH, Kase NG (1994) Clinical gynecologic endocrinology and infertility. Williams and Wilkins, Baltimore, pp 426–434

Stovall DW, Christman GM, Hammond MG, Talbert LM (1992) Abnormal findings on hysterosalpingography – effects on fecundity in a donor insemination program using frozen semen. Obstet Gynecol 80:249–252

Strandell A, Lindhard A, Waldenstrom U, Thorburn J, Janson PO, Hamberger L (1999) Hydrosalpinx and IVF outcome: a prospective, randomized multicentre trial in Scandinavia on salpingectomy prior to IVF. Hum Reprod 14:2762–2769

Taylor AE, Schneyer AL, Sluss PM, Crowley WF (1993) Ovarian failure, resistance, and activation. In: Adashi EY, Leung PCK (eds) The ovary. Raven, New York, pp 629–661

Thonneau P, Ducot B, Spira A (1993) Risk factors in men and women consulting for infertility. Int J Fertil 38:37–43

Udoff LC, Adashi EY (1999) Autocrine/paracrine regulation of the ovarian follicle. Endocrinologist 9:99–106

Van der Poel CL, Cuypers HT, Reesink HW (1994) Hepatitis C virus six years on. Lancet 344:1475–1479

van Leeuwen I, Branch DW, Scott JR (1993) First trimester ultrasonography findings in women with a history of recurrent pregnancy loss. Am J Obstet Gynecol 168:111–114

Venezia R, Zangara C, Knight C, Cittadini E (1993) Initial experience of a new linear everting falloposcopy system in comparison with hysterosalpingography. Fertil Steril 60:771–775

Vercellini P, Maddalena S, DeGiorgi O, Aimi G, Crosignani PG (1998) Abdominal myomectomy for infertility: a comprehensive review. Hum Reprod 13:873–879

Verkauf BS (1983) The incidence and outcome of single-factor, mulitfactorial and unexplained infertiliy. Am J Obstet Gynecol 147:175–181

Watson A, Vandekerckhove P, Lilford R, Vail A, Brosens I, Hughes E (1994) A meta-analysis of the therapeutic role of oil soluble contrast media at hysterosalpingography – a surprising result. Fertil Steril 61:470–477

Wathen NC, Perry L, Lilford RJ, Chard T (1984) Interpretation of single progesterone measurement in diagnosis of anovulation and defective luteal phase: observation of the normal range. Br Med J 288:7–9

WHO Laborhandbuch zur Untersuchung des menschlichen Ejakulats und der Spermien-Zervikalschleim-Interaktion (1999) Übersetzung von: Nieschlag E, Nieschlag S, Bals-Pratsch M, Behre HM, Knuth UA, Meschede D, Niemeier M, Schick A, 4th edn. Springer, Berlin Heidelberg New York

Wildt L, Leyendecker G, Sir Petermann T, Weibeltreber S (1993) Treatment with Naltrexone in hypothalamic ovarian failure – incidence of ovulation and pregnancy. Hum Reprod 8:350–358

Wilcox AJ, Baird DD, Weinberg CR (1999) Time of implantation of the conceptus and loss of pregnancy. N Engl J Med 340:1796–1799

Yeh J, Seibel MM (1987) Artificial insemination with donor sperm: a review of 108 patients. Obstet Gynecol 70:313–316

CHAPTER 15

Testosterone Therapy

15

E. Nieschlag · H. M. Behre

15.1 Indications and Preparations: An Overview

All forms of hypogonadism described in the previous chapters associated with Leydig cell insufficiency require testosterone therapy. In secondary hypogonadism long-term testosterone therapy is also indicated. This is only to be interrupted for GnRH or gonadotropin therapy when offspring are desired.

Male hypogonadism is the main indication for testosterone. Table 15.1 provides an overview of **other possible applications**. Some of these applications are dealt with in other chapters of this volume, for example in constitutionally delayed puberty (Chap. 7), in senescence (Chap. 21), in male hormonal contraception (Sect. 20.4) and in idiopathic male infertility (Chap. 16). In addition, this chapter deals with its use in excessively tall stature (Sect. 15.5) and with its abuse in doping and body-building (Sect. 15.6). Because of its erythropoetic effect testosterone is also licensed for the treatment of aplastic and renal anemia, but lost ground to erythropoetin after the latter was introduced. For treatment of this condition, the reader is referred to textbooks of internal medicine.

Testosterone therapy is indicated when, in cases with androgen deficiency, serum testosterone concentrations drop below 12 nmol/l in the morning (see Chap. 6).

Since we are dealing with hormone replacement therapy, its effectiveness can be measured directly by checking serum testosterone concentrations.

According to international consensus, the major goal of testosterone therapy is to replace testosterone levels at as close to physiological concentrations as is possible (WHO 1992). Furthermore, the **naturally occurring testosterone molecule** should be used for substitution in order to guarantee the broad spectrum of testosterone effects. Available testosterone preparations should be judged according to these criteria.

Table 15.1. Use of testosterone in men

Clinical applications	Hypogonadism, Delayed puberty, Aplastic and renal anemia
Off-label use	Excessive growth
Application under discussion	Senescence
Experimental use	Male contraception
Obsolete application	Idiopathic infertility
Abuse	High-performance athletics and bodybuilding

Certain target organs are able to use testosterone directly, while others must first be converted to 5α-DHT or estradiol in order for them to become effective (see Sect. 3.6.3). To achieve a physiological balance between testosterone and its active metabolites, natural testosterone should be used and not synthetic androgens which are metabolized into other forms (e.g. 19-nortestosterone) or are direct derivatives of the metabolites (e.g. mesterolone). In the same vein there is little purpose in applying estrogens either directly or exclusively to the hypogonadal male. Nor has any rational basis for the use of testosterone precursors such as DHEA or androstendione been established to date. The use of natural testosterone allows all androgen-dependent functions to be induced or maintained in the safest way possible and side effects to be avoided.

Most of the **testosterone preparations** available today for clinical use are old products, in part dating back to the early phase of endocrinological pharmacology. Although these preparations are not ideal, for a long time no new products were developed. This can be partially explained by the fact that hypogonadal patients needing substitution represent a relatively small group and thus are an insignificant market for pharmaceutical companies. The possibility of new indications (e.g. senescence, male contraception) prompted **new developments** and at the present time a series of testosterone preparations is being tested. Although by and large these products are not yet available, some will be discussed here so that the reader may examine the present and future therapeutic options. For the sake of completeness, preparations are also included which are only available for clinical use in some countries, but such information will complete the spectrum of therapeutic possibilities.

At present, one oral, two transdermal and several injectable preparations are available. The experienced physician must select the form most suitable for the patient, considering both his symptoms and phase of life. Often several preparations will have to be tried before finding an optimal choice for the individual patient.

15.2 Pharmacology of Testosterone Preparations

In chemical terms, testosterone is derived from the basic structure of all androgens, i.e. from androstane. It owes its specific biological activity to the keto-group in position 3, the double-bond in position 4 and the hydroxy-group in position 17 of the basic androstane structure (see Fig. 15.1 and Chap. 3). Principally, three modifications of the molecule make testosterone suitable for therapeutic practice:

1. chemical modification of the molecule,
2. esterification in position 17 and
3. various forms of application.

As routes of application are particularly important for clinical purposes, testosterone preparations will be discussed here in these terms. In addition to the modalities described below, nasal, conjunctival or rectal routes of application can be chosen; however, at present these forms play no role in clinical use.

This chapter deals with aspects relevant to androgen therapy. For further reading reference is made to current monographs (Nieschlag and Behre 1998a; Bhasin 1998).

15.2.1 Oral Testosterone Preparations

It would seem obvious to use natural testosterone in the form it is secreted by the testes for substitution therapy. In fact, orally applied free testosterone is well absorbed from the intestine, but is completely metabolized by the liver in the first pass effect, so that it does not reach target organs. About 400 to 600 mg testosterone would have to be given orally, i.e. about 100-fold of the amount normally secreted by the testis daily, in order to exceed the testosterone-metabolizing capacity of the liver and to achieve normal peripheral serum levels. As administering such great amounts of testosterone seems uneconomical and as possible long-term side effects are difficult to evaluate, this form of application never went be-

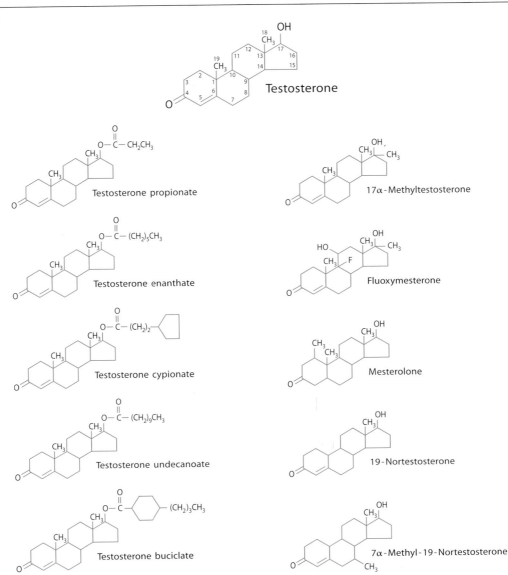

Fig. 15.1. Molecular structures of testosterone and various testosterone preparations

yond the experimental stage (Nieschlag and Behre 1998b).

Testosterone Undecanoate

In order to avoid the first pass effect in the liver after oral application, testosterone was esterified with undecanoic acid in position 17β. This long aliphatic side chain allows resorption of the molecule into the lymph so that testosterone can enter the circulation through the thoracic ducts and via the subclavial vein, thus reaching target organs prior to hepatic metabolism. Resorption is improved if oral testosterone is taken with a meal containing fats.

Testosterone undecanoate is available in 40 mg capsule form with the testosterone being dissolved in oil (Andriol®). As testosterone represents 63% of the molecular weight, one capsule contains about 25 mg testosterone. Maximum serum peaks are attained about 2 to 6 h after ingestion (Schürmeyer 1983; Behre and Nieschlag 1998b). This means that **2 to 4 capsules** spread over the course of a day are required for substitution. Although relatively high testosterone concentrations are given, no long-term side effects or toxic effects have been observed (Gooren 1994).

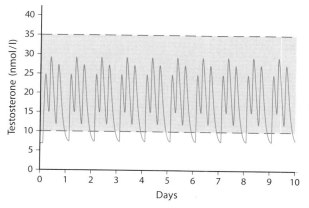

Fig. 15.2. Testosterone serum levels following oral application of 3×40 mg testosterone undecanoate to hypogonadal men (pharmacokinetic computer simulation assuming basal testosterone levels of 7 nmol/l). The gray area indicates the range of testosterone in normal men

Testosterone undecanoate is best suited for substitution therapy when the patient has a residual capacity to secrete testosterone (e. g. Klinefelter patients in the early phase of substitution). Another domain of testosterone undecanoate medication are situations when intramuscular injections cannot be given because of clotting disturbances (e. g. patients on marcumar medication) or the patient cannot attend a physician for the injections (e. g., on holidays). The disadvantage of this therapy lies primarily in the short-lived peaks and troughs in serum testosterone which do not mimic physiological conditions and in the poor predictability of individual resorption patterns (Fig. 15.2).

Methyl Testosterone and Fluoxymesterone

17α-methyl testosterone resulted from attempts started shortly after testosterone synthesis in 1935 to modify the molecule chemically. The methyl group in position 17α protects the testosterone molecule from being metabolized in the liver so that it can reach target organs after oral administration. Long-term use, however, can lead to elevated liver enzymes, as well as to cholostasis and peliosis (for review see Nieschlag 1981).

Fluoxymesterone also contains a methyl group in position 17α in addition to a fluoride atom and hydroxy group. Although this modification makes fluoxymesterone a highly effective oral testosterone preparation, the 17α methyl group makes it liver-toxic as well. For this reason these substances were taken off the market in Germany, first as monosubstances and subsequently their use in combined preparations was prohibited. As they are still available in other countries, attention should be called to their toxic side effects.

In general, 17α-methylation of all androgens (also of anabolic steroids) may cause liver toxicity and therefore these preparations should be considered **obsolete**.

Mesterolone

Mesterolone (Proviron®, Vistimon®) is derived from the 5α-reduced testosterone metabolite 5α-dihydrotestosterone (DHT) and is likewise not subject to hepatic metabolism following oral administration. As a DHT derivative, however, it can only compensate for DHT-dependent functions and not for the immediate effects of testosterone and those following aromatization to estrogens. Thus, it does not develop the full spectrum of testosterone effects which are necessary for hormone replacement therapy and it is therefore **not suitable for substitution in hypogonadism**.

Buccal Administration

The incorporation of testosterone into cyclic dextrins is one of the more recent developments in the field of androgen therapy. Incorporation into this carbohydrate matrix enables testosterone to become soluble in aqueous solutions. As first clinical trials have shown following sublingual or buccal application of testosterone incorporated into cyclodextrins, serum testosterone rises rapidly, but is followed by a similarly rapid decline after the substance dissolves so that multiple daily application is necessary for substitution: the disadvantages are similar to those of testosterone undecanoate (Salehian et al. 1995). Notwithstanding, compared to oral testosterone undecanoate a lower total testosterone dose suffices for substitution. Further clinical trials will show whether this form of substitution has advantages over others.

Incorporating testosterone into polyethylene matrices with limited water-solubility represents a new attempt to develop forms for buccal application: the tablets adhere to the mucosa of the cheek for a number of hours, slowly releasing testosterone into the circulation, thus reaching target organs before metabolism in the liver.

15.2.2 Intramuscular Testosterone Preparations

Testosterone Enanthate

When natural testosterone is injected intramuscularly, its half-life is very short. In order to prolong its effectiveness, testosterone was esterified in position 17 with aliphatic side chains. The duration of half-life depends upon the length and structure of the side chain.

Table 15.2. Pharmacokinetic data of various testosterone preparations

Preparation	Application	"Mean Residence Time" (MRT)	Terminal mean time (t $^1/_2$)
Testosterone undecanoate	p.o.	3.7 hours	1.6 hours
Testosterone propionate	i.m.	1.5 days	0.8 days
Testosterone enanthate	i.m.	8.5 days	4.5 days
Testosterone undecanoate in teaseed oil	i.m.	34.9 days	20.9 days
Testosterone undecanoate in castor oil	i.m.	36.0 days	33.9 days
Testosterone buciclate	i.m.	60.0 days	29.5 days

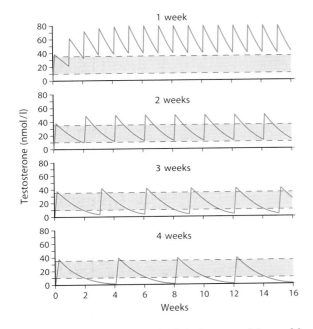

Fig. 15.3. Testosterone serum levels in hypogonadal men following intramuscular injection of 250 mg testosterone enanthate given at intervals of 1, 2, 3, or 4 weeks. The gray area indicates the normal range of testosterone

Intramuscular adminstration of **testosterone enanthate** is the form most widely used in hormone replacement therapy and was introduced in 1952. Its terminal half-life is 4.5 days (Table 15.2). The standard dose is 200–250 mg testosterone enanthate (e.g. Testoviron® Depot 250 mg, Testosterone Depot). As the pharmacokinetics show, supraphysiological serum testosterone concentrations are rapidly achieved and are maintained for several days (Fig. 15.3) (Behre and Nieschlag 1998). Subsequently serum levels gradually decline, passing the lower level of normal on about day 12. Repeated injections, such as are necessary for substitution therapy, produce a "saw-tooth profile" with supraphysiological, physiological and infraphysiological levels following one another depending on the injection interval (Fig. 15.3). While this substitution regimen is adequate to maintain the biological effects of testosterone, the patient finds these extremes disturbing, as general well-being, moods, and sexual activity reflect these patterns. Nonetheless, testosterone enanthate was considered standard therapy for many years.

Other Testosterone Esters

Testosterone cypionate and **testosterone cyclohexanecarboxylate**, available in some countries, have the same pharmacokinetics as testosterone enanthate and, consequently, similar advantages and disadvantages.

Testosterone propionate (Testoviron®) has a short half-life as a consequence of its short side chain (Table 15.2). Initial serum concentrations following i.m. injection may be as high as with testosterone enanthate, but the injections must be repeated every 2–3 days because of its short half-life to achieve full substitution. Because of the necessity for frequent injections testosterone propionate is not suitable for chronic therapy, nor does a combination of testosterone propionate and testosterone enanthate offer any advantage (Behre and Nieschlag 1998).

When **testosterone undecanoate** in oily solution is administered intramuscularly its half-life is significantly longer than that of testosterone enanthate (Table 15.2, Fig. 15.4). Its longer half-life is due not only to the ester itself but also to the vehicle and the volume in which the substance is administered (Behre et al. 1999a). Its longer duration of effectiveness plus the lack of initial peaks in serum testosterone gives it an advantage over testosterone enanthate. Clinical studies in China (Zhang et al. 1998) and our initial experience indicate that good substitution with injection intervals up to 12 weeks can be achieved using this preparation (Nieschlag et al. 1999).

An even flatter testosterone curve with even longer injection intervals can be achieved when **testosterone**

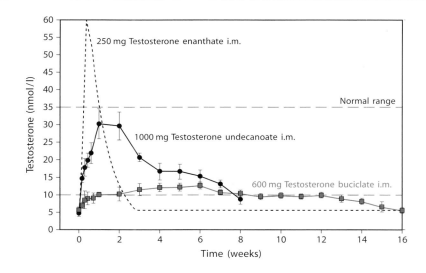

Fig. 15.4. Comparative pharmacokinetics following single intramuscular injections of 250 mg testosterone enanthate, 1000 mg testosterone undecanoate, and 600 mg testosterone buciclate in hypogonadal men. The dotted lines represent the normal range of testosterone

buciclate is applied (Table 15.2, Fig. 15.4). Following a single intramuscular injection of 1000 mg serum values are maintained for about 3 months in the lower normal range. Initial clinical studies demonstrated the effectiveness of this preparation on erythropoesis, anabolism, libido and potency (Behre and Nieschlag 1992; Behre et al. 1996). Should repeated injection intervals confirm the 3-month interval as suitable for routine purposes, this preparation would also represent considerable therapeutic progress.

Testosterone Microspheres

A further attempt to develop a new testosterone depot preparation was made by incorporating testosterone into polylactide-coglycolide microspheres. Initial clinical studies with this modality showed serum testosterone values in the physiological range for about 70 days following a single injection (Bhasin et al. 1992). The matrix of the microspheres is completely biodegradable, similar to resorbable sutures. As the capacity of microspheres for testosterone uptake is very limited, a relatively large volume must be injected. Moreover, manufacturing consistent charges has proved to be a problem so that this preparation continues to remain in an experimental stage.

15.2.3 Transdermal Testosterone Preparations

Trans-Scrotal Testosterone Preparations

Transdermal application of medication has gained in popularity in recent years because of the many advantages it has over conventional forms. In the endocrinological field the transdermal form has become widely

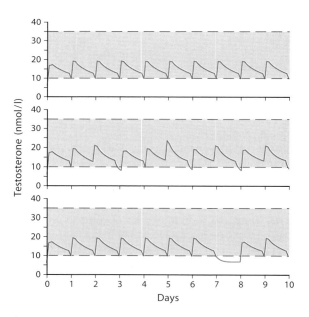

Fig. 15.5. Testosterone serum levels in hypogonadal men following daily scrotal application of 15 mg transscrotal therapeutic system (TTS Testoderm) (pharmacokinetic computer simulation assuming a testosterone secretion of 7 mmol/l). Upper drawing, regular application every 24 h; middle drawing, daily applications with intervals varying ± 2 h; lower drawing, application forgotten on day 7

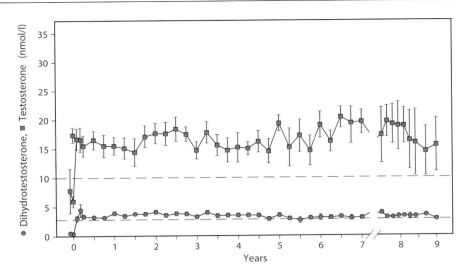

Fig. 15.6. Serum testosterone and DHT in 11 hypogonadal men treated over 10 years with transscrotal testosterone (Testoderm®). The upper broken line indicates the lower limit of normal for testosterone and the lower broken line the upper limit of normal for DHT

used for treating menopausal deficiency symptoms with estrogens. Development of a transdermal system for replacement therapy of hypogonadal men met with difficulties as in hypogonadism testosterone doses in the range of normal production i. e. about 6 mg per day are required, whereas the corresponding dose of estradiol for women lies in the μg-range. Different skin types have differing resorption capacities. Since scrotal skin has high blood circulation extending into the uppermost layers of the epithelial layers (because of its role in physiological temperature regulation), this skin type has especially high resorption capacity (about 40 times higher than the skin of the lower arm). This particularity was used to advantage in developing a trans-scrotal application system.

The **trans-scrotal therapeutic system** (Testoderm®) consists of a 40 or 60 cm² polymere membrane loaded with 10 or 15 mg pure natural testosterone. When these membranes are applied to the scrotum they release enough testosterone into the system to guarantee physiological serum testosterone levels for one day. When the membrane is applied in the morning, physiological daily rhythms of testosterone can be mimicked (Bals-Pratsch 1986; Atkinson et al. 1998) (Fig. 15.5). Daily renewal provides constant serum testosterone levels in the normal range (Fig. 15.6). Patients treated with this form of substitution therapy (for up to 10 years) show very good results (Behre et al. 1999b). Since an "enhancer" is not used, skin irritations rarely occur. In order to guarantee good skin contact, the scrotum must be freed of hair from time to time (scissors or razor).

As scrotal skin has high 5α-reductase activity, part of the testosterone applied there is metabolized to DHT so that serum DHT concentrations are elevated above upper normal levels and the DHT:testosterone quotient is increased. Like testosterone levels, estradiol levels always remain in the normal range. Long-term studies showed that slightly elevated DHT has no negative effect on prostate size (Behre et al. 1994b).

Since only natural testosterone is used in this preparation and since serum levels always remain in the physiological range, this therapy best fulfills the aforementioned criteria for optimal testosterone substitution. Because of the limited area of application, overdosing and abuse are impossible. Furthermore, should it become necessary, substitution therapy can be interrupted immediately, which injectable testosterone preparations do not permit.

Non-Scrotal Transdermal Testosterone Preparations

Following transscrotal forms, **transdermal testosterone patches** were developed which can be applied to non-scrotal skin (e. g. abdominal or upper arm skin) (Androderm®). In order to transport the required amount of testosterone through the skin, these systems are equipped with an "enhancer" which may lead to skin irritation. Two systems must be applied in the evening and worn for 24 hours for hormone replacement therapy. Daily renewal is necessary for chronic substitution (Meikle 1998). In 1999 a further transdermal system was introduced to the American market. Because of its large area, only one system needs to be applied daily. The fact that it bears the same brand name of Testoderm® (although with the addition of TTS) causes confusion. In Europe it will be marketed under the name of Virormon®. As in the transscrotal systems, testosterone values in the normal range and with a physiological circadian profile can be achieved, with DHT and estradiol remaining in the normal range.

Today, the patient is able to choose which form of application he prefers or tolerates better, pharmacokinetics and pharmacodynamics being equal.

A further application form is the use of testosterone gels, which are applied to large skin areas in order to allow sufficient amounts of the hormone to be resorbed. While medical research continues to carry out clinical trials, these preparations are already available on the black market for anabolic steroid users, as a curious side-effect was able to document. A two-year old boy developed precocious puberty (penis length: 8.5 cm!) after prolonged skin contact with his father, who used testosterone gels, and with the father's contaminated bodybuilding equipment (Yu et al. 1999). These cases characterize the major side-effect of androgen-containing gels. Meanwhile a transdermal testosterone gel has been licensed in the USA under the brand name Androgel® and is well suited for the treatment of hypogonadism (Wang et al. 2000).

Transdermal Dihydrotestosterone

In France a further **transdermal preparation** is on the market containing **5α-dihydrotestosterone** (Andractim®). At a concentration of 2.5% the DHT is incorporated into a hydroalcoholic gel from which the DHT penetrates the skin if it is applied to sufficiently large surfaces, e.g. the chest and abdomen. Supraphysiological DHT values are measured in serum. Hypogonadal patients treated in this matter appear to be adequately substituted (Schaison and Couzinet 1998). However, the criticism that is applicable to mesterolone is also valid here, namely that the full spectrum of direct testosterone effects and those mediated by estradiol are not able to be exerted. Moreover, applying a gel over such a large skin surface seems impractical; contact with skin and underwear may cause testosterone uptake and virilization in the female partner (Delanoe et al. 1984).

15.2.4 Testosterone Implants

Testosterone implants are among the oldest testosterone preparations. They consist of pure testosterone molded into cylindrical forms of 12 mm length and 4.5 mm diameter. An implant contains 200 mg. They are implanted through a 0.5–1 cm incision under the abdominal skin under sterile conditions using a trocar. The wound is closed with a bandage or stitches. Patients with a tendency towards infection are given an antibiotic prophylactically. If three to six implants are inserted, slowly declining serum testosterone levels in the normal range

are achieved for 4–6 months (Handelsman 1998). Despite the long-lasting depot effect and the positive serum testosterone levels these products are only available in the UK, in Australia and South Africa. The minor surgery necessary for implantation, an 8.5% extrusion rate (n = 97.3 in 221 patients over a period of 13 years) and bleeding (2.3%) and occasionally infection (0.6%) are limiting factors.

15.3 Monitoring Testosterone Therapy in Hypogonadism

As can be seen from foregoing sections, the "classic" therapy for hypogonadism is administration of 200–250 mg testosterone enanthate (e.g. Testoviron Depot® 250 mg or Testosterone Depot) every 2 to 3 weeks. In addition, testosterone undecanoate p.o. (Andriol®) 2–4 x 40 mg daily is available. Finally, testosterone can also be applied transdermally, whereby one fresh membrane of Testoderm® must be applied daily to the scrotum or one (Virormon®, Testoderm® TTS) or two patches (Androderm®) must be applied daily to the abdominal and/or chest area.

All these forms of testosterone therapy pursue the same goal, namely to provide optimal substitution with testosterone. From its physiological effects and from those resulting from pharmacokinetics and pharmacodynamics various parameters can be measured to determine the effectiveness of testosterone therapy; these will be discussed in the following sections (overview in Table 15.3).

15.3.1 Psyche and Sexuality

A patient's **general well-being and activity** are good parameters to check the effectiveness of replacement therapy. When testosterone levels are adequate, the patient feels active in body and mind, alert and in good spirits, whereas inadequate testosterone levels are accompanied by inactivity, lethargy and depressive moods (Barratt-Connor et al. 1999; Christiansen 1998; Wang et al. 1996).

While loss of **libido and sexual appetite** are signs of reduced testosterone levels, adequate substitution is accompanied by **sexual thoughts and phantasies**. Their frequency correlates with testosterone values. Spontaneous **nightly or morning erections** are signs of good substitution, but even when testosterone values are deficient, erections can still be provoked by visual stimulation. In the normal to slightly subnormal range serum testosterone correlates with the **frequency of ejacula-**

Table 15.3. Criteria for monitoring testosterone substitution

Psychic and sexual parameters	General well-being Intellectual and physical activity Mood Libido Erections Sexual activity
Somatic parameters	Body proportions Body weight Muscle mass and strength Fat distribution Hair pattern (beard, pubes, frontal hair line) Sebum production Voice mutation
Laboratory parameters	Serum testosterone (SHBG, free testosterone, salivary testosterone) Gonadotropins (LH, FSH) DHT, Estradiol Erythropoiesis (hematocrit, erythrocyte count, hemoglobin) (Liver enzymes)
Prostate/seminal vesicles	Ejaculate volume Prostate size / ultrasound results (Palpation and TRUS) PSA in serum Uroflow
Bones	Bone density

tions and sexual intercourse; however, above the lower limit of normal such a correlation no longer exists so that further increase of testosterone will not lead to a further increase in sexual activity. This indicates that in-depth conversation and a sexual diary – at least from time to time – give useful hints for evaluating testosterone therapy. Sexual questionnaires providing information about sexual thoughts and phantasies, appetite, satisfaction with sexuality, frequency of erections and ejaculations can make results of therapy objective (Bals-Pratsch et al. 1986; Behre and Nieschlag 1992; Burris et al. 1992; Carani et al. 1992; Clopper et al. 1993; Cunningham et al. 1990; Morales et al. 1997).

When testosterone values were decreased pharmacologically by GnRH antagonists, it appeared that adequate sexual function was still found in the presence of relatively low and slightly subnormal testosterone values (Bagatell et al. 1994; Behre et al. 1994a), whereas other functions required higher testosterone values. Thus, while the patient's sexuality provides an important parameter for monitoring therapy, it cannot be considered the only one.

15.3.2 Somatic Parameters

Muscle mass and strength increase in hypogonadal patients treated with testosterone and they develop a more virile phenotype (Bhasin et al. 1998). The anabolic effect of testosterone causes **body weight** to increase by about 5%. Thus, body weight, easily monitored, is one of the parameters to be checked routinely. The relative increase of muscle mass concomitant with the loss of fat can be measured, but does not yet belong to standard monitoring of testosterone therapy. Similarly, the distribution of fat over lower abdomen, hips and buttocks, characterized by a feminine pattern in the hypogonadal patient, assumes a masculine type under testosterone treatment.

The development and maintenance of a male **hair pattern** is a good parameter for monitoring testosterone therapy (Randall 1998). **Beard growth** and the frequency of shaving are easily checked. Hair growth in the **upper pubic triangle** especially is an important indicator for adequate testosterone replacement. Whereas women, prepubertal boys and untreated hypogonadal patients have a straight hairline, androgenization is accompanied by the formation of **temporal recession** and, depending on genetic disposition, by **balding**. Some patients consider this a negative effect about which they should be informed prior to therapy. The male hair pattern is of greater importance than its intensity, as the latter is not correlated with serum testosterone values (Knussmann 1992). A well-substituted patient will comment on shaving daily or may develop a full beard. Some predisposed patients may not, however, develop beard growth, which cannot be stimulated by higher testosterone doses.

Hypogonadal patients have prepubertal dry **skin**. Testosterone substitution induces **sebum production** and during the early phases some patients complain about increasing greasiness of skin, especially on the head which makes frequent shampooing necessary. Patients should be informed about these normal symptoms of masculinity. **Acne**, especially on the trunk and, more rarely, facial acne may occur under testosterone enanthate therapy; it may be necessary to reduce the dose or to switch preparations in order to avoid initial supra-physiological peak values.

Gynecomastia may occur when doses of testosterone enanthate are too high. This makes dose reduction necessary. Pre-existing gynecomastia in Klinefelter patients will hardly be influenced by testosterone substitution.

Shortly after initiation of testosterone substitution, patients who have not gone through puberty will experience **mutation of the voice**. This phenomenon reinforces the patient's self-confidence and social adjustment as the gap between chronological and biological age is closed. Being recognized as a man on the basis of the voice is of enormous importance for the patient's self-confidence; this becomes especially obvious from telephone conversations. Once mutation has taken place, the voice provides no further index of testosterone therapy, as larynx size, vocal cord length and thus vocal register are maintained even without further testosterone substitution.

In the course of time patients with prepubertal hypogonadism develop eunuchoid bodily proportions, as the epiphyseal fissures close more slowly than in normal growth. Testosterone substitution initiates a brief growth spurt prior to rapid closure of the fissures and cessation of growth. In these patients bone age of the left hand must be determined before the onset of puberty and periodic determinations of bone age will show when bone maturity is reached. The ratio of armspan to height and trunk height to leg length should be followed until definite bodily proportions are established. Further increase of arm span indicates insufficient testosterone therapy.

15.3.3 Laboratory Parameters

When **serum testosterone concentrations** are used to evaluate testosterone substitution therapy, the pharmacokinetic profile of the various preparations must be considered. Furthermore, for long-term evaluation of testosterone therapy, methods of determining testosterone serum concentrations must be subjected to strict quality control so that reliable values will be available over long periods.

Since for routine evaluation the duration of action of a given preparation is of prime importance, serum testosterone values should be measured immediately before the next application of a testosterone preparation. Especially for oral or transdermal preparations, the exact timepoint of the last application must be noted in order to interpret the results properly.

- For practical purposes, substitution therapy with **testosterone enanthate** should start with 3-week intervals between injections of 250 mg. If values are below normal 3 weeks after injection of testosterone enanthate the injection interval should be reduced. If, however, the values are still in the upper range, the interval may be increased.
- If serum testosterone values are low 2–4 h after ingestion of **testosterone undecanoate**, the patient should be reminded to take the drug with a meal for better resorption. Because of the considerable variation between inter- and intra-individual resorption patterns it is difficult to monitor oral testosterone undecanoate therapy on the basis of serum testosterone values, and other parameters are more important.
- Insufficient skin contact between membrane and scrotum may produce unsatisfactory serum values during **transdermal scrotal testosterone** application. The scrotal surface must be large enough, hair growth, which may impede contact between system and skin, should be checked.
- If subnormal values are measured when non-scrotal systems are used, poor adhesion to the skin (e. g. because of perspiration) or skin irritation may be at fault.

Testosterone may have to be determined repeatedly until the correct form of substitution is found. Once good substitution is established, the patient should be checked at 6 to 12-month intervals with blood samples being taken at the end of a therapy interval.

Basically, the determination of **total testosterone** in **serum** suffices and measuring **free testosterone** i. e. that fraction not bound to sex hormone binding globulin (SHBG) is unnecessary, as free and bound testosterone are well correlated in most instances. **Hyperthyroidism** and medication for **epilepsy** may, however, cause SHBG to increase so that total testosterone also rises. Conversely, extreme **adipositas** leads to a drop in total testosterone. In these cases, SHBG or free testosterone should be measured. The concentration of **testosterone in saliva** can also be used as an indicator for free testosterone. Most laboratories, however, lack sensitive enough methods.

In patients developing therapy-induced gynecomastia simultaneous determination of **estradiol** and testosterone is indicated in order to check for increased conversion to estradiol. In this event, the dose should be reduced or the patient should be switched from testosterone enanthate to testosterone patches.

Whereas **gonadotropins** are of decisive importance to differentiate between primary and secondary hypogonadism, their role in monitoring testosterone therapy for (primary) hypogonadism is less significant. In some forms of primary hypogonadism e.g. anorchia, serum testosterone concentrations and LH but also FSH are correlated relatively well. In these cases, normalization of gonadotropins may occur, especially with testosterone enanthate therapy. In the most frequent form of hypogonadism, the Klinefelter syndrome, however, under testosterone therapy LH and FSH values do not always correlate with serum testosterone values although all other parameters indicate adequate testosterone substitution. Likewise, oral and transdermal testosterone therapy have little influence on gonadotropins. For these reasons, gonadotropins are not very useful for monitoring testosterone therapy and then only in primary hypogonadism.

The slight anemia characteristic of hypogonadal patients disappears under testosterone therapy. Thus, **hemoglobin**, **erythrocyte count** and **hematocrit** are good parameters for monitoring therapy (Jockenhövel et al. 1997). If testosterone doses are too high, hemoglobin, erythrocytes and hematocrit may move into the supraphysiological range and polycythemia may develop. This is particularly true of older patients (Hajjar et al. 1997). In this case, the testosterone must be reduced. If despite adequate substitution anemia persists, other reasons, e.g. iron deficiency must be considered and must then be treated accordingly. At the beginning of testosterone therapy, red blood counts should be performed every 3 months, later at yearly intervals.

The testosterone preparations recommended here have no negative influence on **liver function** even when used chronically (Gooren 1994; Hajjar et al. 1997; Meikle 1998; Behre et al. 1999b) even though some physicians continue to believe so. This idea developed from the obsolete administration of 17α-alkylated anabolic steroids which are indeed liver toxic. This does not apply to natural testosterone. However, monitoring liver function is particularly important in patients with hepatic disease or with hypogonadism caused by general disease. In these cases, additional medication may influence liver function and thus also testosterone metabolism e.g. by increasing SHBG concentrations. This must be considered when evaluating testosterone values. Liver values should be checked at yearly follow-up.

Testosterone influences **lipid metabolism** and the **clotting system**. Although is it difficult to find bioequivalent doses, the effects vary when comparing different preparations (Jockenhövel et al. 1999). Testosterone therapy of hypogonadal patients should cause these parameters to move into the normal range for males and it remains unclear whether an increase in LDL and a decrease of HDL within the limits of normal has any biological significance for the cardiovascular system. Taken together, the pro- and anti-atherogenic effects of testosterone appear to be balanced (von Eckardstein 1998). Patients at risk should be given the preparation least likely to cause pathological alterations of these parameters.

Untreated patients have elevated *leptin* levels which drop into the normal range when testosterone substitution is sufficient (Behre et al. 1997). Current investigations may show whether it can serve as a parameter to monitor effectiveness of substitution.

15.3.4 Prostate and Seminal Vesicles

Under the influence of testosterone therapy, prostate and seminal vesicles of the hypogonadal patient enlarge and assume normal functions (see Chap. 3 and 6) (Behre et al. 1994b). This can best be documented by the increase of **ejaculate volume** into the normal range. Normal ejaculate volume (>2 ml) is a good parameter for measuring the efficacy of testosterone therapy.

Testosterone treatment does not enlarge **prostate volume** over the normal range. This is also true of testosterone enanthate therapy which intermittently achieves supraphysiological serum testosterone values (Fig. 15.7). **PSA** (**prostate specific antigen**) values remain in the normal range and uroflow is not influenced negatively. Rectal examination of the prostate for size, surface and consistency is part of routine monitoring of testosterone therapy.

As **benign prostate hyperplasia** (**BPH**) and **prostate carcinoma** increase with age and thus also the danger of stimulating an existing prostate carcinoma, before testosterone therapy, every patient should be thoroughly examined and, if over 40, the prostate should be checked at least annually.

If possible, rectal palpation should be supplemented by **transrectal ultrasonography** (TRUS) as it allows non-invasive evaluation of the entire organ. **PSA** (prostate spe-

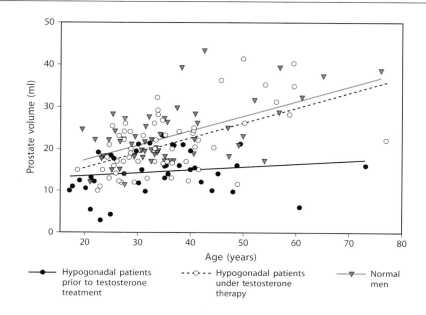

Fig. 15.7. Prostate volume (planimetric determination by transrectal ultrasound) in hypogonadal patients prior to testosterone therapy, in hypogonadal men receiving long-term effective testosterone substitution, and in age-matched normal men

Fig. 15.8. Bone mineral density (BMD), measured by QCT of the lumbar vertebrae during long-term testosterone substitution therapy up to 16 yr in 72 hypogonadal patients. *Circles* indicate hypogonadal patients with first QCT measurement before initiation of testosterone substitution therapy, *squares* show those patients already receiving testosterone therapy at the first QCT. The *dark shaded area* indicates the range of high fracture risk, the *unshaded area* shows the range without significant fracture risk, and the *light shaded area* indicates the intermediate range where fractures may occur (20, 21)

cific antigen) determined in serum and measuring **uroflow** belong to routine monitoring.

When a carcinoma is suspected, the patient must be referred for urologic consultation, in the course of which prostate biopsy may complete the diagnosis.

15.3.5 Bone Mass

Reduced **bone mass** in hypogonadal man can be normalized by testosterone therapy (Chap. 6) (Behre et al. 1997) (Fig. 15.8). In good therapeutic adjustment both cortical as well as trabecular mass increase while vertebral surfaces (in QCT) remain unaltered (Leifke et al. 1998). If, however, testosterone therapy begins too late, predominantly cortical bone mass will increase (Finkel-

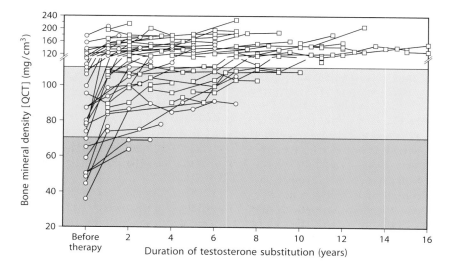

stein 1998; Horowitz et al. 1992); vertebral bone mass can also increase and even normalize in patients in whom testosterone therapy becomes necessary at an advanced age (Behre et al. 1997; Snyder et al. 1999).

> As osteoporosis and risk of fracture compromise the quality of a patient's life, we **measure bone density** before and at 1–2 year intervals in every patient on testosterone therapy. The results are considered when choosing the testosterone dose.

Even if not all patients can be monitored in this matter, at least those with long untreated hypogonadism and older patients should be examined at the time of first diagnosis. If bone density values are pathological, normalization should be documented by further investigations. At the very earliest, increases in bone density can be observed half a year after inception of testosterone therapy. The various diagnostic procedures are discussed in Chap. 6.

15.4 Evaluation of Testosterone Substitution Therapy

Testosterone deficiency is not life-threatening, but it does reduce the **quality of life** drastically and may induce various illnesses (see Chap. 7, 8 and 9). The assumption, often expressed, that testosterone is responsible for shorter life expectancy in men can hardly be tested experimentally. The same long life-span of men castrated prepubertally and of intact men (Nieschlag et al. 1993) supports the theory that factors other than testosterone are responsible for the different life expectancies between the sexes (see also Sect. 8.1.2, Acquired Anorchia). At the very least there is no reason to deny a patient testosterone substitution. Testosterone is characterized by **high therapeutic safety**, supported by the absence of serious long-term side effects following high dose administration as used for excessively tall stature (see Sect. 15.5) and its illegal use in extremely high doses in athletics and by bodybuilders (see Sect. 15.6). The only real contraindications are manifest prostate carcinoma or a very rare mamma carcinoma.

It is difficult to quantify the actual advantage of testosterone substitution therapy. The **improved quality of life** of a patient receiving testosterone therapy is undisputed. Increased self-confidence and satisfaction, confirmed by sexual activities, are factors not be underestimated concerning the patient's social integration. By supporting physical and psychic activity his capacities are increased or maintained; elimination of anemia, strengthening of the skeleton and reduction of risk of fracture prevent invalidity and infirmity.

> Adequate replacement therapy allows the patient to be integrated into society and to enjoy satisfactory quality of life.

Even if one or another patient must be convinced of the usefulness of a suggested therapy because he lacks the imagination to see its advantages, in the long run hardly any patient is willing to forego substitution therapy. Increased public discussion of the effects of testosterone and suggestions from increasing numbers of self-help groups make it easier for patients to formulate their own ideas concerning adequate therapy. It remains the physician's task to guide the patient, to monitor the various parameters and to find optimal therapeutic adjustment for the individual patient.

15.5 Excessive Height

Testosterone deficiency at the time of puberty causes eunuchoid skeletal proportions, whereas normally testosterone induces proportioned body growth by timely induction of epiphyseal maturation. Prior to puberty testosterone can cause closure of the epiphyseal lines and cause small stature, as for example in pubertas praecox. It is possible to take advantage of these facts in order to modify final height in boys predisposed to excessive height (over 2 m). High-dose testosterone administered early can stop growth. Usually, 250 mg testosterone enanthate every week or 500 mg every two weeks are given intramuscularly between the ages of 12–16 years for about one year. The dose to be administered is at least twice that used for substitution. Therapeutic phases that are too short coupled with discontinuance before complete epiphyseal maturity prevents the therapeutic goal from being reached. Before growth ceases, possible therapeutic success can be tested be determining bone age. The sooner therapy is begun, the more effective growth reduction will be. If bone age exceeds 14 years, testosterone is usually without effect (for review see Drop et al. 1998). However, very early therapy should be avoided as precocious puberty with its psychosocial and physical implications would be induced.

Even if testosterone is not licensed for this indication (as in Germany), for many years such treatment was carried out relatively often since the early 1950. It is remarkable that no controlled studies have been performed to test the actual therapeutic effect. For this reason it is also important to question the results of possible long-term effects. During treatment with pharmacological doses of testosterone, testicular development is suppressed and the question arises whether this temporary suppression of the testis and the high doses of testosterone may have untoward effects in the (pre)pubertal patient. A similar question can be raised concerning studies on male contraception based on testosterone, but with the difference that here vertical growth is to be suppressed in an immature patient. After cessation of therapy the endocrine pituitary-gonadal axis quickly returns to normal (Brämswig 1984). Long-term follow-up studies in treated boys showed no anomalies attributable to treatment compared to control populations (van de Waal 1995; Lemcke et al. 1996). No alterations in the cardiovascular system and in serum lipids or in the prostate (volume, sonographic structure and PSA) were observed. Subnormal semen parameters seen relatively frequently in follow-up examinations were attributable to cryptorchidism and varicocele rather than to testosterone therapy (Lemcke et al. 1996). Concerning therapeutic safety, follow-up investigations to date show that the use of relatively high doses of testosterone in puberty remains without long-term side effects.

Even if long-term follow–up investigations do not argue against such therapy, it should be considered that this testosterone therapy accelerates pubertal development with all its psychic and physical consequences. Since psychological reasons for this therapy outweigh any medical considerations, each individual case should be carefully considered and therapy should only be administered in cases of extreme expected height. As the boys (and their parents!) tend to suffer from extreme height predominantly during the growth period, but are later well integrated, adequate medical or psychological counselling towards better adjustment is always indicated. Often such care is sufficient and makes further testosterone therapy superfluous.

15.6 Use and Abuse of Anabolic Steroids

As testosterone has a strong anabolic i.e. protein-building component and induces muscle growth when accompanied by physical exercise, in the 50s and 60s an attempt was made to dissociate the androgenic and anabolic effects by chemically altering the testosterone molecule. As a result, a multitude of so-called **anabolic steroids** were synthesized and some of them were also applied clinically (Kochakian 1976; Kopera 1985). They attempt to make clinical use of the positive effects of testosterone on muscle metabolism, blood formation and bone metabolism, while dispensing with androgenic side effects e.g. virilization in women and children. However, separation of anabolic and androgenic components remained impossible in anabolic steroids.

Extreme physical performance carried out over extended periods causes a drop of testosterone in circulation (e.g. Schürmeyer et al. 1984). Until recently, it was believed that use of androgens by eugonadal athletes would, at the very outside, have placebo effects. Recent investigations were able to show that pharmacological

doses of androgens accompanied by exercise could indeed induce muscle growth (Bhasin et al. 1996, 1998). This, however, does not apply to all androgenic steroids. For the androgen precursor androstenedione, taken by famous baseball players such as Mark McGwire and freely available in the USA as an over-the-counter food supplement, no anabolic effect could be documented (King et al. 1999). Present studies to date failed to confirm any necessity for substitution therapy in high-performance athletics. Nevertheless, the gain in strength and muscle mass induced by testosterone and anabolics led to their abuse by high-performance athletes and body builders. The doses taken are often 10–100 fold higher than those used in replacement therapy (Wilson 1988; Knuth et al. 1989; Schänzer et al. 1998). Testosterone itself, followed by nandrolone (19-nortestosterone), metandienone, stanazolol, methenolone, mesterolone, 17α-methyltestosterone and many other substances are used. Often substances are combined and used in increasing and decreasing regimens ("stacking"). Special attention should be given to this abuse. Because of these high doses androgenic side-effects such as suppression of hypothalamic-pituitary function and spermatogenesis up to azoospermia (Knuth et al. 1989), acne, gynecomastia and fluid retention (and irreversible alterations of voice and clitoris and virilization in women) are well-known side-effects. Furthermore, if (obsolete) 17α-alkylated steroids (stanazolol, 17α-methyltestosterone) are used, liver toxicity with cholostasis, peliosis and even malignant neoplasm may result. Increased aggressiveness has been repeatedly ascribed to anabolic steroids and single cases are always cited as examples. Whether these cases are coincidental, as to be expected in widespread abuse of anabolics or whether there is a causal connection, cannot be determined to date because convincing studies are lacking (Nieschlag 1992).

As a whole, in view of the many substances taken in high doses, serious side-effects rarely occur. If they were more frequent, their use would be self-limiting. In positive terms, the high doses used speak for the low toxicity of testosterone, and androgens have been taken in very high doses and over prolonged periods. Scientific societies and organizations have come out clearly against the use of anabolic steroids in athletics so that their use has become prohibited in competition and its discovery leads to disqualification and disbarring of athletes from competition.

As anabolic steroids do not have the full spectrum of effects of testosterone, and as effective replacement therapy with testosterone preparations is available, anabolic steroids are not indicated for the treatment of male hypogonadism (see negative monographs of the German Federal Health Ministry 1990–1994). Whether knowledge of the androgen receptor and intracellular testosterone metabolism will provide new impulses for the development of more selective androgens remains to be seen.

15.7 References

Atkinson L, Chang Y-L, Snyder PJ (1998) Long-term experience with testosterone replacement through scrotal skin. In: Nieschlag E, Behre HM (eds) Testosterone – action, deficiency, substitution, 2nd edn. Springer, Berlin Heidelberg New York, pp 365–388

Bagatell CJ, Heimann JR, Rivier JE, Bremner WJ (1994) Effects of endogenous testosterone and estradiol on sexual behaviour in normal young men. J Clin Endocrinol Metab 78:711–716

Bals-Pratsch M, Knuth UA, Yoon YD, Nieschlag E (1986) Transdermal testosterone substitution therapy for male hypogonadism. Lancet ii:943–946

Barratt-Connor E, von Mühlen DG, Kritz-Silverstein D (1999) Bioavailable testosterone and depressed mood in older men: the Rancho Bernardo study. J Clin Endocrinol Metab 84:573–577

Behre HM, Nieschlag E (1992) Testosterone buciclate (20-Aet-1) in hypogonadal men: pharmacokinetics and pharmacodynamics of the new long-acting testosterone ester. J Clin Endocrinol Metab 75:1204–1210

Behre HM, Nieschlag E (1998) Comparative pharmacokinetics of testosterone esters. In: Nieschlag E, Behre HM (eds) Testosterone – action, deficiency, substitution, 2nd edn. Springer, Berlin Heidelberg New York, pp 329–348

Behre HM, Böckers A, Schlingheider A, Nieschlag E (1994a) Sustained suppression of serum LH, FSH testosterone and increase of high-density lipoprotein cholesterol by daily injections of the GnRH antagonist cetrorelix over 8 days in normal men. Clin Endocrinol 40:241–248

Behre HM, Bohmeyer J, Nieschlag E (1994b) Prostate volume in testosterone-treated and untreated hypogonadal men in comparison to age-matched normal contrals. Clin Endocrinol 40:341–349

Behre HM, Kliesch S, Leifke E, Link TM, Nieschlag E (1997) Long-term effect of testosterone therapy on bone mineral density in hypogonadal men. J Clin Endocrinol Metab 82: 2386–2390

Behre HM, Abshagen K, Oettel M, Hübler D, Nieschlag E (1999a) Intramuscular injection of testosterone undecanoate for the treatment of male hypogonadism: phase I-studies. Eur J Endocrinol 140:414–419

Behre HM, von Eckardstein S, Kliesch S, Nieschlag E (1999b) Long-term substitution therapy of hypogonadal men with transscrotal testosterone over seven to ten years. Clin Endocrinol 50:629–635

Bhasin S (ed) (1998) The therapeutic role of androgens. Baillières Clin Endocrinol Metab 12(3)

Bhasin S, Swerdloff RS, Steiner B, Peterson MA, Meridores T, Galmirin M (1992) A biodegradable testosterone microcapsule formulation provides uniform eugonadal levels of testosterone for 10–11 weeks in hypogonadal men. J Clin Endocrinol Metab 74:75–83

Bhasin S, Storer TW, Berman N, Callegari C, Clevenger B, Phillips J, Bunnell TJ, Tricker R, Shirazi A, Casaburi R (1996) The effects of supraphysiologic doses of testosterone on muscle size and strength in normal men. N Engl J Med 335:1–7

Bhasin S, Bross R, Storer TW, Casaburi R (1998) Androgens and muscles. In: Nieschlag E, Behre HM (eds) Testosterone – action, deficiency, substitution, 2nd edn. Springer, Berlin Heidelberg New York, pp 209–227

Brämswig JH, Nieschlag E, Schellong G (1984) Pituitary-gonadal function in boys after high-dose testosterone treatment of excessively tall stature. Acta Endocrinol 107:97–103

Bundesgesundheitsamt (1990) Negativ-Monographien zu anabolen Steroiden: Stanozolol (Bundesanzeiger 1990, Nr. 18), Metenolon (Bundesanzeiger Nr. 48, 1990), Oxabolon (Bundesanzeiger Nr. 111, 1990), Androstanolon (Bundesanzeiger Nr. 240, 1990) Nandrolon (Bundesanzeiger Nr. 69, 1993), Clostebol (Bundesanzeiger Nr. 132, 1993), Chlordehydromethyltestosteron (Bundesanzeiger Nr. 72, 1994)

Burris AS, Banks SM, Carter CS, Davidson JM, Sherins RJ (1992) A long-term prospective study of the physiologic and behavioural effects of hormone replacement in untreated hypogonadal men. J Androl 13:297–304

Carani C, Bancroft J, Granata A, Del Rio G, Marrama P (1992) Testosterone and erectile function: nocturnal penile tumescence and rigidity, and erectile response to visual erotic stimuli in hypogonadal men. Psychoneuroendocrinology 17:647–654

Christiansen K (1998) Behavioural correlates of testosterone. In: Nieschlag E, Behre HM (eds) Testosterone – action, deficiency, substitution, 2nd edn. Springer, Berlin Heidelberg New York, pp 107–142

Clopper RR, Voorhess ML, MacGillivray MH, Lee PA, Mills B (1993) Psychosexual behaviour in hypopituitary men: a controlled comparison of gonadotropin and testosterone replacement. Psychoneuroendocrinology 18:149–161

Cunningham GR, Hirshkowitz M, Kroenman SG, Karacan I (1990) Testosterone replacement therapy and sleep-related erections in hypogonadal men. J Clin Endocrinol Metab 70:792–797

de Waal WJ, Vreeburg JTM, Bekkering F, de Jong FH, de Muinck Keizer-Schrama SMPF, Drop SLS, Weber RFA (1995) High-dose testosterone therapy for reduction of final height in constitutionally tall boys: does it influence testicular function in adulthood? Clin Endocrinol 43:87–95

Delanoe D, Fougevrollas B, Meyer L, Thonneau P (1984) Androgenisation of female partners of men on medroxyprogesterone acetate/percutaneous testosterone contraception. Lancet 1:276

Dobs AS, Hoover DR, Chen MC, Allen R (1998) Pharmacokinetic characteristics, efficacy, and safety of buccal testosterone in hypogonadal males: a pilot study. J Clin Endocrinol Metab 83:33–39

Drop SLS, de Waal J, de Muinck Keizer-Schrama SMPF (1988) Sex steroid treatment of constituional tall stature. Endocr Rev 19:540–558

von Eckardstein A (1998) Androgens, cardiovascular risk factors and atherosclerosis. In: Nieschlag E, Behre HM (eds) Testosterone – action, deficiency, substitution, 2nd edn. Springer, Berlin Heidelberg New , pp 229–257

Finkelstein JS, Klibanski A (1990) Effects of androgens on bone metabolism. In: Nieschlag E, Behre HM (eds) Testosterone – action, deficiency, substitution. Springer, Berlin Heidelberg New York, pp 204–215

Gooren LJG (1998) A ten year safety study on the oral androgen testosterone undecanoate. J Androl 15:212–215

Hajjar RR, Kaiser FE, Morley JE (1997) Outcomes of long term testosterone replacement in older hypogonadal males: a retrospective analysis. J Clin Endocrinol Metab 82:3793–3796

Handelsman DJ (1998) Clinical pharmacology of testosterone pellet implants. In: Nieschlag E, Behre HM (eds) Testosterone – action, deficiency, substitution, 2nd edn. Springer, Berlin Heidelberg New York, pp 348–364

Horowitz M, Wishart JM, O'Loughlin PD, Morris HA, Need AG, Nordin BEC (1992) Osteoporosis and Klinefelter-syndrome. Clin Endocrinol 36:113–118

Jockenhövel F, Vogel E, Reinhardt W, Reinwein D (1997) Effects of various modes of androgen substitution therapy on erythropoiesis. Eur J Med Res 2:293–298

Jockenhövel F, Bullmann C, Schubert M, Vogel E, Reinhardt W, Reinwein D, Müller-Wieland D, Krone W (1999) Influence of various modes of androgen substitution on serum lipids and lipoproteins in hypogonadal men. Metabolism 48:590–596

Kelleher S, Turner L, Howe C, Conway AJ, Handelsman DJ (1999) Extrusion of testosterone pellets: a randomized controlled clinical study. Clin Endocrinol 51:469–471

King DS, Sharp RL, Vukovich MD, Brown GA, Reifenrath TA, Uhl NL, Parsons KA (1999) Effect of oral androstenedione on serum testosterone and adaptations to resistance training in young men: a randomized controlled trial. JAMA 281:2020–2028

Knussmann R, Christansen K, Kannmacher J (1992) Relations between sex hormone levels and character of hair and skin in healthy young men. Am J Phys Anthropol 88:59–67

Knuth UA, Maniera H, Nieschlag E (1989) Anabolic steroids and semen parameters in body builders. Fertil Steril 52:1041–1047

Kochakian CD (ed) (1976) Anabolic androgenic steroids. Springer, Berlin Heidelberg New York (Handbook of experimental pharmacology, vol 43)

Kopera H (1985) The history of anabolic steroids and a review of clinical experiences with anabolic steroids. In: Eickelboom FS, van der Vies J (eds) Anabolics in the 80s. Acta Endocrinol [Suppl] 217:11–18

Leifke E, Körner HC, Link TM, Behre HM, Peters PE, Nieschlag E (1998) Effects of testosterone replacement therapy on cortical and trabecular bone mineral density, vertebral body area and paraspinal muscle area in hypogonadal men. Eur J Endocrinol 138:51–58

Lemcke B, Zentgraf J, Behre HM, Kliesch S, Nieschlag E (1996) Long-term effects on testicular function of high-dose testosterone treatment for excessively tall stature. J Clin Endocrinol Metab 81:296–301

Meikle AW (1998) A permeation-enhanced non-scrotal testosterone transdermal system for the treatment of male hypogonadism. In: Nieschlag E, Behre HM (eds) Testosterone – action, deficiency, substitution, 2nd edn. Springer, Berlin Heidelberg New York, pp 389–422

Morales A, Johnston B, Heaton JP, Lundie M (1997) Testosterone supplementation for hypogonadal impotence: assessment of biochemical measures and therapeutic outcomes. J Urol 157:849–854

Nieschlag E (1981) Ist die Anwendung von Methyltestosteron obsolet? Dtsch Med Wochenschr 106:1123

Nieschlag E (1992) Testosteron, Anabolika und aggressives Verhalten bei Männern. Dtsch Ärztebl 89:2967–2972

Nieschlag E, Behre HM (eds) (1998a) Testosterone – action, deficiency, substitution, 2nd edn. Springer, Berlin Heidelberg New York

Nieschlag E, Behre HM (1998b) Pharmacology and clinical use of testosterone. In: Nieschlag E, Behre HM (eds) Testosterone – action, deficiency, substitution, 2nd edn. Springer, Berlin Heidelberg New York, pp 293–328

Nieschlag E, Nieschlag S, Behre HM (1993) Life expectancy and testosterone. Nature 366:215

Nieschlag E, Büchter D, von Eckardstein S, Abshagen K, Behre HM (1999) Repeated intramuscular injections of testosterone undecanoate for substitution therapy of hypogonadal men. Clin Endocrinol 51:757–763

Randall VA (1998) Androgens and hair. In: Nieschlag E, Behre HM (eds) Testosterone – action, deficiency, substitution, 2nd edn. Springer, Berlin Heidelberg New York, pp 169–186

Schaison G, Couzinet B (1998) Percutaneous dihydrotestosterone treatment. In: Nieschlag E, Behre HM (eds) Testosterone – action, deficiency, substitution, 2nd edn. Springer, Berlin Heidelberg New York, pp 423–436

Schürmeyer T, Nieschlag E (1984) Comparative pharmacokinetics of testosterone enanthate cyclohexanecarboxylate as assessed by serum and saliva testosterone in normal men. Int J Androl 7:181–187

Schürmeyer T, Wickings EJ, Freischem CW, Nieschlag E (1983) Saliva and serum testosterone following oral testosterone undecanoate administration in normal and hypogonadal men. Acta Endocrinol 102:456–462

Schürmeyer T, Jung K, Nieschlag E (1984) The effect of a 1100 km run on testicular, adrenal and thyroid hormones. Int J Androl 7:276–282

Salehian B, Wang CH, Alexander G, Davidson T, McDonald V, Berman N, Dudley RE, Ziel F, Swerdloff RS (1995) Pharmacokinetics, bioefficacy and safety of sublingual testosterone cyclodextrin in hypogonadal men: comparision to testosterone enanthate. J Clin Endocrinol Metab 80:3567–3575

Snyder PJ, Peachey H, Hannoush P, Berlin JA, Loh L, Holmes JH, Dlewati A, Staley J, Santanna J, Kapoor SC, Attie MF, Haddad JG Jr, Strom BL (1999) Effect of testosterone treatment on bone mineral density in men over 65 years of age. J Clin Endocrinol Metab 84:1966–1972

Wang C, Alexander G, Berman N, Salehian B, Davidson T, McDonald V, Steiner B, Hull L, Callegari C, Swerdloff RS (1996) Testosterone replacement therapy improves mood in hypogonadal men – a clinical research center study. J Clin Endocrinol Metab 81:3578–3583

Wang C, Berman N, Longstreth JA, Chuapoco B, Hull L, Steiner B, Faulkner S, Dudley RE, Swerdloff RS (2000) Pharmacokinetics of transdermal testosterone gel in hypogonadal men: application of gel at one site versus four sites: J Clin Endocrinol Metab 85:964–969

Wilson JD (1988) Androgen abuse by athletes. Endocr Rev 9:181–199

World Health Organization (1992) Nieschlag E, Wang CH, Handelsman DJ, Swerdloff RS, Wu FCW, Einer-Jensen N, Khanna J, Waites GMH (eds) Guidelines for the use of androgens. WHO, Geneva

Yu YM, Punyasavatsu N, Elder D, D'Ercole AJ (1999) Sexual development in a two-year-old boy induced by topical exposure to testostereone. Pediatrics 104:23

Zhang GY, Gu YQ, Wang XH, Cui YG, Bremner WJ (1998) A pharmacokinetic study of injectable testosterone undecanoate in hypogonadal men. J Androl 19:761–768

CHAPTER 16

Empirical Therapies for Idiopathic Male Infertility

16

E. Nieschlag · E. Leifke

16.1 Definition and Incidence of Male Idiopathic Infertility

The term **"idiopathic infertility"** designates **diagnosis by exclusion**. Only after all other possible causes for infertility have been eliminated can the diagnosis of "idiopathic infertility" be established. Seminal parameters are frequently subnormal and may be associated with elevated serum FSH, indicating spermatogenic failure. Testicular biopsies often show incomplete spermatogenic arrest or focal SCO and fail to provide further information concerning pathogenesis. These patients represent the largest group of men attending fertility clinics (about 30 % at our institute).

The collective diagnosis of "idiopathic infertility" most likely comprises a multitude of different pathogenic mechanisms. One of andrology's most important and exciting tasks is to disclose the workings of these mechanisms und ultimately to eliminate their cause by rational therapy. New points of departure are expected from research on molecular genetics and paracrinological regulation of spermatogenesis; the effects of gonadotropins and sex hormones at the molecular level, microdeletions on the Y chromosome, CFTR-mutations in congenital bilateral aplasia of the vas deferens (CBAVD), the pathology of the androgen receptor and the biology of gametes are examples of such research results (Hansson et al. 1996; Stefanini et al. 1998).

It should be pointed out that the term **idiopathic infertility** has different meanings in andrology and gynecology. In gynecology, the term "female idiopathic infertility" refers to a condition in which clinical examination does not reveal any pathological finding which might explain the infertility of the couple. Here it would be more accurate to speak of **unexplained infertility** (see Chap. 14).

Even in the absence of clearcut pathophysiological concepts explaining the suitability of a given medication for treating idiopathic infertility, numerous pharmacological regimes were and continue to be applied, often for considerable periods of time, both in combined and sequential form. Theses are summarized below as **"empirical therapy"**. The postulate of **evidence-based medicine** following controlled studies is particularly appropriate for the critical evaluation of these therapeutic regimes (see Sec. 1.6).

16.2 Empirical Therapy

16.2.1 hCG/hMG

For want of a rational therapeutic approach to idiopathic infertility it seemed reasonable to apply previously successful endocrine treatment modalities for appropriate indications, i.e. in secondary hypogonadism. Because of the success rate of hCG/hMG treatment in inducing pregnancies in patients with hypogonadotropic hypogonadism and on the hypothesis that elevation of gonadotropins may lead to stimulation of spermatogenesis this regimen was also applied to patients with normogonadotropic fertility disturbances. Numerous open studies tried to demonstrate its effectiveness. Surprisingly, it was used for 2 decades for idiopathic infertility until a critical review concluded that its efficacy remained unproven and that controlled clinical studies were urgently needed (Schill 1986).

A **placebo-controlled, prospective, double-blind and randomized study of hCG/hMG treatment** for normogonadotropic oligoasthenoteratozoospermic men with sperm concentrations below 10^6/ml could not demonstrate any beneficial effect on sperm parameters or pregnancy rates (Knuth et al. 1987). Each change in the treatment group could be matched with a similar change in the placebo group (Fig. 16.1). Such changes would probably have been taken as genuine therapeutic effects if the trial had not been placebo-controlled, emphasizing the importance of placebo for the evaluation of therapeutic benefits in clinical studies.

In conclusion, there is no evidence for benefits of hCG/hMG treatment in normogonadotropic idiopathic infertility.

16.2.2 Pulsatile GnRH

It was suggested that oligoasthenoteratozoospermia in men with elevated serum FSH might be caused by too infrequent GnRH pulses. Thus the term "slow pulsing oligospermia" was introduced into andrology (Wagner and Warsch 1984). A carefully done study has reported slower LH- but normal FSH-pulsatility in men with oligozoospermia compared to controls (Reyes-Fuentes et al. 1996). In addition, the amplified mass of LH and FSH secreted basally as well as after GnRH-injection was higher in infertile men than in controls in this study. It was claimed that GnRH injections administered at a physiologic pulse frequency would improve sperm parameters in these patients. An **uncontrolled study** was able to show that such therapy indeed normalized FSH values, but neither improvements in sperm parameters nor in pregnancy rates were proved (Bals-Pratsch et al. 1989). The hypothesis that elevated FSH values are the cause and not the effect of disturbed spermatogenesis could not be confirmed. The lack of a pathophysiologi-

Fig. 16.1. Results of a placebo-controlled, double-blind, randomized study concerning hCG/hMG treatment for male idiopathic infertility. Columns represent differences in motile sperm after a treatment period of 12 weeks compared to pretreatment values. Patients are grouped according to the extent of the change observed. Stars representing patients with no corresponding "partner" in the verum group. No differences between verum and placebo group can be observed. (Knuth et al. 1987)

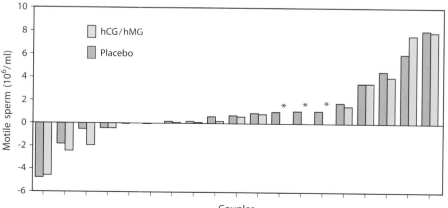

cal concept and therapeutic success make a controlled study with this design superfluous.

16.2.3 Highly Purified and Recombinant FSH

Once highly purified FSH became available for clinical use it was also applied to male infertility. An increase in fertilization and pregnancy rates was reported in men treated with highly purified FSH who had failed to fertilize an oocyte in vitro prior to treatment (Acosta et al. 1992). Although the evidence revealed by these studies is weak because of their uncontrolled design, they gave rise to a series of studies, which were, however, similarly uncontrolled. Only three were randomized and placebo-controlled (Comodo et al. 1996; Kamischke et al. 1998) or just randomized (Matorras et al. 1997). None showed any significant improvement of ejaculate parameters when compared to basal values or to the placebo group. The meta-analysis of all three studies yielded an odds-ratio of 1.45 with respect to the pregnancy rate (Fig. 16.2) so that 22 patients would have to be treated to gain one additional pregnancy (Kamischke and Nieschlag 1999). In view of the high costs and the success rates, marginal if at all, in its present form FSH therapy does not appear justified for idiopathic infertility.

It should be mentioned that improvements in sperm morphology were observed by electron microscopy in one study, unfortunately uncontrolled (Bartoov et al. 1994) and in our study significant increases of testicular volume and sperm DNA condensation were seen. Although the underlying mechanism remains unclear, the results indicate that further investigations on the basic principle are worthwhile, and might help to identify patients responding positively.

Fig. 16.2. Individual (*squares*) and combined (*COR; diamonds*) odds-ratio for pregnancies in randomized controlled studies with highly purified or recombinant human FSH (95% confidence interval). The *broken line* shows the COR. (From Kamischke and Nieschlag 1999)

16.2.4 Androgens

The requirement of testosterone for normal spermatogenesis under physiological conditions led to the use of androgens in the therapy of idiopathic infertility in men, although androgen deficiency could not be demonstrated in these patients. **Mesterolone** especially – a 5α-reduced testosterone derivative – was used for almost 2 decades in andrological practice until a **multicenter, placebo-controlled, double-blind and randomized WHO study** with 246 couples proved its ineffectiveness as no statistically significant increase in pregnancy rates was seen (WHO 1989).

Further publications followed, so that nine randomized, placebo-controlled, double-blind studies could be evaluated in a meta-analysis. With respect to pregnancy rates, in 1205 couples a combined odds-ratio of only 1.02 (Fig. 16.3) resulted. In other words, 359 patients would have to be treated for one additional pregnancy to occur (Kamischke and Nieschlag 1999). Hence, administration of androgens is not warranted in cases of idiopathic male infertility.

Testosterone and its synthetic derivatives suppress the pituitary gonadotropin secretion, thus leading to inhibition of spermatogenesis. A large proportion of patients treated with androgens become azoospermic. This effect of exogenously administered androgens is used for contraceptive trials in males (see Chap. 20). It was believed that in men with idiopathic infertility, spermatogenic activity would be increased following treatment with testosterone, resulting in elevated sperm concentrations compared to pretreatment values (so-called **rebound effect**). This initial speculation, however, could not be confirmed by later clinical studies, neither in patients with idiopathic infertility nor in normal volunteers. All studies were uncontrolled and the pregnancy rates reported were widely scattered. For these reasons this therapy cannot be recommended. However, the initial fear that rebound therapy might lead to hyalinization of the seminiferous tubules was not confirmed.

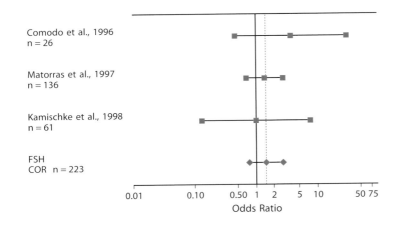

Comodo et al., 1996
n = 26

Matorras et al., 1997
n = 136

Kamischke et al., 1998
n = 61

FSH
COR n = 223

0.01   0.10   0.50 1   2   5   10   50 75
Odds Ratio

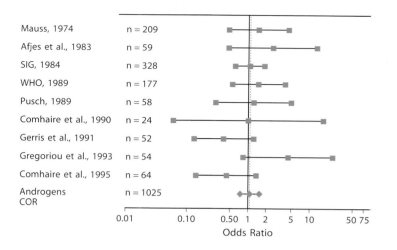

Fig. 16.3. Individual (*squares*) and combined (*COR; diamonds*) odds-ratio for pregnancies in randomized controlled studies with androgens (95% confidence interval). The broken line shows the COR. (From Kamischke and Nieschlag 1999)

Likewise, complete reversibility of suppressed spermatogenesis was observed in volunteers treated with testosterone for contraceptive purposes (see Chap. 20).

To date there is no proof for the effectiveness of oral testosterone undecanoate and thus no rationale for its use. One attempt failed to justify the use of androgens for idiopathic infertility by giving oval **testosterone undecanoate** prior to in-vitro fertilization (Abdelmassih et al. 1992). Here again, the observational data were uncontrolled and could not be confirmed in a later controlled study (Comhaire et al. 1995). A placebo-controlled, double-blind study described an increase in sperm motility when men with idiopathic infertility were treated with testosterone undecanoate as a supplementary agent to tamoxifen treatment (Adamopoulos et al. 1997). However, whether the improvement in sperm motility would be associated with increased pregnancy rates remained uninvestigated.

16.2.5 Antiestrogens and Aromatase Inhibitors

Antiestrogens (e.g. clomiphene, tamoxifen) antagonize estrogenic activity by competitively blocking the estrogen receptor at target sites. Aromatase inhibitors (e.g. testolactone) exert similiar effects by inhibiting aromatase enzyme activity which normally converts androgens to estrogens. Since estrogens suppress pituitary gonadotropin secretion via a negative feedback, both estrogen receptor blockade as well as lowering endogenous estrogen levels will lead to an increase in circulating LH and FSH. On the hypothesis that such an increase would

result in an improvement of spermatogenic activity and sperm concentration, antiestrogens and aromatase inhibiting agents were widely used to treat male idiopathic infertility.

The inefficacy of **aromatase inhibitors** in the treatment of male infertility has been shown by a placebo-controlled, double-blind, randomized trial (Clark and Sherins 1989). For **clomiphene** a more recently performed large multicenter study could not demonstrate any significant differences in the pregnancy rate between treatment and placebo groups (WHO 1992) (Fig. 16.4). In Germany **tamoxifen** is the preferred antiestrogen used in andrological treatment. A recent review clearly pointed out that only 8 out of 29 published studies evaluating the possible benefits of tamoxifen treatment in male infertility were controlled. None of the 8

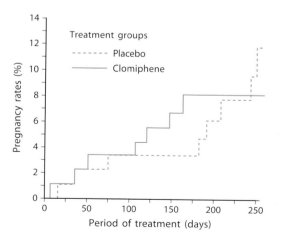

Fig. 16.4. Results of a WHO multicenter study concerning clomiphene for male idiopathic infertility are shown. Cumulative pregnancy rates of couples whose men were either treated with clomiphene (25 mg/d, n = 44) or with placebo (n = 34) are plotted (WHO 1992)

Table 16.1. Randomized studies concerning tamoxifen treatment for idiopathic male infertility (Rolf et al. 1996) (*s* significant, *n.s.* non-significant)

References	Study design	Patients (n)	Dose (mg/day)	Duration of treatment (months)	Sperm concentration (million/ml)	Sperm motility	Sperm morphology	Pregnancy
Willis et al. 1977	single-blind cross-over	16	10	2 placebo, 6 tamoxifen, 4 placebo	n.s.	n.s.	n.s.	?
Török 1985	double-blind	A=27, B=27	A=20, B=placebo	3	n.s.	n.s.	n.s.	A=9 (33%), B=5 (25%)
Ainmelk et al. 1987	random, double-blind cross-over	16	20	3 3	n.s.	n.s.	n.s.	2 after 1 month of therapy
Krause et al. 1992	random	A=39, B=37	A=30, B=placebo	3	n.s.	n.s.	n.s.	5 (13%) in 9 months 3 (8%) in 9 months
Breznik u. Borko 1993	random	A=22, B=20, C=27	A=20, B=25 mg clomiphene, C=placebo	1–7	A: n.s., B: n.s.	A: n.s., B: n.s.	n.s.	A=7 (31,7%), B=5 (15%), C=8 (29,6%) in 4 years
Kotulas et al. 1994	random	A=122, B=117	A=20, B=placebo	3	s.	n.s.	n.s.	?
Maier u. Hiernert 1988	random	A=20, B=20	A=30, B=30, (+150mg testolacton)	3	A: s., B: s., A vers B n.s.	A: n.s., B: n.s.	A: n.s., B: n.s.	A=4 (15%), B=4 (15%)
Maier u. Hiernert 1990	random	A=33, B=34	A=30, B=30, (+600 IE kallikrein)	3	s. (only above 10^6/ml)	A: n.s., B: s.	A: n.s., B: s.	A=4 (12%)

controlled trials could demonstrate a beneficial effect on fertility for the subjects treated with tamoxifen (Rolf et al. 1996) (Table 16.1). A meta-analysis of six studies concluded that at least 29 patients needed to be treated to yield one additional pregnancy (Kamischke and Nieschlag 1999). In addition, in view of potential cancerogenic effects, antiestrogens are not suitable for treating idiopathic infertility (Vandekerckhove et al. 1998a).

16.2.6 Kallikrein

There is no clear pathophysiological or pharmacological concept for kallikrein as a treatment regimen in idiopathic male infertility. Nevertheless, it has been applied in andrological practice for 15 years by now. Originally, improvement of sperm motility was claimed after kallikrein application. Data concerning seminal parameters, including sperm motility as well as pregnancy rates are contradictory. We could not demonstrate that kallikrein effected any significant improvement of seminal parameters and pregnancy rates in a controlled, randomized, placebo-controlled, double-blind trial including 91 couples (Keck et al. 1994). Similar negative results were reported in Japan (Yamamoto et al. 1996). The results were in line with a prospective, placebo-controlled, randomized study done in Israel including 114 couples which showed no improvement in seminal parameters (Glezermann et al. 1993).

All properly designed studies lead to the conclusion that kallikrein – given orally at the doses tested – has no benefical effect on male idiopathic infertility (Vandekerckhove 1998b).

16.2.7 Pentoxyphylline

Pentoxyphylline belongs to the family of methylxanthines. One pharmacological effect is the relaxation of vascular smooth muscles. It is therefore prescribed in vasculatory diseases associated with circulatory disturbances (e.g. intermittent claudication). It has been speculated that in men with idiopathic infertility testicular circulation might be disturbed and would be improved by pentoxyphylline (Heite 1979). However, there is neither evidence for circulatory disturbances in idiopathic infertility nor is there proof for any clear therapeutic effects of pentoxyphylline as an infertility regimen (Wang et al. 1983; Shen et al. 1991).

Apart from oral application pentoxyphylline was used as an in-vitro additive in IVF in order to improve fertilization rates. However, an improvement in fertilization rates in asthenozoospermia, after IVF-failure or in the presence of anti-sperm antibodies has not been clearly demonstrated (for review see Tournaye et al. 1995) (see Chap. 17).

16.2.8 α-blocking Agents

Although no clear pathophysiological concept exists for the use of α-blocking agents in the treatment of male infertility, studies have been performed using such substances (e.g. Gulmez et al. 1991; Yamamoto et al. 1995; Gregoriou et al. 1997). The placebo-controlled studies claimed an improvement in ejaculate volume, sperm concentration and total number of motile sperm (Yamamoto et al. 1995; Gregoriou et al. 1997). However, efficacy in terms of improved pregnancy rates has not been demonstrated. In addition, most of the studies revealed only weak statistical evidence for the conclusion drawn. Further controlled clinical studies are necessary before the efficacy of such treatment can be appropriately evaluated.

16.2.9 Antioxidants

In almost all fields of medicine oxidative damage of proteins and nucleic acids is being discussed as a major contributing factor in pathology such as aging, degenerative diseases, cancer and arteriosclerosis. During the past decade the role of oxidative stress and especially the therapeutic use of antioxidative vitamins has been more widely considered for fertility disturbances (e.g. Dawson et al. 1987; Fraga et al. 1991; Ochsendorf 1999). Although oxidative stress could be damaging to reproduction by affecting spermatogenesis, sperm maturation or storage, reactive oxygen species (ROS) in physiological amounts are required for normal sperm function (Aitken and Fisher 1994; Aitken 1995). For instance, an inverse correlation has been shown between fertilization rate in IVF and the ROS scavenging activities of sperm involved (Yeung et al. 1996). On the other hand, as early as 1926 it was demonstrated that ascorbic acid (vitamin C)-deficient diets result in severe damage of the germinal epithelium in guinea pigs (Lindsay and Medes 1926). Placebo-controlled clinical studies have shown improvement of sperm quality when 200–1000 mg ascorbic acid were given to patients with increased sperm agglutination but without anti-sperm antibodies or to heavy smokers (Dawson et al. 1987, 1992). In addition, controlled studies have been performed for other antioxidants. After a two-month course of **glutathione** application, improvement in sperm motility was reported (Lenzi et al. 1993) and **vitamin E** when given orally for 3 months seems to enhance zona pellucida binding of sperm (Kessopoulou et al. 1995).

At least one study found an increased pregnancy rate after vitamin E administration (Suleiman et al. 1996). However, combined vitamin C and E in a randomized placebo-controlled study failed to show a positive effect on sperm parameters or pregnancy rates (Rolf et al.

1999). Even if patient numbers in studies are small so far, the results encourage further investigation of the concept and initiation of additional therapeutic studies.

16.2.10 Further Substances

Several other substances have been used to treat idiopathic male infertility. **Bromocriptine**, successfully used in hyperprolactinemia, was tried without success in infertility. Lacking a clear concept, recombinant growth hormone was tried, but except for increased ejaculate volume (possibly also increased testosterone), was without effect (Carani et al. 1999). When applying this hormone in men with no pituitary disease it must be considered that increased growth hormone may lead to prostate hypertrophy, as observed in acromegalic patients (Colao et al. 1999).

Substances used empirically include interferon-α, mast cell blockers and antihistamines (ketotifen), angiotensin-converting enzyme (ACE) inhibitors (captopril), α-receptor blockers (bunazosin) and zinc salts; no convincing data have been produced to date for the beneficial use of these substances.

16.3 Therapeutic Guidelines

In summary, pharmacological approaches to the therapy of male idiopathic infertility have been highly disappointing. Although a variety of drug regimens has been offered for clinical practise no single regimen mentioned above turned out to have any significant effect on pregnancy rates in controlled clinical studies. This overview emphasizes the importance of well-designed **controlled clinical studies** for the evaluation of therapeutics in andrology (Kamischke and Nieschlag 1999). Until a given therapeutic regimen has proven its benefits in controlled clinical studies, it should not be prescribed for general practise and physicians should be guided by the following principle:

> Any therapy in male infertility is to be considered experimental as long as it has not proven its efficacy in controlled clinical studies. Therapeutic regimens without evidence for their efficacy should only be applied in clinical studies.

This principle demands great **discipline** from the physician who may be urged towards therapeutic intervention by the patient's suffering and expectations. In addition, **consensus** among the medical profession is necessary to prevent untimely use of unproven therapies so

that **spontaneous** pregnancies are not ascribed to these therapies by grateful patients.

At present attention previously given to empirical forms of therapy is waning in the face of clinical success enjoyed by techniques of **assisted fertilization**. Pharmacological approaches to male idiopathic infertility are becoming less important. In particular, **ICSI** is proving to be beneficial in cases of severe oligoasthenozoospermia and even in azoospermia (see Chap. 17). Assisted fertilization is proving anew the adage that intensive therapy of female reproductive functions is the best treatment for male infertility, summarized in the following principle:

> Every therapy for male infertility must be accompanied by optimization of the female reproductive functions. This is especially valid when no effective treatment is available for disturbed male fertility.

Empirical therapies which have remained without success so far must not prevent the search for effective treatments of male infertility. The success of assisted reproduction notwithstanding, most patients would prefer to conceive their children in privacy and not in the laboratory and would prefer a cause-related therapy for their illness. In addition, especially when the costs for assisted reproduction are not assumed by insurers, there is much demand for medication which is reimbursable or at least less costly than assisted reproduction. This pressure must not give rise to hasty prescribing but should motivate researchers to carry out more intensive research.

16.4 References

Aafjes JH, van derVijver JC, Brugman FW, Schenck PE (1983) Double-blind cross over treatment with mesterolone and placebo of subfertile oligozoospermic men: value of testicular biopsy. Andrologia 15:531–535

Abdelmassih R, Dhont M, Comhaire F (1992) Pilot study with 120 mg Andriol treatment for couples with a low fertilization rate during in-vitro fertilization. Hum Reprod 7:267–268

Acosta A, Khalifa E, Oehninger S (1992) Pure human follicle stimulating hormone has a role in the treatment of severe male infertility by assisted reproduction: Norfolk's total experience. Hum Reprod 7:1067–1072

Adamopoulos DA, Nicopoulou S, Kapolla N, Karamertzanis M, Andreou E (1997) The combination of testosterone undecanoate with tamoxifen citrate enhances the effects of each agent given independently on seminal parameters in men with idiopathic oligozoospermia. Fertil Steril 67:756–762

Ainmelk Y, Belisle S, Carmel M, JP Tetrault (1987) Tamoxifen citrate therapy in male infertility. Fertil Steril 48:113–127

Aitken RJ (1995) Free radicals, lipid peroxidation and sperm function. Reprod Fertil Dev 7:659–668

Aitken RJ, Fisher H (1994) Reactive oxygen species generation and human spermatozoa: the balance of benefit and risk. BioEssays 16:259–267

Bals-Pratsch M, Knuth UA, Hönigl W, Klein HM, Bergmann M, Nieschlag E (1989) Pulsatile GnRH-therapy in oligozoospermic men does not improve seminal parameters despite decreased FSH levels. Clin Endocrinol 30:549–560

Bartoov B, Har-Even D, Eltes F, Lederman H, Lunenfeld E, Lunenfeld B (1994) Sperm quality of subfertile males before and after treatment with human follicle-stimulating hormone. Fertil Steril 61:727–734

Breznik R, Borko E (1993) Effectiveness of antiestrogens in infertile men. Arch Androl 31:43–48

Carani C, Granata AR, De Rosa M, Garau C, Zarrilli S, Paesano L, Colao A, Marrama P, Lombardi G (1999) The effect of chronic treatment with GH on gonadal function in men with isolated GH deficiency. Eur J Endocrinol 140:224–230

Clark R, Sherins RJ (1989) Treatment of men with idiopathic oligozoospermic infertility using the aromatase inhibitor testolactone. Results of a double-blinded, randomized, placebo-controlled trial with crossover. J Androl 10:240–347

Colao A, Marzullo P, Piezia S, Ferone D, Giaccio A, Cerbone G, Pivonello R, Di Somma C, Lombardi G (1999) Effect of growth hormone (GH) and insulin-like growth factor I on prostate diseases: an ultrasonographic and endocrine study in acromegaly, GH deficiency, and healthy subjects. J Clin Endocrinol Metab 84:1986–1991

Comhaire FH (1990) Treatment of idiopathic testicular failure with high-dose testosterone undecanoate: a double blind pilot study. Fertil Steril 54:689–693

Comhaire F, Schoonjans F, Abdelmassih R, Gordts S, Campo R, Dhont M, Milingos S, Gerris J (1995) Does treatment with testosterone undecanoate improve the in-vitro fertilizing capacity of spermatozoa in patients with idiopathic testicular failure (results of a double-blind study)? Hum Reprod 10:2600–2602

Comodo F, Vargiu N, Farina M (1996) Double-blind FSH-HP/Placebo treatment of severe male factor related infertility: effect on sperm parameters and IVF/ICSI outcome. ESHRE abstract book S41

Dawson EB, Harris WA, Rankin WE, Charpentier LA, McGanity WJ (1987) Effect of ascorbic acid on male fertility. Ann NY Acad Sci 498:312–323

Dawson EB, Harris WA, Teter MC, Powell LC (1992) Effect of ascorbic acid supplementation on the sperm quality of smokers. Fertil Steril 58:1034–1039

Fraga CG, Motchnik PA, Shigenaga MK, Helbock HJ, Jacob RA, Ames BN (1991) Ascorbic acid protects against endogenous oxidative DNA damage in human sperm. Proc Natl Acad Sci USA 88:11003–11006

Gerris J, Comhaire F, Hellemans P, Peeters K, Schoonjans F (1991) Placebo controlled trial of high dose Mesterolone treatment of male infertility. Fertil Steril 55:603–607

Glezermann M, Huleihel M, Lunenfeld E, Soffer Y, Potashnik G, Segal S (1993) Efficacy of kallikrein in the treatment of oligozoospermia and asthenozoospermia: a double-blind trial. Fertil Steril 60:1052–1056

Gregoriou O, Papadias C, Gargaropoulos A, Konidaris S, Kontogeorgi Z, Kalampokas E (1993) Treatment of idiopathic infertility with testosterone undecanoate. A double blind study. Clin Exp Obstet Gynecol 20:9–12

Gregoriou O, Vitoratos N, Papadias C, Gargaropoulos A, Konidaris S, Giannopoulos V, Chryssicopoulos A (1997) Treatment of idiopathic oligozoospermia with an alpha-blocker: a pla-cebo-controlled double-blind trial. Int J Fertil Womens Med 42:301–305

Gulmez I, Tatlisen A, Karacagil M, Kesekci S (1991) Seminal parameters of ejaculates collected successively with sixty minute interval in infertile men: effect of combination of prazosin and terbutaline on these parameters. Andrologia 23:167–169

Hansson V, Levy FO, Taskén K (eds) (1996) Signal transduction in testicular cells. Springer, Berlin Heidelberg New York (Ernst Schering Research Foundation Workshop, Suppl 2)

Heite HG (1979) The effect of Trental on spermiographic parameters, a clinical study in patients with reduced fertility. Fertil Steril 20 [Suppl 1]:38–42

Kamischke A, Nieschlag E (1999) Analysis of medical treatment of male infertility. Hum Reprod 14 [Suppl 1]:1–23

Kamischke A, Behre HM, Bergmann M, Simoni M, Schäfer T, Nieschlag E (1998) Recombinant human follicle-stimulating hormone for treatment of male idiopathic infertility: a randomized, double-blind, placebo-controlled, clinical trial. Hum Reprod 13:596–603

Keck C, Behre HM, Jockenhövel F, Nieschlag E (1994) Ineffectiveness of kallikrein in treatment of idiopathic male infertility: a double-blind, randomized, placebo-controlled trial. Hum Reprod 9:325–329

Kessopoulou E, Russel JM, Powers HJ, Cooke ID, Sharma KK, Barratt CLR, Pearson MJ (1995) A double-blind randomized placebo cross-over controlled trial using the antioxidant vitamin E to treat reactive oxygen species associated male infertility. Fertil Steril 64:825–831

Knuth UA, Hönigl W, Bals-Pratsch M, Schleicher G, Nieschlag E (1987) Treatment of severe ologozoospermia with hCG/hMG. A placebo-controlled double-blind trial. J Clin Endocrinol Metab 65:1081–1087

Kotulas IG, Cardamakis E, Michopoulos J, Mitropoulos D, Dounis A (1994) Tamoxifen treatment in male infertility. Effect on spermatozoa. Fertil Steril 61:911–914

Krause W, Holland-Moritz H, Schramm P (1992) Treatment of idiopathic oligozoospermia with tamoxifen. A randomized controlled study. Int J Androl 15:14–18

Lenzi A, Culasso F, Gandini L, Lombardo F, Dondero F (1993) Placebo-controlled, double-blind, cross-over trial of glutathione therapy in male infertility. Hum Reprod 8:1657–1662

Lindsay B, Medes G (1926) Histological changes in the testis of the guinea-pig during scurvy and inanition. Am J Anat 37:213–230

Maier U, Hiernert G (1988) Tamoxifen and kallikrein in therapy of oligoasthenozoospermia. Results of a randomized study. Eur Urol 14:447–449

Maier U, Hiernert G (1990) Tamoxifen and kallikrein in therapy of oligoasthenozoospermia. Results of a randomized study. Eur Urol 17:223–225

Matorras R, Perez C, Corcostegui B, Pijoan JI, Ramon O, Delgado P, Rodriguez-Escudero FJ (1997) Treatment of the male with follicle-stimulating hormone in intrauterine insemination with husband's spermatozoa: a randomized study. Hum Reprod 12:24–28

Mauss J (1974) Ergebnisse der Behandlung von Fertilitätsstörungen des Mannes mit Mesterolon oder einem Placebo. Arzneimittelforschung 24:1338–1341

Nieschlag E (1994) Clinical relevance and irrelevance of molecular and cellular research on the testis. In: Verhoeven G, Habenicht UF (eds) Molecular and cellular endocrinology of the testis. Springer, Berlin Heidelberg New York, pp 273–292

Ochsendorf FR (1999) Infections in the male genital tract and reactive oxygen species. Hum Reprod Update 5:399–420

Pusch H (1989) Oral treatment of oligozoospermia with testosterone-undecanoate: results of a double blind study. Arch Androl 2:479–486

Reyes-Fuentes A, Chavarria ME, Carrera A, Aguilera G, Rosado A, Samojlik E, Iranmanesh A, Veldhuis JD (1996) Alterations in pulsatile luteinizing hormone and follicle-stimulating hormone secretion in idiopathic oligoasthenospermic men: assessment by deconvolution analysis – a clinical research center study. J Clin Endocrinol Metab 81:524–529

Rolf C, Behre HM, Nieschlag E (1996) Tamoxifen bei männlicher Infertilität. Analyse einer fragwürdigen Therapie. Dtsch Med Wochenschr 121:33–39

Rolf C, Cooper TG, Yeung CH, Nieschlag E (1999) Antioxidant treatment of patients with asthenozoospermia or moderate oligoasthenozoospermia with high-dose vitamin C and vitamin E: a randomized, placebo-controlled, double-blind study. Hum Reprod 14:1028–1033

Schill W-B (1986) Medical treatment of male infertility. In: Insler V, Lunenfeld B (eds) Infertility: male and female. Churchill Livingstone, Edinburgh, pp 533–573

Scottish Infertility Group (SIG) (1984) Randomized trial of mesterolone versus vitamin C for male infertility. Br J Urol 56:740–744

Shen M-R, Chiang P-H, Yang R-C, Hong C-Y, Chen S-S (1991) Pentoxifylline stimulates human sperm motility both in vitro and after oral therapy. Br J Clin Pharmacol 31:711–714

Stefanini M, Boitani C, Galdieri M, Geremia R, Palombi F (eds) (1998) Testicular function: from gene expression to genetic manipulation. Springer, Berlin Heidelberg New York (Ernst Schering Research Foundation Workshop, Suppl 3)

Suleiman SA, ElaminAli M, Zaki ZMS et al (1996) Lipid peroxidation and human sperm motility: protective role of vitamin E. J Androl 17:530–537

Török L (1985) Treatment of oligozoospermia with tamoxifen (open and controlled studies). Andrologia 17:497–501

Tournaye H, Devroey P, Camus M, Van der Linden M, Janssens R, Van Steirteghem A (1995) Use of pentoxifylline in assisted reproductive technology. Hum Reprod 10 [Suppl 1]:72–79

Vandekerckhove P, Lilford R, Hughes E (1998a) The medical treatment of idiopathic oligo/asthenospermia: anti-oestrogens (clomiphene or tamoxifen) versus placebo or no treatment. In: Lilford R, Hughes E, Vandekerckhove P (eds) Subfertility module of the Cochrane database of systematic reviews. Cochrane Library. The Cochrane Collaboration, Issue 2. Update Software, Oxford

Vandekerckhove P, Lilford R, Hughes E (1998b) Kinin enhancing drugs for male infertility. In: Lilford R, Hughes E, Vandekerckhove P (eds) Subfertility module of the Cochrane database of systematic reviews. Cochrane Library. The Cochrane Collaboration, Issue 2. Update Software, Oxford

Wagner ROF, Warsch F (1984) Pulsatile LHRH therapy of "slow pulsing oligospermia": indirect evidence for a hypothalamic origin of the disorder. Acta Endocrinol (Copenh) 105 [Suppl 264]:142–145

Wang C, Chan CW, Wong KK, Yeung KK (1983) Comparison of the effectiveness of placebo, clomiphene citrate, mesterolone, pentoxyfylline and testosterone rebound therapy for the treatment of idiopathic oligospermia. Fertil Steril 40:358–365

Willis KJ, London DR, Bevis MA, Butt WR, Lynch SS, Holder G (1977) Hormonal effects of tamoxifen in oligospermic men. J Endocrinol 73:171–178

WHO Task Force on the Diagnosis and Treatment of Infertility (1989) Mesterolone and idiopathic male infertility: a double-blind study. Int J Androl 12:254–264

WHO Task Force on the Prevention and Management of Infertility (1992) A double-blind trial of clomiphene citrate for the treatment of idiopathic male infertility. Int J Androl 15:299–307

Yamamoto M, Hibi H, Mijake K (1995) Comparison of the effectiveness of placebo and α-blocker therapy for treatment of idiopathic oligozoospermia. Fertil Steril 63:396–340

Yamamoto M, Katsuno S, Hibi H, Miyake K (1996) The lack of effectiveness of kallikrein in the treatment of idiopathic oligozoospermia: a double-blind, randomized, placebo-controlled study. Jpn J Fertil Steril 41:1–6

Yeung CH, De Geyter C, De Geyter M, Nieschlag E (1996) Production of reactive oxygen species by and hydrogen peroxide scavenging activity of spermatoza in an IVF program. J Assist Reprod Genet 13:495–500

CHAPTER 17

Assisted Fertilization

C. De Geyter · M. De Geyter · D. Meschede · H. M. Behre

17.1 Assisted Fertilization as a Treatment of Infertility

Even the most intensive diagnostic protocol cannot identify all factors contributing to infertility. Only in a few instances can treatment which eliminates all factors causing infertility be carried out. Such treatment would be, however, preferable, because it is effective in the long range. Examples of such causal treatment of infertility are the use of dopaminergic drugs in hyperprolactinemia, the pulsatile administration of GnRH in hypogonadotropic hypogonadism and, not least, the microsurgical reconstruction of the Fallopian tubes or the efferent seminal ducts.

Neither in gynecology nor in andrology can the causes of infertility be treated adequately in a majority of patients, so that instead a number of **treatment strategies** have been developed to deal with childlessness exclusively as a **symptom**, without removing the cause of infertility itself. Most of these strategies can be summarized by the term "**assisted fertilization**". The major disadvantage of any form of assisted fertilization is its short-term efficacy, because the therapeutic effect of assisted fertilization is active only during the treatment cycle itself. If this treatment cycle proves to be unsuccessful or if infertility recurs after delivery of a healthy baby, the entire treatment must be repeated.

Notwithstanding this major disadvantage, today the majority of infertile couples can be treated with one of the many techniques of assisted fertilization currently available. The tremendous development of assisted fertilization in recent years can be best illustrated by the introduction of **intracytoplasmic sperm injection** (**ICSI**) for the treatment of couples suffering from **male infertility**. Nowadays, nearly all cases of male infertility can be potentially treated by some method of assisted fertilization.

17.2 Methods of Assisted Fertilization

Assisted fertilization comprises various treatment modalities, which can be differentiated by more or less stringent control over the processes of fertilization and by the degree of invasiveness. For the purpose of this chapter the various forms of assisted fertilization are subdivided into three major groups:

- **Insemination** denotes a group of techniques in which the sperm are transferred into the female partner by various methods. Insemination aims at increasing the concentration of fertile spermatozoa in the vicinity of the oocyte within the Fallopian tube around the time of ovulation.
- **In vitro fertilization** (IVF) fertilization does not take place in the Fallopian tube of the female partner. Before ovulation the oocyte is removed from the mature follicle and cultured in an artificial environment in which fertilization and early embryonic development can take place. The probability of IVF can be influenced not only by the addition of higher numbers of motile spermatozoa to the oocytes, but also by the selection of mature oocytes. Thereafter, this treatment permits visual registration of successful fertilization and normal embryonic development, thereby enabling the physician to assess, to some degree, the fertility status and the prognosis of the individual couple.
- In **intracytoplasmic sperm injection** (ICSI) a single vital spermatozoon is placed into the oocyte by penetrating it, through all its investments, with a micropipette. ICSI enables successful fertilizations not only despite severe abnormalities in motility, morphology and capacitation process of the injected spermatozoa, but also despite functional and anatomical anomalies of the testes, the epididymis and the efferent ducts.

17.3 Insemination

17.3.1 Spontaneous Conception Rate in the Infertile Couple

Any treatment of infertility is effective only if its pregnancy rate exceeds the conception rate in the untreated infertile couple. The **spontaneous conception** rate is determined by various factors, the most important being the duration of infertility (Léridon and Spira 1984). It is during the first three ovulatory cycles after inception of unprotected sexual intercourse that the highest conception rates per cycle are observed: 20–25 % (Spira 1986; Hull 1992). In subsequent cycles the rate of naturally occurring pregnancies steadily decreases, so that after

twelve months the pregnancy rate may vary between 0.75 and 3.97 % per cycle (Crosignani et al. 1991).

Nevertheless, because any infertility treatment may be protracted owing to the necessity of repeated treatment trials of assisted fertilization, spontaneously occurring pregnancies are not uncommon. In our own patient population 141 patients under treatment with assisted fertilization were observed over a period of 24 months and the cumulative spontaneous conception rate was 12.1 %. Therefore, in order to assess the real therapeutic efficacy of the various methods of assisted fertilization, the success rates should be compared with the cumulative spontaneous conception rate during the same time interval (Glass and Ericsson 1979; Collins et al. 1983).

Prognostically favorable findings in the patient's history are previous intact pregnancies with the same partner, the age of the female partner and the duration of infertility (Collins et al. 1995). Conversely, endometriosis, tubal factors and male infertility all are prognostically unfavorable for future childbearing (Collins et al. 1995). Although the parameters of **conventional semen analysis** bear hardly any relationship to the physiology of sperm capacitation and fertilization, they are correlated with male fertility. The probability of spontaneous conception is severely reduced in the presence of reduced ejaculate volume, a low percentage of normal sperm morphology, reduced concentration of sperm in the seminal plasma and in the presence of high numbers of immotile spermatozoa (Bonde et al. 1998). Another factor determining the degree of infertility and the efficacy of assisted fertilization is the combination of multiple infertility factors in both partners. For example, the therapeutic efficacy of heterologous insemination in male infertility is higher in male patients suffering from azoospermia than in patients with only abnormal semen quality (Emperaire et al. 1982). This difference can only be explained by differences in the **fertility status of the female partner**.

17.3.2 Intravaginal and Intracervical Insemination (ICI)

This form of assisted fertilization represents the earliest method of insemination. With these techniques some anatomical barriers in the vagina and in the cervix of the female partner (cervical infertility) and disturbances of sperm deposition in the male partner (hypospadias, retrograde ejaculation, impotentia coeundi) can be overcome (Allen et al. 1985).

During intravaginal or **intracervical insemination** 1–2 ml of freshly collected or cryopreserved and thawed semen is deposited in the vagina or in the cervical canal by the use of a catheter connected to a syringe (Fig. 17.1). Besides the liquefaction of the semen, which occurs spontaneously after thirty minutes of incubation at

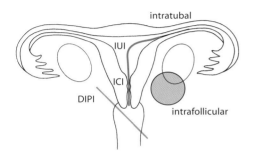

Fig. 17.1. Graphic presentation of the different techniques of insemination: intracervical (*ICI*), intrauterine (*IUI*), intratubal, direct intraperitoneal (*DIPI*), intrafollicular

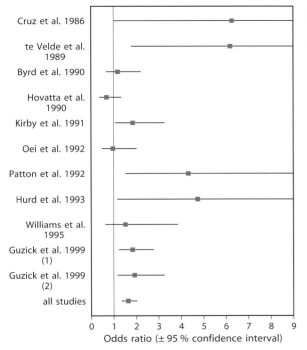

Fig. 17.2. The odds ratio (and the 95% confidence interval, calculated on the chi-squared test according to Pearson, Mantel and Haenszel) of successful IUI compared with other techniques of insemination in several prospective studies. In most studies IUI was more successful in achieving pregnancies (odds ratio >1) than other methods. This is especially so when the results of all studies are combined. (*1*) ovulation induction with gonadotropins, (*2*) insemination in the untreated menstrual cycle

room temperature, no particular manipulation or preparation of the semen is necessary, so that this treatment does not require any laboratory equipment. Special care should be taken not to introduce any semen into the uterine cavity, because the prostaglandins contained in the seminal plasma may cause painful contractions of the myometrium. To prevent contact of the semen with the vaginal milieu, which owing to its acidity is hostile to sperm, the semen sample can be separated from the vagina with a cap fitted on the portio of the cervix immediately after the cervical insemination. After about six hours this cap can be removed by the patient herself.

In recent years intravaginal and intracervical inseminations have been replaced largely by intrauterine insemination (IUI) because of the higher efficacy of the latter. In several controlled studies, the therapeutic efficacy of IUI was compared with intracervical and intravaginal insemination and the former was found to be significantly superior in most studies (Cruz et al. 1986; Byrd et al. 1990; Patton et al. 1990; Hurd et al. 1993; Williams et al. 1995; Fig. 17.2). With intrauterine insemination higher sperm numbers can be brought into the uterine cavity and into the Fallopian tubes (Ripps et al. 1994). It has been claimed that in intracervical insemination the reservoir function of the cervix ensures a longer-lasting availability of living spermatozoa than in intrauterine insemination, but after intrauterine insemination an intense retrograde migration of sperm into the cervix was also observed, refuting this argument (Ripps et al. 1994).

17.3.3 Intrauterine Insemination (IUI)

In intrauterine insemination 0.2 to 0.5 ml of a washed sperm sample is introduced with a fine catheter connected to a syringe into the uterine cavity of a periovulatory patient. The aim of this technique is to achieve a higher concentration of motile spermatozoa within the lumen of the Fallopian tube in order to increase the probability of fertilization. One particular modification of intrauterine insemination involves the **perfusion** of a larger volume of a prepared sperm sample (4 ml) over a period of 4 minutes into the uterine cavity, to ensure the attachment of a larger number of spermatozoa to the mucosa of the Fallopian tube (Kahn et al. 1993a). Another method to increase further the number of motile spermatozoa in the uterine cavity and in the Fallopian tubes in order to improve the pregnancy rate consists of repeating IUI on two subsequent days (12 and 34 hours after ovulation induction: Ragni et al. 1999) or before and after ovulation (Silverberg et al. 1992).

In recent years the therapeutic efficacy of intrauterine insemination has been drastically improved by adopting techniques which were originally conceived for IVF. Mainly the development of new methods of sperm preparation and improvements in the monitoring and stimulation of follicular development have upgraded IUI.

In several studies the therapeutic efficacy of IUI was compared with the success rate of other forms of assisted fertilization, mainly with IVF, and with the spontaneous conception rate. The cumulative pregnancy rate of IUI is significantly better than the spontaneous conception rate in some patients suffering from male infertility (te Velde et al. 1989; Kirby et al. 1991; Guzick et al. 1999).

The efficacy of IUI appears ineffective in male immunological infertility (Francavilla et al. 1992). In patients with sperm concentration below 1×10^6/ml after preparation the prognosis of IUI is unfavorable. In comparison with more invasive and more costly treatments, such as in IVF, the pregnancy rate of one single treatment trial with IUI is worse (Mills et al. 1992; Goverde et al. 2000), but the cumulative pregnancy rate of up to four treatment trials with IUI is comparable (Peterson et al. 1994). In couples suffering from male and unexplained infertility, the efficacy of six consecutive treatments with IUI is comparable to the efficacy of a single treatment of IVF, involving, however, lower financial costs (Goverde et al. 2000) Therefore, it is important to explain to the patients that IUI must not be considered as one single treatment, but rather as a series of successive trials.

IUI is performed easily, requires minimal equipment and and remains practically **without complications**. Infections after IUI, such as endometritis or pelvic inflammatory disease, are observed extremely rarely. In 5–17 % of the cases IUI may cause some minor discomfort in the lower abdomen (Allen et al. 1985), but this may also be caused by ovulation. The induction of antisperm antibodies was detected in 4–10 % of patients treated with IUI (Horvath et al. 1989b; Moretti-Rojas et al. 1990; Friedman et al. 1991; Kahn et al. 1993b). Considering the similar prevalence of antisperm antibodies in untreated infertile patients (Horvath et al. 1989b), the possibility of such an immunological reaction after IUI appears to be clinically insignificant.

17.3.4 Intratubal Insemination (ITI)

In several animal species it was shown that, in addition to the cervix, a second sperm reservoir exists in the isthmic part of the Fallopian tube (see also Chap. 4). Based on these findings, the technique of **intratubal insemination** was invented to transfer washed spermatozoa beyond the isthmic portion of the Fallopian tube in order to achieve a higher sperm concentration within the ampulla, where fertilization normally occurs (Jansen and Anderson 1987). However, controlled studies demonstrated that with intratubal insemination the pregnancy rate is no better than with IUI (Oei et al. 1992; Hurd et al. 1993).

17.3.5 Direct Intraperitoneal Insemination (DIPI)

In **direct intraperitoneal insemination** the posterior vaginal pouch is punctured with a needle connected to a syringe containing the prepared sperm suspension, and 0.2–2 ml of this is injected into the peritoneal cavity (Forrler et al. 1986). The spermatozoa can be transported into the lumen of the Fallopian tube by the ciliary movement of the mucosal cells covering the abdominal infundibulum of the oviduct. By DIPI, not only the cervix but also the isthmic part of the Fallopian tube is circumvented, as both are considered to be obstacles for defective spermatozoa.

This method can be applied only to patients with intact Fallopian tubes and was first used predominantly in couples suffering from unexplained and cervical infertility, later also in male infertility. This form of insemination has been considered as an alternative approach to GIFT (gamete intrafallopian transfer) which is technically much costlier and more invasive (Asch et al. 1984). Using controlled randomized settings, the pregnancy rate of direct intraperitoneal insemination was not better than the pregnancy rate of timed natural intercourse (Campos-Liete et al. 1992) or of IUI (Hovatta et al. 1990). This technique may still be used in women with a severe cervical stenosis which cannot be passed without damage to the endometrium. No induction of antisperm antibodies could be demonstrated as a consequence of this method of insemination.

17.3.6 Intrafollicular Insemination

In **intrafollicular insemination** several mature cumulus-oocyte complexes are recovered by transvaginal ultrasound-guided puncture of all but one preovulatory ovarian follicle. After selection of the most mature cumulus-oocyte complexes, these are mixed with 0.03–0.5 ml of the previously prepared sperm suspension and are then inserted during the same transvaginal ultrasound-guided puncture into one mature ovarian follicle. The rationale of **intrafollicular insemination** is based on the hypothesis that in direct intraperitoneal insemination or in gamete intrafallopian transfer the sperm suspension becomes diluted rapidly, so that the actual number of fertile spermatozoa in the vicinity of the oocyte is low. Within the boundaries of a mature ovarian follicle, the inseminated spermatozoa have sufficient time to bind firmly to the zona pellucida of the inserted oocytes before the rupture of the follicle releases the oocytes into the Fallopian tube (Lucena et al. 1991; Zbella et al. 1992). Furthermore, as in IVF, multiple cumulus-oocyte complexes can be selected according to morphological criteria (Werner-von der Burg et al. 1993). This method was further supported by the finding of some factors present in follicular fluid (e. g. progesterone) which may physiologically stimulate both capacitation and the acrosome reaction of spermatozoa.

In a prospective cohort study involving 50 couples only one pregnancy could be achieved (Nuojua-Huttonen et al. 1995), so this technique does not seem to be of any benefit compared to other forms of insemination.

17.4 In Vitro Fertilization and Related Techniques

17.4.1 In Vitro Fertilization (IVF)

The basic characteristic of IVF, distinguishing it from other procedures of assisted fertilization, is that the physiological process of fertilization takes place **outside the body** of the patient in an artificially constructed environment. For this purpose, one or more oocytes are recovered from preovulatory ovarian follicles and subsequently coincubated in a defined culture medium together with motile spermatozoa previously separated from the seminal plasma, immotile spermatozoa and non-spermatozoal cells. After identification of successful fertilization, either at the pronuclear stage, at an early cleavage stage or at the later blastocyst stage, the embryos are placed in the uterine cavity for nidation in the endometrium and pregnancy.

IVF was originally introduced for the treatment of tubal infertility caused either by occlusion of the Fallopian tubes or by impairment of their function (Edwards 1981). However, soon after its successful introduction, its potential value for the treatment of male infertility became an issue of intensive debate. In IVF motile sperm are added to one or more extra-corporal egg cells in culture medium. Extra-corporal fertilization allows early visualization of the result of the fertilization process and selection of those oocytes which are fertilized.

In contrast to all existing forms of artificial insemination, IVF offers the possibility of **inseminating the oocytes with a predetermined and constant number of motile sperm**, permitting the interaction of oocytes with supraphysiogical numbers of motile spermatozoa during a relative long period of undiluted coincubation (Oehninger et al. 1988). In those patients in whom only few spermatozoa are available, the oocyte and the sperm are coincubated in a small volume to improve their interaction (Van der Ven et al. 1987). As a result of the hormonal stimulation of the ovaries, causing more follicles to mature, more oocytes can be inseminated and possibly fertilized; this procedure aims to improve the pregnancy rate despite the low overall fertilization rate in couples suffering from male infertility (Ramsewak et al. 1990). However, more recent studies have disproved the potential advantages of IVF in the treatment of male infertility. First, the prolonged coincubation of sperm and oocytes is associated with a significantly reduced pregnancy rate compared with a coincubation time of 4–5 hours (Dirnfeld et al. 1999). The presence of an excessive concentration of spermatozoa around the oocyte for conventional IVF is also associated with reduced pregnancy rates compared with ICSI (Kastrop et al. 1999; Benoff et al. 1999). In addition, the enzymatic removal of the cumulus oophorus does not improve the fertilization rate in cases with abnormal sperm quality (Mahadevan and Trounson 1985).

Although IVF can be performed with some success with naturally matured oocytes, it has become widespread practice to carry out this treatment in combination with **hormonal stimulation of the ovaries**, so that **multiple oocytes** become available for IVF. The improved pregnancy rate of IVF in hormonally stimulated cycles results mainly from the replacement of several fertilized oocytes. Ovarian stimulation also provides a better assessment of the events controlling follicular maturation, in turn leading to the collection of more mature oocytes with high developmental capacity. Furthermore, ovarian stimulation compensates for clinical and subclinical defects in the follicular development of some patients. The risk of multiple pregnancies, which became increasingly evident in demographic studies during the late eighties and nineties represents the major disadvantage of replacing more than one embryo. Currently, there is an increased trend to replace fewer embryos per cycle (Bergh et al. 1999). The general improvement in ovarian stimulation protocols and culture conditions, the possibility of embryo selection in some countries (Staessen et al. 1993; Roest et al. 1997) and the development of blastocyst culture (Milki et al. 1999) have enabled many treatment centers to replace only two embryos per cycle without lowering pregnancy rates. Recently, it was demonstrated that multiple pregnancies can be avoided almost completely by the replacement of only one embryo per cycle without reduction of the overall pregnancy rate (Vilska et al. 1999; Gerris et al. 1999). However, the success of these studies depended on the selection of those embryos with the highest developmental capacity and on cryopreservation of the others. The legal and ethical discussion concerning the possibility of surplus embryos has not been solved yet.

The results of conventional IVF in couples suffering from idiopathic male infertility have been disappointing.

In couples treated only because of male infertility the success rates of IVF were the lowest of all (Tournaye et al. 1992a; Tan et al. 1992a). The results of IVF in male infertile patients did not appear to be better than the **spontaneous conception rate** during a six-month waiting period (Soliman et al. 1993). Nowadays, intracytoplasmic sperm injection has replaced conventional IVF in the treatment of couples suffering from idiopathic male infertility.

Conventional IVF has not only been used in male idiopathic infertility, but also in more defined forms of male infertility. Conventional IVF was performed in patients suffering from ejaculatory disturbances caused by neuropathy in diabetes mellitus or by neural tube defects. In some patients suffering from retrograde ejaculation or in patients with occlusion of the vas deferens, motile spermatozoa were recovered surgically from the vas deferens or from the epididymis (**MESA, microsurgical epididymal sperm aspiration,** Temple-Smith et al. 1985). Motile spermatozoa were also aspirated from the testis for IVF and fertilizations, but no pregnancies were achieved (**TESE, testicular sperm extraction,** Hirsh et al. 1993a).

In general, very low pregnancy rates resulted from conventional IVF with spermatozoa collected from the epididymis (11.1%: Bladou et al. 1991; 8.9%: Hirsh et al. 1994). More potentially fertilizing spermatozoa were collected from the proximal portion of the epididymis or from the efferent ducts than from the more distal portion, which is apparently in contradiction to established common knowledge about the physiology of the unobstructed epididymis (see Chap. 4, Silber et al. 1988). Several pregnancies have also been reported after conventional IVF using cryopreserved and thawed spermatozoa in azoospermic patients previously treated with chemo- or radiotherapy because of malignant tumors (Davis et al. 1990; Tournaye et al. 1991; Khalifa et al. 1992) (see Chap. 18). Since the rapid development of **intracytoplasmic sperm injection (ICSI),** conventional IVF has become obsolete in these particular forms of male infertility.

Whereas the decision to perform ICSI rather than IVF is obvious in many situations, the choice may become difficult in many borderline cases. In couples with normozoospermic semen but suffering from tubal infertility, the fertilization rates obtained with IVF were similar to those observed after ICSI (Aboulghar et al. 1996; Staessen et al. 1999). However, the frequency of complete fertilization of all oocytes was much higher after ICSI (e.g. 12.5%) than after IVF (3.6%, Staessen et al. 1999). The dilemma of performing conventional IVF or, alternatively, ICSI, still largely relies on **conventional semen analysis.** The **predictive accuracy** of conventional semen analysis for the results of IVF was determined prospectively and reached 77% for the prediction of an inadequate fertilization rate and 95% for the prediction of a sufficient fertilization rate (Duncan et al. 1993). Obviously, successful fertilization in IVF can be predicted on one basis of conventional semen analysis, but not the lack of fertilization. Using **computer-assisted sperm motion analysis (CASA)** and based on the sperm mo-

tion parameter "**curvilinear velocity**" (VCL), patients with high fertilization and pregnancy rates in IVF could be well identified prospectively. Although men with sperm swimming at low curvilinear velocity achieved significantly lower pregnancy rates in their partners, the total absence of fertilization could not be predicted with CASA (De Geyter et al. 1998). At present, none of the available sperm function tests can reliably predict the absence of fertilizing ability.

17.4.2 Gamete Intra-Fallopian Transfer (GIFT)

In contrast to the biologically inert culture medium used for IVF, the tubal environment may be better suited for supporting the processes of sperm capacitation, fertilization and early embryonic development. Therefore, the technique of **intra-Fallopian transfer of gametes** was developed as an alternative to both IVF and IUI (Asch et al. 1984, Fig. 17.3).

In GIFT, ovarian stimulation is performed using protocols similar to IVF, but mature oocytes are collected by laparoscopy only. Based on the morphological assessment of the cumulus oophorus and the corona radiata or, if possible, by the visualization of the first polar body, two to four mature oocytes are selected and incubated for a short time under cultured conditions. During the same laparoscopy, these selected cumulus-oocyte complexes are brought together with the previously prepared sperm suspension and are then inserted by a catheter through the abdominal **infundibulum** into the ampulla of one intact Fallopian tube, where fertilization can take place.

The major advantage of GIFT, compared with IVF, is that fertilization can take place within the tubal environment, which is thought to support this process better. The shorter incubation time of the oocytes and the simpler handling of the gametes require less laboratory

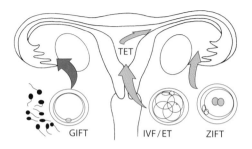

Fig. 17.3. Graphic presentation of the different methods of replacement of gametes or embryos: in vitro fertilization (IVF) and replacement of the embryos into the uterine cavity, gamete intra-Fallopian transfer (*GIFT*), zygote intra-Fallopian transfer (*ZIFT*), tubal embryo transfer (*TET*)

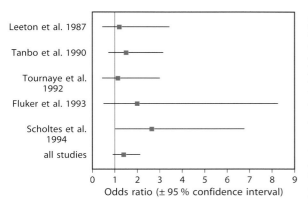

Fig. 17.4. The odds ratio (and the 95% confidence interval, based on the chi-squared test according to Pearson, Mantel and Haenszel) of IVF compared with GIFT, ZIFT and TET was calculated using the data from several prospective studies. In most studies the pregnancy rate of IVF was superior to those of other treatment modalities (odds ratio >1), especially when the data of all studies are compiled

equipment and expertise, making GIFT a cheaper alternative to IVF. In comparison with IUI, GIFT allows a more intensive ovarian stimulation and the selection of mature cumulus-oocyte complexes without the uncontrolled risk of high-grade multiple pregnancies.

Originally, GIFT was developed for the treatment of couples suffering from **unexplained infertility**, but soon it was used in **male infertility** too. However, in prospective-controlled studies, GIFT did not prove to be more successful than conventional IVF in the treatment of unexplained and male infertility (Leeton et al. 1987; Tanbo et al. 1990; Fig. 17.4). A decisive disadvantage of GIFT is the lack of information about the occurrence of fertilization in the couples in whom GIFT did not lead to pregnancies. Nowadays, this technique has been largely abandoned and replaced by IVF and ICSI.

17.4.3 Intra-Fallopian Transfer of Zygotes (ZIFT) or Pronucleate-Stage Oocyte Transfer (PROST)

In order to combine the advantage of GIFT, permitting early embryonic development within the physiological environment of the Fallopian tube, with the advantage of IVF, in which information about the fertilization process is acquired, **intra-Fallopian transfer of zygotes (ZIFT)** was developed (Devroey et al. 1986). Simultaneously, and based on the same reasoning as for ZIFT, an analogous method, the transfer of **pronucleate-stage oocytes** into the Fallopian tube (PROST), was introduced into assisted fertilization (Yovich et al. 1987). In both methods two operations have to be performed on the same patient in two consecutive days. Oocytes are collected by ultra-

sound-guided vaginal puncture of the preovulatory follicles after ovarian stimulation and are then coincubated overnight with motile spermatozoa. The next morning pronuclei are identified as a sign of successful sperm penetration. Two to three oocytes in the pronucleate stage or zygotes may then be replaced during laparoscopy through the abdominal infundibulum into the lumen of the Fallopian tube.

Both ZIFT and PROST were developed for couples suffering from unexplained and male infertility (Palermo et al. 1989b). Although very high pregnancy rates were achieved, the therapeutic advantage of these complex treatments, compared with conventional IVF, could not be proven in prospective randomized studies (Fig. 17.4; Tanbo et al. 1990; Tournaye et al. 1992b; Fluker et al. 1993). The main disadvantage of both treatments is the high financial cost and the physical burden for the patient, because two invasive operations are performed on subsequent days. Both techniques have now been largely abandoned.

17.4.4 Tubal Embryo Transfer (TET)

Transvaginal/transuterine transfer of embryos into the Fallopian tube was introduced to reduce the physical burden of the patient caused by ZIFT (Diedrich et al. 1991). Using specially designed flexible catheters, the isthmo-ampullar lumen of the oviduct can be reached via the vagina and the uterine cavity (Jansen and Anderson 1987), avoiding both laparoscopy and general anesthesia. This type of catheterization can be performed as an outpatient procedure in most patients without any need of narcotics or analgesia. However, in a prospective randomized study, this treatment did not result in significantly better pregnancy rates than conventional IVF (Scholtes et al. 1994). The pregnancy rate may be occasionally compromised by the damage of the endometrium caused by difficult catheterization in some patients. This technique has now been abandoned.

17.5 Micro-assisted Fertilization

In recent years the treatment of **male infertility** was revolutionized by the rapid development of **micro-assisted fertilization**, which was motivated both by the lack of a treatment of most causes of male infertility and by the low success rate of conventional IVF in these patients.

The rapid development of the various methods of micro-assisted fertilization in the past was characterized by the stepwise circumvention of all processes involving

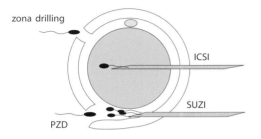

Fig. 17.5. Graphic presentation of the different methods of micro-assisted fertilization: *zona drilling*, partial zona dissection (*PZD*), subzonal sperm injection (*SUZI*), intracytoplasmic sperm injection (*ICSI*)

sperm capacitation and fertilization (Fig. 17.5). The results achieved by the different methods of micro-assisted fertilization clearly demonstrated that only those techniques in which the physiological sequences of fertilization were most effectively bypassed achieved the highest pregnancy rates.

Micro-assisted fertilization developed out of conventional IVF. Therefore, micro-assisted fertilization also requires adequate stimulation of the ovaries, the collection of mature oocytes from preovulatory follicles and the replacement of fertilized oocytes into the uterine cavity of the patient. All techniques of micro-assisted fertilization differ from conventional IVF by the necessity of preparing the oocytes from the surrounding cells of the **cumulus oophorus** and of the **corona radiata**. This is achieved in part enzymatically with **hyaluronidase**, in part mechanically using a fine bore micropipette. Preparation of the freshly collected oocytes prior to insemination allows better identification of the maturity stage of the oocyte (by visualization of the polar body) and improves the selection of high quality oocytes (by judgement of the texture and color of the cytoplasm). The oocyte's chances of successful fertilization and implantation are impaired if the polar body appears fragmented, if the perivitelline space is widened and in the presence of abnormal cytoplasmic inclusions (Xia 1997).

17.5.1 Previously Used Techniques of Micro-assisted Fertilization

The technique of zona drilling was developed because the **zona pellucida** was initially considered the most difficult obstacle to successful fertilization in patients with abnormal sperm quality (see Chap. 4). Fertilization was therefore facilitated by boring a small hole into the zona pellucida. After insemination of these pretreated oocytes with high concentrations of motile spermatozoa, individual spermatozoa were able to slip through the hole, to complete the acrosome reaction in the perivitelline space and to fuse with the membrane of the oocyte.

Various techniques of boring a hole in the zona pellucida of human oocytes were developed with time. The earliest method consisted of applying small amounts of an acid solution or a proteolytic substance to the zona pellucida with a micropipette. Later, the zona pellucida was partially vaporized with a fine laser beam. Although higher fertilization rates were achieved than with conventional IVF, the pregnancy rate with zona drilling remained extremely low. The technique used was later adopted for improvement of the implantation rate by opening the zona pellucida prior to embryo replacement: "**assisted hatching**" (see Sec. 17.9).

In order to enhance further the penetration of motile spermatozoa into the perivitelline area, larger openings in the zona pellucida than those made in zona drilling were produced by the **partial dissection of the zona pellucida** (PZD) from the vitelline membrane. This is achieved by first slightly aspirating the oocyte onto a holding pipette. Then the zona is punctured tangentially with a microneedle. By removing the microneedle at a right angle to the oocyte, the zona is torn and dissected from the membrane of the oocyte.

In **subzonal sperm injection** (SUZI) one or more motile spermatozoa are inserted with a micropipette into the perivitelline space between the zona pellucida and the membrane of the oocyte. Until the development of ICSI the subzonal injection of multiple spermatozoa was the most effective method of micro-assisted sperm injection in severe male infertility. In patients suffering from abnormal sperm quality not only the binding of capacitated sperm to the zona pellucida is hampered, but also the acrosome reaction and fusion with the vitelline membrane of the oocyte are disturbed. Thus, subzonal sperm injection was more successful when several motile spermatozoa were injected into the perivitelline space. Experience with the subzonal injection of several motile spermatozoa demonstrated that in the human system not only the zona pellucida, but also the vitelline membrane utilizes a protective mechanism against the penetration of supernumerary spermatozoa, so that the rate of polyspermy remains low. Nowadays, this technique has been largely replaced by ICSI.

17.5.2 Intracytoplasmic Sperm Injection (ICSI)

In this procedure a micropipette injects a single vital spermatozoon through the zona pellucida and the vitelline membrane into the cytoplasm of a mature oocyte.

For this purpose, the vitality of sperm is usually identified by observation of sperm movement and some selection is possible according to morphology and progres-

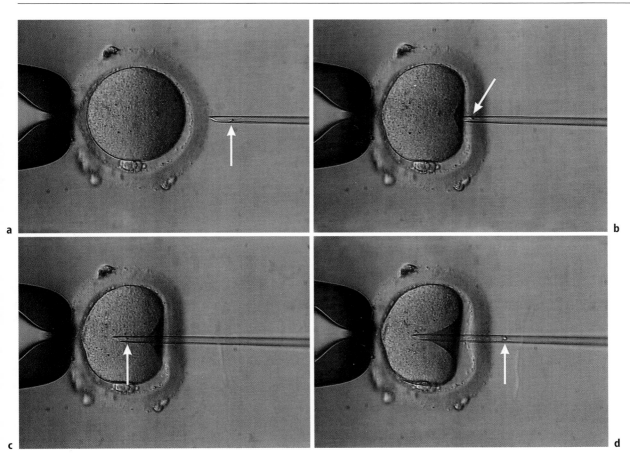

a   b

c   d

Fig. 17.6 a–d. Injection of one motile spermatozoon into the cytoplasm of an oocyte (ICSI). **a** The spermatozoon is captured by the injection micropipette, which is then directed to the oocyte fixed on a holding pipette. **b** Penetration of the zona pellucida. **c** Penetration of the vitelline membrane of the oocyte. **d** Aspiration of some cytoplasm into the injection pipette before the spermatozoon is transmitted into the oocyte

sive motility, but not based on genotypic properties. The spermatozoon is first immobilized and then aspirated with its head towards the tip of the micropipette.

The oocyte must be aspirated onto the tip of a holding pipette and will be held fixed in a position in which the polar body is visible at its upper or lower pole, in order to avoid damage to the meiotic spindle during the injection (Fig. 17.6). Various studies have demonstrated that fertilization and pregnancy rates are higher when the polar body and the beveled bore of the micropipette are directed towards the lower pole of the oocyte (Nagy et al. 1995; Van der Westerlaken et al. 1999). During the injection process first the zona pellucida and then the vitelline membrane are penetrated, both of which may display a high degree of elasticity. To ascertain the rupture of the oocyte's membrane prior to placement of the

spermatozoon into the cytoplasm, the membrane, together with some cytoplasm are aspirated into the micropipette. This allows the vitelline membrane to close the opening immediately, thereby reducing the risk of atresia or parthenogenetic activation (Nagy et al. 1995).

To facilitate drawing of the sometimes highly motile spermatozoa into the micropipette, the prepared spermatozoa may be incubated in culture medium supplemented with the macromolecule **polyvinylpyrrolidone** (PVP). Owing to the viscosity of the medium, the velocity of the capacitating sperm becomes lower. Individual spermatozoa are immobilized by touching them with the micropipette, thereby opening their membrane. Systematic studies have demonstrated that more injected oocytes are activated when the spermatozoon's membrane is opened mechanically (Dozortsev et al. 1995; Van den Bergh et al. 1995). The oocyte can only be activated if one or more cytoplasmic factors are liberated from the spermatozoon's equatorial segment into the injected oocyte. The cascade of events caused by these factors results in the pulsatile secretion of calcium ions from the oocyte over a period of approximately 30 minutes. The pulsatile excretion of calcium ions eventually leads to activation of the oocyte, to decondensation of the spermatozoon's DNA and to the formation of both pronuclei. One of the sperm factors responsible for this process has been identified (**oscillin**, Parrington et al. 1996).

Because the timing of the penetration of the spermatozoon into the oocyte is exactly known in ICSI, the exact timing of the various steps of fertilization can be determined (Payne et al. 1997):

- Extrusion of the second polar body after approximately 2.5 hours
- Appearance of the female pronucleus after approximately 5 hours
- Appearance of the male pronucleus a few minutes later
- Collateral approximation of both pronuclei after approximately 7 hours.

The probability of activation and further development of the injected oocyte depends on its quality, which can be partially estimated by assessing its morphology (Xia 1997). Other important factors in the success rate of ICSI are the experience of the technician involved (Van der Westerlaken et al. 1999) and the technique itself (Nagy et al. 1995; Van der Westerlaken et al. 1999). Approximately 10 % of all injected oocytes become atretic after the procedure (Nagy et al. 1995). It must be assumed that the meiotic spindle is not always located in the vicinity of the polar body and that in some oocytes it may be damaged (Hewitson et al. 1999). Nevertheless, the normal diploid fertilization rate in ICSI seems to be similar to that in conventional IVF.

The prevalence of parthenogenetic activation may be higher in ICSI then in IVF (11.5 %, Sultan et al. 1995). 2.5–6.5 % of all injected oocytes fail to extrude the second polar body, so that three pronuclei develop subsequently (digynic triploidy, Grossmann et al. 1997). In oocytes of rhesus monkeys treated by ICSI, it was demonstrated that the spermatozoon's DNA decondenses unevenly, compared with the gradual decondensation of the sperm DNA in IVF (Hewitson et al. 1999). The DNA close to the acrosome, which also contains the X chromosome, is the last to become decondensed. It has been suggested that this may be responsible for the slightly higher prevalence of gonosomal abnormalities in the offspring after ICSI (Luetjens et al. 1999).

> **Intracytoplasmic sperm injection** by far exceeds all other forms of micro-assisted fertilization in the limited number of motile sperm needed for successful fertilization and in the apparent absence of any correlation between sperm (dys)-function and the fertilization rate.

The high efficacy of ICSI greatly extended the spectrum of treatable abnormalities in male fertility. The success rate of ICSI in male infertile couples is not limited by the conventional semen characteristics such as concentration, progressive motility or percentage normal morphology, nor by the degree of physiological maturation in the testis and the epididymis, nor by the exhibition of capacitation by the spermatozoa. Even the presence of motion in spermatozoa as a sign of vitality is not essential for the success of ICSI, as in patients with complete lack of sperm motility, due to defects of the axonemal apparatus in the sperm tail, vitality can be demonstrated by the swelling of sperm in a hypotonic solution.

The first report of a pregnancy with this technology (Palermo et al. 1992) was followed by a rapid succession of more extended clinical experience (Palermo et al. 1993; Van Steirteghem et al. 1993a; Van Steirteghem et al. 1993b; Tsirigotis et al. 1994; Tucker et al. 1995), all demonstrating the high therapeutic efficacy of ICSI in the treatment of couples suffering from **severe male infertility** (Table 17.1). ICSI has been applied successfully in a high diversity of sperm dysfunctions:

- Severe forms of idiopathic male infertility in which capacitation and fertilization are highly unlikely to occur: such as severe **hypergonadotropic oligoasthenoteratozoospermia**, in which occasionally only few motile spermatozoa can be recovered from the ejaculate.
- Organic causes of male infertility in which the absence or loss of function of various anatomic parts of the male genital tract causes infertility: **obstructive azoospermia** with sperm recovered from the epididymis or from a testis biopsy (Tournaye et al. 1994a). In hypergonadotropic azoospermia sperm can be retrieved from multiple testis biopsies (Devroey et al. 1994; Silber et al. 1995; Yemini et al. 1995; Jezek et al. 1998). In **retrograde ejaculation** sperm may be recovered from the bladder (Gerris et al. 1994). In longstanding paralysis sperm can be collected by electroejaculation (Chung et al. 1998).
- In azoospermic patients, in whom no mature spermatozoa can be detected even in testicular tissue, successful treatments have been performed with haploid spermatids (Fishel et al. 1995) and even with diploid secondary spermatocytes (Sofikitis et al. 1998). In the latter the injected oocyte was again penetrated with the micropipette 1–2 hours later to induce the second meiotic division of the injected spermatocyte. This process resulted in the extrusion of another polar body which contained the haploid chromosome complement of the injected spermatocyte.
- Rare and sporadic forms of male infertility which are probably caused by mutations, such as **globozoospermia** (Lundin et al. 1994; Bourne et al. 1995; Liu et al. 1995; Catt et al. 1996) and total sperm immotility

Table 17.1. Results with ICSI

Method	Reference	Oocytes activated/injected	%	Pregnancies per cycle	%
ICSI	Aboulghar et al. 1996	400/572	69.9	19/58	32.8
vs. IVF[a]		477/736	64.8	18/58	31.0
ICSI	Tsirigotis et al. 1994	71/127	55.9	5/12	41.7
ICSI	Tucker 1995	192/485	39.6	13/50	26.0
ICSI	Palermo et al. 1995	1142/1923	59.4	84/227	37.0
MESA/ICSI[b]	Tournaye et al. 1994a	71/127	55.9	5/12	41.7
MESA/ICSI[b]	Silber et al. 1994	80/197	41.6	8/17	47.0
PESA/ICSI[b]	Rosenlund et al. 1998	321/511	62.8		
TESE/ICSI	Silber et al. 1995	86/185	46.5	5/12	41.7
TESE/ICSI[c]	Balaban et al. 1999	646/898	71.9	35/73	47.9
TEFNA/ICSI[d]	Lewin et al. 1999	154/406	37.9	18/111	16.2

[a] Results of a prospective study in couples suffering from tubal infertilty but with normozoospermic semen to compare the efficacy of IVF and ICSI.
[b] Patients with obstructive azoospermia only.
[c] TESE, performed one day before oocyte collection and ICSI. The tissue was coincubated with recombinant FSH.
[d] Patients with testicular azoospermia only.

(Nijs et al. 1996; Casper et al. 1996; Liu et al. 1997; Kahraman et al. 1997). In these rare occasions the fertilization rate after ICSI seemed to be lower than the usual, which varies between 60–70 %.

The ICSI can be performed successfully with **frozen-thawed** spermatozoa from tumor patients in whom sperm quality was often already impaired in the original ejaculate and who could not be treated successfully with earlier treatment modalities (Agarwal et al. 1996; see Chap. 18). ICSI can also be performed with sperm from cryopreserved testicular tissue, so that the repetition of all invasive procedures of sperm collection such as testicular biopsy can be avoided.

Although the decision to perform ICSI is obvious in many situations, the exact spermatological criteria for its use have not yet been established.

Intracytoplasmic sperm injection as a treatment for male infertility reaches its limitation in at least three different clinical entities:

- Significant lower fertilization and implantation rates were reported in couples treated because of hypergonadotropic azoospermia and in whom sperm has to be retrieved from testicular tissue (Aboulghar et al. 1997; Vanderzalmen et al. 1997).
- In some cases of globozoospermia surprisingly low fertilization rates were reported (Liu et al. 1995; Battaglia et al. 1997; Tasdemir et al. 1997).

- In necrozoospermia, in which all seminal spermatozoa had lost their vitality because of some degenerative process, ICSI is not successful with ejaculated spermatozoa (Tournaye et al. 1996). However, the collection of spermatozoa from the testicles may be helpful under these circumstances.

Whereas in most spermatological situations ICSI presents as a highly effective method to induce successful fertilizations, the probability of pregnancy largely depends on factors determined by the female partner.

The results of ICSI are mainly influenced by the age of the female partner (Abdelmassih et al. 1996), by the ovarian response to the hormonal stimulation (Alrayyes et al. 1997) and by the quality of the oocytes (Alikani et al. 1995; Xia et al. 1997). Although the oocytes can indeed be successfully fertilized with ICSI, the pregnancy rates remain disappointing after their replacement into older recipients. Obviously, the therapeutic efficacy of ICSI seems to be limited to the process of fertilization only, whereas the probability of pregnancy depends on the quality of embryo replacement and of the hormonal environment in the recipient. Therefore, if the desired pregnancy does not occur despite successful fertilization induced by ICSI, the female partner, already carrying most of the therapeutic burden, might easily be placed in the position of being blamed for the failure of treatment.

17.6 Collection and Preparation of Sperm for Assisted Fertilization

17.6.1 Collection of Semen for Assisted Fertilization

Usually, semen can be collected for assisted fertilization by masturbation after a **period of abstinence** of 2–7 days, as recommended by the World Health Organization (WHO 1999, see also Chap. 6). In oligozoospermic patients the number of spermatozoa collected can be increased by prolonging the period of abstinence and/or by the production of more than one ejaculate prior to semen preparation (Tur-Kaspa et al. 1990; Cooper et al. 1993).

Sometimes, owing to a **pathological or psychological blockade**, semen cannot be collected by masturbation. In some of these cases semen may collected in a **condom** during natural sexual intercourse, provided the condom is not coated with a spermicidal substance. In patients suffering from **impotence** caused by paralysis in the segments ThXI-LII, ejaculation can also be induced by **vibration** or by **electroejaculation**. Although these procedures are effective in 90% of the patients, in some patients sperm may also be collected surgically by **aspiration** from the longitudinally incised **vas deferens** after scrotal incision (Hirsh et al. 1993b; Hovatta and von Smitten 1993).

In **male immunological infertility** or in patients with viscous semen, special care must be taken for appropriate collection of the semen sample. Sperm preparation can be facilitated by collecting the semen into 2 ml of equilibrated culture medium in order to reduce not only the **agglutination** of sperm, but also to limit the binding of antibodies to the sperm surface during liquefaction. In some cases, dissociation of agglutinated sperm can also be achieved by the addition of **proteolytic enzymes**. For this purpose various enzymes have been tested: chymotrypsin, trypsin and papain. These enzymes can be added to the sperm suspension in an albumin-free culture medium for up to twenty minutes without damage (Pattinson et al. 1990). However, the medium containing the enzyme should be washed away before insemination to prevent any interference of the proteolytic enzyme with the interaction between the gametes.

In patients suffering from **retrograde ejaculation**, three different methods can be used for sperm collection for assisted fertilization.

- First, **antegrade ejaculation** may be achieved by the administration of specific drugs, such as **alpha-adrenergic** substances (phenylpropanolamine, oxedrine)

or **anticholinergics** (bromopheniramine) (Kamischke and Nieschlag 1999).

- An alternative consists of collecting the freshly ejaculated sperm from the bladder through a catheter. Because of the acidity and the high osmolarity of the urine, adequate preparation of the patient is necessary to protect the sperm before and after ejaculation. Before ejaculation the bladder should be emptied and rinsed with 10 ml of the culture medium. Before ejaculation the urine may be alkalinized by oral intake of a high-dose sodium bicarbonate (1–4 g).

- A third method consists of the microsurgical aspiration of motile spermatozoa through a longitudinal incision in the vas deferens.

In **obstructive azoospermia** sperm is collected from a microsurgically incised tubule of the epididymis by aspiration into a capillary ("**microsurgical epididymal sperm aspiration**", MESA) (Silber et al. 1994, 1995). Usually motile spermatozoa are not found immediately and several incisions into the epididymis have to be made, first in the distal portion of the cauda epididymidis, and then more proximally, until motile spermatozoa can be recovered. In most patients suffering from long-standing obstructive azoospermia motile spermatozoa are not recovered from the cauda epydidimidis, but rather from the more proximal portion of the epididymis. The concentration of the spermatozoa recovered from an obstructed epididymis may vary, but motility is usually below 20% (Hirsh et al. 1994; Tournaye et al. 1994a). This time-consuming procedure can also be performed one day before oocyte collection. At present, there is a trend towards collecting the spermatozoa from the testes rather than from the epididymis, because the former is much more time-consuming and costly than the latter. Single cell gel electrophoresis of DNA from testicular sperm seems to be more stable than of DNA from epididymal sperm (Steele et al. 1999), but prospective clinical trials comparing both methods are still lacking.

Sperm can be recovered for ICSI not only from the vas deferens and the epididymis, but also from the testis itself. For this purpose one (in **obstructive azoospermia**) or up to nine tissue samples (in **hypergonadotropic azoospermia**, Devroey et al. 1994; Silber et al. 1995) can be removed from the testis, in which viable spermatozoa can be sought for ICSI ("**testicular sperm extraction**", TESE). Even in severe testicular atrophy with highly elevated serum FSH levels some of the seminal tubules may contain localized spermatogenesis, from which viable spermatozoa can be collected for ICSI. Viable spermatozoa can be identified by slight or more intensive motility at 200- to 400-fold magnification with an inverted microscope and isolated from the tissue with a micropipette. In order to extract single vital spermatozoa from the connective tissue, the biopsy may be minced mechanically or treated enzymatically (collagenase and trypsin-inhibitor, Salzbrunn et al. 1996). For better planning, the testicular biopsy may be performed on the day before oocyte collection, prepared and cultured overnight (Hu et al. 1999). The addition of recombinant FSH to the cultured testicular tissue (25 IU/l) signficantly improves the fertilization rate, the implantation rate and even the pregnancy rate (Balaban et al. 1999). Because it is sometimes difficult and time-consuming to search for individual spermatozoa in the biopsied and minced testicular tissue, an alternative method was recently presented in which testicular germ cells were isolated from frozen-thawed biopsies treated with collagenase.

In testis-related azoospermia the couples must be informed about the risk of not finding spermatozoa in the collected biospies (40–50 %). However, the probability of positive retrieval of vital spermatozoa can be reliably predicted from detailed histological study of the testicular biopsy (Jezek et al.1998). In order to avoid unnecessary ovarian stimulation of the female partner followed by oocyte retrieval, the concept of **Cryo-TESE** was developed (Fisher et al. 1996). In Cryo-TESE several biopsies are taken from both testes prior to any treatment of the female partner. One biopsy of each testis is examined histologically and the presence or absence of spermatogenesis is recorded. Two biopsies are prepared both mechanically and enzymatically and the presence of vital spermatozoa is recorded. The remaining biopsies are cryopreserved.

In 76.9 % of all biopsies the presence of spermatozoa can be detected histologically (Schulze et al. 1999). The prediction of finding spermatozoa in the frozen-thawed biopsies based on the histological proof of foci with active spermatogenesis in single testicular tubules was incorrect in only 2.9 % of all cases. In 0.7 % of all biopsies **testicular cancer or carcinoma in situ** was detected (Schulze et al. 1999). The fertilization rate, the implantation rate and the pregnancy rate did not differ after ICSI performed with sperm retrieved from freshly collected testis biopsies or from previously cryopreserved biopsies (Ben-Yosef et al. 1999).

The collection of sperm by simple percutaneous puncture of the epididymal tubule ("**percutaneous epididymal sperm aspiration**", PESA, Craft et al. 1995) or from the testis ("**testicular fine needle sperm aspiration**", TEFNA, Friedler et al. 1997) and subsequent aspiration with a syringe has also been described. The advantage of these techniques is that the sperm collection for ICSI can be performed not only faster but also without the costly equipment needed for MESA or TESE. The number of aspirated spermatozoa seems to be lower with PESA and with TEFNA than with alternative, more invasive techniques. At the moment, no prospective randomized study has been performed to compare the clinical benefits of the available methods.

17.6.2 Preparation of Sperm for Assisted Fertilization

Before the actual processing of the semen sample can be started, the semen must be liquefied by simple incubation at room temperature for 30 minutes.

A subsequent washing procedure of the semen is required, because **seminal plasma** can be toxic both for the sperm itself, as well as for the oocytes, even at low concentration (Kanwar et al. 1979). Furthermore, bacteria may be present in the semen, which, after insemination into the genital tract of the female partner or after insemination in vitro, may proliferate and cause damage. Seminal plasma also contains high concentrations of prostaglandins, which, after their introduction into the uterine cavity, may induce paroxysmal and painful contractions of the myometrium. The preparation of the semen not only separates the spermatozoa from the surrounding seminal plasma, but the proportion of highly motile and normally formed spermatozoa is increased and the process of capacitation is also induced. Recently, methods have been developed to enhance the **selection of spermatozoa** with particular genetic features (such as X and Y spermatozoa for the prevention of sex-chromosome linked diseases).

Based on the different physical principles the various methods of sperm preparation are divided into four groups:

- **filtration**,
- **swim-up**,
- **density grade centrifugation**,
- **flow cytometry**.

In most methods of sperm preparation, semen is first liquefied by simple incubation and the fraction containing the spermatozoa is then separated from the seminal plasma by centrifugation. After discarding the supernatant one of the preparation procedures listed above can be initiated.

Filtration

Filtration of spermatozoa on a column preloaded with **glasswool** (Paulson and Polakoski 1977) or with **glass beads** (Daya et al. 1987) has found widespread acceptance. The suspension containing the spermatozoa freed from the seminal plasma is loaded onto a vertically positioned column, which is prefilled with either 15 mg of glass wool (microfibercode 112) or with 1 g of glass beads (each of 75 to 150 μm diameter). Before adding the sperm suspension the column is rinsed with culture medium to remove potential toxic substances and to equilibrate the content of the column. The sperm suspension is then added on top of the column, flows downward and a highly motile fraction of spermatozoa can be gathered dropwise from the column and used for assisted fertilization. Immotile spermatozoa, leucocytes and round cells tend to adhere to the glass or remain trapped in the mesh, in contrast to the motile spermatozoa which readily pass through the column.

The filtration of sperm has the advantage of rapidly achieving a high yield of progressively motile spermatozoa. In this regard sperm filtration with columns loaded with glass wool seems to be as effective as the swim-up-method (Van der Ven et al. 1988; Katayama et al. 1989) or as density gradient centrifugation (Rhemrev et al. 1989). The loss of spermatozoa during the filtration process seems to be low and the duration of the processing is particularly short (10 minutes). The results of IVF with filtered sperm are comparable to those achieved with swim-up sperm (Van der Ven et al. 1988; Katayama et al. 1989).

The main disadvantage of the filtration method, particularly if glass wool is used for filtration, is the lack of standardization of the glass wool mesh and the resulting variability of the filtration results.

Swim-up

Swim-up is a method most widely used for sperm preparation in assisted fertilization (Lopata et al. 1976). It is based on the principle that the most motile and capable spermatozoa can swim vigorosly upwards against gravity into a layer of culture medium positioned on top of the sperm pellet. A fraction of highly motile sperm free of seminal plasma and leucocytes can be collected after 60 to 90 minutes of incubation. The significance of swim-up for sperm preparation is further enhanced by the finding that those properties needed for the penetration of motile sperm into the supernatant are the same required for the **penetration into cervical mucus** and for the **actual fertilization of oocytes** (De Geyter et al. 1988). Thus the concentration of sperm after swim-up is also correlated with the results of assisted fertilization. In contrast to earlier reports, no selection of Y chromosome bearing spermatozoa can be achieved with the swim-up-procedure (Han et al. 1993).

The main disadvantage of the swim-up-method is the low recovery rate of motile spermatozoa, especially in cases with severe abnormalities of the original semen sample. The yield of spermatozoa can be improved by prolonging the duration of incubation, by slightly tilting the culture tube and by using several tubes for parallel swim-up (so-called "multiple-tube swim-up").

Nevertheless, in comparison to other methods of sperm preparation such as density gradient centrifugation and filtration, swim-up is characterized by better motility and relatively higher numbers of normally formed spermatozoa (Englert et al. 1992). In one prospective controlled study the results of IVF were not significantly influenced by the method of sperm preparation (Englert et al. 1992). Although the swim-up-procedure is time-consuming, it is technically easy to perform, requires little laboratory equipment and is highly reproducible when performed by different technicians.

Density Gradient Centrifugation

With density gradient centrifugation, motile and normally formed spermatozoa are separated not only by centrifugal force, but also by differences in the density of individual cells. The density of living spermatozoa is known to differ from that of degenerated or dead spermatozoa. To achieve a separation with density gradient centrifugation the washed sperm suspension is layered onto a column comprising several layers of a colloid suspension of different density and subsequently centrifuged. For this purpose **Percoll** can be used, which contains **colloidal particles made of silicone** with diameters between 15 and 30 nm. These particles are coated with the biologically inert **polyvinylpyrollidone** (Pharmacia, Uppsala, Sweden).

In the column containing various layers of different density colloidal particles not only vital and dead spermatozoa but also leucocytes and spermatozoa can be separated during centrifugation. Various modifications and compositions of the solutions containing the colloidal particles have been designed: continuous density gradients (Berger et al. 1985), discontinuous density gradients (Guérin et al. 1989) and discontinuous density gradients in small volume (mini-Percoll, Ord et al. 1990). For the establishment of continuous density gradients ultracentrifugation must be performed ($>100{,}000$ g) which is more suitable for the separation of small-sized particles such as viruses and mitochondria. Therefore, for the separation of the relatively larger sized spermatozoa, discontinuous density gradients are predominantly used. The enriched fraction containing motile spermatozoa can be recognized easily as a discrete turbid band in the area between 85 % and 100 % of the Percoll suspension. In patients with extremely abnormal sperm quality and with very reduced sperm numbers the preparation of semen samples with the mini-Percoll-column might be helpful, since it can be performed on a volume of only 0.9 ml.

Although density gradient centrifugation yields more motile spermatozoa than the swim-up-method, the impact of both methods on the results of conventional IVF is controversial. In a controlled prospective study, the fertilization rates after both preparation methods were not significantly different (Englert et al. 1992; Byrd et al. 1994). However, in another controlled study the fertilization rate after density gradient centrifugation appeared to be significantly better than after swim-up (Jaroudi et al. 1993). Nevertheless, the results of infertility treatment may depend more on the inherent fertility of both partners than on the method of sperm preparation itself.

Compared with the swim-up method (at least 60 minutes), sperm preparation with density gradient centrifugation (20 minutes) is less time-consuming. Density gradient centrifugation is not associated with any enrichment of Y chromosome-carrying spermatozoa (Vidal et al. 1993). Furthermore, the risk of inflammation caused by colloidal silicone particles in the genital tract of the patients after insemination was ruled out experimentally (Pickering et al. 1989). Because of its contamination with endotoxins the use of Percoll itself is not recommended for the preparation of sperm. However, other density gradient systems have become available for this purpose.

Sperm Selection by Flow Cytometry

Parallel to the development of **preimplantation diagnostics** in the early embryo, interest in the **selection** of spermatozoa containing certain genetic features to prevent hereditary diseases has grown. The first step consists of the separation of spermatozoa containing the Y chromosome from those carrying the X chromosome to prevent X chromosome-dependent illnesses even before fertilization. In certain patients an abnormally high number of diploid spermatozoa may be responsible for repeated miscarriages. Further miscarriages may be prevented by separating diploid from haploid spermatozoa before insemination and fertilization. This can be achieved by means of flow cytometry and selection of spermatozoa previously marked with a fluorescent dye, which allows the distinction of spermatozoa based on the quantity of DNA in their genome. For example, spermatozoa with an X chromosome contain approximately 3% more DNA than spermatozoa carrying a Y chromosome.

With flow cytometry a sufficient number of motile spermatozoa can be selected rapidly enough to be used in assisted fertilization (Johnson et al. 1993). Several pregnancies have been achieved using this method in IUI, in conventional IVF and in ICSI, mainly for the prevention of X chromosome-linked genetic diseases (Fugger et al. 1998). Although this method of sperm selection can be abused to manipulate the sex of the newborn, in the near future it may become of utmost importance for the prevention of inborn diseases. The risk of alterations in the DNA structure induced by the fluorescent dyes has been excluded in extensive animal research.

Processing of Sperm for ICSI

In extreme oligoasthenoteratozoospermia or in sperm aspirated from the epididymis (MESA), small-volume density gradients, such as the mini-Percoll, can be used for sperm preparation (Ord et al. 1990). In some patients treated with ICSI, often only isolated motile spermatozoa are available and no adequate separation can be performed. In these cases one simple washing of the sample consisting of centrifugation and discharge of the supernatant fluid and resuspension of the pellet of spermatozoa, can sufficiently clean the sample of debris.

To facilitate catching single motile spermatozoa with the micropipette, the viscosity of the culture medium may be increased by the addition of a high concentration of the biologically inert **polyvinylpyrrolidone** (8 g/100 ml culture medium), a macromolecule with a molecular weight of 360,000 kD. Any alleged mutagenic action of polyvinylpyrrolidone possibly entering the oocyte during the intracytoplasmic injection has been ruled out experimentally (Ray et al. 1995).

ICSI can also be performed successfully with immotile but vital spermatozoa (Nijs et al. 1996; Casper et al. 1996; Liu et al. 1997). Because vitality of the sperm cannot be recognized by cellular movements, the integrity of the spermatozoon's membrane is used to prove its vitality. This can be achieved with the hypoosmotic swelling test. For this purpose the sperm are incubated in culture medium previously diluted 1:1 (v/v) with distilled water. A typical swelling of the tail of the sperm indicates its vitality. The sperm will recover when transferred with the micropipette into the native culture medium before ICSI.

17.6.3 Treatment of Spermatozoa in Culture

As well as the selection of fertile spermatozoa by using different methods of sperm preparation, changing the composition of the culture medium surrounding the spermatozoa also improves the results of assisted fertilization.

For this purpose various chemical substances are added to the culture in order to stimulate sperm motility: **2-deoxyadenosine** (Aitken et al. 1986), **pentoxiphylline** (Yovich et al. 1990) and **caffeine** (Imoedemhe et al. 1992). These substances act as inhibitors of phosphodiesterase, which is associated with an increase of the intracellular concentration of cAMP. It has been demonstrated that after addition of each of these substances to the seminal plasma or to the culture medium, the motility, velocity and extent of hyperactivation rate can be increased significantly (Imoedemhe et al. 1992; Ka et al. 1994). However, despite these obvious changes in sperm motion, fertilization and pregnancy rates were not improved (Tournaye et al. 1994b; Dimitriadou et al 1995). A further disadvantage was that at least for caffeine, a dose-dependent embryo-toxicity was demonstrated (Imoedemhe et al. 1992).

Besides the addition of defined **chemical substances** to the culture medium, sperm function is also improved by **coculture** of the spermatozoa with epithelial cells in vitro. These attempts were motivated by the observation that in various animal species the function of the spermatozoa seems to be influenced by direct contact with the mucosal cells lining the lumen of the oviduct. Experimental evidence demonstrated that both the motility of sperm and the extent of hyperactivation of cultured spermatozoa can be increased by contact with various cells in coculture (Wetzels et al. 1991; Guérin et al. 1991; Pearlstone et al. 1993; Chen et al. 1994). However, the impact of coculture of spermatozoa with other cell lines on the outcome of assisted fertilization has not yet been determined. To a large extent, the cells of the **cumulus oophorus** and of the **corona radiata** remain in contact with the spermatozoa overnight during conventional IVF and may be considered to function as a useful coculture system (Mansour et al. 1995).

17.7 Ovarian Follicular Development, Ovarian Stimulation, Ovulation Induction and Oocyte Collection

17.7.1 Monitoring of Ovarian Follicular Development and Ovarian Stimulation for Insemination

The therapeutic efficacy of insemination not only results from an increased number of motile spermatozoa in the lumen of the Fallopian tube, but also from the exact timing of ovulation, with which insemination must be optimally synchronized. Both the observation of the changes occurring during a natural menstrual cycle leading to ovulation and the active induction of ovulation have been used for this purpose.

The preovulatory surge of the **endogenous luteinizing hormone (LH)** was determined in natural menstrual cycles or after a mild ovarian stimulation with clomiphene citrate to predict ovulation and was shown to be equivalent to the active induction of the ovulation with **human chorionic gonadotropin (hCG)** (Martinez et al. 19; Zreik et al. 1999).

To determine endogenous LH, simple urinary sticks with a color indicator were developed for practical use at home. Insemination is performed 16 to 28 hours after the initial rise of LH. In patients stimulated with gonadotropins, the amplitude of the endogenous preovulatory LH secretion is usually reduced or absent, so that in these patients ovulation should always be induced exogenously with hCG. Insemination is performed 36–40 hours after administration of hCG.

Several prospective studies have convincingly demonstrated that the pregnancy rate from insemination was correlated proportionally with the quality of support of follicular maturation (Ho et al. 1992; Peterson et al. 1994; Cohlen et al. 1998; Guzick et al. 1999). Therefore, the pregnancy rate following insemination after stimulation of the **ovaries with gonadotropins** was the highest. The higher pregnancy rate in these patients results not only from an increased number of induced ovulations, but also from compensation of subclinical abnormalities in follicular development by exogenous gonadotropins. However, the most important disadvantage of gonadotropin stimulation is the higher rate of **multiple pregancies**. The rapidly increasing prevalence of multiple pregnancies in many countries during the last decade has been induced by modern reproductive medicine and imposes a heavy burden on many obstetric and neonatal units. As multiple pregnancies are frequently associated with complications, often leading to prematurity, the far-reaching consequences are of major financial and emotional concern to our society. The risk of multiple pregnancy can be reduced significantly by low-dosed gonadotropin administration and/or by the preovulatory aspiration of supernumerary follicles (De Geyter et al. 1996). Any insemination should be cancelled in the presence of more than three follicles with a diameter of at least 14 mm. Furthermore, gonadotropin stimulation of the ovaries may be confounded by the **ovarian hyperstimulation syndrome**, which is a potentially life-threatening complication. The severe form of the ovarian hyperstimulation syndrome is rare in patients treated with insemination, compared with treatment cycles for IVF or ICSI, because of the generally lower doses of gonadotropins used in the former group.

17.7.2 Ovarian Stimulation for IVF and ICSI

Soon after introduction of IVF for the treatment of infertility it was found that the pregnancy rate was correlated directly with the **number of embryos replaced**. A multitude of different treatment protocols for the stimulation of ovarian follicular development were developed over time and were correlated with the results of assisted fertilization.

Originally follicular development was stimulated with **clomiphene citrate** with or without **human urinary gonadotropins**, but 25–30% of the treatment cycles had to be abandoned because of premature luteinizations or ovulations. Therefore, treatment with gonadotropins was increasingly combined with long-acting GnRH-analogues in order to down-regulate the endogenous gonadotropin secretion and to prevent the preovulatory release of LH. In a large-scale prospective investigation it was demonstrated that down-regulation with **long-acting GnRH-analogues** is associated with a significant increase in the pregnancy rate (Tan et al. 1992b). Co-treatment with GnRH-analogues enhances the recruitment of a larger number of ovarian follicles and can also be used to reduce the number of treatments with assisted fertilization during weekends. However, the major **disadvantage** is the higher consumption of gonadotropins, thereby considerably increasing the cost of the treatment and the higher risk of the **ovarian hyperstimulation syndrome** (7%, Bergh and Lundkvist 1992). The number of **multiple pregnancies** can be limited to 15–20% by the replacement of a maximum of three embryos in one treatment cycle.

In most patients ICSI cannot be performed effectively without the use of ovarian stimulation, since only 55% of the oocytes become subsequently activated and up to 15% become atretic after injection. In ICSI, as in conventional IVF, the most commonly used protocol of ovarian stimulation consists of previous desensitization of the pituitary with long-acting GnRH-analogues followed by administration of gonadotropins. Only in adequately stimulated cycles can a sufficient number of oocytes in metaphase II, suitable for injection, be collected.

In contrast to conventional IVF, the assessment of oocytes is easier and more complete in ICSI, because prior to injection, the oocytes must be freed from the surrounding cumulus and coronal cells. Not only accurate assessment of the stage of meiotic development is possible by visualization of the germinal vesicle and the polar body, but also the texture and the color of the cytoplasm, the vitelline membrane and the zona pellucida may be used to select the oocytes suitable for injection and likely to develop successfully.

In contrast to conventional IVF, in which the fertilization rate is determined by the fertilizing capacity of sperm and the number of motile spermatozoa added to the oocytes (De Geyter et al. 1992), the activation rate of the injected oocytes in ICSI seems to be more dependent on the quality of follicular development and oocyte maturation.

17.8 Methods of Oocyte Collection

Surgical laparoscopy was one of the basic techniques contributing to the successful introduction of IVF during the 1970s (Steptoe 1970), because it gave the physician easier and less traumatic access to the ovaries to collect oocytes than laparotomy. Laparoscopy remains, however, an invasive technique and it usually requires general anesthesia. The major disadvantage of laparoscopy for oocyte collection, especially in IVF, is the difficult access to the ovaries in some patients suffering from extensive adhesions in the peritoneal cavity. The need for insufflating carbon dioxide into the peritoneum may lower the pH in the direct environment of the oocytes, and thereby reduce their developmental ability.

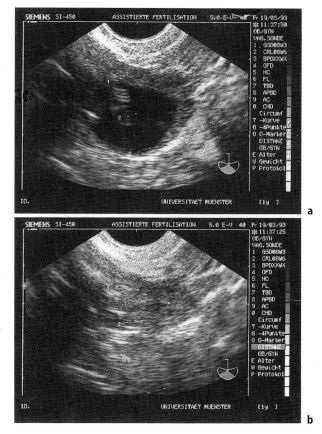

a

b

Fig. 17.7. For ultrasound-guided collection of oocytes a hollow needle is first inserted transvaginally into the antrum of a mature ovarian follicle. Then the content of the follicle is aspirated into a culture tube. In the aspirated follicular fluid the cumulus oophorus-oocyte complex can be identified rapidly under a stereomicroscope

Laparoscopy was one of the basic techniques which contributed to the successful introduction, not only of IVF, but also of GIFT and of ZIFT.

The collection of oocytes for assisted fertilization was greatly facilitated by **ultrasound-guided transvaginal puncture of the follicles,** which can usually be performed without intensive anesthetics, even in patients with extensive peritoneal adhesions. Ultrasound-guided transvaginal puncture of preovulatory follicles with a hollow needle is essentially an outpatient procedure, which in most treatment centers has largely replaced surgical laparoscopy for the collection of oocytes. Three main properties of the ovary enabled the development of this procedure: first, the ovaries are usually located directly behind the vagina. Secondly, the ovaries are hardly sensitive to pain. And thirdly, owing to the plasticity of the organ, the follicles can be emptied one by one by slight movement of the needle, thereby avoiding repeated transvaginal punctures (Fig. 17.7). In general, ultrasound-guided puncture of ovarian follicles is performed in patients previously sedated with diazepam 5 mg, pentazocin 30 mg, and midazolam 5 mg, or under general anesthesia with midazolam 5 mg and ketamine intravenously (0.5 mg/kg body weight).

The complication rate of this procedure is extremely low: abdominal bleeding is found in less than 0.8% of the patients (Dicker et al. 1993), infections in 0.24% (Dicker et al. 1993) to 0.3% of the patients (Bergh and Lundkvist 1992). In order to avoid infectious complications, cystic structures of the ovaries, especially those associated with endometriosis, should not be punctured inadvertently.

17.9 Assisted Hatching

The capacity of the embryo to implant after IVF or ICSI is generally as low as 10–20%. This low embryonic implantation rate is caused by genetic abnormalities in less then half of the replaced embryos. Implantation may also be impaired by mechanical obstacles such as the zona pellucida, which is known to become hardened during in vitro culture and may interfere with the hatching process, in which the blastocyst escapes from the zona pellucida. Additionally, the development of some embryos generated with IVF or ICSI may lag behind normal embryo development in the Fallopian tube, also causing difficulties during the hatching process.

The techniques developed for "zona drilling" and "partial zona dissection", originally conceived to improve fertilization rates in couples suffering from male infertility, were modified to improve the implantation rate. The method essentially consists of making a hole in

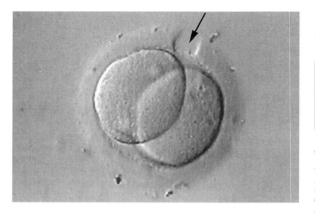

Fig. 17.8. For "assisted hatching", performed immediately before embryo replacement into the uterine cavity, the zona pellucida is opened (*arrow*) with a laser beam or with a locally applied acid solution. This technique was modified from two micro-assisted fertilization methods, "zona drilling" and "partial zona dissection" and aims at improving the implantation rate of the embryos

the zona pellucida of approximately the same diameter as the thickness of the zona pellucida itself (Fig. 17.8). Assisted hatching was first performed with a locally applied acid solution, later also with a laser beam.

Assisted hatching was considered helpful in women with an abnormally thick zona pellucida (>15 μm) and in embryos with fragmented blastomeres (Cohen et al. 1992). However, the therapeutic efficacy of assisted hatching remains to be established in large-scale prospective studies. A significantly higher prevalence of **monozygotic twinning** was observed after assisted hatching in one study (Hershlag et al. 1999).

17.10 Embryo Transfer

The embryos resulting from successful IVF are placed in the genital tract of the patient for later implantation, usually in the uterine cavity. **Uterine placement of embryos** is a procedure causing no pain and is nowadays performed within a few minutes as part of a routine gynecological investigation.

After visualization of the cervix with a speculum, the anterior portion of the cervix is clamped with a forceps. Under slight traction a catheter is introduced into the cervical canal. Then the embryos are aspirated, along with a small drop of cultured medium (approximately 10 μl), into a fine teflon catheter. This fine catheter is then inserted carefully through the previously positioned broader catheter into the uterine cavity (about 6 cm depth) (Fig. 17.9). Although embryo transfers are usually performed blindly, recent findings indicate that ultrasound-guided insertion of the catheter may significantly improve the results of IVF and ICSI (Kan et al. 1999). Not only the low volume of fluid introduced along with the embryos is important, but also carrying out the procedure in an absolutely atraumatic fashion. After a few minutes the patient is allowed to stand up and to leave the unit.

> The optimal technique of embryo transfer is one of the most important factors contributing to consistently high pregnancy rates in IVF and ICSI.

The complication rate of intrauterine embryo transfer is very low. In rare cases endometritis may occur. The replaced embryos may slip into the Fallopian tube, causing **ectopic** pregnancies especially in patients with widened tubal diameters (sactosalpinx). Ectopic pregnancies, mainly tubal pregnancies, are observed in approximately 6% of the pregnancies achieved with IVF. In a multicenter prospective randomized study it was demonstrated that for women with bilateral hydrosalpinges visible in ultrasound, implantation and pregnancy rates can be

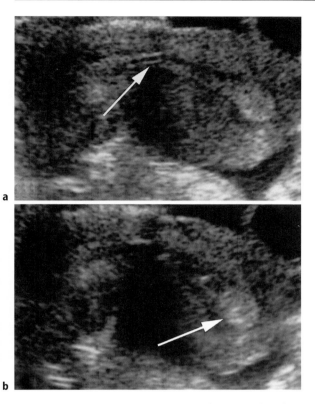

a

b

Fig. 17.9 a, b. Sonographic presentation of the transfer of an embryo into the uterine cavity. **a** Tip of the replacement catheter guided through the cervical canal into the uterine cavity. **b** The tip of the catheter is situated in the upper part of the uterine cavity. The embryos are situated in a droplet of culture medium surrounded by two air bubbles and by two additional droplets of culture medium

improved significantly by laparoscopic excision of the diseased Fallopian tube prior to assisted reproduction (Strandell et al. 1999).

Occasionally, stenosis of the cervical canal may constitute an insurmountable obstacle to the replacing of embryos. In some of these cases atraumatic embryo transfer can still be achieved by dilatation of the cervical canal during menstruation prior to ovarian stimulation. In other patients, embryo transfer can be performed successfully by transmyometrial injection through the anterior wall of the uterus into the endometrium (Kato et al. 1993).

17.11 Cryopreservation of Oocytes in the Pronucleate Stage

The German Embryo Protection Act stipulates that in each treatment cycle with IVF or ICSI not more than three oocytes may be fertilized and replaced after devel-

opment into the embryo stage. If more than three oocytes are fertilized with IVF or ICSI, they can be cryopreserved in the pronucleate stage prior to completion of the fertilization process. When pregnancy does not occur in the treatment cycle with fresh oocytes, the cryopreserved oocytes may be thawed and replaced, thereby avoiding repeated ovarian stimulation and oocyte collection.

Cryopreservation of oocytes in the pronucleate stage must be carried out prior to the approximation of both pronuclei, about 20 hours after in vitro insemination in IVF or after the ICSI procedure. The pronucleate oocytes are first dehydrated at room temperature in a series of solutions in order to prevent crystallization of water within the oocyte during the freezing process, which may cause extensive damage. Before starting the freezing protocol the pronucleate oocytes, surrounded by cryoprotectant, are inserted into plastic straws. After sealing and coding the straws, cryopreservation is performed in liquid nitrogen, usually in an automated system, which controls the freezing process at a predetermined pace. At –6 to –7°C seeding is induced, after which crystallization occurs, avoiding possible damage to the oocytes. Long-term cryopreservation follows by transferring the straws into tanks filled with liquid nitrogen (below –140°C).

Replacement of the thawed pronucleate oocytes takes place after their development into the early embryonic stage. This is usually performed in the natural menstrual cycle, after treatment with clomiphene citrate or after preparation of the endometrium with estradiol valerate followed by micronized progesterone. The survival rate of the thawed oocytes varies between 75–90%, but the pregnancy rates appear to be much lower than those observed during the treatments with fresh oocytes (Al-Hasani et al. 1996; Hoover et al. 1997; Macas et al. 1998). Neither increased prevalence of malformations nor of developmental abnormaties have been been observed among children conceived after replacement of frozen-thawed pronucleate oocytes (Ludwig et al. 1999)

17.12 Genetic Counselling in Assisted Fertilization

All patients who consider assisted reproduction and whose fertility problem has a genetic basis should undergo formal genetic counselling. The same recommendation is made when the patients' medical history or the family history suggest specific genetic risk factors.

Some centers have included genetic counselling in the standard protocol for all ICSI candidates even when no specific genetic risks are evident.

Table 17.2

Important questions concerning genetic history	Repeated miscarriages or stillbirths in the patient or among relatives?
	Congenital abnormalities, hereditary diseases in the couples or among their relatives?
	Are there other couples in the family suffering from infertility?
	Consanguinity of the couple or of their parents?
Indications for chromosome analysis	Repeated miscarriage in the patients or among their relatives.
	Previous stillbirth (especially when malformations were present, or the cause of fetal death was unclear).
	History of malformations or other congenital disorders in the patients or their relatives (indication for karyotyping to be assessed on an individual basis).
	Other couples in the family suffering from infertility.
	Planned intracytoplasmic sperm injection (ICSI).

It is not usual that infertile patients routinely undergo genetic counselling prior to **homologous insemination** or **conventional IVF**. Planning **intracytoplasmic sperm injection** is a different situation. There are two main reasons why genetic counselling and testing may be generally advisable prior to ICSI:

> Intracytoplasmic sperm injection per se may carry genetic risks for children conceived with this technique.

Possible genetic risks associated with the ICSI technique have been the subject of considerable debate. However so far, all concerns of this kind are purely hypothetical or were based on laboratory data with questionable relevance for the clinical setting. For example, it was argued that ICSI could inhibit a natural selection process against genetically aberrant male germ cells. The point has also been raised that mechanical manipulation of the gametes might disturb the first mitotic divisions of the embryo (Hewitson et al. 1999). It has also been hypothesized that ICSI with surgically retrieved sperm could interfere with the genomic "imprinting" of the spermatozoal genome (Tycko et al. 1997). The empirical data from prenatal and pediatric follow-up studies argue against a significant adverse effect arising from any of these mechanisms on children conceived with ICSI support. As currently available follow-up data are not yet sufficient for a definite evaluation, it appears prudent to inform patients that the genetic risk potential of ICSI is still the subject of research.

> Fertility problems that require ICSI have a genetic basis more frequently than infertility amenable to less invasive treatment modalities.

- Four to 5% of men and 6–7% of women enrolled in ICSI programs have an abnormal karyotype.
- Severe oligozoospermia and azoospermia are classical indications for ICSI. Patients presenting with either of these findings have a 3–5% prevalence rate of Y chromosomal microdeletions.
- MESA / TESE with consecutive ICSI is the treatment modality of choice for congenital bilateral absence of the vas deferens (CBAVD) and bilateral ejaculatory duct obstruction. Approximately 85% of men presenting with either of these variants of obstructive azoospermia carry mutations in the cystic fibrosis (CFTR) gene.
- In about 1% of men treated with ICSI, the fertility problem is one facet of a syndrome type of disorder.
- 2% of patients enrolled for ICSI are affected with non-reproductive, potentially heritable disorders, e.g. congenital heart disease, cleft lip and palate etc. This rate slightly exceeds the baseline prevalence (1%) of such disorders among fertile controls.

Hereditary disorders are not more common in the **families** of patients with severe impairments of fertility than in the families of fertile controls. Thus, there is no evidence for a familial genetic makeup that would predispose a sibship to both infertility and congenital diseases (Meschede et al. 2000).

As a **minimum requirement**, genetic diagnostics prior to ICSI should encompass a careful documentation of the personal, medical and family history (including the construction of a pedigree) and karyotyping of both partners. In cases of unexplained azoospermia or severe oligozoospermia, testing for Y chromosomal microdeletions is advisable (see Chap. 8). Other tests, such as mutation screening in the CFTR gene in patients with CBAVD are performed when suggested by the clinical situation.

Table 17.3. Prevalence of major congenital malformations in children born after ICSI compared with children born after natural conception or IVF

References	ICSI children (n)	Rate of malforma-tion after ICSI	Control children (n)	Malformations in controls
Palermo et al. 1996	578	1.6%	–	–
Bonduelle et al. 1998a	1,987	2.3%	–	–
Bowen et al. 1998	89	4.5%	80[a]	5.0%
Ludwig et al. 1998	270	3.7%	–	–
Hamori and Antoni 1999	570	3.8%	–	–
Loft et al. 1999	721	2.2%	–	–
Rossin-Amar 1999	2,322	2.4%	6,655[b]	1.8%
Sutcliffe et al. 1999b	207	4.3%	214[a]	3.7%
Wennerholm et al. 1999	1,187	4.4%	–	–

[a] Children born after natural conception.
[b] Children born after IVF.

It would be ideal if every couple considering micro-assisted reproduction underwent **formal genetic counselling**. This would also provide a well-structured framework for discussing the developmental data from the follow-up of ICSI children. The question of prenatal diagnosis can also be raised early in the therapeutic process. If routine genetic counselling is not possible, the physician in charge of therapy should at least check the points listed in Table 17.2 and order the appropriate genetic laboratory tests.

17.13 Pregnancy-related and Pediatric Aspects of Assisted Fertilization

The rate of congenital malformations among **children born after conventional in vitro fertilization (IVF)** is not higher than in naturally conceived controls (MRC Working Party 1990). Also, their cognitive and psychosocial development runs a normal course (Cederblad et al. 1996). Preliminary data suggest that the incidence of cancer does not exceed the baseline rate in the general population (Doyle et al. 1999).

Intracytoplasmic sperm injection actively intervenes in the process of fertilization and is therefore biologically more invasive than insemination or conventional IVF. This is one of the reasons why ICSI has been suspected to be particularly risk-laden in genetic terms. Both to confirm or disprove of this suspicion requires large and long-term follow-up studies. The developmental data pubished at the time of this writing do not allow definite conclusions about the genetic risk potential of ICSI. On the other hand, it should be clearly stated that

all studies available so far show no or only **minor differences between ICSI children and controls:**

- From 1.6–4.5% of ICSI children are born with a **major congenital malformation** (Table 17.3). The corresponding rate in children conceived naturally or through conventional IVF is 1.8–5.0% in those studies that included an internal control cohort. Thus, clearly the rate of major malformations in ICSI children does not exceed the baseline prevalence. Claims to the contrary have been derived from studies (e.g. Kurinczuk and Bower 1997) that used historical control cohorts. This design is prone to methological errors, and the value of such studies is dubious.

- **Chromosomal data** after ICSI treatment were almost exclusively generated in the prenatal setting, i.e. through chorionic villus sampling or amniocentesis. It is therefore difficult to compare the reported aberration rates with data obtained through serial karyotyping of newborns. Another point to consider is the comparatively advanced age of women pregnant by ICSI, which predisposes their children to aneuploidy. Given these methodological problems, one is left with a probably slight increase in the chromosomal aberration rate after ICSI as a currently reasonable, but not definitely proven working hypothesis.

- With a prevalence of approximately 1% abnormalities of the **sex chromosomes** appear to be somewhat more common in ICSI than in natural pregnancies. It is important to note that most gonosomal aneuploidies are clinically benign (Meschede and Horst 1997). Similar considerations apply to a second category of chromosomal aberrations that occur more commonly in ICSI pregnancies, i.e. balanced structural aberrations of the autosomes which are inherited from one of the parents. However, there are also several reports of trisomies 13, 18 or 21 or unbalanced structural anomalies. So far it is not possible to judge whether the incidence of these clinically grave aneuploidies is higher than usual.

- Two studies reported normal **psychomotor and cognitive development** of ICSI children (Bonduelle et al. 1998b; Sutcliffe et al. 1999a), whereas another report claimed a mild developmental delay of the ICSI-conceived cohort (Bowen et al. 1998). Given these contradictory findings, no definite conclusions can be drawn, even though the evidence for normal psychomotor development appears stronger. In none of these studies were children followed up for more than the first two years of life.

- Prior to puberty no clinical or laboratory parameter allows later **fertility** or infertility to be predicted. Therefore, at present we have no information concerning the prevalence of fertility problems in the adult after ICSI. Indirect evidence comes from the high prevalence of genetic aberrations in ICSI-treated patients (see Sec. 17.12) and the not so rare familial aggregation of male infertility (Meschede et al, in press). These findings suggest that ICSI children could be at increased risk for compromised fertility later in life.

17.14 Prenatal Diagnosis after Assisted Reproduction

There are no special aspects to prenatal diagnosis in **pregnancies conceived through homologous insemination or conventional IVF.** Invasive and non-invasive tests are applied in the same manner as in natural pregnancies. Preliminary evidence suggests that triple serum marker screening (α-fetoprotein, hCG, estriol) for Down syndrome has yielded increased (falsely) positive results after IVF (Milunsky 1998).

Given the slightly increased rate of chromosomal aberrations after **ICSI** (see Sec. 17.13), all women pregnant following this procedure should be offered **invasive prenatal diagnosis** by chorionic villus sampling or amniocentesis. A detailed high-resolution ultrasound scan at a specialized institution is also recommended. However, any decision of a women pregnant following ICSI not to undergo prenatal tests must be respected (Meschede et al. 1998). Meticulous care should be taken to document the offer of prenatal diagnosis.

In weighing the pros and cons of prenatal diagnosis in an ICSI pregnancy, the following points are of particular relevance:

- **Advanced maternal age.** Usually defined as a maternal age of ≥35 years at the expected date of confinement. Approximately 25% of women treated with ICSI are in this age group. As is well-known, there is a positive correlation between maternal age and the risk for a fetal numerical chromosome aberration, in particular trisomy 21.

- **Proven chromosomal anomaly.** If one of the partners carries a chromosomal aberration, invasive prenatal diagnosis usually is recommended. However, every case merits individual consideration. A human geneticist should devise the optimal strategy for prenatal diagnosis.

- **Y chromosomal microdeletion.** This type of genetic aberration is passed on to every son of the carrier. In the authors' opinion, a paternal Y chromosome microdeletion does not justify invasive prenatal diagnosis.

- **Mutation in the CFTR gene.** Carriership for mutations in the CFTR gene in both partners of a couple conveys a high risk for cystic fibrosis in their offspring. While this situation is a clear indication for prenatal diagnosis, carriership for a CFTR mutation in only one of the partners is not.

- **Syndrome disease.** A syndrome type of disorder and other potentially hereditary conditions present in one of the partners may or may not be an indication for prenatal diagnosis. A human geneticist should be consulted.

- **Parental consanguinity.** This is common in certain ethnic groups, e.g. patients from Turkey or the Middle East. Genetic counselling is advisable. The actual risk purported by parental consanguinity depends on the family history and how closely related the two partners are.

Certain monogenic and chromosomal disorders can be diagnosed in vitro in the pre-implantation embryo (Verlinsky and Kuliev 1999). Whether or not **preimplantation genetic diagnosis** (PGD) is permitted under the German Embryo Protection Act is an unresolved issue. If legal, this technique would be an option for couples treated with conventional IVF or ICSI. During the interval between fertilization and intrauterine transfer their embryos are stored in vitro and thereby easily accessible to a diagnostic procedure. In principle, PGD can be used to diagnose almost any monogenic disorder, e.g. cystic fibrosis or Duchenne muscular dystrophy. It is an absolute precondition that the parental mutation(s) are known. A chromosomal abnormality carried by one of the partners is another potential indication for PGD. Finally, PGD is now advocated as a means of improving the efficacy of IVF or ICSI in women who, owing to their advanced reproductive age, have a poorer chance of getting pregnant (Templeton et al. 1996). In this scenario PGD is used to select those embryos for transfer which are free of the common aneuploidies (Reubinoff and Shushan 1996), possibly resulting in improved pregnancy rates for these reproductively "old" patients.

17.15 References

Abdelmassih R, Sollia S, Moretto M, Acosta AA (1996) Female age is an important parameter to predict treatment outcome in intracytoplasmic sperm injection. Fertil Steril 65: 573–577

Aboulghar MA, Mansour RT, Serour GI, Amin YM, Kamal A (1996) Prospective controlled randomized study of in vitro fertilization versus intracytoplasmic sperm injection in the treatment of tubal factor infertility with normal semen parameters. Fertil Steril 66:753–756

Aboulghar MA, Mansour RT, Serour GI, Fahmy I, Kamal A, Tawab NA, Amin YM (1997) Fertilization and pregnancy rates after intracytoplasmic sperm injection using ejaculate semen and surgically retrieved sperm. Fertil Steril 68:108–111

Agarwal A, Shekarriz M, Sidhu RK, Thomas AJ Jr (1996) Value of clinical diagnosis in predicting the quality of cryopreserved sperm from cancer patients. J Urol 155:934–938

Aitken RJ, Mattei A, Irvine S (1986) Paradoxical stimulation of human motility by 2-deoxyadenosine. J Reprod Fertil 78: 515–527

Akhondi MA, Chapple C, Moore HDM (1997) Prolonged survival of human spermatozoa when co-incubated with epididymal cell cultures. Hum Reprod 12:514–522

Al-Hasani S, Ludwig M, Gasteiger F, Küpker W, Sturm R, Yilmaz A, Bauer O, Diedrich K (1996) Comparison of cryopreservation of supernumerary pronuclear human oocytes obtained after intracytoplasmic sperm injection (ICSI) and after conventional in-vitro fertilization. Hum Reprod 11: 604–607

Alikani M, Palermo G, Adler A, Bertoli M, Blake M, Cohen J (1995) Intracytoplasmic sperm injection in dysmorphic human oocytes. Zygote 3:283–288

Allen NC, Herbert CM, Maxson WS, Rogers BJ, Diamond MP, Wentz AC (1985) Intrauterine insemination: a critical review. Fertil Steril 44:569–580

Alrayyes S, Fakih H, Khan I (1997) Effect of age and cycle responsiveness in patients undergoing intracytoplasmic sperm injection. Fertil Steril 68:123–127

Anderson RA, Kinniburgh D, Baird DT (1999) Preliminary experience of the use of a gonadotrophin-releasing hormone antagonist in ovulation induction/in-vitro fertilization prior to cancer treatment. Hum Reprod 14:2665–2668

Asch RH, Ellsworth LR, Balmaceda JP, Wong PC (1984) Pregnancy after translaparoscopic gamete intrafallopian transfer. Lancet 2:1034–1035

Balaban B, Urman B, Sertac A, Alatas C, Aksoy S, Mercan R, Nuhoglu A (1999) In-vitro culture of spermatozoa induces motility and increases implantation and pregnancy rates after testicular sperm extraction and intracytoplasmic sperm injection. Hum Reprod 14:2808–2811

Battaglia DE, Koehler JK, Klein NA, Tucker MJ (1997) Failure of oocyte activation after intracytoplasmic sperm injection using round-headed sperm. Fertil Steril 68:118–122

Benoff S, Cooper GW, Paine T, Hurley IR, Napolitano B, Jacob A, Scholl GM, Hershlag A (1999) Numerical dose-compensated in vitro fertilization inseminations yield high fertilization and pregnancy rates. Fertil Steril 71:1019–1028

Ben-Yosef D, Yogev L, Hauser R, Yavetz H, Azem F, Yovel I, Lessing JB, Amit A (1999) Testicular sperm retrieval and cryopreservation prior to initiating ovarian stimulation as the first line approach in patients with non-obstructive azoospermia. Hum Reprod 14:1794–1801

Berger T, Marrs RP, Moyer DL (1985) Comparison of techniques for selection of motile spermatozoa. Fertil Steril 43:268–273

Bergh T, Lundkvist Ö (1992) Clinical complications during in-vitro fertilization treatment. Hum Reprod 7:625–626

Bergh T, Ericson A, Hillensjö T, Nygren K-G, Wennerholm U-B (1999) Deliveries and children born after in-vitro reproduction in Sweden 1982–95: a retrospective cohort study. Lancet 354:1579–1585

Bladou F, Grilo JM, Rossi D, Noizet A, Gamerre M, Erny R, Luciani JM, Serment G (1991) Epididymal sperm aspiration in conjunction with in-vitro fertilization and embryo transfer in cases of obstructive azoospermia. Hum Reprod 6:1284–1287

Bonde JPE, Ernst E, Jensen TK, Hjollund NH, Kolstad H, Henriksen TB, Schelke T, Giwercman A, Olsen J, Skakkebaek NE (1998) Relation between semen quality and fertility: a population-based study of 430 first-pregnancy planners. Lancet 352:1172–1177

Bonduelle M, Aytoz A, Wilikens A, Buysse A, van Assche E, Devroey P, van Steirteghem AC, Liebaers I (1998a) Genetic problems and congenital malformations in 1987 ICSI children. Hum Reprod 13 (Abstract Book 1):108–109

Bonduelle M, Joris H, Hofmans K, Liebaers I, Van Steirteghem AC (1998b) Mental development of 201 ICSI children at 2 years of age. Lancet 351:1553

Bourne H, Liu DY, Clarke GN, Baker GHW (1995) Normal fertilization and embryo development by intracytoplasmic sperm injection of round-headed acrosomeless sperm. Fertil Steril 63:1329–1332

Bowen JR, Gibson FL, Leslie GI, Saunders DM (1998) Medical and developmental outcome at 1 year for children conceived by intracytoplasmic sperm injection. Lancet 351:1529–1534

Byrd W, Bradshaw K, Carr B, Edman C, Odom J, Ackerman G (1990) A prospective randomized study of pregnancy rates following intrauterine and intracervical insemination using frozen donor sperm. Fertil Steril 53:521–527

Byrd W, Drobnis EZ, Kutteh WH, Marshburn P, Carr BR (1994) Intrauterine insemination with frozen donor sperm: a prospective randomized trial comprising three different sperm preparation techniques. Fertil Steril 62:850–856

Callahan TL, Hall JE, Ettner SL, Christiansen CL, Greene MF, Crowley WF Jr (1994) The economic impact of multiple-gestation pregnancies and the contribution of assisted-reproduction techniques to their incidence. N Engl J Med 331:244–249

Campos-Liete E, Insull M, Kennedy SH, Ellis JD, Sargent I, Barlow DH (1992) A controlled assessment of direct intraperitoneal insemination. Fertil Steril 57:168–173

Casper RF, Meriano JS, Jarvi KA, Cowan L, Lucato ML (1996) The hypo-osmotic swelling test for selection of viable sperm for intracytoplasmic sperm injection in men with complete asthenozoospermia. Fertil Steril 65:972–976

Catt JW, Ryan JP, Pike IL, Porter R, Saunders DM (1996) Successful pregnancy after fertilization using intracytoplasmic sperm injection of sperm lacking acrosomes. Aust NZ J Obstet Gynecol 36:61–62

Cederblad M, Friberg B, Ploman F, Sjöberg NO, Stjernqvist K, Zackrisson E (1996) Intelligence and behaviour in children born after in-vitro fertilization treatment. Hum Reprod 11:2052–2057

Chen HF, Ho HN, Chen SU, Lien YR, Chao KH, Lin HR, Huang SC, Lee TY, Yang YS (1994) Co-culture with Vero cell monolayer maintains the motility of asthenozoospermic semen samples. Hum Reprod 9:1276–1280

Chung PH, Palermo G, Schlegel PN, Veeck LL, Eid JF, Rosenwaks Z (1998) The use of intracytoplasmic sperm injection with electroejaculates from anejaculatory men. Hum Reprod 13:1854–1858

Cohen J, Alikani M, Trowbridge J, Rosenwaks Z (1992) Implantation enhancement by selective assited hatching using zona drilling of human embryos with poor prognosis. Hum Reprod 7:685–691

Cohlen BJ, te Velde ER, van Kooij RJ, Looman CWN, Habbema JDF (1998) Controlled ovarian hyperstimulation and intrauterine insemination for treating male subfertility: a controlled study. Hum Reprod 13:1553–1558

Collins JA, Wrixon W, Janes LB, Wilson EH (1983) Treatment-independent pregnancy among infertile couples. N Engl J Med 309:1201–1206

Collins JA, Burrows EA, Willan AR (1995) The prognosis for live birth among untreated infertile couples. Fertil Steril 64: 22–28

Cooper TG, Keck C, Oberdieck U, Nieschlag E (1993) Effects of multiple ejaculations after extended periods of sexual abstinence on total, motile and normal sperm numbers, as well as accessory gland secretions, from healthy normal and oligozoospermic men. Hum Reprod 8:1251–1258

Craft I, Tsirigotis M, Bennett V, Taranissi M, Khalifa Y, Hogewind G, Nicholson N (1995) Percutaneous epididymal sperm aspiration and intracytoplasmic sperm injection in the management of infertility due to obstructive azoospermia. Fertil Steril 63:1038–1042

Crosignani PG, Walters PE, Soliani A (1991) The ESHRE multicentre trial on the treatment of unexplained infertility: a preliminary report. Hum Reprod 6:953–958

Cruz RI, Kemmann E, Brandeis VT, Becker KA, Beck M, Beardsley L, Shelden R (1986) A prospective study of intrauterine insemination of processed sperm from men with oligoasthenospermia in superovulated women. Fertil Steril 46:673–677

Davis OK, Bedford JM, Berkeley AS, Graf MJ, Rosenwaks Z (1990) Pregnancy achieved through in vitro fertilization with cryopreserved semen from a man with Hodgkin's lymphoma. Fertil Steril 53:377–378

Daya S, Gwatkin RBL, Bissessar H (1987) Separation of motile human spermatozoa by means of a glass bead column. Gamete Res 17:375–380

De Geyter Ch, Bals-Pratsch M, Dören M, Yeung CH, Grunert JH, Bordt J, Schneider HPG, Nieschlag E (1988) Human and bovine cervical mucus penetration as a test of sperm function for in-vitro fertilization. Hum Reprod 3:948–954

De Geyter Ch, De Geyter M, Castro E, Bals-Pratsch M, Nieschlag E, Schneider HPG (1996) Experience with transvaginal ultrasound-guided aspiration of supernumerary follicles for the prevention of multiple pregnancies after ovulation induction and intrauterine insemination. Fertil Steril 65:1163–1168

De Geyter Ch, De Geyter M, Koppers B, Nieschlag E (1998) Diagnostic accuracy of computer-assisted sperm motion analysis. Hum Reprod 13:2512–2520

Devroey P, Braeckmans P, Smitz J, Van Waesberghe L, Wisanto A, Van Steirteghem A, Heytens L, Camu F (1986) Pregnancy after translaparoscopic zygote intrafallopian transfer in a patient with sperm antibodies. Lancet 1:1329

Devroey P, Liu J, Nagy Z, Tournaye H, Silber SJ, Van Steirteghem AC (1994) Normal fertilization of human oocytes after testicular sperm extraction and intracytoplasmic sperm injection. Fertil Steril 62:639–641

Dicker D, Ashkenazi J, Feldberg D, Levy T, Dekel A, Ben-Rafael Z (1993) Severe abdominal complications after transvaginal ultrasonographically guided retrieval of oocytes for in-vitro fertilization and embryo transfer. Fertil Steril 59:1313–1315

Diedrich K, Bauer O, Werner A, Van der Ven H, Al-Hasani S, Krebs D (1991) Transvaginal intratubal embryo transfer: a new treatment of male infertility. Hum Reprod 6:672–675

Dimitriadou F, Rizos D, Mantzavinos T, Arvaniti K, Voutsina K, Prapa A, Kanakas N (1995) The effect of pentoxiphylline on sperm motility, oocyte fertilization, embryo quality, and pregnancy outcome in an in vitro fertilization program. Fertil Steril 63:880–886

Dirnfeld M, Bider D, Koifman M, Calderon I, Abramovici H (1999) Shortened exposure of oocytes to spermatozoa improves in-vitro fertilization outcome: a prospective, randomized, controlled study. Hum Reprod 14:2562–2564

Doyle P, Bunch KJ, Beral V, Draper GJ (1999) Cancer incidence in children conceived with assisted reproduction technology. Lancet 352:452–453

Dozortsev D, Rybouchkin A, De Sutter P, Dhont M (1995) Sperm plasma membrane damage prior to intracytoplasmic sperm injection: a necessary condition for sperm nucleus decondensation. Hum Reprod 10:2960–2964

Duncan WW, Glew MJ, Wang XJ, Flaherty SP, Matthews CD (1993) Prediction of in vitro fertilization rates from semen variables. Fertil Steril 59:1233–1238

Edwards RG (1981) Test-tube babies, 1981. Nature 293:253–256

Emperaire JC, Gauzère-Soumireu E, Audebert AJM (1982) Female fertility and donor insemination. Fertil Steril 37:90–93

Englert Y, Van den Bergh M, Rodesch C, Bertrand E, Biramane J, Legreve A (1992) Comparative auto-controlled study between swim-up and Percoll preparation of fresh semen samples for in-vitro fertilization. Hum Reprod 7:399–402

Fishel S, Green S, Bishop M, Thornton S, Hunter A, Fleming S, Al-Hassan S (1995) Pregnancy after intracytoplasmic injection of spermatid. Lancet 345:1641–1642

Fischer R, Baukloh V, Naether OGJ, Schulze W, Salzbrunn A, Benson DM (1996) Pregnancy after intracytoplasmic sperm injection of spermatozoa extracted from frozen-thawed testicular biopsy. Hum Reprod 11:2197–2199

Fluker MR, Zouves CG, Bebbington MW (1993) A prospective randomized comparison of zygote intrafallopian transfer and in vitro fertilization-embryo transfer for nontubal factor infertility. Fertil Steril 60:515–519

Forrler A, Dellenbach P, Nisand I, Moreau L, Cranz C, Clavert A, Rumpler Y (1986) Direct intraperitoneal insemination in unexplained and cervical infertility. Lancet 2:916

Francavilla F, Romano R, Santucci R, Marrone V, Corrao G (1992) Failure of intrauterine insemination in male immunological infertility in cases in which all spermatozoa are antibody-coated. Fertil Steril 58:587–591

Friedler S, Raziel A, Strassburger D, Soffer Y, Komarovsky D, Ron-El R (1997) Testicular sperm retrieval by percutaneous fine needle sperm aspiration compared with testicular sperm extraction by open biopsy in men with non-obstructive azoospermia. Hum Reprod 12:1488–1493

Friedman AJ, Juneau-Norcross M, Sedensky B (1991) Antisperm antibody production following intrauterine insemination. Hum Reprod 6:1125–1128

Fugger EF, Black SH, Keyvanfar K, Schulman JD (1998) Births of normal daughters after MicroSort sperm separation and intrauterine insemination, in-vitro fertilization, or intracytoplasmic sperm injection. Hum Reprod 13:2367–2370

Gerris J, Van Royen E, Mangel-Schots K, Joostens M, De Vits A (1994) Pregnancy after intracytoplasmic sperm injection of metaphase II oocytes with spermatozoa from a man with complete retrograde ejaculation. Hum Reprod 9:1293–1296

Gerris J, De Neubourg D, Mangelschots K, Van Royen E, Van de Meerssche M, Valenburg M (1999) Prevention of twin pregnancy after in-vitro fertilization or intracytoplasmic sperm injection based on strict embryo criteria: a prospective randomized clinical trial. Hum Reprod 14:2581–2587

Glass RH, Ericsson RJ (1979) Spontaneous cure of male infertility. Fertil Steril 31:305–308

Golombok S, Brewaeys A, Cook R, Giavazzi MT, Guerra D, Mantovani A, van Hall E, Crosignani PG, Dexeus S (1996) The European study of assisted reproduction families: family functioning and child development. Hum Reprod 11:2324–2331

Goverde AJ, McDonnell J, Vermeiden JP, Schats R, Rutten FF, Schoemaker J (2000) Intrauterine insemination or in-vitro fertilisation in idiopathic subfertility and male subfertility: a randomised trial and cost-effectiveness analysis. Lancet 355:13–18

Grossmann M, Calafell JM, Brandy N, Vanrell JA, Rubio C, Pellicer A, Egozcue J, Vidal F, Santaló J (1997) Origin of triplonucleate zygotes after intracytoplasmic sperm injection. Hum Reprod 12:2762–2765

Guérin JF, Mathieu C, Lornage J, Pinatel MC, Boulieu D (1989) Improvement of survival and fertilizing capacity of human spermatozoa in an IVF programme by selection on discontinuous Percoll gradients. Hum Reprod 4:798–804

Guérin JF, Ouhibi N, Regnier-Vigouroux G, Menezo Y (1991) Movement characteristics and hyperactivation of human sperm on different epithelial cell monolayers. Int J Androl 14:412–422

Guzik DS, Carson SA, Coutifaris C, Overstreet JW, Factor-Litvak P, Steinkampf MP, Hill JA, Mastroianni L, Buster JE, Nakajima ST, Vogel DL, Canfield RE (1999) Efficacy of superovulation and intrauterine insemination in the treatment of infertility. National Cooperative Reproductive Medicine Network. N Engl J Med 340:177–183

Hamori M, Antoni K (1999) Chromosomal anomalies and malformations after ICSI without the use of PVP. Hum Reprod 14 (Abstract Book 1):58–59

Han TL, Flaherty SP, Ford JH, Matthews CD (1993) Detection of X- and Y-bearing human spermatozoa after motile sperm isolation by swim-up. Fertil Steril 60:1046–1050

Hershlag A, Paine T, Cooper GW, Scholl GM, Rawlinson K, Kvapil G (1999) Monozygotic twinning associated with mechanical assisted hatching. Fertil Steril 71:145–146

Hewitson L, Dominko T, Takahashi D, Martinovich C, Ramalho-Santos J, Sutovky P, Fanton J, Jacob D, Monteith D, Neuringer M, Battaglia D, Simerly C, Schatten G (1999) Unique checkpoints during the first cell cycle of fertilization after intracytoplasmic sperm injection in rhesus monkeys. Nat Med 5:431–433

Hirsh A, Montgomery J, Mohan P, Mells C, Bekir J, Tan SL (1993a) Reproduction by testicular sperm with standard IVF techniques. Lancet 2:1237–1238

Hirsh AV, Mills C, Tan SL, Bekir J, Rainsbury (1993b) Pregnancy using spermatozoa aspirated from the vas deferens in a patient with ejaculatory failure due to spinal injury. Hum Reprod 8:89–90

Hirsh AV, Mills C, Bekir J, Dean N, Yovich JL, Tan SL (1994) Factors influencing the outcome of in-vitro fertilization with epididymal spermatozoa in irreversible obstructive azoospermia. Hum Reprod 9:1710–1716

Ho PC, So WK, Chan YF, Yeung WHB (1992) Intrauterine insemination after ovarian stimulation as a treatment for subfertility because of subnormal semen: a prospective randomized controlled trial. Fertil Steril 58:995–999

Hoover MS, Baker BS, Check JH, Lurie D, Summers D (1997) Clinical outcome of cryopreserved human pronuclear stage embryos resulting from intracytoplasmic sperm injection. Fertil Steril 67:621–624

Horvath PM, Beck M, Bohrer MK, Shelden RM, Kemmann E (1989) A prospective study on the lack of development of antisperm antibodies in women undergoing intrauterine insemination. Am J Obstet Gynecol 160:631–637

Hovatta O, von Smitten K (1993) Sperm aspiration from vas deferens and in-vitro fertilization in cases of non-treatable anejaculation. Hum Reprod 8:1689–1691

Hovatta O, Kurunmäki H, Tiitinen A, Lähteenmäki P, Koskimies AI (1990) Direct intraperitoneal or intrauterine insemination and superovulation in infertility treatment: a randomized study. Fertil Steril 54:339–341

Hu Y, Maxson WS, Hoffman DI, Ory SJ, Licht MR, Eager S (1999) Clinical application of intracytoplasmic sperm injection using in vitro cultured testicular spermatozoa obtained the day before egg retrieval. Fertil Steril 72:666–669

Hughes EG, Fedorkow DM, Daya S, Sagle MA, Van de Koppel P, Collins JA (1992) The routine use of gonadotropin-releasing hormone agonists prior to in vitro fertilization and gamete intrafallopian transfer: a meta-analysis of randomized controlled trials. Fertil Steril 58:888–896

Hull MGR (1992) Infertility treatment: relative effectiveness of conventional and assisted conception methods. Hum Reprod 7:785–796

Hurd WW, Randolph Jr. JF, Ansbacher R, Menge AC, Ohl DA, Brown AN (1993) Comparison of intracervical, intrauterine, and intratubal techniques for donor insemination. Fertil Steril 59:339–342

Imoedemhe DAG, Sigue AB, Pacpaco ELA, Olazo AB (1992) The effect of caffeine on the ability of spermatozoa to fertilize mature human oocytes. J Ass Reprod Genet 9:155–160

Jansen RPS, Anderson JC (1987) Catheterisation of the fallopian tubes from the vagina. Lancet 2:309–310

Jaroudi KA, Carver-Ward JA, Hamilton CJCM, Sieck UV, Sheth KV (1993) Percoll semen preparation enhances human oocyte fertilization in male-factor infertility as shown by a randomized cross-over study. Hum Reprod 8:1438–1442

Jezek D, Knuth UA, Schulze W (1998) Successful testicular sperm extraction (TESE) in spite of high serum follicle stimulating hormone and azoospermia: correlation between testicular morphology, TESE results, semen analysis and serum hormone values in 103 infertile men. Hum Reprod 13:1230–1234

Johnson LA, Welch GR, Keyvanfar K, Dorfmann A, Fugger EF, Schulman JD (1993) Gender preselection in humans? Flow cytometric separation of X and Y spermatozoa for the prevention of X-linked diseases. Hum Reprod 8:1733–1739

Kahn JA, Sunde A, Koskemies A, von Düring V, Sordal T, Christensen F, Molne K (1993a) Fallopian tube sperm perfusion (FSP) veresus intra-uterine insemination (IUI) in the treatment of unexplained infertility: a prospective randomized study. Hum Reprod 8:890–894

Kahn JA, Sunde A, von Düring V, Sordal T, Remen A, Lippe B, Siegel J, Molne K (1993b) Formation of antisperm antibodies in women treated with Fallopian tube sperm perfusion. Hum Reprod 8:1414–1419

Kahraman S, Özgür S, Alatas C, Aksoy S, Balaban B, Evrenkaya T, Nuhoglu A, Tasdemir M, Biberoglu K, Schoysman R, Vanderzwalmen P, Nijs M (1996) High implantation and pregnancy rates with testicular sperm extraction and intracytoplasmic sperm injection in obstructive and non-obstructive azoospermia. Hum Reprod 11:673–676

Kahraman S, Isik AZ, Vicdan K, Özgür S, Özgün OD (1997) A healthy birth after intracytoplasmic sperm injection by using immotile testicular spermatozoa in a case with totally immotile ejaculated spermatozoa before and after Percoll gradients. Hum Reprod 12:292–293

Kamischke A, Nieschlag E (1999) Treatment of retrograde ejaculation and anejaculation. Hum Reprod Update 5:448–474

Kan AKS, Abdalla HI, Gafar AH, Nappi L, Ogunyemi BO, Thomas A, Ola-ojo OO (1999) Embryo transfer: ultrasound-guided versus clinical touch. Hum Reprod 14:1259–1261

Kanwar KC, Yanagimachi R, Lopata A (1979) Effects of human seminal plasma on fertilizing capacity of human spermatozoa. Fertil Steril 31:321–327

Kastrop PMM, Weima SM, Van Kooij RJ, Te Velde ER (1999) Comparison between intracytoplasmic sperm injection and in-vitro fertilization (IVF) with high insemination concentration after total fertilization failure in a previous IVF attempt. Hum Reprod 14: 65–69

Katayama KP, Stehlik E, Jeyendran RS (1989) In vitro fertilization outcome: glass wool-filtered sperm versus swim-up. Fertil Steril 52:670–672

Kato O, Takatsuka R, Asch RH (1993) Transvaginal-transmyometrial embryo transfer: the Towako method; experiences of 104 cases. Fertil Steril 59:51–53

Kay VJ, Coutts JRT, Robertson L (1993) Pentoxyphylline stimulates hyperactivation in human spermatozoa. Hum Reprod 8:727–731

Khalifa E, Oehninger S, Acosta AA, Morshedi M, Veeck L, Bryzyski RG, Muasher SJ (1992) Successful fertilization and pregnancy outcome in in-vitro fertilization using cryopreserved/thawed spermatozoa from patients with malignant diseases. Hum Reprod 7:105–108

Kirby CA, Flaherty SP, Godfrey BM, Warnes GM, Matthews CD (1991) A prospective trial of intrauterine insemination of motile spermatozoa versus timed intercourse. Fertil Steril 56:102–107

Kurinczuk JJ, Bower C (1997) Birth defects in infants conceived by intracytoplasmic sperm injection: an alternative interpretation. Br Med J 315:1260–1266

Leeton J, Roger P, Caro C, Healy D, Yates C (1987) A controlled study between the use of gamete intrafallopian transfer (GIFT) and in vitro fertilization and embryo transfer in the management of idiopathic and male infertility. Fertil Steril 48:605–607

Léridon H, Spira A (1984) Problems in measuring the effectiveness of infertility therapy. Fertil Steril 41:580–586

Lewin A, Reubinoff B, Poratz-Katz A, Weiss D, Eisenberg V, Arbel R, Bar-el H, Safran A (1999) Testicular fine needle aspiration: the alternative method for sperm retrieval in non-obstructive azoospermia. Hum Reprod 14:1785–1790

Liu J, Nagy Z, Joris H, Tournaye H, Devroey P, Van Steirteghem AC (1995) Successful fertilization and establishment of pregnancies after intracytoplasmic sperm injection in patients with globozoospermia. Hum Reprod 10:626–629

Liu J, Tsai Y-L, Katz E, Compton G, Garcia JE, Baramki TA (1997) High fertilization rate obtained after intracytoplasmic sperm injection with 100 % nonmotile spermatozoa selected by using a simple modified hypo-osmotic swelling test. Fertil Steril 68:373–375

Loft A, Petersen K, Erb K, Mikkelsen AL, Grinstedt J, Hald F, Hinkdjaer J, Nielsen KM, Lundstrom P, Gabrielsen A, Lenz S, Hornnes P, Ziebe S, Ejdrup HB, Lindhard A, Zhou Y, Nyboe Andersen A (1999) A Danish national cohort of 730 infants born after intracytoplasmic sperm injection (ICSI) 1994–1997. Hum Reprod 14:2143–2148

Lopata A, Patullo MJ, Chang A, James B (1976) A method for collecting motile spermatozoa from human semen. Fertil Steril 27:677–684

Lucena E, Ruiz JA, Mendoza JC, Lucena A, Arango A (1991) Direct intrafollicular insemination: case report. J Reprod Med 36:525–526

Ludwig M, Ghasemi M, von Gizycki U, Al-Hasani S, Küpker W, Felberbaum R, Diedrich K (1998) Auswertung der Daten von 310 Schwangerschaften und 270 geborenen Kindern nach IVF/ICSI. Arch Gynecol Obstet 261 [Suppl 1]: Abstract P3.06.11

Ludwig M, Al-Hasani S, Felberbaum R, Diedrich K (1999) New aspects of cryopreservation of oocytes and embryos in assisted reproduction and future perspectives. Hum Reprod 14 [Suppl 1]:162–185

Luetjens CM, Payne C, Schatten G (1999) Non-random chromosome positioning in human sperm and sex chromosome anomalies following intracytoplasmic sperm injection. Lancet 353:1240

Lundin K, Sjögren A, Nilsson L, Hamberger L (1994) Fertilization and pregnancy after intracytoplasmic microinjection of acrosomeless spermatozoa. Fertil Steril 62:1266–1267

Mahadevan MM, Trounson AO (1985) Removal of the cumulus oophorus from the human oocyte for in vitro fertilization. Fertil Steril 43:263–267

Mansour RT, Aboulghar MA, Serour GI, Abbas AM, Elattar I (1995) The life span of sperm motility and pattern in cumulus coculture. Fertil Steril 63:660–662

Martinez AR, Bernardus RE, Voorhorst FJ, Vermeiden JPW, Schoemaker J (1991) Pregnancy rates after timed intercourse or intrauterine insemination after human menopausal gonadotropin stimulation of normal ovulatory cycles: a controlled study. Fertil Steril 55:258–265

Meschede D, Horst J (1997) Sex chromosomal anomalies in pregnancies conceived through intracytoplasmatic sperm injection – a case for genetic counselling. Hum Reprod 12:1125–1127

Meschede D, Lemcke B, Stüssel J, Louwen F, Horst J (1998) Strong preference for non-invasive prenatal diagnosis in women pregnant through intracytoplasmic sperm injection (ICSI). Prenat Diagn 18:700–705

Meschede D, Lemcke B, Behre HM, De Geyter Ch, Nieschlag E, Horst J (2000) Clustering of male infertility in the families of couples treated with intracytoplasmatic sperm injection. 15:1604–1608

Milki A, Fisch JD, Behr B (1999) Two-blastocyst transfer has similar pregnancy rates and a decreased multiple gestation rate compared with three-blastocyst transfer. Fertil Steril 72:225–228

Mills MS, Eddowes HA, Cahill DJ, Fahy UM, Abuzeid MIM, McDermott A, Hull MGR (1992) A prospective controlled study of in-vitro fertilization, gamete intra-Fallopian transfer and intrauterine insemination combined with superovulation. Hum Reprod 7:490–494

Milunsky A (1998) Multianalyte maternal serum screening for chromosomal defects. In: Milunsky A (ed) Genetic disorders and the fetus. Johns Hopkins University Press, Baltimore, pp 702–749

Moretti-Rojas I, Rojas FJ, Leisure M, Stone SC, Asch RH (1990) Intrauterine inseminations with washed human spermatozoa does not induce formation of antisperm antibodies. Fertil Steril 53:180–182

MRC Working Party on Children Conceived by In Vitro Fertilization (1990) Births in Great Britain resulting from assisted conception, 1978–1987. Br Med J 300:1229–1233

Nagy ZP, Liu J, Joris H, Bocken G, Desmet B, Van Ranst H, Vankelecom A, Devroey P, Van Steirteghem AC (1995) The influence of the site of sperm deposition and mode of oolemma breakage at intracytoplasmic sperm injection on fertilization and embryo development rates. Hum Reprod 10:3171–3177

Nijs M, Vanderzwalmen P, Vandamme B, Segal-Bertin G, Lejeune B, Segal L, van Roosendaal E, Schoysman R (1996) Fertilizing ability of immotile spermatozoa after intracytoplasmic sperm injection. Hum Reprod 11:2180–2185

Norman RJ, Payne D, Matthews CD (1995) Pregnancy following intracytoplasmic sperm injection (ICSI) of a single oocyte in a natural cycle. Hum Reprod 10:1626–1627

Nuojua-Huttunen S, Tuomivaara L, Juntunen K, Tomás C, Kauppila A, Martikainen H (1995) Intrafollicular insemination for the treatment of infertility. Hum Reprod 10:91–93

Oehninger S, Acosta AA, Morshed M, Veeck L, Swanson RJ, Simmons K, Rosenwaks Z (1988) Corrective measures and pregnancy outcome in in vitro fertilization in patients with severe sperm morphology abnormalities. Fertil Steril 50:283–287

Oei ML, Surrey ES, McCaleb B, Kerin JF (1992) A prospective, randomized study of pregnancy rates after transuterotubal and intrauterine insemination. Fertil Steril 58:167–171

Olivennes E, Alvarez S, Bouchard P, Fanchin R, Salat-Baroux J, Frydman R (1998) The use of a GnRH antagonist (Cetrorelix) in a single dose protocol in IVF-embryo transfer: a dose finding study of 3 versus 2 mg. Hum Reprod 13:2411–2414

Ord T, Patrizio P, Marello E, Balmaceda JP, Asch RH (1990) Mini-Percoll: a new method of semen preparation for IVF in severe male factor infertility. Hum Reprod 5:987–989

Palermo G, Devroey P, Camus M, De Grauwe E, Khan I, Staessen C, Wisanto A, Van Steirteghem AC (1989) Zygote intra-Fallopian transfer as an alternative treatment for male infertility. Hum Reprod 4:412–415

Palermo G, Joris H, Devroey P, Van Steirteghem AC (1992) Pregnancies after intracytoplasmic sperm injection of single spermatozoon into an oocyte. Lancet 340:17–18

Palermo G, Joris H, Derde MP, Camus M, Devroey P, Van Steirteghem AC (1993) Sperm characteristics and outcome of human assisted fertilization by subzonal insemination and intracytoplasmic sperm injection. Fertil Steril 59:826–835

Palermo GD, Cohen J, Alikani M, Adler A, Rosenwaks Z (1995) Intracytoplasmic sperm injection: a novel treatment for all forms of male factor infertility. Fertil Steril 63:1231–1240

Palermo GD, Colombero LT, Schattman GD, Davis OK, Rosenwaks Z (1996) Evolution of pregnancies and initial follow-up of newborns delivered after intracytoplasmatic sperm injection. JAMA 276: 1893–1897

Parrington J, Swann K, Shevchenko VI, Sesay AK, Lai FA (1996) Calcium oscillations in mammalian oocytes by a factor obtained from rabbit sperm. Nature 379:364–368

Pattinson HA, Mortimer D, Curtis EF, Leader A, Taylor PJ (1990) Treatment of sperm agglutination with proteinolytic enzymes. I. Sperm motility, vitality, longevity and successful disagglutination. Hum Reprod 5:167–173

Patton PE, Burry KA, Thurmond A, Novy MJ, Wolf DP (1992) Intrauterine insemination outperforms intracervical insemination in a randomized, controlled study with frozen, donor semen. Fertil Steril 57:559–564

Paulson JD, Polakoski KL (1977) A glass wool column procedure for removing extraneous material from the human ejaculate. Fertil Steril 28:178–181

Payne D, Flaherty SP, Barry MF, Matthews CD (1997) Preliminary observations on polar body extrusion and pronuclear formation in human oocytes using time-lapse video cinematography. Hum Reprod 12:532–541

Pearlstone AC, Chan SYW, Tucker MJ, Wiker SR, Wang C (1993) The effects of Vero (Green monkey kidney) cell coculture on the motility patterns of cryopreserved human spermatozoa. Fertil Steril 59:1105–1111

Peterson CM, Hatasaka JJ, Jones KP, Poulson AM Jr, Carrell DT, Urry RL (1994) Ovulation induction with gonadotropins and intrauterine insemination compared with in vitro fertilization and no therapy: a prospective, nonrandomized, cohort study and meta-analysis. Fertil Steril 62:535–544

Pickering SJ, Fleming TP, Braude PR, Bolton VN, Gresham GAG (1989) Are human spermatozoa separated on a Percoll density gradient safe for therapeutic use? Fertil Steril 51:1024–1029

Ragni G, Maggioni P, Guermandi E, Testa A, Baroni E, Colombo M, Crosignani PG (1999) Efficacy of double intrauterine insemination in controlled ovarian hyperstimulation cycles. Fertil Steril 72:619–622

Ramsewak SS, Cooke ID, Li TC, Kumar A, Monks NJ, Lenton EA (1990) Are factors that influence oocyte fertilization also predictive? An assessment of 148 cycles of in vitro fertilization without gonadotropin stimulation. Fertil Steril 54:470–474

Ray BD, Howell RT, McDermott A, Hull MGR (1995) Testing the mutagenic potential of polyvinylpyrrollidone and methyl cellulose by sister chromatid exchange analysis prior to use in intracytoplasmic sperm injection procedures. Hum Reprod 10:436–438

Reubinoff BE, Shushan A (1996) Preimplantation diagnosis in older patients. To biopsy or not to biopsy? Hum Reprod 11:2071–2078

Rhemrev J, Jeyendran RS, Vermeiden JPW, Zaneveld LJD (1989) Human sperm selection by glass wool filtration and two-layer, discontinuous Percoll gradient centrifugation. Fertil Steril 51:685–690

Ripps BA, Minhas BS, Carson SA, Buster JE (1994) Intrauterine insemination in fertile women delivers larger numbers of sperm to the peritoneal fluid than intracervical insemination. Fertil Steril 61:398–400

Roest J, van Heusden AM, Verhoeff A, Mous HVH, Zeilmaker GH (1997) A triplet pregnancy after in vitro fertilization is a procedure-related complication that should be prevented by replacement of two embryos only. Fertil Steril 67:290–295

Rosenlund B, Westlander G, Wood M, Lundin K, Reismer E, Hillensjö T (1998) Sperm retrieval and fertilization in repeated percutaneous epididymal sperm aspiration. Hum Reprod 13:2805–2807

Rossin-Amar B, Safi A, Pouly JL, de Mouzon J (1999) Analysis of babies conceived by ICSI. Comparison with babies born after conventional in-vitro fertilization or natural conception. Hum Reprod 14 (Abstract Book 1):79–80

Salzbrunn A, Benson DM, Holstein AF, Schulze W (1996) A new concept for the extraction of testicular spermatozoa as a tool for assisted fertilization (ICSI). Hum Reprod 11:752–755

Scholtes MCW, Roozenburg BJ, Verhoeff A, Zeilmaker GH (1994) A randomized study of transcervical intrafallopian transfer of pronucleate embryos controlled by ultrasound versus intrauterine transfer of four- to eight-cell embryos. Fertil Steril 61:102–104

Schulze W, Thoms F, Knuth UA (1999) Testicular sperm extraction: comprehensive analysis with simultaneously performed histology in 1418 biopsies from 766 subfertile men. Hum Reprod 14 [Suppl 1]:82–96

Silber SJ, Balmaceda J, Borrero C, Ord T, Asch R (1988) Pregnancy with sperm aspiration from the proximal head of the epididymis: a new treatment for congenital absence of the vas deferens. Fertil Steril 50:525–528

Silber SJ, Van Steirteghem AC, Liu J, Nagy Z, Tournaye H, Devroey P (1995) High fertilization and pregnancy rate after intracytoplasmic sperm injection with spermatozoa obtained from testicle biopsy. Hum Reprod 10:148–152

Silverberg KM, Johnson JV, Olive DL, Burns WN, Schenken RS (1992) A prospective, randomized trial comparing two different intrauterine insemination regimens in controlled ovarian hyperstimulation cycles. Fertil Steril 57:357–361

Sofikitis N, Mantzavinos T, Loutradis D, Yamamoto Y, Tarlatzis V, Miyagawa I (1998) Ooplasmic injections of secondary spermatocytes for non-obstructive azoospermia. Lancet 351:1177–1178

Soliman S, Daya S, Collins J, Jarrell (1993) A randomized trial of in vitro fertilization versus conventional treatment for infertility. Fertil Steril 59:1239–1244

Spira A (1986) Epidemiology of human reproduction. Hum Reprod 1:111–115

Staessen C, Janssenswillen C, Van Den Abbeel E, Devroey P, Van Steirteghem AC (1993) Avoidance of triplet pregnancies by elective transfer of two good quality embryos. Hum Reprod 8:1650–1653

Staessen C, Camus M, Claesen K, De Vos A, Van Steirteghem A (1999) Conventional in-vitro fertilization versus intracytoplasmic sperm injection in sibling oocytes from couples with tubal infertility and normozoospermic semen. Hum Reprod 14:2474–2479

Steele EK, McClure N, Maxwell RJ, Lewis SEM (1999) A comparison of DNA damage in testicular and proximal epididymal spermatozoa in obstructive azoospermia. Mol Hum Reprod 5:831–835

Steptoe PC (1970) Laparoscopic recovery of preovulatory human oocytes after priming of ovaries with gonadotrophins. Lancet 1:683–689

Strandell A, Lindhard A, Waldenström U, Thorburn J, Janson PO, Hamberger L (1999) Hydrosalpinx and IVF outcome: a prospective, randomize multicentre trial in Scandinavia on salpingectomy prior to IVF. Hum Reprod 14:2762–2769

Sultan KM, Munné S, Palermo GD, Alikani M, Cohen J (1995) Chromosomal status of uni-pronuclear human zygotes following in-vitro fertilization and intracytoplasmic sperm injection. Hum Reprod 10:132–136

Sutcliffe AG, Taylor B, Li J, Thornton S, Grudzinskas JG, Lieberman BA (1999a) Children born after intracytoplasmic sperm injection: population control study. Br Med J 318:704–705

Sutcliffe AG, Taylor B, Li J, Thornton S, Grudzinskas JG, Lieberman BA. (1999b) United Kingdom study of children born after intracytoplasmic sperm injection. Hum Reprod 14 (Abstract Book 1):10

Tan SL, Royston P, Campbell S, Jacobs HS, Betts J, Mason B, Edwards RG (1992a) Cumulative conception and livebirth rates after in-vitro fertilization. Lancet 1:1390–1394

Tan SL, Kingsland C, Campbell S, Mills C, Bradfield J, Alexander N, Yovich J, Jacobs HS (1992b) The long protocol of administration of gonadotropin-releasing hormone agonist is superior to the short protocol for ovarian stimulation for in vitro fertilization. Fertil Steril 57:810–814

Tanbo T, Dale PO, Abyholm T (1990) Assisted fertilization in infertile women with patent Fallopian tubes. A comparison of in-vitro fertilization, gamete intra-Fallopian transfer and tubal embryo stage transfer. Hum Reprod 5:266–270

Tasdemir I, Tasdemir M, Tavukcuoglu S, Kahraman, Biberoglu K (1997) Effect of abnormal sperm head morphology on the outcome of intracytoplasmic sperm injections in humans. Hum Reprod 12:1214–1217

Temple-Smith PD, Southwick GJ, Yates CA, Trounson AO, De Kretser DM (1985) Human pregnancy by in vitro fertilization (IVF) using sperm aspirated from the epididymis. J In Vitro Fert Embryo Transfer 2:119–122

Templeton A, Morris JK, Parslow W (1996) Factors that affect outcome of in-vitro reproduction treatment. Lancet 348:1402–1406

te Velde ER, van Kooy RJ, Waterreus JJH (1989) Intrauterine insemination of washed husband's spermatozoa: a controlled study. Fertil Steril 51:182–185

Tournaye H, Camus M, Bollen N, Wisanto A, Van Steirteghem AC, Devroey P (1991) In vitro fertilization techniques with frozen-thawed sperm: a method for preserving the progenitive potential of Hodgkin patients. Fertil Steril 55:443–445

Tournaye H, Devroey P, Camus M, Staessen C, Bollen N, Smitz J, Van Steirteghem AC (1992a) Comparison of in-vitro fertilization in male and tubal infertility: a 3 year survey. Hum Reprod 7:218–222

Tournaye H, Devroey P, Camus M, Valkenburg M, Bollen N, Van Steirteghem AC (1992b) Zygote intrafallopian transfer or in vitro fertilization and embryo transfer for the treatment of male factor infertility: a prospective randomized trial. Fertil Steril 58:344–350

Tournaye H, Devroey P, Liu J, Nagy Z, Lissens W, Van Steirteghem AC (1994a) Microsurgical epididymal sperm aspiration and intracytoplasmic sperm injection: a new effective approach to infertility as a result of congenital absence of the vas deferens. Fertil Steril 61:1045–1051

Tournaye H, Janssens R, Verheyen G, Camus M, Devroey P, Van Steirteghem AC (1994b) An indiscriminate use of pentoxyphylline does not improve in-vitro fertilization in poor fertilizers. Hum Reprod 9:1289–1292

Tournaye H, Liu J, Nagy Z, Verheyen G, Van Steirteghem AC, Devroey P (1996) The use of testicular sperm for intracytoplasmic sperm injection in patients with necrozoospermia. Fertil Steril 66:331–334

Tsirigotis M, Yang D, Redgment CJ, Nicholson N, Pelekanos M, Craft IL (1994) Assisted fertilization with intracytoplasmic sperm injection. Fertil Steril 62:781–785

Tucker MJ (1995) Micromanipulative and conventional insemination strategies for assisted reproductive technology. Am J Obstet Gynecol 172:773–778

Tur-Kaspa I, Dudkiewicz A, Confino E, Gleicher N (1990) Pooled sequential ejaculates: a way to increase the total number of motile sperm from oligozoospermic men. Fertil Steril 54:906–909

Tycko B, Trasler J, Bestor T (1997) Genomic imprinting: gametic mechanisms and somatic consequences. J Androl 18:480–486

Van den Bergh M, Bertrand E, Biramane J, Englert Y (1995) Importance of breaking a spermatozoon's tail before intracytoplasmic injection: a prospective randomized trial. Hum Reprod 10:2819–2820

Van der Westerlaken LAJ, Helmerhorst FM, Hermans J, Naaktgeboren N (1999) Intracytoplasmic sperm injection: position of the polar body affects pregnancy rate. Hum Reprod 14:2565–2569

Van der Ven HH, Hoebbel K, Al-Hasani S, Diedrich K, Krebs D (1987) Befruchtung menschlicher Eizellen in Kapillarröhrchen mit sehr geringen Spermatozoenzahlen. Geburtsh Frauenheilkd 47:630–635

Van der Ven HH, Jeyendran RS, Al-Hasani S, TÅnnerhoff A, Hoebbel K, Diedrich K, Krebs D, Perez-Palaez M (1988) Glass wool column filtration of human semen: relation to swim-up procedure and outcome of IVF. Hum Reprod 3:85–88

Vanderzwalmen P, Zech H, Birkenfeld A, Yemini M, Bertin G, Lejeune B, Nijs M, Segal L, Stecher A, Vandamme B, van Roosendaal E, Schoysman R (1997) Intracytoplasmic sperm injection of spermatids retrieved from testicular tissue: influence of testicular pathology, type of selected spermatids and oocyte activation. Hum Reprod 12:1203–1213

Van Steirteghem AC, Nagy Z, Joris H, Liu J, Staessen C, Smitz J, Wisanto A, Devroey P (1993a) High fertilization and implantation rates after intracytoplasmic sperm injection. Hum Reprod 8:1061–1066

Van Steirteghem AC, Liu J, Joris H, Nagy Z, Janssenswillen C, Tournaye H, Derde MP, Van Assche E, Devroey P (1993b) Higher sucess rate by intracytoplasmic sperm injection than by subzonal insemination. Report of a second series of 300 consecutive treatment cycles. Hum Reprod 8:1055–1060

Verlinsky Y, Rechitsky S, Verlinsky O, Ivachnenko V, Lifchez A, Kaplan B, Moise J, Valle J, Borkowski A, Nefedova J, Goltsman E, Strom C, Kuliev A (1999) Prepregnancy testing for single-gene disorders by polar body analysis. Genet Test 3:185–190

Vidal F, Moragas M, Català V, Torelló MJ, Santaló J, Calderón G, Gimenez C, Barri PN, Egozcue J, Veiga A (1993) Sephadex filtration and human serum albumin gradients do not select spermatozoa by sex chromosome: a fluorescent in-situ hybridization study. Hum Reprod 8:1740–1743

Vilska S, Tiitinen A, Hyden-Granskog C, Hovatta O (1999) Elective transfer of one embryo results in an acceptable pregnancy rate and eliminates the risk of multiple birth. Hum Reprod 14:2392–2395

Werner-von der Burg W, Coordes I, Hatzmann W (1993) Pregnancy following intrafollicular gamete transfer. Hum Reprod 8:771–774

Wennerholm U-B, Bergh C, Hamberger L, Nilsson L, Wikland M (1999) Obstetric and perinatal outcome of pregnancies following intracytoplasmic sperm injection. Hum Reprod 14 (Abstract Book 1):57–58

Wetzels AMM, Bastiaans BA, Goverde HJM, Janssen HJG, Rolland R (1991) Vero cells stimulate human sperm motility in vitro. Fertil Steril 56:535–539

WHO (1999) Laborhandbuch zur Untersuchung des menschlichen Ejakulates und der Spermien-Zervikalschleim-Interaktion, 4th edn. Springer, Berlin Heidelberg New York

Williams DB, Moley KH, Cholewa C, Odem RR, Willand J, Gast MJ (1995) Does intrauterine insemination offer an advantage to cervical cap insemination in a donor insemination program? Fertil Steril 63:295–298

Xia P (1997) Intracytoplasmic sperm injection: correlation of oocyte grade based on polar body, perivitelline space and cytoplasmic inclusions with fertilization rate and embryo quality. Hum Reprod 12:1750–1755

Yemini M, Vanderzwalmen P, Mukaida T, Schoengold S, Birkenfeld A (1995) Intracytoplasmic sperm injection, fertilization, and embryo transfer after retrieval of spermatozoa by testicular biopsy from an azoospermic male with testicular tubular atrophy. Fertil Steril 63:1118–1120

Yovich JL, Blackledge DG, Richardson PA, Matson PL, Turner SR, Drager R (1987) Pregnancies following pronuclear stage tubal transfer. Fertil Steril 48:851–857

Yovich JM, Edirisinghe WR, Cummins JM, Yovich JL (1990) Influence of pentoxiphylline in severe male factor infertility. Fertil Steril 53:715–722

Zbella EA, Tarantino S, Wade R (1992) Intrafollicular insemination for male factor infertility. Fertil Steril 55:442–443

Zreik TG, García-Velasco JA, Habboosh MS, Olive DL, Arici A (1999) Prospective, randomized, crossover study to evaluate the benefit of human chorionic gonadotropin-timed versus urinary luteinizing hormone-timed intrauterine inseminations in clomiphene citrate-stimulated treatment cycles. Fertil Steril 71:1070–1074

CHAPTER 18

Cryopreservation of Human Semen

18

S. KLIESCH · A. KAMISCHKE · E. NIESCHLAG

Malignant diseases in children and adults can be cured by surgery, chemo- or radiotherapy in a high percentage of cases, resulting in increased survival rates. In those patients where this is not possible, an increase of disease-free intervals may be achieved by adequate therapeutic strategies. Therefore the implications for long-term toxicity and delayed results of therapeutic intervention become more and more important. Chemo- or radiotherapy as well as surgical intervention have a tremendous influence on male reproductive functions. Their negative influence on reproduction depends on the therapeutic modalities, the substances and dosages chosen and can be irreversible.

> Cryopreservation of semen represents a preventive, concomitant therapeutic option of oncological patients that offers the chance of maintaining reproductive abilities.

The following chapter provides a review of the present state of technology, practicability and limits of cryopreservation of human spermatozoa. Its aim is to encourage physicians and health care providers to consider the needs of a patient's life quality in respect to his family planning and fertility on a long-term basis and to include these topics when counselling the patient and planning therapy.

18.1 History of Cryopreservation of Human Semen

The first observation that human sperm can preserve their motility after freezing and thawing was made by Spallanzani in 1776. In the middle of the 19th century the idea arose to establish a sperm bank for cattle breeding. At nearly the same time the possibility of freezing soldiers' semen was considered with the purpose of enabling their wives to bear their children, should they die during war. Serious attempts to improve the technical requirements of the cryopreservation of semen were performed in the first half of the 20th century (Jahnel 1938; Shettles 1940; Hoagland and Pincus 1942; Sherman

1963). Great improvements were achieved by introducing the first cryoprotective substance, glycerin, into the cryopreservation process to protect spermatozoa during freezing (Polge et al. 1942). By this invention sperm function could be preserved. Shortly after that, the first successful fertilization and pregnancy with cryopreserved semen was reported (for review see Byrd et al. 1990).

18.2 Analysis and Preparation of Semen Samples for Cryopreservation

The liquefied ejaculate is analyzed according to the guidelines of the World Health Organization (WHO 1999) (see Chap. 6). The standard parameters sperm concentration, total number of sperm, sperm morphology and motility prior to cryopreservation give important information for later use of the semen in assisted fertilization procedures. In addition, sperm function tests can be performed, such as the hypo-osmotic swelling (HOS) test to investigate whether the sperm membrane remains intact. However, no correlation between hypo-osmotic swelling and sperm quality after cryopreservation could be established (Chan et al. 1993).

The eosin test as an indicator of vital sperm may be useful to demonstrate the percentage of vital sperm after cryopreservation. A selection of motile sperm prior to cryopreservation by swim-up procedures does not lead to an improvement of sperm quality after cryopreservation in comparison to cryopreservation of unselected, native ejaculates. However, investigating ejaculates of healthy volunteers demonstrated that by modifying the cryopreservation procedure and sperm selection by swim-up prior to cryopreservation the results of sperm morphology obtained after freezing and thawing could be improved (Péréz-Sanchez et al. 1994). It still remains unclear whether sperm morphology is of importance for successful artificial fertilization in humans.

During the **process of freezing** spermatozoa are exposed to extreme temperature changes that result in damaged sperm morphology and function by changing the states of aggregation at extracellular and intracellular levels. Dehydration results in shrinkage of the cell and the extra- and intra-cellular formation of ice crystals leads to impairment of electrolyte concentrations of spermatozoa and to disruption of sperm membrane permeability (Hammerstedt et al. 1990; Watson et al. 1992).

Ice crystals will cause intracellular lesions and cell death during thawing. Therefore **cryoprotective media** are added to the ejaculate prior to the freezing process. They are based either on egg yolk mixed with glucose and fructose or consist of culture media, human serum albumin, glycerin and additional kallikrein. These cryoprotective media are used to prevent cell shrinkage by influencing the ion exchange of the cells and reducing ice crystal formation (e.g. glycerol and sorbitol, which are sperm membrane-penetrating cryoprotective substances). Cryoprotective substances that do not penetrate the sperm membrane (e.g. human serum albumin and additions based on egg yolk) are protective by binding to and stabilizing the cell membrane (Watson et al. 1992). Experimentally, antioxidants (vitamin E), substances forming calcium chelates such as EDTA, or derivatives of phosphatidylcholine (platelet-activating factor) and derivatives of methylxanthine (pentoxyfylline) are used for cryopreservation of spermatozoa (Alvarez and Storey 1993; Wang et al. 1993). Moreover, novel techniques aimed at improving post-thaw sperm motility by varying concentrations of what are being attempted (Morris et al. 1999).

18.3 Cryopreservation Techniques

After liquefaction at $37°C$ the sterile ejaculate is carefully mixed with the same volume of a cryoprotective medium (volume/volume) (e.g. Steritec™, Steripharm, Berlin, Germany; TEST-Yolk buffer, freezing medium, Irvine Scientific, Irvine, CA, USA). The diluted semen sample is transferred to straws under sterile laboratory conditions. Each straw has a maximum volume of 300 µl and consists of a plastic material that offers optimal temperature distribution during cooling. A maximum of 12 straws can be stored in one cryo-cassette. The cryo-cassettes are cooled using a computerized, automated cryo-machine (e.g. Planer Kryo 10-Serie II, Messer Griesheim, Krefeld, Germany, ICEcube™ 1810, Tec-Lab, Hedel, Netherlands) to offer standardized cryopreservation conditions.

Inadequate **freezing and thawing conditions** may lead to cell shrinkage, osmotic cell lesions and ice crystal formation. Therefore freezing and thawing times should be well adjusted (Hammerstedt et al. 1990; Watson et al. 1992). Most groups work with stepwise freezing. Shortly after reaching the freezing point of water, extracellular ice crystal formation begins at about $-5°C$, and at about $-15°C$ to $-80°C$ intracellular ice crystal formation occurs (Hammerstedt et al. 1990). There are no uniform guidelines available for the optimal freezing time to be chosen between $0°C$ to $-80°C$. In principle, cooling leads to increased cell shrinkage by dehydration if it is performed too rapidly, while it promotes ice crystal formation if it is performed too slowly. A freezing velocity of 8 to $21°C$ per minute is used by most groups working with cryopreservation of human semen. After $-196°C$ is reached the cryopreserved semen samples are **stored in liquid nitrogen**.

When semen samples are later thawed, **thawing velocity** should be adapted to freezing velocity (Hammerstedt et al. 1990; Watson et al. 1992). At our institute we use the programmed cryo-machine which is initially cooled to –196°C, and afterwards thawing is performed in reverse o the freezing programme. Other institutions choose room temperature or a water bath warmed to 37°C for thawing. After cryopreservation is performed we recommend thawing a small aliquot of the sample to analyze sperm motility. This information may be helpful for later use of the sperm during assisted fertilization techniques.

Surgically retrieved spermatozoa (either epididymal or testicular) are placed in a special medium for transportation and further preparation, are then mixed with cryoprotective substances and finally cryopreserved and stored in liquid nitrogen. The ampoules for storage vary from laboratory to laboratory. Usually for epididymal probes the above-mentioned "straws" are used whereas for testicular probes small tubes suitable for sterile cryopreservation are employed (Salzbrunn et al. 1996).

18.4 Storage of Cryopreserved Semen Samples

Only little information is available about whether long-term storage of cryopreserved semen samples using modern cryo-techniques leads to a decrease of sperm quality. Smith and Steinberger (1973) were able to show that storing for longer than 36 months results in a decrease of sperm motility. However, no systematic or prospective studies exist that investigate the influence of modern standardized cryopreservation techniques on the maintenance of sperm quality during long-term storage. So far, results and experience with cryopreserved semen are based on investigations with sperm of normal healthy donors. However, these results are not fully applicable to oncological patients because these patients already show limitations of sperm concentration, motility and morphology prior to antitumor therapies.

Based on the assumption that most oncological patients will undergo aggressive chemo- or radiotherapy after cryopreservation of their ejaculates, they will wait a certain period of time following treatment before becoming involved in family planning. It is probable that at least a **five-year period** may pass until these patients use their cryopreserved semen for assisted fertilization. Adequate counselling in respect to the chances of inducing a pregnancy by means of assisted reproduction using cryopreserved semen samples remains difficult. So far, from the published data on pregnancies and deliveries of children of oncological patients conceived after insemination or in vitro-fertilization with cryopreserved sperm stored for up to 9 years after freezing, it may be concluded that the time of storage itself does not significantly influence the later use of cryopreserved semen samples (Köhn and Schill 1988; Sanger et al. 1992).

Long-term storage of semen samples may be undertaken in the institution performing cryopreservation. Constant storage temperatures must be guaranteed; they should not be endangered by repeated opening of the containers of liquid nitrogen. Long-term storage may also be performed in a commercial cryobank. Patients who decide on long-term storage sign a contract with the institution performing long-term storage that may be continued or cancelled on a yearly basis. The minimum costs of cryo-storing per year are about 300 EURO in Germany and usually must be paid by the patient. In very exceptional cases costs may be paid by the health insurance. If the semen sample is needed to perform assisted fertilization, it can be sent to the doctor on the patient's authorization.

18.5 Indications for Cryopreservation of Semen

> Cryopreservation of semen is a preventive therapeutic option to preserve the fertilizing capability in patients with malignancies. By early detection and improved therapeutic concepts the survival rates of oncological patients who become ill at a young age, e.g. with testicular tumors, Hodgkin disease and leukemia, have been increased.

These diseases strike most of the patients at a time when family planning has not started or is not yet finished. At this critical point of time, individual reproductive function may have a high impact on life quality. Of the 681 oncological patients (mean age 28 years) presenting for cryopreservation of their semen between 1987 and 1999, only 183 (27%) were already married and only 86 men (12%) had already fathered at least one child (62 patients) or two and more children (24 patients) before they became ill.

The extent of impairment of gonadal function by chemo- or radiotherapy cannot definitely be predicted and the possibility of testicular function recovering depends on the therapeutic intervention itself, the dosages applied and the individual susceptibility of the patient (Brämswig et al. 1990; Kreuser et al. 1992; Behre et al. 1994; Kliesch et al. 1996; Palmieri et al. 1996). Until now it has not been possible to protect testicular function from the toxic effects of chemo- and radiotherapy; a retrograde ejaculation after retroperitoneal lymphadenectomy can be treated with some medical effort, but impotentia generandi resulting from radical surgery (e.g. radical prostatectomy) cannot be treated at all in respect to fertility.

Prophylactic cryopreservation of semen offers the chance of preventing the hazardous effects of disease and therapy on fertility and may contribute to the per-

Tabelle 18.1. Indications and frequency of cryopreservation (of 718 consecutive patients of the Institute of Reproductive Medicine of the University, Münster, Germany)

Diagnosis	Number of patients (%)
Testicular tumors	377 (52)
Hodgkin disease/ Non-Hodgkin disease	143 (20)
Leukemias	63 (9)
Bone tumors	50 (7)
Other malignancies	48 (7)
Benign diseases	37 (5)

sonal stabilization of the mainly young patients in this critical and acute situation. Most patients deciding in favor of cryopreservation of semen are patients with malignant diseases. Others seek cryopreservation because the extent of their disease is not yet clear, or potentially toxic treatments have to be performed because of benign diseases that may damage testicular function (Table 18.1). An average of 2 to 3 semen samples per patient are frozen in our institute.

Moreover, the cryopreservation of surgically sampled spermatozoa for use in assisted fertilization techniques has become increasingly important in recent years. In cases with non-reconstructable obstruction and in patients with primary testicular failure, epididymal sperm aspiration and testicular extraction of spermatozoa, in combination with cryopreservation, have become routine procedures in reproductive centers.

Cryopreservation of sperm plays an increasing role in establishing internal and external **quality control** systems in andrology (Cooper et al. 1992; Neuwinger et al. 1999). This aspect, however, will not be discussed in the present chapter, nor will the use of cryopreserved donor semen for heterologous assisted fertilization that is practiced in various countries depending on currently applicable laws (Critser 1995).

18.5.1 Oncological Diseases in Adults

In patients with testicular tumors or other malignancies (e.g. Hodgkin disease, leukemia) impairment of testicular function is known. However, the underlying causes of reduced fertility in relation to the malignant disease are not understood (Hansen et al. 1991; Viviani et al. 1991) (see Chap. 12). Our own patients revealed reduced semen parameters with oligoasthenozoospermia in 60% of men with testicular tumors, 44% men with lymphatic or leukemic diseases and 35% of patients with different solid tumors (Fig. 18.1) prior to cryopreservation. A total of 34 patients showed azoospermia; 73 patients had sperm concentrations below 1 million/ml; in 299 patients normal sperm concentrations were found. However, reduced sperm concentrations do not play the most important role in predicting the success of assisted fertilization procedures (Palermo et al. 1992) (see Chap. 17).

Fig. 18.1. Age and sperm concentrations of 683 patients with malignancies at the time of cryopreservation. Note logarithmic scale. The lower normal limit for sperm concentration is 20 million sperm/ml (*broken line*). (Up dated and modified from: Kliesch et al. 1996)

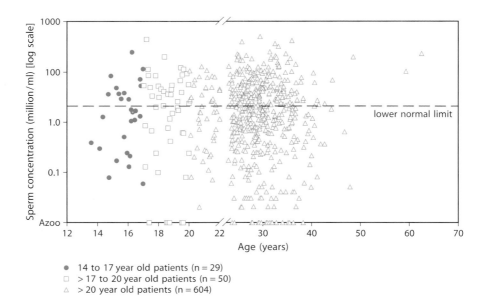

- 14 to 17 year old patients (n = 29)
- > 17 to 20 year old patients (n = 50)
- > 20 year old patients (n = 604)

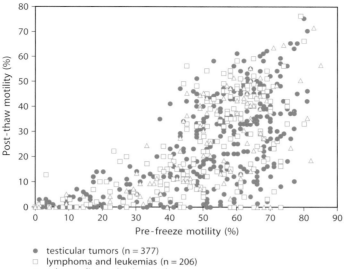

Fig. 18.2. Sperm motility prior to (*x-axis*) and after freezing and thawing (*y-axis*) in patients with different oncological diseases at the time of cryopreservation of semen. The lower normal limit for the pre-freeze progressive sperm motility is 50 %

Sperm motility is particularly impaired by the cryopreservation process (Fig. 18.2). While the mean progressive motility of sperm in oncological patients is about 40 %, we notice a significant drop of sperm motility to a mean of 16 % immediately after freezing and thawing an aliquot, independent of the underlying disease and the patients' age (Keck and Nieschlag 1993; Kliesch et al. 1996). The better the pre-freeze sperm motility is (Fig. 18.2), the better post-thaw motility tends to be. As sperm motility is regarded as one of the important parameters for increasing success rates in insemination and in vitro-fertilization therapies (De Geyter et al. 1992), this decrease of sperm motility due to the cryopreservation itself, may explain the often unsuccessfully performed insemination or in vitro-fertilization cycles. However, with respect to intracytoplasmic sperm injections (ICSI) the proportion of motile sperm is not as relevant. In ICSI treatment sperm motility is used as an indicator for vitality of sperm to be selected for microinjection (see Chap. 17).

18.5.2 Oncological Diseases in Childhood

Cryopreservation cannot only be offered successfully to adults but also to juvenile patients with malignancies. Prior to and after cryopreservation, 14 to 17 year-old boys show semen parameters that are comparable to 18 year-old boys, independent of the underlying oncological disease (Kliesch et al. 1996). Although chemotherapy protocols used in childhood have become less harmful, the prognosis concerning gonadal toxicity and impairment of gonadal function on a long-term basis remains difficult and depends on the chemotherapeutic combinations used. Those therapies not using alkylating substances (e. g. adriamycin, vincristine, methotrexat) induce persistent azoospermia during adulthood after childhood treatment in up to 16 % of treated patients.

When cisplatin-based chemotherapies are used, a mean of 37 % of cured patients remain azoospermic during adulthood. If alkylating substances (e. g. cyclophosphamide or procarbazine) are used during childhood cancer treatment, infertility may result in 68 % of the treated patients during adulthood (for review see Kliesch et al. 1996). Whether the possibility of sampling gonadal tissue in oncologically ill (prepubertal) boys prior to toxic treatment will offer a real chance for later re-transplantation to regain fertility, depends on future research developments. So far, first experimental attempts have been made to establish germ cell transplantation techniques (for review see Bahadur and Ralph 1999; Schlatt et al. 1999).

The preventive aspect of cryopreservation of sperm in respect to long-term life quality, including potential paternity, should be considered when counselling the very young patient and his parents prior to treatment which may prove toxic to the gonads.

18.5.3 Cryopreservation Prior to Vasectomy and after Vasovasostomy

Cryopreservation of sperm may be seriously considered for patients who will undergo vasectomy as no hormonal, reversible contraceptive device comparable to the female pill is available for men (Djerassi and Leibo 1994). Vasectomy is an invasive and often irreversible contraceptive method (see Chap. 20). The patient and his female partner have to make a definite decision on their family planning. Daily clinical work, however, demonstrates that suddenly changed circumstances of the patients' lives (death of a child or the female partner, new partnership with the desire to have children) give rise to the wish to reverse vasectomy and to perform microsurgical vasovasostomy or vasoepididymostomy. For these patients cryopreserved semen might offer the chance to father a child by means of assisted fertilization in case of unsuccessful or impossible refertilization. After successful vasovaso- or vasoepididymostomy the risk exists that patency of the ducts may not be permanent, resulting in obstruction. Therefore the patients should be offered the possibility to cryopreserve either intraoperatively aspirated spermatozoa or ejaculated semen after successful refertilization. In about one third of patients intraoperative sperm aspiration is successful in collecting motile sperm that may be used for later microinjection therapy if refertilization fails (Belker and Bergamini 1997). However, the additional costs must be critically discussed with the patient.

18.5.4 Cryopreservation in Patients with Spinal Cord Injury

A minor, less extensively considered patient group is that with lesions of the spinal cord. Up to 95% of patients lose their ability to ejaculate. By rectal electric stimulation ejaculations may be performed and semen may be successfully used for assisted fertilization. As electrostimulation is inconvenient and much depends on interdisciplinary and logistic cooperation between patient and physicians, cryopreservation offers an advantage to collect semen samples for later use in artificial fertilization treatment (Chung et al. 1995).

18.5.5 Cryopreservation of MESA and TESE Samples

In the context of andrologically relevant microsurgery, microsurgical epididymal sperm aspiration (MESA) (or in some cases percutaneous epididymal sperm aspiration, PESA) offers the chance to provide sperm from patients with obstructive azoospermia who cannot be successfully treated by reconstructive microsurgery, namely vasovasostomy or vasoepididymostomy. Patients with post-infectious obstructive azoospermia, as well as patients with congenital bilateral aplasia of the vas deferens or abnormalities of the epididymides, belong to this treatment group (Craft and Tsirigotis 1995). Aspirated sperm not used for fertilization techniques can be cryopreserved and may be used for further treatment cycles in assisted fertilization. Cryopreservation of surgically obtained sperm specimens may prevent another invasive attempt. Experience with the quality of these cryopreserved samples has shown that with fresh, as well as with cryopreserved epididymal sperm, microinjection therapy may be performed successfully. However, it is also known that post-thaw motility of epididymal sperm is significantly decreased and pregnancy rates are lower compared to microinjection therapy with fresh spermatozoa (Palermo et al. 1999).

In addition to epididymal sperm, testicular sperm from patients with severe oligoasthenozoospermia/hypergonadotropic azoospermia with testicular dysfunction due to focal Sertoli-cell-only-syndrome or incomplete arrest of spermatogenesis may be used after testicular sperm aspiration or extraction (TESE) from surgically obtained testicular tissue in combination with the intracytoplasmic sperm injection technique (ICSI) (Devroey et al. 1995; Silber et al. 1995). Patients should be offered the possiblity of cryopreserving unused testicular tissue for later preparation in further treatment cycles. The experience in recent years with TESA or TESE itself, as well as with that of cryopreserved testicular tissue has proved to be an effective treatment option for infertile azoospermic men. Overall, in up to 70% of azoospermic men, spermatozoa may be extracted from testicular tissue (Jezek et al. 1998). However, pregnancy rates vary – depending on the center and, especially, depending on the severity of spermatogenic impairment – between 10 and 30% (Friedler et al. 1997). The chances for fertilization and pregnancy achieved with testicular sperm are much higher when single spermatozoa are found in the sediment of the patient's ejaculate (Palermo et al. 1999).

18.6 Assisted Fertilization with Cryopreserved Sperm

Information on sperm quality of cryopreserved samples used for assisted fertilization is variable. No systematic information on the number of treatment cycles, methods of gynecological therapy and the total number of treated andrological patients is available. Between 1983 and 1992 a total of 117 pregnancies and 115 births after insemination or in vitro-fertilization with cryopreserved semen samples of oncological patients were published (Sanger et al. 1992). In Germany another two centers provided data on cryopreserved semen samples of oncological patients. They reported on 136 cryopreserved specimens collected between 1974 and 1988, including those from 8 patients who used their cryopreserved sperm for assisted fertilization after a period of up to 5 years (Köhn and Schill 1988; Holland-Moritz and Krause 1990).

Simultaneously with the further development of the techniques of assisted reproduction (insemination, in vitro-fertilization, microinjection), chances of inducing a pregnancy increased because of the improvement in sperm quality by better freezing techniques and improved preservation of sperm function. Therefore the "minimal criteria" for sperm to be cryopreserved (e.g. post-thaw motility of at least 10%, sperm concentration >10 million/ml) (Köhn and Schill 1988; Keck and Nieschlag 1993) that were generally accepted several years ago have become irrelevant in view of microinjection therapy.

Until now, however, existing cryo-depots have only rarely been used. Altogether 42% of the patients of the Institute of Reproductive Medicine store their semen samples on a long-term basis. Over a period of 12 years, 25 out of 414 patients (6%) used their depots either for insemination, in vitro-fertilization or microinjection therapies. The cryopreserved spermatozoa were used in 39 treatment cycles. A total of 14 pregnancies resulted of which five failed to carry to term. A triplet pregnancy was achieved, resulting in a live birth of twins. One third of treatment cycles was performed after ICSI was offered at the end of 1994. Twenty-seven cycles with ICSI resulted in fertilization and 12 pregnancies of which four were aborted. Reports concerning the use of cryopreserved semen from oncological patients for ICSI therapy are still rare, possibly due to the short period of time since introduction of the technique (Lass et al. 1998; Naysmith et al. 1998). The introduction of microinjection therapy will definitely contribute to the more successful use of cryopreserved semen samples of oncological patients.

18.7 Genetic Risks of Using Cryopreserved Spermatozoa

The question whether an increased genetic risk exists for the offspring of patients suffering from malignancies or treated by oncological chemo- or radiotherapy remains difficult to answer. In principle two different aspects are to be considered. One aspect refers to the risk arising from the malignant disease itself and possibly mutagenic effects of chemo- and radiotherapy. The second aspect involves the possible risk of a genetically determined disease in the offspring when using assisted fertilization techniques with cryopreserved spermatozoa.

The available cytogenetic investigations in spermatozoa from patients after chemo- or radiotherapy show a significantly increased proportion of structural chromosomal anomalies in comparison to controls (Genescà et al. 1990; Rousseaux et al. 1993). However, these in vitro results are not supported by **clinical data** that might suggest increased rates of anomalies in children born.

With respect to the clinical aspect of a potentially increased genetic risk, no case-control studies exist that could provide reliable answers to these questions.

However, the documented data of IVF centers and the data obtained from offspring of oncological patients both indicate that no increased genetic risk and no increased risk for malformation exists that could result from the underlying oncological disease or the applied assisted fertilization technique with cryopreserved spermatozoa (Sanger et al. 1992; Dodds et al. 1993; Rufat et al. 1994; Schenker and Ezra 1994).

In addition, the problem of familial cancer risk exists and should lead to the recommendation to offer any cancer patient genetic counselling prior to fertilizing therapies.

18.8 Problems and Limitations of Cryopreservation

Counselling of patients in respect to cryopreservation takes place at a point in time when the physical and psychological integrity of the patient is disturbed. In view of the acute and stressful situation (confrontation with diagnosis and treatment) it seems difficult for both patient and doctor to consider the relative importance of cryopreservation to preserve progenitive ability with repect to the long-term quality of life. Especially for juvenile patients, this counselling requires a high degree of involvement and willingness to break taboos and to discuss problems of sexuality and fertility. Notwithstanding, cryopreservation may contribute to the patient's personal stability in an acute and oppressive situation.

One **methodological problem of cryopreservation** is insufficient preparation of the ejaculate with reduced quality contributing to further decrease of sperm quality and function by the process of freezing. These methodological shortcomings render the later use of cryopreserved spermatozoa for assisted fertilization difficult. Consequently, the cryopreservation of semen only preserves the ability to produce offspring if the oncological patient is offered a high technical standard of assisted reproduction in qualified interdisciplinary reproductive centers with optimal gynecological treatment options for the female partner. Moreover, there is need for discussion of ethical questions arising from the fact that cryopreservation depots and thus preservation of potential paternity is set up for patients who may die (see Chap. 22). While destruction of cryo-depots is contractually defined if the patient dies, the use of semen samples of incurably ill patients confronts doctor, patient and the patient's female partner with a situation that is neither regulated nor – at least so far – thoroughly discussed.

In summary, the cryopreservation of human sperm offers a preventive, pre-therapeutic possibility of preserving progenity in oncological patients prior to toxic therapies that can impair gonadal function. Moreover, cryopreservation may be used in patients who undergo micro-surgical therapies during assisted fertilization treatment (MESA, TESE). In combination with intracytoplasmic sperm injection and in vitro-fertilization the cryopreserved semen may be successfully used for fertilization. Chances of inducing pregnancy in the female partner have been improved and continue to increase by using modern techniques of assisted fertilization.

18.9 References

Alvarez JG, Storey BT (1993) Evidence that membrane stress contributes more than lipid peroxidation to sublethal cryodamage in cryopreserved human sperm: glycerol and other polyols as sole cryoprotectant. J Androl 14:199–208

Bahadur G, Ralph D (1999) Gonadal tissue cryopreservation in boys with paediatric cancers. Hum Reprod 14:11–17

Belker AM, Bergamini DA (1997) The feasibility of cryopreservation of sperm harvested intraoperatively during vasectomy reversals. J Urol 157:1292–1294

Brämswig JH, Heimes E, Heiermann W, Schlegel W, Nieschlag E (1990) The effects of different cumulative doses of chemotherapy on testicular function. Results in 75 patients treated for Hodgkin's disease during childhood or adolescence. Cancer 65:1298–1302

Byrd W, Bradshaw K, Carr B, Edman C, Odom J, Ackerman G (1990) A prospective randomized study of pregnancy rates following intrauterine and intracervical insemination using frozen donor sperm. Fertil Steril 53:521–527

Chan SYW, Pearlstone A, Uhler M, Tucker M, Greenspoon R, Leung A, Wang C (1993) Human spermatozoal tail hypo-osmotic swelling test, motility characteristics in hypotonic saline, and survival of spermatozoa after cryopreservation. Hum Reprod 8:717–721

Chung PH, Yeko TR, Mayer JC, Sanfor EJ, Maroulis GB (1995) Assisted fertility using electroejaculation in men with spinal cord injury – a review of literature. Fertil Steril 64:1–9

Cooper TG, Neuwinger J, Bahrs S, Nieschlag E (1992) Internal quality control of semen analysis. Fertil Steril 58:172–177

Craft I, Tsirigotis M (1995) Debates: simplified recovery, preparation and cryopreservation of testicular spermatozoa. Hum Reprod 10:1623–1627

Critser JK (1995) Therapeutic insemination by donor I: a review of its efficacy. Reprod Med Rev 4:9–17

De Geyter C, De Geyter M, Schneider HPG, Nieschlag E (1992) Subnormal sperm parameters in conventional semen analysis are associated with discrepancies between fertilization and pregnancy rates in in vitro fertilization and embryo transfer. Int J Androl 15:485–491

Devroey P, Liu J, Nagy Z, Goossens A, Tounaye H, Camus M, Van Steirteghem A, Silber S (1995) Pregnancies after testicular sperm extraction and intracytoplasmic sperm injection in non-obstructive azoospermia. Hum Reprod 10:1457–1460

Dodds L, Marrett LD, Tomkins DJ, Green B, Sherman G (1993) Case-control study of congenital anomalies in children of cancer patients. Br Med J 307:164–168

Friedler S, Raziel A, Soffer Y, Strassburger D, Komarovsky D, Ron-El R (1997) Intracytoplasmic injection of fresh and cryopreserved testicular spermatozoa in patients with non-obstructive azoospermia – a comparative study. Fertil Steril 68:892–897

Genescà A, Benet J, Caballín MR, Miró R, Germà JR, Egozcue J (1990) Significance of structural chromosome aberrations in human sperm: analysis of induced aberrations. Hum Genet 85:495–499

Hammerstedt RH, Graham JK, Nolan JP (1990) Cryopreservation of mammalian sperm: what we ask them to survive. J Androl 11:73–88

Hansen PV, Glavind K, Panduro J, Pedersen M (1991) Paternity in patients with testicular germ cell cancer: pretreatment and post-treatment findings. Eur J Cancer 27:1385–1389

Hoagland H, Pincus G (1942) Revival of mammalian sperm after immersion in liquid nitrogen. J Gen Physiol 25:337–339

Holland-Moritz H, Krause W (1990) Inanspruchnahme von Sperma-Kryodepots bei Tumorpatienten. Hautarzt 41:204–206

Jahnel F (1938) Über die Widerstandsfähigkeit von menschlichen Spermatozoen gegenüber starker Kälte. Klin Wochenschr 17:1273–1274

Jezek D, Knuth UA, Schulze W (1998) Successful testicular sperm extraction (TESE) in spite of high serum follicle stimulating hormone and azoospermia: correlation between testicular morphology, TESE results, semen analysis and serum hormone values in 103 infertile men. Hum Reprod 13:1230–1234

Keck C, Nieschlag E (1993) Kryokonservierung von Spermien als Zeugungsreserve für onkologische Patienten. Internist 34:775–780

Kliesch S, Behre HM, Jürgens H, Nieschlag E (1996) Cryopreservation of semen from adolescent patients with malignancies. Med Ped Oncol 26:20–27

Köhn FM, Schill WB (1988) Kryospermabank München – Zwischenbilanz 1974–1986. Hautarzt 39:91–96

Kreuser ED, Klingmüller D, Thiel E (1992) Diagnostik und Prognose gonadaler Toxizität nach Chemotherapie und Bestrahlung. Dtsch Med Wochenschr 117:1810–1817

Lass A, Akagbosu F, Abusheikha N, Hassouneh M, Blayney M, Avery S, Brinsden P (1998) A programme of semen cryopreservation for patients with malignant disease in a tertiary infertility centre: lessons from 8 years' experience. Hum Reprod 13:3256–3261

Morris GJ, Acton E, Avery S (1999) A novel approach to sperm cryopreservation. Hum Reprod 14:10132–1021

Naysmith TE, Blake DA, Harvey VJ, Johnson NP (1998) Do men undergoing sterilizing cancer treatment have a fertile future? Hum Reprod 13:3250–3255

Neuwinger J, Behre HM, Nieschlag E (1990) External quality control in the andrology laboratory: an experimental multicenter trial. Fertil Steril 54:308–314

Palermo G, Joris H, Devroey P, Van Steirteghem AC (1992) Pregnancies after intracytoplasmatic injection of single spermatozoon into an oocyte. Lancet 340:17–18

Palermo GD, Schlegel PN, Hariprashad JJ, Ergün B, Mielnik A, Zaninovic N, Veeck LL, Rosenwaks Z (1999) Fertilization and pregnancy outcome with intracytoplasmic sperm injection for azoospermic men. Hum Reprod 14:741–748

Péréz-Sanchez F, Cooper TG, Yeung CH, Nieschlag E (1994) Improvement in quality of cryopreserved human spermatozoa by swim-up before freezing. Int J Androl 17:115–119

Polge C, Smith AU, Parkes AS (1942) Revival of spermatozoa after vitrification and dehydration at low temperatures. Nature 164–167

Rousseaux S, Sèle B, Cozzi J, Chevret E (1993) Immediate rearrangement of human sperm chromosomes following in-vivo irradiation. Hum Reprod 8:903–907

Rufat P, Olivennes F, de Mouzon J, Dhean M, Frydman R (1994) Task force report on the outcome of pregnancies and children conceived by in vitro fertilization (France: 1987 to 1989). Fertil Steril 61:324–330

Salzbrunn A, Benson DM, Holstein AF, Schulze W (1996) A new concept for the extraction of testicular spermatozoa as a tool for assisted fertilization (ICSI). Hum Reprod 11:752–755

Sanger WG, Olson JH, Sherman JK (1992) Semen cryobanking for men with cancer – criteria change. Fertil Steril 58:1024–1027

Schenker JG, Ezra Y (1994) Complications of assisted reproductive techniques. Fertil Steril 61:411–422

Schlatt S, Rosiepen G, Weinbauer GF, Rolf C, Brook PF, Nieschlag E (1999) Germ cell transfer into rat, bovine, monkey and human testes. Hum Reprod 14:144–150

Sherman JK (1963) Improved methods of preservation of human spermatozoa by freezing and freeze drying. Fertil Steril 14:723–729

Shettles LB (1940) The respiration of human spermatozoa and their response to various cases and low temperature. Am J Physiol 128:408–415

Silber SJ, Van Steirteghem AC, Liu J, Nagy Z, Tournaye H, Devroey P (1995) High fertilization and pregnancy rate after intracytoplasmic sperm injection with spermatozoa obtained from testicle biopsy. Hum Reprod 10:148–152

Smith KD, Steinberger E (1973) Survival of spermatozoa in a human sperm bank. J Am Med Assoc 223:774–774

Viviani S, Ragni G, Santoro A, Perotti L, Caccamo E, Negretti E, Valagussa P, Bonadonna G (1991) Testicular dysfunction in Hodgkin's disease before and after treatment. Eur J Cancer 27:1389–1392

Wang R, Sikka SC, Veeraragavan K, Bell M, Hellstrom WJG (1993) Platelet activating factor and pentoxifylline as human sperm cryoprotectants. Fertil Steril 60:711–715

Watson PF, Critser JK, Mazur P (1992) Sperm preservation: fundamental cryobiology and practical implications. In: Templeton AA, Drife JO (eds) Infertility. Springer, Berlin Heidelberg New York, pp 101–114

WHO Laborhandbuch zur Untersuchung des menschlichen Ejakulates und der Spermien-Zervikalschleim-Interaktion (1999). Übersetzt von: Nieschlag E, Nieschlag S, Bals-Pratsch M, Behre HM, Knuth UA, Meschede D, Niemeier M, Schick A, 4th edn. Springer, Berlin Heidelberg New York

CHAPTER 19

The Psychology of Fertility Disorders

R. OBERPENNING · F. OBERPENNING · F. A. MUTHNY

19.1 A Survey of Psychological Research into Infertility

In the past two decades, reproductive medicine has made a huge leap forward. The World Health Organization (WHO) reckons annually with approx. 2 million new infertile couples. Today the traditional methods such as surgery, hormone treatments and inseminations are being supplemented by in vitro fertilization (IVF), intracytoplasmic sperm injection (ICSI), microsurgical epididymal sperm aspiration (MESA) and by TESE (testicular sperm extraction).

According to Pöhler (1992), the **decision to have invasive infertility therapy** can be seen as an expression of a strong motivation towards self-realization and a conscious decision regarding parenthood. Other authors see a "structurally conditional offer of denial" which hampers coping with limited treatment modalities of unwanted childlessness (Hölzle 1987). The majority of unintentionally childless couples have unrealistically high expectations at the beginning of their medical reproductive treatment (Eckert et al. 1998; Goldschmidt et al. 1997). Thus a relatively high number of couples in the third cycle of treatment discontinue the therapy although relatively good rates of pregnancy are achieved in this cycle (Land et al. 1997). In contrast to these are the patients who, in spite of a bad prognosis, can see no alternative to a child of their own and engage in "**doctor shopping**" (Strauß 1996). They are considered especially problematical in expert circles as they find it very difficult to cope with their unfulfilled desire to have a child and can hardly see any alternative life perspectives. Turkish couples who have migrated equally fail to see an alternative to having a child of their own because of their system of values (Yüksel et al. 1999).

Essentially, the following themes are emphasized in the psychological literature on unwanted childlessness:

- The psychic preconditions for unwanted childlessness,
- the psychic results/effects of unwanted childlessness in view of the many different medical reproductive techniques,
- the role of psychosocial factors in the indication/contraindication of therapies,

- the effects of psychotherapeutic interventions,
- the further psychosocial developments after treatment for infertility, especially the development of parents and children after IVF and ICSI.

19.1.1 Psychological Conditions of Unwanted Childlessness

When the psychological studies on the conditions of unwanted childlessness are broken down, personality-psychological, psycho-dynamic, stress-theoretical and psycho-biological approaches can be distinguished. At the end of the fifties and the middle of the sixties, **personality-psychological approaches**, which saw infertility in connection with certain personality traits of those concerned, were dominant among psychological investigations on unwanted childlessness (Sturgis et al. 1957). Thus, for example, a greater number of psycho-vegetative complaints was contributed by infertile couples and childless marital partners were characterized as mainly depressive, fearful and inhibited personalities. Comparative psychological investigations on fertile and infertile couples in the seventies and eighties expressed reservations towards the concept of "psychogenic infertility" or refused to attribute male/female infertility to certain personality traits or emotional disorders (Seibel and Taymor 1982). Thus, in a recent pilot study by Seikowski et al. (1998) on 100 male patients of the andrological department at the University of Leipzig, it was discovered that sperm motility and sperm morphology were greatly reduced in hypochondriac patients. They do, however, at the same time point out that their statistical approach was very uninformative because it failed to record the individual reaction patterns of each participant to stressful situations.

Wright et al. (1989), in their review on infertile patients with depressive disorders, came to the conclusion that **psychological characteristics are no useful predictor of infertility**. Further investigations on the psychic characteristics of childless couples wishing offspring should, according to Brähler (1993), rather **aim to prevent** infertility. Thus, immigrant **Turkish couples** are recommended to use invasive methods cautiously as they frequently wish to have children at a very young age. Due to a lower average level of general education and lack of sexual education these patients particularly have difficulties in comprehending the necessary diagnostic and therapeutic procedures. Comprehensive counselling – preferably in the couple's native language – seems to be a valid approach for this group of patients, since reported **spontaneous pregnancy rates are relatively high** (Yüksel et al. 1999).

Psychodynamic investigations are based on psychoanalytical theory and see the suppression of psychic conflicts as the central factor in the conditional connection with infertility. On special consideration of the relationship of couples who may be described as clingingly symbiotic (Stauber 1979, 1989), unwanted childlessness appears as the common symptom of a couple to protect themselves against other psychic problems (Goldschmidt and De Boor 1976). While these and similar investigations contain stimulating ideas on innerpsychological conflicts as possible conditions of infertility, they frequently remain fixated on the problems of the woman, ignore the man and do not adequately, but rather speculatively, explain the **interactive relationship between the psychic and the somatic** (Bents 1985; Ulrich 1988). Thus, it can be observed on the basis of improved medical diagnostics that the concept of psychogenic sterility has dropped from a former 50% (Eisner 1963) to under 5% (Bettendorf 1989) today.

The **theory** of infertility based **on stress** works from the premise that, with longer-lasting pressure of stress, various functions of the organism are restricted and a **subjectively experienced stress situation** can lead to infertility by a disturbance of endocrinological functions. Schuermann (1948) and Stieve (1952) had already indicated that serious psychic stress stimuli such as, for example, death sentences, war events and captivity and internment in concentration camps are associated with anatomically recognizable change of the sex hormones and can reduce sperm production. This was the impetus for research of male infertility based on the stress theory. Subsequent studies distinguished the connection between stress and infertility according to the kind of stress (e.g. pressure in the private or professional sphere) and ejaculation results (Stauber 1979; Poland et al. 1986). The study of Matzen et al. (1998) is also worth mentioning in this context as, contrary to their expectations, it noted a higher regularity in the circadian rhythm of activity as well as in the pattern of sleep quality in idiopathically infertile men in comparison to the control group.

All in all, however, the question was never posed throughout these investigations whether or not there was a connection between personality pre-conditioned behavioral dispositions, on the one hand, and biological parameters such as the sperm count and quality, on the other hand caused by certain **strategies of coping with stress**.

Psychobiological investigations take up this notion of the stress theory and attempt to ascertain the psychic factors which are part of the stress reaction of the organism. In the mid eighties, Hellhammer et al. (1985) carried out investigations on the possible **connection between personality and infertility**. The surprising result was that the infertile men displayed personality traits such as self-confidence, extraversion and social competence, whereas those with personality traits such as depressivity, introversion and social anxiety showed better fertility parameters (Hubert et al. 1985). Stress-induced infer-

Table 19.1. Studies on the conditions of unwanted childlessness. *SVF* Questionnaire on coping with stress, *REP* Repertory-Grid-TEST, *ILE* Inventory of life events, *FAPK* Questionnaire on assessing psychosomatic pathological picture, *FPI* Freiburg Personality Inventory, *U-Questionnaire* Uncertainty Questionnaire, *SRM* (Social-Rhythm-Metric-Diary), *CCR* Curve of Complaint Record

Authors	Group	Method	Results
Deipenwisch et al. (1994)	25 infertile men, 25 fertile men	Questionnaire (e.g. SVF,REP)	No difference
Greimel et al. (1992)	18 men with pathological ejaculate findings, 10 men with pathol. genital findings, 36 healthy men	Interview, Questionnaire (e.g. ILE), spermiogram	Stress primarily restricts quality of sperm
Hellhammer et al. (1985)	117 men	Questionnaire (e.g. FPI, U-questionnaire), Ratings on partnership situtation, spermiogram	Self-confidence, extraversion and social competence negatively connected with male fertility parameters.
Hubert et al. (1985)	101 infertile men	Questionnaire (e.g. FAPK), spermiogram	Depressive, introverted and socially insecure men show better fertility parameters.
Matzen et al. (1999)	20 idiopathic infertile men, 38 healthy men	Diary (SRM), Pittsburgh-Sleep-Diary	Greater regularity of daily activity rhythm, Better sleep quality.
Seikowski et al. (1998)	100 men from infertility consultation	Spermiogram, CCR-questionnaire	Connection between hypochondria/ananchasm and restricted motility and morphology.

tility is connected with specific forms of coping with stress (**coping**) and with specific personality traits. In a more recent investigation on men with idiopathic infertility in comparison to a control-group of fertile males, no greater tendency to active coping was found (Deipenwisch et al. 1994). Active coping exists when individuals do not avoid stress situations, but rather work on them and possibly change them so that they are less stressful. Even if active coping with infertility is seen as generally helpful and relieving, empirical certainty of this association is still lacking (Pook et al. 1999).

Greimel et al. (1992) found in their investigation that men with idiopathic infertility indicated significantly more pressure factors at work and more individual stress than the men for whom an organic reason for their pathological semen quality was presumed. The men with idiopathic infertility also reported significantly more life-events (e.g. sicknesses, deaths, financial losses) than the men with an organic reason, or the healthy control-group. In summary, Table 19.1. shows individual investigations which examined the psychic conditions of unwanted childlessness more closely, including men.

19.1.2 Psychological Effects of Unwanted Childlessness

It may be ascertained from the literature on the psychic effects of unwanted childlessness that there are considerable discrepancies between the statements of the researchers: the psychic effects depend on the psychological orientation (e.g. psychoanalysis, behavioral or cognitive psychology), the cause of infertility (of the woman, the man or of both partners) and how great the desire for children is. It is, however, in the majority of cases clearly confirmed that infertility represents a stressful life event. A comparative investigation by Kedem et al. (1990) with 107 infertile and 30 fertile men showed that the infertile men had lower self-esteem, greater fear and more symptoms (interpreted as stress-indicators) than the fertile ones. The question whether these psychic stress symptoms are to be understood as a cause or a reaction cannot be answered by their investigation.

In a study on childless couples in the Federal Republic of Germany it was confirmed that consciously and involuntarily childless couples experience **social discrimination**, leading to considerable social pressure that must be dealt with on the individual, partnership-related and social level. The **model** by Guttormsen (1992) based on **how persons cope with the diagnosis of infertility** or sterility proposes eight phases ranging from shock, denial, anger about not becoming pregnant, guilt and embarrassment, isolation, depression, sorrow and, finally, acceptance of the diagnosis. According to Onnen-Isemann (1998), unintentionally childless couples do not experience each of these phases, they skip one or the other. The fact that the couples eliminate the important phase of accepting the diagnosis of infertility and begin treatment directly results in considerably greater strain placed on these couples by medical treatment.

With regard to couple dynamics, van Keep and Schmidt-Elmendorff (1974) noted that within a period of observation of 9 years the divorce rate among involuntarily childless couples was about 7 % higher than in marriages with children. In a post-investigation on couples with heterologous insemination Goebel and Lübke (1987) found the highest rate of divorce among those couples who failed to have children, either by treatment, adoption or by spontaneous pregnancy. In contrast to this, an investigation on IVF couples discovered that after completing treatment the couples assessed their conjugal bliss more highly than before, regardless of whether treatment had beeen successful or not (Leiblum et al. 1987). The first retrospective study concerned with the different coping strategies of 281 IVF or ICSI couples (Beutel et al. 1987) showed that, independent of the type of treatment, women were significantly more subject to depression than a normal reference population or their husbands. The men in the ICSI/MESA/TESE groups felt more responsible for the infertility and to a greater extent restricted in their daily sense of satisfaction with life, due in part to stressful infertility treatment. Altogether, the investigation identified the following risk groups for depression:

- Unsuccessfully or repeatedly treated couples,
- couples with lower socio-economic status,
- couples with foreign nationality,
- couples in which the male partner is not very supportive of his female partner.

An important psychological impact within IVF/ICSI treatment for both partners is **uncertainty** during egg cell harvesting, fertilization, embryo transfer and when awaiting results of the pregnancy test. This uncertainty is accompanied by ambivalent feelings, emotional distress and positive feelings such as hope and familiarity. Thus, **informing the couple realistically and as quickly as possible** of the results of the examination can reduce stress (Boivin et al. 1998).

In recent years the view that unwanted childlessness, or **fertility restriction** among couples, is to be seen as **multi-factorial** (Strauß 1991) and has commanded in-

creasing attention. The results of psychological investigations carried out with standardized tests and control groups show no, or merely unessential, differences between fertile couples and those with fertility disorders with regard to pressure and possible partnership conflicts (Dunkel-Schetter and Lobel 1991; Eckert et al. 1998; Gagel et al. 1998).

19.2 The Psychology of Fertility Disorders in Males

It is generally accepted today that almost half the couples with an unfulfilled wish for children suffer from disturbances on the male side (cf. Chap. 1). Some of the more recent treatment methods, such as MESA/TESE, allow for a treatment of the couple whose wish for children has not been fulfilled and who manifest a serious infertility disorder. Indeed, in the future these methods allow us to hope that men will be considered to a greater extent (cf. Bents 1985) in the psychological research on infertility.

It is well known that men find it much more unpleasant than women to speak about their fertility problem outside their partnership (Brand 1989). Furthermore, scientific access to the infertile man is greatly hindered by the fact that he can only be treated to a limited extent by medication. Since spontaneous pregnancies can occur even with a sperm concentration of under 10^6/ml (Knuth and Nieschlag 1985), it is to be hoped that doctors dealing with these cases display optimism so that an infertile man may feel less responsible for his wife's failure to become pregnant.

Investigations on more recent methods of treatment in cases of serious male fertility disorders indicate that nowadays the man feels a greater responsibility for childlessness and perceives the method of treatment, especially MESA/TESE as stressful (Beutel et al. 1999). The results of Stauber et al. (1985), who report on men's **guilty feelings towards their partner**, who normally bears the greater burden of therapy, speak for the greater involvement of infertile men in therapeutic treatments. As already mentioned, studies of cases in which the cause of infertility lies with the male, show greater emotional pressure on the man (Nachtigall 1992; Beutel et al. 1999), especially on those men who are vulnerable for stress situations in general and who deal with them by using coping strategies of avoidance (such as resignation). Moreover, it is more difficult for these men to seek social support for dealing with their unfulfilled desire for children (Band et al. 1998). Men who are solely responsible for infertility display more negative attitudes to sexuality, especially if they manifest an OAT syndrome (Fischer et al. 1996).

A further investigation, likewise concerned with male and female diagnosis-dependent forms of coping, showed that subfertile men seemed relatively "submis-

Table 19.2. Studies on the effects of unwanted childlessness. *SCL-90-R*: Self-Report Symptom-Inventory, *FEKB*: Questionnaire to establish forms of coping with disease, *REP*: Repertory-Grid-Test, *HSCL*: Hopkins Symptom Check List, *SVF*: Questionnaire on coping with stress, *STAI*: State-Trait-Fear-Inventory

Authors	Group	Method	Results
Berg et al. (1991)	104 couples with primary infertility	Questionnaire (e.g. SCL-90-R)	Infertile women have no higher distress levels than their husbands. No gender differences in the emotional stress factors "marital contentment" and "sexual contentment". Masculinity associated with less emotional stress and greater marital contentment in both sexes.
Bernt et al. (1992)	8 functionally sterile couples, 10 couples with andrological sterility, 8 couples with tubal sterility	Questionnaire (e.g. SCL-90-R)	Wives of subfertile men bear the emotional burden of the treatment. The healthy partners are always the dominant ones. Andrologically caused sterile couples stand out because of wives' dominance.
Beutel et al. (1999)	281 former IVF/ICSI couples	Questionnaire (e.g. D-S)	ICSI treatment additionally stressful for the man. Women more depressive than normopopulation or husband
Boivin et al. (1998)	40 IVF/ICSI couples	Diary notes	Uncertainty in the treatment cycle is the important psychological determinate; occurrence of emotional distress as well as positive feelings such as hope and affection for one another.
Grimmig et al. (1992)	30 infertile couples, 24 voluntary non-parents	Ratings, questionnaire (e.g. REP, Questionnaire on bodily perception)	No difference between self and ideal self in the experimental and control group. Men of the study group appear more self-confident and attractive than men in comparative group.
Kedem et al. (1990)	107 infertile men, 30 fertile men	Questionnaire (e.g. HSCL, Attributional Style Questionnaire), Ratings	Infertile men report less self-esteem, higher levels of fear and psycho-somatic complaints.
Knorre (1981)	57 infertile couples, 15 fertile couples	Interview	More sexual disharmony in male infertility.
Nachtigal et al. (1992)	6 couples with male infertility, 19 couples with female infertility, 11 couples with male/female infertiliy	Interview	Male infertility associated with emotional impairment as e.g. lower self-esteem.
Stanton (1992)	61 infertile women, 52 infertile men (among them 52 couples)	Interview, questionnaire (e.g. SCL-90-R)	83% of men vs. 45% of women presume that they display more appropriate coping strategies e.g. for dealing with infertility than other members of their sex. 51% of men and 47% of women see no differences in the effectivity of their coping strategies.
Stauber et al. (1985)	68 couples with male infertility	Questionnaire (e.g. Giessen Test)	Tendency to depressive mood swings. Negative social resonance in the women as well as the men.
Strauß et al. (1991)	103 IVF couples	Questionnaire (e.g. SVF, STAI, Giessen Test)	44% of women and 14% of men report reduction of sexual desire after sexual activities, about 47% of men report reduction in frequency of sexual contacts.
van Keep & Schmidt, Elmendorff (1974)	75 infertile couples	Interview	Deterioration of marital bliss from moment when sterility diagnosed, but fewer extra marital-associations

sive" (Giessen Test), less involved and interested, as well as less frightened than their fertile wives. The authors presume that the subfertile men are so well able to keep their fear at bay and to distance themselves from their infertility problem because their healthy partner bears the emotional burden of the treatment (Bernt et al. 1992). Other authors assume that the principal problem of the infertile/subfertile men consists in their relationship to their unhappy wife and their stressful married life (Greil et al. 1989). The results of Meyer and Felder (1998), however, show how important a **happy partnership** seems to be in coping with unwanted childlessness during IVF treatment. The couples who were categorized as "happy partnerships" have better forms of communication at their disposal, pursue more satisfying leisure activities, and the men in this group were seen as being significantly under less pressure throughout treatment. According to the authors, these men do not give such extreme priority to realizing their desire to have children and can thus probably face the various steps of treatment in a more relaxed fashion.

Investigations concerned with the **cognitive comparative processes** of infertile couples concluded that the majority of infertile men deploy downwardly directed cognitive comparative processes towards other infertile men (Stanton 1992). This implies that men affected by infertility presume that they have at their disposal better stress-coping strategies than other men concerned. Whether this cognitive form of coping means that men feel less threatened by infertility cannot as yet be properly assessed.

Altogether, however, it may be said that the emotional pressure on men does not seem to be any less than that on women, when the cause of infertility is ascribed to them (Berg 1991; Connolly et al. 1987). Furthermore, it is important to consider that in standardized tests, men tend to present themselves in a much better light by showing mostly higher levels on the so-called lie scales (Lalos et al. 1985; Harrison et al. 1986) which deal with the psychic effects of unwanted childlessness (Table 19.2).

19.3 Psychosexual Development

As psychosexual development and the gender role identity of men and women may be connected with coping with infertility, we deal with the various psychosexual development theories of psychology in this section. First of all, however, a definition of the terms of gender identity/ role may be taken from Money (1994):

> **Gender identity** means maintenance, unity and continuation of one's own individuality as a male,

female or androgynous person to a more or less greater degree, especially as experienced in one's self-awareness or behavior. **Gender role** is everything that a person says or does to show others or him/herself to which extent he/she is male, female or androgynous; this includes sexual and erotic sensitivity and reaction, but is not restricted to that.

This definition makes it clear according, to Money (1994), that gender identity is the personal experience of gender role; gender role, on the other hand, is the public manifestation of gender identity.

It is indisputable that the psychosexual development of man plays a significant role in taking on the gender role, or identification and the developmental tasks connected with that. Thus, unsuccessful psychosexual phases of development are seen as the cause or condition of certain **personality disorders** in adulthood.

It is common to all psychological theories related to assumption and development of gender role that cognitive, motivational and emotional factors are involved, if in different ways. At present, three different theoretical methods of explanation exist. A detailed presentation and discussion of the theories can be found in Trautner (1991).

Gender Role Identification According to Freud

The boy assumes his gender role, according to Freud, in three stages of development (Oerter 1987). At first the mother is the primary love object of the boy, whereby at the same time he forms a fear of the rival father so that he feels, having discovered that girls do not have a penis, threatened with being castrated by his father if he desires his mother as a love object. In order not to lose the mother as a love object, the boy then identifies with his father (defensive identification or **identification with the aggressor**). In the end the boy gives his mother up as a love object and directs his sexual desire towards other women.

The girl, having recognized that she does not have a penis, develops **penis envy**. The mother, who likewise does not have a penis, is valued less by the girl; the latter turns towards the father in rivalry with her mother. However, the fear of losing her motherly love causes the girl to turn again to her mother by identifying with her. The affective relationship to the people they relate most closely to, in other words the parents, is regarded within the oedipal phase as decisive for the development of gender role.

Confirmation Theory According to Mischel

According to Mischel (1971) the **principles of reinforcement**, **blotting out and discrimination** are applied as they were conceived for the development of behavior in general. The theory of reinforcement of the development of gender role presumes that parents, and other persons they are closely related to, form the gender role behavior of children by rewarding (positive reinforcement) typical gender behavior and punishing (negative reinforcement) untypical gender behavior (blotting out). Accordingly, parents reward their sons for self-assertive and confident behavior but ignore their silly games. Daughters, on the other hand, are encouraged to be caring and dependent in their behavior and are punished for aggressive, dominant behavior.

Gender Role Identification According to Kohlberg

According to Kohlberg (1974), the basic premise for successful **gender role identification** is that the child recognizes what is expected from his/her role gender. This step is introduced by learning the verbal description "boy" and "girl". Accordingly the child, having recognized its own gender role, generally at the age of 5–6 years, actively chooses among the modes of behavior in his/her surroundings which, in his/her opinion, are suitable. Kohlberg calls this self-categorization a "cognitive reality judgement". He assumes that cognitive development and gender role development are parallel. As every child experiences different socialization in his development, Kohlberg's theory is directed towards individual gender role identification. Thus identification with the parents is a result and not, as in the psychoanalytical theory of Freud, a cause. Gender identity is the basis for the gender role attitudes of the child and later adult. Kohlberg also stresses that there are characteristic gender differences which, to his mind, occur because the male role is more highly valued and is granted more prestige. This is demonstrated, for example, by the fact that among boys at the age of 6–7 years, their own gender role preference reaches its height.

The Androgyny Concept

The androgyny concept presumes that gender role identity has two dimensions, that is, a **masculinity and, distinct from it, a femininity dimension** (Alfermann 1993). The result of this is that a person can attribute masculine as well as feminine traits to him/herself. Masculinity no longer automatically means the exclusion of femininity. It is accepted nowadays that a person who displays masculine and feminine traits has a better concept of him/herself and feels better psychically. The mascu-line component is, however, seen as responsible for psychic health.

In a longitudinal investigation, Trautner (1992) noted that the educational ideal in children and parents bears strong androgynous characteristics. Nevertheless, androgyny seems to be an advantage for today's women, who, more than in the past, occupy "male professions" and leading positions in which self-assertiveness is demanded. Even today an increase in femininity for men is still seen as less advantageous (Alfermann 1993).

Infertility and Gender Identity Role

Infertile couples who display higher levels of masculinity seem less under pressure and more content in their partnerships. At the same time, men with higher levels of **masculinity** show greater sexual contentment in their partnership even if without issue. **Femininity** also proves to be a good predictor of greater partnership and sexual contentment in both sexes in an involuntarily childless marriage (Berg et al. 1991). Roos and Cohen (1987) found fewer psychological problems in the face of stress factors among individuals with higher levels of masculinity. Infertile couples in whom the cause of infertility is on the man's side, however, display fewer problem-solving strategies than those couples among whom infertility is on the female or on both sides. It is also clear that at the end of the treatment men develop greater fear in connection with infertility problems, perhaps presuming that other men doubt their manliness, thus threatening their gender role identity as typically "male" (Connolly et al. 1992). An investigation on the **self-image and body-concept** of childless men who are not happy with their state shows clearly that they see themselves as more unattractive than the men in the control-groups of "spontaneous fathers" or "voluntarily non-fathers". The women of the investigation group considered mothers to be more self-confident than themselves and voluntarily childless women were assessed as even more self-confident (Grimmig et al. 1992). Thus Edelman et al. (1994) found that a reduced sexual self-image is accompanied by increased pressure in both infertile men and women. Because of their **socialization**, women need parenthood to a greater degree for their identity. For men, on the other hand, their professional career is more frequently relevant to their self-esteem. As a result of differing socialization, conflicts frequently arise because women believe that men do not desire a child as strongly. In contrast, women talk much more to those around them about their childlessness (Liebmann-Smith 1987), perhaps explaining why women experience greater social support than their male partners (Abbey et al. 1991).

19.4 Psychosocial Aspects of the Desire for Children

Although the birth rate in Germany is among the lowest in the world, family and parents are mentioned as essentials in surveys of young and adult people (Schneider 1991). The first family survey carried out by the Federal Ministry for Youth, Family, Women and Health showed that there was a positive connection between the number of children in the **family of origin** and the number of children born and desired (based on 10,043 persons questioned aged between 18 and 55 years). With increased education the number of children desired rises; the number of children born, however, drops (Löhr 1992). The desire for children and the decision to have a child are two different phenomena. Thus one may desire to have a child in childhood, but one may concretely decide to have one only at a later point of time.

According to Onnen-Isemann (1995), couples initially seem merely to postpone their desire for children, and she sees this in connection with women's **professional interests** and their concept of a maternal role. **Procrastinating the fulfilment of the desire for children** bears the danger, however, that, due to the decreasing conception rates among older couples, couples may remain childless. In the former German Democratic Republic (GDR) most women, regardless of their level of education had their first child in relatively young years. Brähler et al. (1998) presume that, for the near future, a drastic increase in unwanted childlessness is to be expected, because following the reunion of the formerly divided Germany, the ex-GDR adapted to western standards. Thus **women's interest in having** a child is determined by their **professional interest**, whereas men's interest in children is independent of their professional interest, which is why men consider a larger number of children to be desirable (Könnecke et al. 1998).

In their study on the **motives** for wanting children among men who were unintentionally childless and at the onset of medical treatment, they found that patients with a bad prognosis displayed a more strongly formulated desire to have children than patients with a good prognosis, regardless of whether they were aware of the andrological findings. Altogether, these men expected emotional stabilization and personal reevaluation from producing offspring. According to Pöhler and Weiland (1998), investigating 56 couples from an IVF program, men try significantly more frequently than women to ward off the hurt and sorrow accompanying childlessness by withdrawing from social communication and thus behave in a more reserved fashion and show less kindness to their wife.

In investigations on developmental psychology, parenthood is listed as a normative transition in the course of life (Gloger-Tippelt 1988). According to the developmental psychologist, Erikson (1976), coping or not coping with a psychosocial task dictates whether an individual takes a good or bad course in his/her development: the mature adult needs to have the feeling that he is needed. Therefore, if pregnancy does not occur, the individual or couple may experience a crisis in their development. Gagel et al. (1998) see an opportunity, as well as a risk, to fulfil the respective requirements in the "crisis". In their work on partnership, pregnancy and early childhood development, after the desire for a child has been fulfilled by IVF, they distinguish between phases of

- personality and partnership crisis,
- sterility crisis,
- IVF-crisis,
- pregnancy and birth crisis,
- family crisis,

although these cannot be clearly separated from one another. According to Brähler and Brähler (1992), infertility is assessed as the worst critical life event, followed by divorce and the death of a close relative or friend. The motivation for wanting offspring is also shaped by the upbringing of the parents and by society's attitudes, in the case of non-parenthood social pressure can affect the self-esteem of a couple negatively. When infertile couples are asked about their desire to have children, they normally mention the motives listed in Table 19.3.

The motives given indicate a desire to exist not only for oneself and for one's partner. Frequently the motives for pregnancy are ambivalent; in addition to the desire for a child, there is the fear of the associated burdens and restrictions (c.f. Frick-Bruder 1989, 1991). As well as the "primary" decision to have a child at all, the involuntarily childless couples have to decide whether, and to what extent, medical help must be sought. Throughout this discussion, however, it is frequently forgotten that the desire for a child may first of all be seen as something quite natural (Lukesch 1983; Pöhler 1992).

For a long time investigation of the **male's desire for children** was neglected. According to psychoanalytical theory, this desire has its origin in the oedipal phase. Kühler (1989) writes on the psychology of the male's desire for children:

"The desire for children must twice be rejected in early childhood by the boy (= wanting to bear children himself), the other time it is the oedipal desire for children (= to have a child with his mother). This enormous effort at suppression could help to explain why a wish to have children of their own is so inaccessible to them."

Mertens (1994) emphasizes what an effort of sacrifice in narcissistic and oedipal-incestuous terms the boy must make when he renounces his own desire to bear children and why wanting to be technically, scientifically and artistically productive is so important for many men's male self-esteem. Many unconscious wishes

Table 19.3. Motives of desire for children according to Lalos et al.(1985)

Philosophical motives	Hope for immortality through children of one's own Securing human survival Meaning of life God's will
Sociocultural motives	Satisfaction of social needs Status improvement of woman or man Interpersonal motives Confirmation of relationship by pregnancy Child as expression of couple's love
Intrapsychic motives	Confirmation of one's own sexual identity Replacement for another lost person Understanding and identifying with one's own parents Reliving one's own childhood Sign of independence

Table 19.4. Male motives for desire for children according to Diamond (1991)

Sublimated wishes to be dependent	Satisfaction of one's own desire for children by identification with child Securing one's own manliness – by identification with the fatherliness of one's own father.
Desire for the continuity of one's self	Challenges by the child lead to an increase in the responsibility, consideration and empathy of the man.
Desire to extend the partnership	Alleviation or cancellation in partnership of fulfilment of aim experienced
Wish to identify with one's own parents	Aim of resuscitating one's own parents, e.g. the grandchild is supposed to give back to his/her own parents what was taken from them.

which may be "behind" the manifest desire for children among men; these include the following (Diamond 1991; Table 19.4):

Social Network and Infertility

Important components of social support include the affective aspect (providing emotional warmth), the activity-related aspect (offering concrete support) and the cognitive aspect (giving advice). Couples lacking an intact social network usually have more problems in overcoming their infertility crisis. Women display greater emotional stability and ability to adapt socially if they perceive their partner as reliable and trusting (McEwan et al. 1987; Beutel 1999). Whether sufficient social support of the partner has a positive effect on the man with a fertility disorder and accordingly prevents psychic disturbances can, owing to a lack of investigations on this theme, not yet be answered.

Talks with relatives about their unwanted childlessness are usually considered unhelpful by an infertile couple. Although couples want more informative counselling from the physician providing IVF therapy, they rarely express the wish for more elaborate psychological measures (Hölzle 1990; Strauß and Ulrich 1991). Moreover, **couples' unwillingness to reveal a diagnosis of infertility** prevents them from taking up the offers of social support available. Male infertility tends to be concealed much more, especially if heterologous insemination was performed. Thus 34 out of 40 couples concealed the fact that they were having heterologous insemination even from closest members of their families and only two of 26 "successful" couples were firmly determined to speak openly about how their child was conceived. The reasons given for this are:

- The infertile man's fears of a break with his parents.
- Fantasies of the men that the child could later prefer the biological father.
- The couple's own feelings of inadequacy related to their infertility.

The husbands particularly wished to keep the heterologous insemination secret, while their wives were more likely to accept disclosure (Schilling 1995).

19.5 Psychogenic Sexual Disorders

In a survey article on the **prevalence of sexual functional disorders** in the general population Spector and Carey (1990) found that 4–9 % of men report on difficulties associated with erection, 4–10 % of all cases of unwanted childlessness on absent or delayed ejaculations, 36–38 % on premature ejaculations and 5–10 % of the women on problems with orgasm. Amelar et al. (1977, cited in Strauß 1991) estimate that 10 % of all cases of unwanted childlessness can be ascribed to the sexual disorders of the male partner. Until about 15 years ago, 80 % of cases of erectile dysfunction were regarded as psychogenic. More recent urological studies have shown, however, that in 80 % of cases erectile dysfunction has an organic cause in which vascular and neuropathic disorders dominate (Roth et al. 1993). Unger et al. (1995), nevertheless warn about making physiological variations or deviations pathological by means of refined techniques of investigation. They point out large overlap of physiological findings among disturbed and undisturbed men in the few controlled investigations that have been made (see detailed review in Chap. 10). In this context, however, it ought to be considered that biased selection occurs when primary health care physicians refer patients to a urologist or sexual therapist (Gnirss-Bormert et al. 1995).

Before establishing male psychogenic sexual disorders, **detailed somatic diagnosis** is always required. This includes establishing general physical condition, hormonal and vascular status, drug history and neurological, urological and andrological status. For differential diagnosis (organic vs. psychic causes), nocturnal and/or morning erections are of greatest significance (e. g. Procci et al. 1983). Penile rigidity can be determined by means of special measuring devices. Differentiating more finely between psychogenic and organic causes is made possible by additional audiovisual stimulation of the patient during which penile rigidity is measured (Steffens et al. 1993). Technical-mechanical aspects of the disorder should not be overemphasized (Unger et al. 1995). If questions regarding nocturnal spontaneous erections, erections during masturbation and other non-coital practices or with other partners are answered affirmatively, this may be seen as sufficient grounds for a psychogenic sexual disturbance.

Establishing psychogenic versus somatogenic categories is performed merely for practical reasons. It should, however, be presumed that a sexual dysfunction in man or woman is based on a multiplicity of factors. Every sexual dysfunction is considered primary if it occurs in every sexual contact. It is considered secondary if there has been at least one sexual contact without a corresponding sexual symptom. Secondary erectile dysfunction occurs more frequently than the primary form and has a better prognosis.

It was, however, shown in a validation study of "Marital Satisfaction Inventory" by Schröder et al. (1994) that even a partnership described as happy was not entirely devoid of **sexual discontent**. This study indicated that 50 % of men living in happy partnerships were discontent with single factors. They name as reasons for their sexual dissatisfaction:

- Discontent regarding the frequency of sexual contacts,
- discontent regarding communication about sexual needs,
- lack of variety.

In recent times a **change in the sexuality** of marital relations has been ascertained. Thus women seek therapeutic help above all because of disturbed libido and men because of erectile disorders (Buddeberg et al. 1994).

Psychogenic Sexual Disorders in Infertile Couples

Findings on the sexual behavior of infertile couples imply a somewhat increased prevalence of sexual problems among them, but the latter are more than likely to be a result of infertility treatment (Ulrich 1988). Among the factors which may lead to sexual dysfunction of a psychogenic nature are situational sources of friction, partnership conflicts, fears related to expectations and to failure, as well as possible intrapsychic conflicts.

Among the **situational causes** of friction as well as **fears regarding expectations and failure** are e. g. rationally planned sexuality for the middle of the menstrual cycle, ejaculation generated by masturbation in the doctor's practice for semen analysis, and IVF. Sexual problems seem to develop to a greater extent in couples who have taken part in IVF treatment. Thus in two thirds of 200 IVF couples Freeman et al. (1985) found that these enjoyed their sexuality less.

In **partnership conflicts** a sexual functional disorder on the part of the man during infertility diagnosis or therapy can be an expression of the conflict of dominance towards the partner who so wants his child.

Thus in their investigation relating to the coping behavior and couple structure of sterile couples, Bernt et al.(1992) found that infertile married men tended to have dominant partners. Findings of interviews with 157 couples with fertility disorders showed that they see themselves as less sexually attractive and report less sexual contentment within their relationship (Andrews et al 1992). In an investigation on 103 IVF couples it was shown that, in contrast to 44 % of the women, only 14 % of the men displayed a clear loss of libido. The decrease in sexual intercourse was, nevertheless, almost equally frequent in both gender groups (Strauß and Ulrich 1991). Kedem et al.(1990) found a higher rate of sexual

Table 19.5. Sexual function disorders at different stages of the sexual interaction (according to Arentewicz and Schmidt 1993)

Stages	Problems in the Man	Problems in the Woman
1. Sexual Approach	**Sexual Aversion:** passive indifference, feeling pestered, feelings of disgust, fear of "failure" or the like: avoidance behavior	
2. Sexual Stimulation	**Erection Disorders:** erection not sufficiently lasting or strong for satisfactory sexual intercourse.	**Arousal Disorders:** arousal not sufficiently lasting or strong for satisfactory sexual intercourse.
3. Insertion of Penis Coitus	–	**Vaginism** (vaginal cramp) Insertion of penis through cramped narrowing of introitus not possible at all or only with pain.
	Painful Sexual Intercourse (Dyspareunia): burning, stinging, itching in the genital area; in women also labor-like pains during orgasm	
4. Orgasm	**Premature Ejaculation:** seminal discharge even before intromission, during insertion or immediately afterwards.	
	Ejaculation fails to occur: inspite of full erection and intensive stimulation, no seminal discharge.	
	Ejaculation without satisfaction: Seminal discharge without pleasure and feeling of orgasm	**Orgasm without satisfaction:** "physiological" orgasm without feelings of pleasure or experiencing orgasm
5. Postorgasmic reaction	**Post-orgasmic disgruntlement:** irritation, inner restlessness, sleeplessness, bursts of crying, ill-feeling in genital area etc.	

dysfunction among men whose partner showed greater medical infertility problems.

The **intrapsychic conflicts** considered to be the cause of male sexual function disorder of psychogenic origin can be seen in analogy to the psychosexual developmental phases of Freud. Accordingly, a sexual function disorder in the man can protect him from unavoidable disappointment, arising from feelings of neglect by non-fulfilment of his needs in the oral phase. Disturbances in the anal phase may, in the adult man, cause sexual fears (e.g. fear of losing control over one's body), including aversion to sexual intercourse. Unsuitable methods of child rearing such as transmission of feelings of shame and guilt may also be seen as responsible for sexual function disorders of psychogenic origin. Thus Fahrner (1993) presumes that functional sexual disorders are the expression of repressed or misguided development, especially of sexuality or in general, of the personality.

Table 19.5 presents a survey of the possible sexual function disorders in the various phases of the sexual cycle of reaction, in which men of infertile couples are especially concerned with stages 1 and 2.

Sexual Anamnesis

A couple consulting a physician regarding fertility ought to be asked about their sexuality at the first consultation. It is, however, a basic precondition that the **relationship between the physician and the couple be based on sufficient trust.** Questions about sexuality signal to the couple that the doctor is prepared to speak to them about such matters and to choose, commensurate with their education, the appropriate level of diction (Crombach-Seeber and Crombach 1980). It is not sufficient to inquire only about the frequency of sexual intercourse, even if this is an important factor in the woman's failure to become pregnant (maximum rate of conception at a coitus frequency of 3–4 times per week (MacLeod et al. 1955)).

The **significance of the sexual history** is still greatly underestimated, particularly since a large percentage of unintentionally childless couples do not have sexual intercourse on the fertile days. Many of these couples have no knowledge of the connection between the menstrual cycle and fertility, or they may, because of a lack of desire or certain ambivalence, not cohabitate at the optimal point of time (Yüksel et al. 1999; cf. also Zinser et al. 1997).

The physician should also enquire whether the couple enjoys sex or whether their sexuality (e.g. desire, frequency of coitus, ability to have an erection, experienced satisfaction etc.) has changed with time. Since examination of the female partner is important for establishing a diagnosis of sexual dysfunction, it ought, if at all possible, be carried out (Schwarzer et al. 1992).

If the couple mentions sexual difficulties or problems, these must be taken seriously. It is important that the doctor ask concrete questions such as, "Perhaps you could tell me simply when you last had sex or slept together, what was good and where the problems arose?" "What did you think, do, feel afterwards?" "Is this the first time this problem has arisen or have you often had such experiences?" "How do you personally explain these difficulties to yourself?" In such a talk the doctor ought to give accepting, encouraging signals by means of gestures, miming, posture and eye contact. The physician must be able to speak without prejudice or inhibition about sexual matters; only then can he get an infertile couple with sexual function disorders to speak about aspects which have shameful connotations. Should such a sexual anamnesis reveal that possibly a more serious, psychogenic sexual disturbance, e.g. impotentia coeundi, makes conception impossible, it will be necessary to refer the couple to a sexual therapist. Otherwise the danger exists that the problem be veiled by insemination or IVF/ICSI treatment and not be dealt with causally.

Men with potency disorders of psychic origin also frequently have **great expectations with regard to organic-somatic therapeutic possibilities** (Schwarzer et al. 1992). Tiefer (1993) speaks in this connection of a "**medicalization of male sexuality.**" A fear of failure, which is subject to a self-reinforcement mechanism, is mostly at the bottom of sexual problems. Failure to have an erection on the part of a man and sexual lack of interest on the part of a woman towards her husband usually leads to sexual avoidance in the relationship. The partner capable of functioning sexually must accept that the one bearing the symptoms withdraws to protect him/herself from possible injury (Buddeberg et al. 1994).

Men with erectile dysfunction usually feel deeply hurt. Men with psychogenic erection disorders are often discontent with their partnership. They frequently experience their partner as more demanding than do patients with somatogenic sexual disorders. Often men experience the quality of their relationship as dependent on their potency, while women see their sexual reactivity rather as dependent on the quality of their relationship (Gnirss-Bormet et al. 1995).

PLISSIT-Model for Coping with Sexual Problems

The PLISSIT-Model of Annon (1987) may help the physician to decide whether he can treat the couple or the male/female patient with sexual function disorders or whether he ought to refer him/her to a sexual therapist (Table 19.6). It comprises four consultative steps, the first three of which the physician can frequently conduct in the office with couples who have slight sexual function disorders, as not every psychically caused erection disorder requires comprehensive psychotherapy.

Interventions of Steps P and LI are quite clearly within the physician's area of competence, Step SS is partly so, as it demands more special sexological knowledge. Step IT, in contrast, demands quite special sexual therapeutic knowledge which normally only a sexual therapist possesses.

Table 19.6. PLISSIT-Model for coping with sexual problems

P-Permission	The physician indicates, directly or indirectly, that he is ready to speak to the couple about sexual questions and problems.
LI-Limited Information	The physician gives the couple with fertility disorder useful information in connection with sexual problems. He gives e.g. information on possible side-effects of prescribed hormonal medication, results of studies on losses of libido which can be seen as temporary or the like.
SS Specific Suggestions	The physician can, even if he has no special therapeutic experience, make some recommendations to the couple in the hope that they will solve the couple's sexual problem (e.g. information from books, pointing to corresponding video tapes on the theme "Sexuality Disorder in Partnership", available e.g. from ProFamilia or from bookshops).
IT-Intensive Therapy	In more serious sexual problems the form of psychotherapy is based on the underlying problem. In partner problems a behavior-therapeutic or psychotherapeutic partner therapy is indicated; in problems connected basically with the patient's personality (e.g. fears), a psychoanalytical therapy may be attempted. In sexual function disorders (e.g. ejaculatio praecox, ejaculatio retarda), Masters and Johnson's, Helen Kaplan's as well as Arentewicz and Schmidt's sexual therapy has proven useful. The success rates of sexual therapies are given as 30–80% (Steffens et al. 1993).

19.6 Role of Clinical and Psychosocial Factors in the Indication or Contraindication of Therapies

Proponents of the psychosomatic approach such as Frick-Bruder (1989) and Stauber (1987) are critical of the unconsidered use of medical reproduction techniques. They are in favor of advocating IVF or insemination treatment only when the couple has overcome the infertility crisis and can accept their sterility. Nevertheless, coping with infertility is never a finally concluded process, according to Knorre (1990), who has had much experience with involuntarily childless couples. The fact that the couple consulting for infertility wishes to be examined only physically is also understandable because new techniques in reproductive medicine have reduced the category of idiopathic infertility to levels hardly over 5 % (Bettendorf 1989), in contrast to former levels of 50 % (Eisner 1963). It may therefore be expected that couples who are psychically heavily overburdened are reinforced in their frequently striking **defense mechanisms** such as rationalizing, sublimating and idealizing their desire for children. Whether uncovering defense mechanisms through psychotherapy is to be preferred to a forced sterility treatment must be decided from case to case. Many somatic criteria are usually cited as clinical criteria of indication and contraindication for assisted fertilization. Psychosocial criteria play a comparatively marginal role.

Stauber (1986) and Kentenich et al. (1987) have listed **psychosomatic contraindications** for assisted fertilization such as IVF treatment, which seem to be understood as a protection against more acute psychic damage, particularly of mother and child. Among these are:

- Psychosis of one of the partners,
- serious neurotic depression of one partner,
- ambivalent desire for children,
- maintaining the partnership by the desired child,
- idiopathic infertility.

It seems questionable to include the "ambivalent desire for children" as a contraindication to assisted fertilization since this can also be seen as mature analysis. An "exaggerated" desire to have children which is, according to Stauber (1991), characterized by extreme pressure of suffering (a child is required at all costs and renouncing parenthood seems impossible) is, on the other hand, a controversial relative contraindication for assisted fertilization (Maier-Kirstatter and Ditz 1994).

It is frequently also difficult for the physician consciously to recognize or deal with the psychological problem of the infertile couple because of achievement-orientated reproductive medicine. The pressure on doctors to achieve is analyzed by Knorre (1990) as "the fear of the doctor to fail with regard to a seemingly slight problem" (compared with the immutability of a fatal disease). It is argued that psychologists ought to be fully integrated in a medical reproduction team and to make it their task, besides offering psychotherapeutic support for the involuntarily childless couples, to advise medical personnel. This concerns how decisions are made for or against treatment of infertility, as well as supervising physicians and others within the medical reproduction team. Strauß and Ulrich (1990) have indicated how unfavorable and paradoxical a situation has arisen as a result of the development of medical reproductive technology, which has eliminated the emotions of the childless couple.

19.6.1 Possibilities and Limitations of Psychotherapy

In their postal survey of gynecologists in private practice, Bengel et al. (1994) noted that 35 % were in favor of psychosocial care throughout the total period of treatment, 40 % wanted psychosocial care during medical interventions, 42 % during the waiting periods and 53 % estimated the greatest need to be psychosocial care in the event of unsuccessful treatment. The basic condition for psychological or psychotherapeutic intervention in childless couples always ought to be the couple's own motivation. Even if psychosocial care is being increasingly demanded by physicians and psychologists, it must be considered that childless couples wanting children tend, at the beginning of infertility treatment, to show rather little motivation for therapy (Strauß 1991). Thus, in **explanatory brochures**, it is suggested, as e. g. in the context of IVF treatment that psychosocial aspects of treatment, the possibilities of success and the medical aspects be more highly stressed than heretofore. For the couple this form of receiving information, aside from the physician's consultation, could be a first step towards taking up an offer of psychosocial support (Strauß and Ulrich-Fehlau 1994). Moreover, the retrospective study by Souter et al. (1998) on 1366 former patients in England seeking offspring showed that only suitable **techniques of communication** could achieve a high level of satisfaction among infertile patients. Thus, a large number of the women interviewed had hoped for more of a say in the medical process of decision making. The physician in charge ought to give the patients greater opportunity to ask questions and to report in detail (orally and in writing) about the effects and side-effects of treatment. The relatively high proportion of drop-outs, especially in the third cycle of treatment (Land et al. 1997), can probably be prevented by detailed and honest information on the treatment and its side-effects.

Moreover, **steps towards self-help** before and during medical interventions such as IVF, the use of relaxation cassettes in one's own private surroundings, attending self-help groups in which leisure activities take place in

Table 19.7. Guide to establishing the psychosocial situation of the infertile couple during consultation with the physician or psychologist (central themes to be discussed)

Couple anamnesis/couple's history	• Getting to know one another, development of couple's relationship • Motivation of couple for wanting to have children • Specific role splitting within the couple's relationship • Changes in the couple's relationship because of diagnosis of infertility
Subjective theories	• Subjective assessment of the cause of childlessness • Possible reproaches (e.g. because of former abortions, infections etc.) • Fantasies about the unborn child
Sexuality	• Contentment with present sex life • Frequency and quality of sexual intercourse • Gender role identity as male/female etc. • Importance of sexuality for the relationship • Possible changes in sexuality because of unfulfilled desire for children
Psychosomatic aspects and processes of coping with unwanted childlessness (how does the couple deal with it emotionally and mentally in concrete actions and in their relationship?)	• Typical psychic complaints such as depression, fear etc. • Psychosomatic complaints such as tension headaches, sleep disorders, stomach complaints etc.
One's own body image and health behavior	• Relationship to and attitude to one's own body (e.g. health behavior in general and in stress situations, subjective evaluation of bodily defects such as a small breasts, penis etc.)
Social situation	• Economic conditions • Professional situation/contentment • Social/emotional support by e.g. friends, acquaintances, closest family members • Leisure behavior
Alternatives to desire for children	• Attitude to adoption/fostering • Considering possible professional/social compensations • Further life aims with or without a child

the company of similarly affected people, ought to be recommended to the couple more often.

Psychological problems of a pathological nature occur in about 20% of involuntarily childless couples (Connolly et al. 1992). Many decisions are demanded of the couple, for example:

- with whom they discuss the treatment,
- when they undergo special fertility treatment,
- at which point they wish to end the treatment,
- what kind of infertility treatment they would accept and which not,
- which alternatives are worth considering if their desire for children is not fulfilled.

It is not surprising that conflicts and tension arise in this connection. During psychotherapy it seems to be particularly important to offer the childless couple support in coping with their experiences of loss as well as dealing with typical conflicts of decision-making.

Conway and Valentine (1987) name the following nine losses which infertile couples must deal with:

- loss of fantasy about having a family,
- loss of genetic continuity,
- loss of self-image as a fertile person,
- loss of experience of pregnancy or birth,
- loss of experience of breast feeding,
- loss of participation in the next family generation,
- loss of further relationships,
- loss of experience of parenthood,
- loss on the part of other family members (e.g. as potential grandparents).

Ideally speaking, the physician in charge and the psychotherapist, as well as the couple, ought to decide together whether psychotherapeutic intervention should take place before, during or after fertility treatment. The perspectives of those concerned may indeed differ with regard to experience and point of view. Thus, older nurses and physicians from medical centers for reproduction might assess the emotional and physical burden of infertile patients as lower than their younger colleagues (Kopitzke et al. 1991).

In this context it is interesting to note the observation of Kemeter (1989), who said that in his institution 25 out of 53 patients at whose first contact there was a psychologist present did not return for further treatment, whereas if there were no psychologist present, only about 18 % of patients stayed away. An essential reason for the greater drop-out rate may be that the presence of the psychologist compelled them to confront their emotions and, with that, the ambivalences which frighten the patient and make him/her insecure. Similar reactions are also known among patients with chronic illnesses (Muthny and Koch 1989), where patients insist upon somatic explanations of their disease and may also see psychosocial possibilities of treatment as psychiatric stigmatization. It is important to emphasize the routine character of the psychologist's participation (e.g. in the routine procedures of a center), the patient's voluntary involvement and the guarantee of discretion.

Table 19.7 lists areas which should be addressed and discussed with the infertile couple by the doctor/psychologist in the fertility consultation to develop a comprehensive overview of their psychic and social situation.

19.6.2 Aims of Psychotherapeutic Intervention

The aim is, first and foremost, to support the couple rather than to uncover conflicts between partners. In concrete terms it is necessary to offer the couples psychological support during physically and emotionally difficult treatment. In addition, possible ways of dealing with their fertility disorder ought to be discussed; here the therapist ought to make the couple aware of biographical influences which frequently unconsciously affect treatment. Often the motivation to have a child is connected to earlier experiences of loss and separation as well as present pressures (Wischmann et al. 1998). In recent times **short-term therapies** are increasingly being carried out for involuntarily childless couples. From the very first session, the therapist focuses on areas in which the client is already successful, thus boosting his/her potential for self-reinforcement. No attempt is made to explain the problem comprehensively because in the theory of short-term therapy it is presumed that the solution itself is its best explanation. The following outlines possible psychotherapeutic procedures aimed at childless couples (Atwood and Dobkin 1992).

- Acceptance of the infertility crisis,
- acquisition of suitable styles of communication,
- transmission of information (e.g. surgery, perspectives for success),
- new definition of the infertility problem (e.g. with help of metaphors),
- clarifying the effects of infertility on partnership, family, friends, profession, etc.,

- making the couple conscious of the fact that occurrence of pregnancy does not lie within their control,
- making the couple conscious of special helpful situations or alternative rewards (e.g. questions such as: "Is it true that you always think of infertility?"),
- new definition of the couple's actual situation,
- offering future perspectives.

At the end of therapy the couple decide for themselves how important the fertility problem now is for them. Its importance has, indeed, frequently decreased.

19.6.3 Psychosocial Effect of Treatment

A study carried out (Bents 1991) on 15 infertile couples showed that 5 of 15 previously infertile patients had become pregnant four months after the end of the behavioral-therapeutic couple therapy according to Hahlweg et al. (1982). In addititon, an increase in sperm count, an improvement in communication between the couple, as well as a reduction in fear were noted among the men. Brandt and Zech (1991) report on the effects of short-term psychotherapy (3–4 sessions) before IVF treatment of 15 female patients. A pregnancy was ascertained in seven of the patients. Stewart et al.(1992) succeeded in greatly improving infertile patients' knowledge of infertility and its cause, marital communication and communication strategies in general, in the course of an 8-week group therapy offered once weekly for 2 hours. Surprisingly, no negative effects of therapy are reported in the literature. At present it is difficult to say which kind of therapy (e.g. psychoanalytical, behavioral, client-centered psychotherapy) is most effective since not enough investigations have been carried out. To this end controlled prospective studies would be required.

As a matter of principle, psychotherapeutic intervention should be offered to the couple as a unit. However, should one of the partners refuse, individual therapeutic therapy sessions may be considered. Not without reason does Schuhrke (1993) end her article surveying psychic problems in the medical treatment of infertility, with a call for the desire for children on the part of involuntarily childless couples not to be considered pathological. Thus the recently evaluated focal counselling concept of Strauß et al. (1999) was unable to show any clear effects of treatment. By and large, however, counselling was positively assessed by the participants in the therapy. In addition, the subjective wish for offspring, especially those of the women, was reduced. Moreover, the counselling had a visible effect on the participants to the extent that, in addition to medical treatment, they included other alternatives, such as new partnerships, intensifying professional and social activities, adoption/fostering in an attempt to fulfill their desire to have children.

19.6.4 Psychosocial Development after Infertility Treatment

Although, presently an estimated 1% of first-born children in western industrial countries result from assisted reproduction and although an increase in these numbers is to be expected by further development of reproductive techniques such as ICSI, the desire for children can only be realized by maximally 20% of all couples treated, often indeed after several **unsuccessful IVF-cycles** (Bindt et al. 1998). Involuntary renunciation of biological offspring after several IVF experiments signifies a lower sense of life satisfaction for many couples, but especially women (Leiblum et al. 1998), even if the marital and sexual relationship of the couple can be regarded as integral. The fact that these couples need psychosocial support in dealing with this crisis cannot be disputed. The physician/therapist should particularly support these couples in dealing with their undesired childlessness and help them to work out future life prospects.

> A follow-up investigation on how content infertile and fertile couples are with life clarifies what restrictions newly-gained parenthood may imply for the man and woman. The results show how important it is to explain to fertile and infertile couples that parenthood may, for both sexes, be connected (at least temporarily) with reduced marital as well as sexual contentment (Abbey et al. 1994).

Nevertheless, **how does a couple's relationship develop after successful medical treatment for disturbed fertility?** The investigation by Bindt et al. (1998) on 38 IVF couples and their children compared a control group with spontaneous pregnancies and showed that the couples with IVF children overall displayed a marked reduced ability to be aware of their own inner conflicts; they could deal with them only by projection, i.e. they attribute them to third parties. During pregnancy, the majority of IVF mothers reported marked **anxiety about whether their pregnancy would last**, which sometimes led to fitting out of the children's room only after the birth of the child. Men, on the other hand, frequently spoke about **fears regarding physical impairment** of an ICSI child. While these fears are understandable, serious physical handicaps in ICSI children do not seem to be any more frequent than in the normal population (Palermo et al.1996).

According to **subjective theories of IVF parents**, behavioral abnormalities in their children, such as sleep disturbances and states of unrestlessness in the first year are connected with the manner of their conception (Bindt et al. 1996). Within this sample survey, however, there was a relatively high proportion (12.5%) of children with handicaps, which the affected parents did not relate to the way they were conceived. Unaffected IVF parents tended to assume causal connections. The parent-child relationship in these families developed rather favorably, a result which is confirmed by Gibson et al. (1998). Nevertheless, greater concern about the well-being of the child in the first year was obvious among the IVF mothers, which can probably be related to the time before the desire for a child was fulfilled. Altogether, the review by van Bahlen (1998) on IVF children indicates that the **mothers and fathers of these children are distinguished by exceptional parental competence and warmth.**

Whether these positive parental conditions apply to a successful **parent-child-relationship** for **multiple births**, especially triplet births, remains to be seen in further studies. According to Bindt et al. (1998), parents of **twins** and **triplets** had underestimated the number of prenatal complications as well as the psychosocial pressures, particularly the social isolation of the mother. Cook et al. (1998), when investigating IVF parents and their twin offspring, found that raising twins subjected them to greater stress than that experienced by the control group. Parental, especially maternal, pressures related to bringing up triplets seem to be particularly great. In their prospective study over a period of two and four years, Garel et al. (1997) found that the mothers felt greatly to very greatly emotionally strained throughout the whole period of investigation. Most of them complained about stress situations with regard to educating children (dealing with childish aggressions and conflicts related to closeness and distance of their three children) as well as about the increased fatigue resulting from bringing up three children together. Of the 11 mothers, four indicated high levels of depression and took sedative drugs. Upon questioning after four years, four mothers said spontaneously that they regretted having had triplets because of the degree of psychic as well as physical strain. Even if this investigation is based on only a small sample, the great strain on families with multiple children remains clear. These families require – at least until their children go to kindergarden – adequate social support from family members, friends or from professional helpers such as child minders, babysitters or an au-pair. The latter cannot normally be financed by average families over a longer period of time.

These results show how important it is to have a social worker in the team providing reproductive care. This worker can make the expectant parents aware of the psychosocial and financial strains they will face and can indicate possibilities and assistance for relief. Well-informed parents can thus take precautions in advance for adequate childcare, thereby allowing a more carefree pregnancy as well as parent-child bonding without complications.

Help from outside, especially from authorities such as the youth welfare departments, may be provided to couples who decide in favor of taking a child by means of **adoption or fostering**. Women can decide more easily in favor of adoption/fostering than men. Men seem to have greater problems of acceptance with regard to raising a non-genetic child (Leiblum et al. 1998). The basic condition for beginning adoption or fostering proceedings is the couple's mutual decision to take a child. Adoption may not be seen as an alternative to a biological child. An unfulfilled desire for a child should be worked out by this time so that the couple is as free as possible to form a healthy parent-child relationship and can dedicate themselves without prejudice or bias to the adopted child. Couples who are deeply unhappy when assisted reproduction fails should not see adopting or fostering as the only possible next step towards their aim. The hurt felt by such a couple because of the woman's failure to become pregnant is altogether too great (von Schelling 1994).

19.6.5 Future Prospects and Psychological Research

Nowadays unwanted childlessness is clearly seen as resulting from a large number of factors. Recent comparative investigations of fertile and infertile couples mainly conclude that there are no significant differences between them. Studies concerned with the psychological differences between fertile and infertile men also come to similar conclusions. Nevertheless, it must be considered that infertile men tend to behave and express themselves in the context of what is socially more desirable than do women. Concepts related to stress-theory with regard to how male infertility occurs and is maintained are, on the other hand, well substantiated (Hurst and Dye 1999). Unwanted childlessness frequently represents a critical life event which is connected with the development of the gender role identity, the social group pressure couples have experienced and their social network. Even if women are integrated in the medical-therapeutic process to a greater extent than men, the men often suffer just as much from their unwanted childlessness as the women. Investigations on the male desire for children indicate that it is not less marked than that of the female. The strategies for solving conflicts used to cope with unwanted childlessness seem to be less appropriate in partnerships where the cause of infertility is on the male side. Gender role identity as typically male is rather a disadvantage in coping with unwanted childlessness. Men have greater problems than their wives in speaking about infertility. Thus to a lesser extent they experience social support which would reduce their stress.

Men, to a greater extent than women, wish to conceal their infertility. This latter fact is made abundantly clear in the context of psychological investigations on heterologous insemination. The majority of childless couples who would like to have children want to undergo medical treatment of a purely organic nature. Their motivation for psychological discussion is relatively slight at the beginning of treatment. Fears and prejudices of the patients towards psychologists, who might possibly prevent medical treatment, are inferred as the reasons for this. Moreover, it is presumed because of their own pressure of achievement, as well as little knowledge of psychology, that the psychological criteria are not sufficiently recognized by experts in reproduction.

Making physicians more aware of the psychic problems and worries of couples receiving treatment, as well as of couples in whom a pregnancy occurred, seems worthwhile (e.g. in the form of psychological training, supervision and Balint groups). Experts in reproductive medicine should pay particular attention to foreign couples, as well as to couples expecting multiple babies, ultimately leading to improved competence in discussion and knowledge about alternative offers of assistance. For this reason, too, routine deployment of social workers and psychologists to centers of reproductive medicine and practices is recommended, providing relief to the couple seeking children as well to the medical staff.

Essential issues of research have not been properly explored to date. Dealing concretely with the following psychosocial themes seems important:

- Classifying lay theories of unwanted childlessness and their prognostic validity regarding the course, success or failure of treatment.
- Investigating the processes of decision-making among couples for or against sterility treatment.
- Establishing how unwanted childlessness is coped with, compared inter-culturally.
- Establishing the life and future prospects of couples after unsuccessful treatment for infertility.
- Elaborating specific offers of support for patients treated unsuccessfully.
- Comparative investigation on the efficacy of couple, group and individual therapy with involuntarily childless patients.
- Elaborating communication training and group concepts for childless couples.
- Developing concepts of further education and psychological treatment manuals for the practice of the physician dealing with infertility.
- Long-term studies of the physical and psychic development of parents and children after assisted reproduction proceedings, with special emphasis on pregnancies with multiple issue.

19.7 References

Abbey A, Andrews FM, Halman LJ (1991) The importance of social relationships for infertile couples' well-being. In: Stanton L, Dunkel-Schetter C (eds) Infertility: perspectives from stress and coping research. Plenum, New York, pp 61–86

Abbey A, Andrews FM, Halman LJ (1994) Infertility and parenthood. Does becoming a parent increase well-being? J Con Clin 62:398–403

Alfermann D (1993) Androgynie. In: Schorr A (eds) Handwörterbuch der angewandten Psychologie. Die angewandte Psychologie in Schlüsselbegriffen. Deutscher Psychologen Verlag, Bonn, pp 15–17

Andrews F, Abbey A, Halman L (1992) Is fertility-problem stress different? The dynamics of stress in fertile and infertile couples. Fertil Steril 57:13–121

Annon JS (1987) Einfache Verhaltenstherapie bei sexuellen Problemen. In: Swanson JM, Forres KA (eds) Die Sexualität des Mannes. Deutscher Ärzteverlag, Cologne, pp 250–271

Arentewicz G, Schmidt G (1993) Sexuell gestörte Beziehungen. Springer, Berlin Heidelberg New York

Atwood JD, Dobkin S (1992) Storm clouds are coming. Ways to help couples reconstruct the crisis of infertility. Hum Sci Press 14:385–402

Band DA, Edelmann RJ, Avery S, Brinsden PR (1998) Correlates of psychological distress in relation to male infertility. Br J Health Psycho 3:245–256

Bengel J, Mahle-Napp C Stegie R (1994) Aus ärztlicher Sicht. Psychosozialer Versorgungsbedarf bei Fertilitätsstörungen. Sexualmedizin 1:7–10

Bents H (1985) Psychology of male infertility – a literature survey. Int J Androl 8:325–336

Bents H (1991) Verhaltenstherapeutische Paartherapie bei Kinderwunschpatienten. Jahrb Med Psychol 5:144–155

Berg BJ, Wilson JF, Weingartner PJ (1991) Psychological sequelae of infertility treatment: the role of gender and sex-role identification. Soc Sci M 33:1071–1080

Bernt H, Bernt WD, Tacke S (1992) Sterilität – Frauensache? Bewältigungsverhalten und Paarstruktur von sterilen Paaren verschiedener Diagnosegruppen. Psychother Psychosom Med Psychol 42:236–241

Bettendorf G (1989) Idiopathische Sterilität. In: Bettendorf G, Brochwoldt M (eds) Reproduktionsmedizin. Fischer, Stuttgart

Beutel M, Kupfer J, Kirchmeyer P; Kehde S, Köhn FM, Schroeder-Printzen I, Gips H, Herrero HJG, Weidner W (1999) Treatment-related stresses and depression in couples undergoing assisted reproductive treatment by IVF or ICSI. Andrologia 31:27–35

Bindt C, Berger M, Ohlsen K (1998) Psychosomatische Aspekte zur Elternschaft und kindlichen Entwicklung. In: Brähler E, Goldschmidt S (eds) Psychosoziale Aspekte von Fruchtbarkeitsstörungen. Huber, Bern, pp 104–113

Boivin J, Shoog-Svanberg A, Andersson, Skoog-Svanberg A, Hjelmstedt, Collins A, Bergh T (1998) Psychological reactions during in-vitro fertilization: similar response pattern in husbands and wives. Hum Reprod 13:3262–3267

Brähler E, Brächler C (1992) Psychische Probleme unfruchtbarer Paare. Psychomed 4:43–47

Brähler E (1993) Fruchtbarkeitsstörungen – Trends in der psychosomatischen Forschung. Psychother Psychosom Med Psychol 43:298–303

Brähler E, Felder H, Strauß B (1998) Psychologische Aspekte von Fruchtbarkeitsstörungen. Psychomed 10:196–203

Brand HJ (1989) The influence of sex differences on the acceptance of infertility. J Reprod Infant Psycho 7:129–131

Brandt KH, Zech H (1991) Auswirkungen von Kurzzeitpsychotherapie auf den Erfolg in einem in-vitro-Fertilisierung/Embryotransfer-Programm. Med Wochenschr Wien 1/2:17–19

Buddeberg C, Bass B, Gnirss-Bornet, R (1994) Die lustlose Frau – der impotente Mann. Zur sexuellen Beziehungsdynamik in ehelichen Zweierbeziehungen. Familiendynamik 19:266–279

Connolly KJ, Edelmann RJ, Cooke ID, Robson J (1992) The impact of infertility on psychological functioning. J Psychosom 36:459–468

Conway P, Valentine D (1987) Reproductive losses and grieving. J Soc Work Hum Sex 6:43–63

Cook R, Bradley S, Golombok S (1998) A preliminary study of parental stress and child behaviour in families with twins conceived by in-vitro fertilization. Hum Reprod 13:3244–3246

Crombach-Seeber B, Crombach G (1980) Wie spreche ich mit meinem Patienten? Formale und inhaltliche Richtlinien für die ärztliche Gesprächsführung. Sexualmedizin 12:488–492

Deipenwisch U, Hilse R, Oberpenning F, Nieschlag E, Sader M (1994) Persönlichkeit und Streßverarbeitungsstrategien von ungewollt kinderlosen Männern. Fertilität 10:118–121

Diamond MD (1991) Der werdende Vater: Psychoanalytische Ansichten über den vergessenen Elternteil. In: Friedman RM, Lerner L (eds) Zur Psychoanalyse des Mannes. Springer, Berlin Heidelberg New York, pp 39–63

Dunkel-Schetter C, Lobel M (1991) Psychological reactions to infertility. In: Stanton AL, Dunkel-Schetter C (eds) Infertility. Perspectives from stress and coping research. Plenum, New York

Eckert H, Sobeslavsky I, Held HJ (1998) Psychische Merkmale bei Paaren mit unerfülltem Kinderwunsch vor IVF. In: Brähler E, Goldschmidt S (eds) Psychosoziale Aspekte von Fruchtbarkeitsstörungen. Huber, Bern, pp 27–50

Edelmann RJ, Connolly KJ (1986) Psychological aspects of infertility. Br J Med Psychol 59:209–219

Edelmann RJ, Humphrey M, Owens DJ (1994) The meaning of parenthood and couples' reaction to male infertility. Br J Med Psychol 67:291–299

Eisner BG (1963) Some psychological differences between fertile and infertile women. J Clin Psyc 19:391–395

Erikson EH (1976) Identität und Lebenszyklus. Suhrkamp, Frankfurt

Fahrner EM (1993) Sexuelle Störungen. In: Schorr A (ed) Handwörterbuch der Angewandten Psychologie. Deutscher Psychologen Verlag, Bonn, pp 632–637

Fischer C, Rohde A, Klaßen R, Marneros A, Dietrich K (1996) Einstellung zu Sexualität, Schwangerschaft und Geburt bei männlichen Patienten einer Kinderwunschsprechstunde. Z Med Psycho 4:176–1985

Freeman E, Boxer A, Rickels K, Tureck R, Mastrioanni L (1985) Psychological evaluation and support in a program of in vitro fertilization and embryo transfer. Fertil Steril 43:48–53

Frick-Bruder V (1989) Das infertile Paar In: Bettendorf G, Breckwoldt M (eds) Reproduktionsmedizin. Fischer, Stuttgart, pp 399–406

Frick-Bruder V (1991) Schwanger um jeden Preis? Sexualmedizin 20:238–242

Gagel DE, Ulrich D, Pastor VS, Kentenich H (1998) Partnerschaft, Schwangerschaft und frühe Kindesentwicklung nach durch IVF-erfülltem Kinderwunsch im Vergleich zu Familien mit natürlich gezeugten Kindern. In: Brähler E, Goldschmidt S (eds) Psychosoziale Aspekte von Fruchtbarkeitsstörungen. Huber, Berlin, pp 113–125

Garel M, Salobir C, Blondel B (1997) Psychological consequences of having triplets: a 4-year follow-up study. Fertil Steril 67:1162–1165

Gibson FL, Ungerer JA, Leslie GI, Saunders DM, Tennant CC (1998) Development, behaviour and temperament: a prospective study of infants conceived through in-vitro fertilization. Hum Reprod 13:1727–1732

Gloger-Tippelt G (1988) Die Entwicklung des Konzept "eigenes Kind" im Verlauf des Übergangs zur Elternschaft In: Bräher E, Meyer A (eds) Partnerschaft, Sexualität und Fruchtbarkeit. Beiträge aus Forschung und Praxis. Springer, Berlin Heidelberg New York, pp 57–69

Gnirrs-Bormet R, Sieber M, Buddeberg C (1995) Sexualmedizinische Diagnostik und Therapie von Erektionsstörungen in einer Spezialsprechstunde. Z Sexualforsch 8:12–23

Goebel P, Lübke F (1987) Katamnestische Untersuchung an 96 Paaren mit heterologer Insemination. Geburtsh Fr 47:636–640

Goldschmidt O, De Boor C (1976) Psychoanalytische Untersuchung funktionell steriler Paare. Psyche 30:899–923

Goldschmidt S, Unger U, Seikowski K, Brähler E (1997) Psychologische Aspekte von Fruchtbarkeitsstörungen. Ein Überblick zum Forschungsthema. Z Med Psycho 3/4:117–130

Greil A, Porter K, Leitko T (1989) Sex and intimacy among infertile couples. J Psychol Hum Sex 2:117–138

Grimmig RE, Jaiser F, Pfründer D (1992) Selbstbild und Körpererleben bei unfreiwilliger Kinderlosigkeit. Psychother Psychosom Med Psychol 42: 253–259

Guttormsen G (1992) Unfreiwillige Kinderlosigkeit: ein Familienproblem. Praxis Kinderpsychol Kinderpsychiat 41:247–252

Hahlweg K, Schindler R, Revenstorf D (1982) Partnerschaftsprobleme. Springer, Berlin Heidelberg New York

Hellhammer DH, Hubert W, Freischem CW, Nieschlag E (1985) Male infertility: relationships among gonadotropins, sex steroids, seminal parameters and personality attitudes. Psychos Med 47:58–66

Hölzle C (1987) Kinderlosigkeit als Krise. Reproduktionsmedizin als Retting In: Zipfel G (ed) Reproduktionsmedizin. Die Enteignung der weiblichen Natur. Konkret Literatur-Verlag, Hamburg, p 22f

Hölzle C (1990) Die psychische Bewältigung der In-vitro-Fertilisation – eine empirische Studie zu Kinderwunsch und Streßverarbeitungsmechanismen von Sterilitätspatientinnen. Literaturverlag, Münster

Hubert W, Hellhammer DH, Freischem CW (1985) Psychobiological profiles in infertile men. J Psychosom 2:161–165

Hurst KM, Dye L (1999) Streß und männliche Subfertilität. In: Brähler E, Felder H, Strauß B (eds) Fruchtbarkeitsstörungen. Hogrefe, Göttingen, pp 27–42 (Jahrbuch der Medizinischen Psychologie 17.)

Kedem P, Mikulincer M, Nathanson YE (1990) Psychological aspects of male infertility. Br J Med Ps 63:73–80

Kemeter P (1989) Praxis der IVF im Rahmen der Sterilitätsbehandlung In: Mohr J, Schuber CH, Jürgensen O (eds) Management der Unfruchtbarkeit. Springer, Berlin Heidelberg New York

Kentenich H, Hölzle C, Schimiady H, Stauber M (1987) Am schlimmsten ist das Warten. Sexualmedizin 16:364–370

Knorre P (1981) Zur sexuellen Entwicklung und zum Sexualverhalten steriler Ehepartner. Geburtsh Fr 41:301

Knorre P (1990) Fertilität und Infertilität aus psychosomatischer Sicht In: Brähler E, Meyer A (eds) Jahrbuch der medizinischen Psychologie. Springer, Berlin Heidelberg New York, pp 3–14

Knuth UA, Nieschlag E (1985) Endokrinologische Aspekte der männlichen Infertilität. Gynäkologe 18:63–69

Könnecke R, Küchenhoff J, Riesbeck M, Ermel S, Schilling S (1998) Kinderwunsch-Motive ungewollt kinderloser Männer. In: Brähler E, Goldschmidt S (eds) Psychosoziale Aspekte von Fruchtbarkeitsstörungen. Huber, Bern, pp 163–188

Kohlberg L (1974) Zur kognitiven Entwicklung des Kindes. Suhrkamp, Frankfurt

Kopitzke EJ, Berg BJ, Wilson JF, Owens D (1991) Physical and emotional stress associated with components of the infertility investigation: perspectives of professionals and patients. Fertil Steril 55:1137–1143

Kühler T (1989) Zur Psychologie des männlichen Kinderwunsches. Ein kritischer Literaturbericht. Deutscher Studien-Verlag, Weinheim

Land JA, Courtar DA, Evers JLH (1997) Patient dropout in an assisted reproductive technology program: implications for pregnancy rates. Fertil Steril 68:278–281

Leiblum S, Kemman E, Lane M (1987) The psychological concomitants of in vitro fertilization. J Psychosom Obstet Gynaecol 6:165–178

Leiblum SR, Aviv A, Hamer R (1998) Life after infertility treatment: a long-term investigation of marital and sexual function. Hum Reprod 13: 3569–3574

Liebman-Smith J (1987) In pursuit of pregnancy. How couples discover, cope with and resolve their infertility problems. Market, New York

Löhr, H (1992) Kinderwunsch und Kinderzahl. In: Bertram H (ed) Die Familie in Westdeutschland. Stabilität und Wandel familialer Lebensformen. (DJI: Familien-Survey 1). Leske und Budrich, Opladen

MacLeod J, Gold RZ, McLane CM (1955) Correlation of the male and female factors in human infertility. Fertil Steril 6:112

Mai FMM, Rump EE (1972) Are infertile men and women neurotic? Aust J Psyc 24:83–86

Maier-Kirstätter C, Ditz S (1994) Psychosomatische Aspekte bei Diagnostik und Therapie der Sterilität. In: Runnebaum B, Rabe T (eds) Gynäkologische Endokrinologie und Fortpflanzungsmedizin, vol 2. Springer, Berlin Heidelberg New York, pp 202–203

Matzen K, Pook M, Schnapper U, Krause W, Florin I (1999) Tages-Aktivitäts-Rhythmik und Schlafqualität bei idiopathisch infertilen Männern. In: Brähler E, Felder H, Strauß B (eds) Fruchtbarkeitsstörungen. Hogrefe, Göttingen, pp 165–174 (Jahrbuch der Medizinischen Psychologie 17)

McEwan KL, Costello CB, Taylor PJ (1987) Adjustment to infertility. J Abn Psych 96:108–116

Mertens W (1994) Zur Psychoanalyse des männlichen Kinderwunsches und des Vaterwerdens. In: Mertens W (ed) Entwicklung der Psychosexualität und der Geschlechtsidentität, vol 2. Kohlhammer, Stuttgart, pp 189–190

Meyer F, Felder H (1998) Das Erleben einer In-Vitro-Fertilisationsbehandlung unter Berücksichtigung der Paarbeziehung. In: Bräher E, Goldschmidt S (eds) Psychosoziale Aspekte von Fruchtbarkeitsstörungen. Huber, Bern, pp 50–63

Mischel W (1971) Introduction to personality. Holt, Rinehart & Winston, New York

Money J (1994) Zur Geschichte des Konzepts Gender Identity Disorder. Z Sexualforsch 7:20–34

Muthny FA, Koch U (1989) Künftige Aufgabenfelder des Psychosomatikers bei chronischen körperlichen Erkrankungen. Psychoätiologischer Spurensucher oder Diener der Organmedizin. In: Speidel H, Strauß B (eds) Zukunftsaufgaben der psychosomatischen Medizin. Springer, Berlin Heidelberg New York, pp 119–132

Nachtigall R, Becker G, Wozny M (1992) The effects of gender-specific diagnosis on men's and women's response to infertility. Fertil Steril 57:113–121

Naeve-Herz R (1988) Kinderlose Ehen. Juventa, Weinheim

Oerter R (1987) Psychosexuelle Identifikation nach Freud. In: Oerter R, Montada L (eds) Entwicklungspsychologie. Psychologie-Verlags-Union, Munich, pp 231–232

Onnen-Isemann C (1998) Ungewollte Kinderlosigkeit und ihre Auswirkungen auf die Ehebeziehung. In: Brähler E, Goldschmidt S (eds) Psychosoziale Aspekte von Fruchtbarkeitsstörungen. Huber, Bern, pp 10–26

Palermo GD, Colombero LT, Schattman GL, Davis OK, Rosenwak Z (1996) Evolution of pregnancies and initial follow-up of newborns delivered after intracytoplasmic sperm injection. J Am Med A 276:1893–1897

Pöhler K (1992) Medizinpsychologische Aspekte der Sterilitätsbehandlung durch In-vitro-Fertilisation. PhD thesis, University of Halle

Pöhler K, Weiland G (1998) Die Bedeutung sozialen Kompetenzerlebens und emotionaler Bindung für die Bewältigung von Fruchtbarkeitsstörungen. In: Brähler E, Goldschmidt S (eds) Psychosoziale Aspekte von Fruchtbarkeitsstörungen. Huber, Bern, pp 125–140

Poland ML, Giblin PT, Ager JW, Moghissi KS (1986) Effect of stress on semen quality in semen donors. Int J Fertil 31:229–231

Pook M, Buschen-Caffier B, Schnapper U, Speiger K, Krause W, Florin I (1999) Kognitionen bei Infertilität: Entwicklung und Validierung eines Fragebogens (KINT). Diagnostica 45:104–113

Procci W, Goldstein DA, Kletzky OA (1983) Impotence in uremia. In: Levy NB (ed) Psychonephrology 2. Plenum, New York, pp 235–246

Roos PE, Cohen LH (1987) Sex role and social support as moderators of life stress adjustment. J Pers Soc Psychol 52:576–585

Roth St, Semjonow A, Rathert P (1993) Potenz und Reproduktion. In: Roth St, Semjonow A, Rathert P (eds) Klinische Urologie. Springer, Berlin Heidelberg New York, pp 76–97

Schilling G (1995) Zur Problematik familiärer Geheimnisse am Beispiel der heterologen Insemination. Psychother Psychosom Med Psychol 45:16–23

Schneider NF (1991) Warum noch Ehe? Betrachtungen aus austauschtheoretischer Perspektive. Z Familienforsch 3:49–72

Schröder S, Hahlweg K, Hank G, Klann N (1994) Sexuelle Unzufriedenheit und Qualität der Partnerschaft (befriedigende Sexualität gleich gute Partnerschaft)? Z Klin Psychol 23:178–187

Schuerman H (1948) Über die Zunahme männlicher Fertilitätsstörungen und über die Bedeutung psychischer Einflüsse für die zentralnervöse Regulation der Spermiogenese. Med Klin 13:366–368

Schuhrke B (1993) Psychische Probleme bei der medizinischen Unfruchtbarkeitsbehandlung und ihre Bewältigung: ein Überblick. Verhaltensmod Verhaltensmed 14:244–270

Schwarzer JU, Kropp W, Kockott G, Poland D (1992) Befragung der Partnerin bei erektiler Impotenz. Ein wichtiges Diagnostikum. Sexualmedizin 21:7–11

Seibel MM, Taymor ML (1982) Emotional aspects of infertility. Fertil Steril 37:137–145

Seikowski K, Glander HJ, Schingnitz U, Wagner D (1998) Psychopathogenetische Aspekte der Subfertilität des Mannes. In: Brähler E, Goldschmidt S (eds) Psychosoziale Aspekte von Fruchtbarkeitsstörungen. Huber, Bern, pp 151–163

Souter VL, Penney G, Hoptin JL, Templeton AA (1998) Patient satisfaction with the management of infertility. Hum Reprod 13:1831–1836

Spector JP, Carey MP (1990) Incidence and prevalence of the sexual dysfunctions: a critical review of the empirical literature. Arch Sex Behav 19:389–408

Stanton A (1992) Downward comparison in infertile couples. Bas Appl Ps 13:389–403

Stauber M (1979) Die Psychosomatik der sterilen Ehe. Grosse, Berlin

Stauber M, Maaßen V, Dincer C, Spielmann H (1985) Extrakorporale Fertilisation – psychosomatische Aspekte In: Jürgensen O, Richter D (eds) Psychosomatische Probleme in der Psychologie und Geburtshilfe (1984). Springer, Berlin Heidelberg New York, pp 163–168

Stauber M (1986) Zur Psychosomatik der modernen Reproduktionsmedizin. Prax Psychother Psychosom 31:7–15

Stauber M (1987) Ein Kind um jeden Preis – psychosomatische Aspekte. Arch Gynecol Obstet 242:136–138

Stauber M (1989) Psychosomatische Aspekte der Sterilität. In: Bettendorf G, Breckwoldt M (eds) Reproduktionsmedizin. Fischer, Stuttgart, pp 390–398

Steffens J, Jünnemann KP, Derouet H, Weidner W (1993) Diagnostik und Therapie der erektilen Dysfunktion. Urologe (B) 33:6–12

Stewart DE, Boydell KM, McCarthy K, Swerdlyk S, Redmond C, Cohrs W (1992) A prospective study of the effectiveness of brief professionally-led support groups for infertility patients. Int J Psy Med 22:173–182

Stieve H (1952) Der Einfluß des Nervensystems auf Bau und Tätigkeit der Geschlechtsorgane des Menschen. Thieme, Stuttgart

Strauß B, Ulrich D (1990) Zur psychologischen Betreuung von Sterilitätspatienten. Aufgaben, Probleme und konzeptionelle Überlegungen. In: Brähler E, Meyer A (eds) Psychologische Probleme in der Reproduktionsmedizin. Springer, Berlin Heidelberg New York, pp 127–143

Strauß B (1991) Psychosomatik der Sterilität und der Sterilitätsbehandlung. Enke, Stuttgart

Strauß B, Ulrich D (1991) Psychologische Betreuung von Sterilitätspatienten. In: Brähler E, Meyer A (eds) Jahrbuch der Medizinischen Psychologie, vol 5. Springer, Berlin Heidelberg New York, pp 127–143

Strauß B, Ulrich-Fehlau P (1994) Patientenaufklärung im Rahmen einer IVF/ET-Behandlung. Eine Inhaltsanalyse schriftlicher Informationsbroschüren. Fertilität 10:48–53

Strauß B (1996) Doctor-Shopping in der Fertilitätsmedizin. Arch Gynäkol 259:24–32

Strauß B, Städing G, Hepp U, Mettler L (1999) Fokale Beratungskonzepte in der Fertilitätsmedizin. In: Bräher E, Felder H (eds) Jahrbuch der Medizinischen Psychologie 17. Hogrefe, Göttingen, pp 272–290

Sturgis SH, Taymor ML, Morris T (1957) Routine psychiatric interviews in a sterility investigation. Fertil Steril 8:521–526

Tiefer L (1993) Über die fortschreitende Medikalisierung männlicher Sexualität. Z Sexualforsch 6:119–131

Trautner HM (1991) Lehrbuch der Entwicklungspsychologie, vol 2. Theorien und Befunde. Hogrefe, Göttingen

Trautner HM (1992) Entwicklung von Konzepten und Einstellungen zur Geschlechterdifferenzierung. Bildung Erziehung 45:47–62

Ulrich D (1988) Zur Psychosomatik des unerfüllten Kinderwunsches: Literaturübersicht. In: Brähler E, Meyer A (eds) Partnerschaft, Sexualität und Fruchtbarkeit. Springer, Berlin Heidelberg New York, pp 101–113

Unger U, Brähler E (1995) Psychosomatik männlicher Potenzstörungen. Psychomed 7:231–235

Wright, J, Allard M, Lecours A, Sabourin S (1989) Psychosocial distress and infertility: A review of controlled research. Int J Fertil 34:126–142

van Bahlen F (1998) Development of IVF-children. Dev Rev 18:30–46

von Schelling C (1994) Wir wollen ein Kind adoptieren. Mosaik Verlag, Munich

Wischmann T, Stammer H, Gerhard I, Verres R (1998) Belastende Lebensereignisse und Paarbeziehungsmuster bei Paaren mit idiopathischer Sterilität – erste Ergebnisse aus der Paarberatung und -therapie in der "Heidelberger Kinderwunsch-Sprechstunde". In: Brähler E, Goldschmidt S (eds) Psychosoziale Aspekte von Fruchtbarkeitsstörungen. Huber, Bern, pp 63–78

Yüksel E, Gacinski L, Kentenich H (1999) Besondere Aspekte in der Betreuung steriler türkischer Paare in der Migration. In: Brähler E, Felder H, Strauß B (eds) Fruchtbarkeitsstörungen. Hogrefe, Göttingen, pp 291–302 (Jahrbuch der Medizinischen Psychologie 17)

Zinser K, Pook H, Florin I, Krause W, Tuschen-Caffier B (1997) Psychotherapie bei idiopathischer männlicher Infertilität. Unveröffentlichter Vortrag beim Workshop "Psychologie der Infertilität". Marburg, 18.1.1997

CHAPTER 20

Male Contribution to Contraception 20

E. Nieschlag · H. M. Behre · U. Engelmann · U. Schwarzer

20.1 Requirements and Perspectives

E. Nieschlag

> Making contraceptive methods available to men is one of the tasks of andrology. Such methods are necessary both to maintain stable populations in industrial nations, as well as to diminish population growth in developing countries (see Chap. 17).

20.1.1 Population Growth and Contraception

On October 12, 1999, the world population exceeded the 6 billion mark and even conservative prognoses estimate that **8 billion** will populate the earth by 2020 (Fig. 20.1). Developing countries bear the onus of this enormous population growth, while the population of industrial nations is largely stable. The population explosion creates hardly surmountable ecological and economic problems. India can be taken as an example, where one sixth of the world's population occupies 2.5 % of the earth's land surface, and where uncontrolled pop-

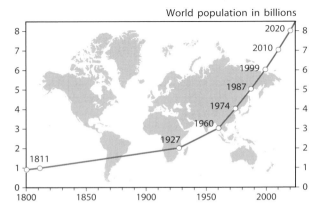

Fig. 20.1. Rapid growth of world population since the middle of the 20th century and its projection into the current century

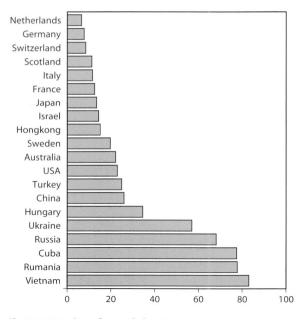

Fig. 20.2. Number of annual abortions per 1000 women in various countries (Alan Guttmacher Institute 1999)

ulation growth wipes out the country's economic progress, which has in part been spectacular. Medical progress has decisively lowered mortality, particularly of children, and ever more people reach reproductive age. Life expectancy has increased, largely due to effective medical intervention. In contrast, medicine offers only limited possibilities of adjusting reproduction to altered social and cultural life circumstances. Thus even today abortion, considered ethically and culturally unacceptable in many countries, is used for "family planning". As a consequence, of the approximately 910,000 conceptions taking place daily, of which about 50% are unplanned and 25% unwanted, **150,000 are terminated daily worldwide by abortion.** Of these terminations, 500 end lethally for the woman (WHO 1992). Comparative investigations have shown unequivocally that the highest numbers of abortions are performed in those countries where effective contraceptive methods are not available (Fig. 20.2). Thus the Netherlands and (formerly West) Germany have the lowest rate, while the formerly eastern block states, Vietnam and Cuba have the highest numbers. The example of Russia illustrates this reciprocal relationship: just prior to the dissolution of the old Soviet empire the rate of legal abortions was 127 per 1,000 women. With the fall of the Iron Curtain the use of modern contraceptives rose rapidly and the abortion rate fell to 68 per 1,000 in 1996. The low birth rates in western industrial nations which are of decisive importance for their stability are largely due to contraceptive methods.

20.1.2 Global Goal of WHO: Reproductive Health

Deeply aware of the situation, WHO introduced the concept of "Reproductive Health" as its goal in this area. **Reproductive health** means that reproductive processes and functions should take place under conditions of "complete physical, mental and social well-being" and signifies not only freedom from disease and from possible disturbances of reproductive functions. A child, once conceived, should have optimal conditions for undisturbed gestation and birth as well as for healthy childhood and development. Reproductive health implies the possibility of realizing the desire for offspring, as well as of controlling and planning fertility. **Contraceptive methods for men and women** are considered essential components of strategies which should lead to a high standard of reproductive health worldwide.

20.1.3 Acceptibility of Male Contraception

Recently public interest in male methods for contraception has notably grown. It is increasingly expected that men share with their partners not only the advantages but also the risks of family planning. Recent discussions concerning the micropill and oral contraceptives containing cyproterone acetate have cast a sudden light on the potential risks of contraceptive methods, even those which have been commercially available for longer periods. As risks tend to increase with duration of use, sharing contraception between men and women would reduce dangers for each partner. Population conferences such as Mexico (1993) and Cairo (1994) explicitly called for new male contraceptive methods.

Worldwide **more than one quarter of all couples practicing contraception rely on male methods**, albeit with varying preferences (Fig. 20.3) and the proportion of men practicing contraception is increasing. In the Netherlands the percentage of vasectomized men whose wives were of reproductive age rose from 2 to 10% from 1975 to 1995 and from 8 to 15% in the USA. It is to be expected that the percentage of men willing to practice contraception varies between cultures and with methods available. According to a survey in Hongkong and Shanghai half the men interviewed were willing to take a daily contraceptive pill; in Edinburgh and Capetown two thirds were willing to do so (Anderson and Baird 1997). After almost 40 years of female oral contraception, the attitude of men towards **new** methods of male contraception has changed. German surveys also showed men willing to use pharmacological contraceptive methods.

World

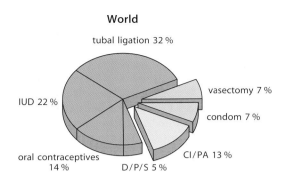

Germany

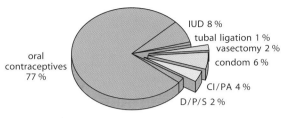

Fig. 20.3. Use of contraceptive methods worldwide (*left*) and in Germany (*right*). *D/P/S* diaphragms, cervical cap, spermicides etc. *CI/PA* coitus interruptus, periodic abstinence (UN Population Division, New York, 6/1998)

20.1.4 Possibilities

In general men's willingness to contribute to contraception can be considered to be high. However, before men accept such a contraceptive method certain prerequisites must be fulfilled. The method should:

1. be as **effective** as comparable female methods.
2. be **acceptable** to both partners.
3. be rapidly **effective**,
4. be **free of side-effects** and especially be without influence on masculinity, libido and potency,
5. be **without influence** on progeny,
6. be **reversible** in regard to fertility,
7. be easily **available** and financially **affordable**.

These criteria provide guidelines for evaluating existing methods and experimental innovations. Basically these methods can be characterized as follows (Table 20.1):

1. **those preventing sperm transport into the female genital tract,**
2. **those suppressing spermatogenesis** or
3. **those preventing sperm maturation.**

All existing methods belong to the first group, whereas current research concentrates on influencing germ cell development and maturation.

> The possibilities of effective and reversible contraception are limited to female methods. Periodic abstinence, the **condom** and **coitus interruptus**, as relatively unsafe methods, or **vasectomy**, as a method with limited reversibility, are **available to the male.**

The distribution of male and female methods used worldwide and for example in Germany shows (Fig. 20.3) that basically only a narrow spectrum of methods is actively available. All pharmacological methods derive from **one** principle, namely **hormonal contraception**. The danger of overdependence on this method becomes apparent when one considers a possibly drastic reduction in its use. This should provide sufficient

Table 20.1. Methods for male contraception

Strategy	Methods In use	Experimental development
Prevention of sperm migration	Periodic abstinence, Coitus interruptus, Condom Vasectomy	Vas occlusion
Suppression of spermatogenesis	–	Hormones, Gossypol, Ultrasound, Heat
Prevention of sperm maturation	–	Nitroimidazole derivates, Tripterygium wilfordii

impulse to search for new methods. As no male pharmacological method for contraception yet exists, research in this field remains a major task.

Existing and experimental methods are described in the following section.

20.2 Existing Methods

E. Nieschlag

20.2.1 Coitus interruptus

The criteria given in section 20.1.4 can be used to evaluate existing and new methods for male contraception. The method practiced longest, **coitus interruptus**, has the additional advantage of being completely free of side-effects, requires nothing additional and costs nothing. It does, however, require dexterity and self-discipline and reduces sexual pleasure. Moreover, **its failure rate is high**, as a pregnancy occurs in 18 out of 100 couples during the first year of practice.

20.2.2 Periodic Abstinence

Periodic abstinence, on which the various methods of **natural family planning** (NFP) are based, limits sexual activity to so-called "safe days" on which the likelihood of conception is low. Even if this method relies on observations based on the female cycle, it does require a male contribution as spontaneity and intercourse must be foregone for relatively long phases of the cycle. The methods' safety increases with the number of days of abstinence from intercourse. On average a large number of failures is presumed in which 20 of 100 couples per year conceive (Trussel et al. 1990). In a German women's hospital 38 of 87 (=45%) women gave birth after pregnancies occurring despite contraception based on "safe days" (Knuth and Mühlenstedt 1992). If a portable monitoring device (Persona®) is used to indicate days on which abstinence is to be practiced by measuring LH and estrone-3-glucuronide in urine the pregnancy rate drops to 12% (Bonnar et al. 1999). On average 13 days within a cycle must be considered "unsafe" or other contraceptive methods must be used.

When evaluating coitus interruptus and periodic abstinence it must be considered that despite their low effectiveness, in demographic terms these methods may contribute to population control, even if the risk of pregnancy remains high for the individual couple.

20.2.3 Condoms

The condom is the oldest barrier method available today. Early Egyptian drawings show men wearing condoms. In 1200 BC fishbladders were used at the Minoan court to prevent disease and pregnancies. In 1564 the Italian anatomist Fallopio described linen bags saturated with medication to be used to avoid venereal disease. In the 17th century condoms were first used in England for birth control. It is not certain whether the name derives from the English physician Condom, who was active at the court of Charles II from 1660 to 1685 and who recommended lamb intestines for contraception. The method was quickly exported to France and became widely used in Paris. They were known there as "capote anglaise", while in England they were called "French letters". The latex-based condom was made possible by the American Charles Goodyear (1800–1860) after he invented the process of vulcanization. The first large-scale manufacturer was Julius Fromm, who produced 150,000 condoms daily in 1920. At present the condom continues to be manufactured from latex. Alternative materials are under development; WHO/HRP issued guidelines for their manufacturing (1997). Polyurethane condoms, undergoing clinical trials, continue to be unsuitable (Frezieres et al. 1999). Since 1996 condoms sold in the European Community must fulfill quality requirements as prescribed in the Euronorm 600 (EN 600).

Even if manufacturing is subject to quality control, in 7–13% of cases the condom may tear during intercourse (Russell-Brown et al. 1992). The older the condom, the higher the risk of damage (Steiner et al. 1992). Apparently sexual practice also plays a role as some couples always report a higher rate of tearing than others as seen in trials with motivated and experienced couples who had no problems with tearing (Rosenberg and Waugh 1997).

Reports on contraceptive effectiveness of the condom show considerable variation. In general, it is assumed that 12 out of 100 couples will conceive during the first year of condom use (Trussel 1990). This is considerably better than the 85% of conceptions arising from unprotected intercourse, but ranges far behind the 3% probably achieved by female oral contraceptive methods. In addition, effectiveness drops if condoms are used for a longer timespan. This depends not only on technical defects of the product but on the fact that condoms must be used in direct connection with the sexual act and require constant motivation and attention. For this reason many couples in stable relationships consider condoms only as a temporary contraceptive method.

The acceptability of condoms varies greatly with socio-cultural factors. It is estimated that in Japan almost four fifths of couples practicing contraception use condoms. In Africa, however, their use is less than 1% of couples when the woman is between 15 and 44 years. In Germany at present about one quarter of couples of reproductive age rely on condoms (Fig. 20.3).

Since the biginning of the AIDS epidemic and the call for "safe sex" the condom has gained greatly in popularity as a means of preventing the risk of infection. Their effectiveness in preventing HIV infections, however, is notably less than that of preventing pregnancies. This is not surprising in view of the technical failure rate and in view of the fact that the danger of infection exists not only at the time of ovulation but during every sexual act. Meta-analyses conclude that the failure rate in the prevention of HIV infections is about 31% (Weller 1993) to 50% (April et al. 1993). Thus the protective effect of the condom against this highly lethal disease must be considered inadequate.

20.2.4 Vasectomy and Refertilization

U. Engelmann, U. Schwarzer

Vasectomy

History of Vasectomy. It is impossible to date the earliest vasectomy. At the end of the 19th century such operations were not performed for sterilization, but for other medical indications. At the time of the earliest vasectomies it was believed that severing the vas deferens would improve prostate disease, heal impotence or extend life expectancy. Vasectomy was advocated in the sense of a "fountain of youth" (Isnardi 1896; Wolfers and Wolfers 1974).

Eugenic aspects also played an important role among the indications for sterilization, as did elements of **social control** as advocated by Ochsner (1899) and Sharp (1902). In the 20s and 30s a series of nations passed laws justifying sterilization for eugenic reasons. Along with the other cruelties practiced by the Third Reich, compulsory sterilization for eugenic reasons achieved worldwide notoriety following the end of World War II. This resulted in the abrogation of the legal basis for eugenic sterilization in most states. Some states, however, maintained these laws and some later tried to apply them. Drake et al. (1999) describe the varied history of vasectomy and its indications changing over the course of time.

Vasectomy as a means of contraception became popular in the 60s, first in the USA, then in Europe and Third World nations. Countries with particularly rapid population growth like India and Thailand (Nirapathpongporn et al. 1990) established vasectomy camps and, according to Smith et al. (1985), in the USA sterilization was the form of fertility control most frequently chosen by married couples over 30 years of age. According to a

survey, in Germany a frequency of about 50,000 vasectomies per year can be extrapolated (Deindl 1990).

Social and Demographic Relevance. Countries with high birth rates should be considered apart from industrial nations. Contraceptive vasectomy is not popular in all developing countries, in some it plays no role at all. In India and China, and, to a lesser extent, in Korea, Sri Lanka and Bangladesh vasectomy is widely performed (Ross and Huber 1983). Generally, sterilization in the male always **competes directly with corresponding measures in the female**, i. e. tubal ligation, which ironically has become increasingly popular because of improved techniques, although vasectomy was always technically simple (Ross and Huber 1983). In any event, the introduction of **minimal invasive "no scalpel" techniques** serves to make vasectomy much more acceptable (Liu and Li 1993; Reynolds 1994). They are based on percutaneous electrocoagulation or chemical denaturing of the vas, or specialized puncture instruments which are used to minimize surgical trauma.

Particular ethical considerations concerning male sterilization apply in developing countries (Rizvi et al. 1995) and explain the current preference for female over male sterilization (3:1) with the rationale that vasectomy is hardly reversible and thus unpopular. New high technology such as sperm cryopreservation is only available in wealthy countries.

In the USA about 25% of eligible couples rely on sterilization for birth control, with distinct differences between black and white populations: among Caucasians vasectomy and tubal ligation are performed about equally, among blacks tubal ligation is clearly preferred (Forste et al. 1995). In the USA vasectomized men generally have above average education, their family planning is complete and they learned about methods of vasectomy in newspapers or magazines (Kohli 1973). In England only minimal differences between social classes were found with respect to the acceptance of vasectomy (Wright et al. 1977).

In Germany Schirren (1983) above all drew attention to the subject of vasectomy, to indications for the intervention and to its possible complications. In 1983 he propagated the opinion, then still widely held, that vasectomy represented an irrevocable intervention which, if performed without sufficient consultation with one's partner and "among friends", could be considered a "dangerous undertaking". Considerable consequences for the personality structure of the man and thus for the partnership were postulated. On the contrary, it could be demonstrated that men who were prepared to undergo vasectomy live in relationships stressing partnership. Under certain conditions, positive and beneficial effects for a relationship are to be expected (Goebel et al. 1987). This influences patient selection made by counselling and operating physicians and in Germany, predominantly men living in stable relationships are vasectomized. In German-speaking countries the number of vasectomized men varies: in Germany 422 men per million inhabitants and year are vasectomized; in Austria the number is only 81 (Engelmann 1990).

Indications for Vasectomy. In contrast to formerly held but still widely accepted opinions, we believe that the indication for contraceptive vasectomy is easily established.

> Every man of legal age and able to give consent may decide in favor of vas ligation or occlusion for the purpose of sterilization.

No special medical or social indication is necessary. But many physicians performing vasectomy require certain preconditions, mostly to provide backup-support for the physician. In such cases, for example, a certain number of children are required, a stable relationship with written consent given by the partner is desired; finally, the chances for refertilization are deliberately and falsely minimized. These measures represent a bias concerning the affected persons; only those highly determined to undergo vasectomy will be accepted. This procedure may be understandable, but it is not directed to the responsible citizen and patient. He has the right to objective counselling about the chances and risks concerning the intervention he wishes. Well-meaning, but false-negative counselling of the patient must not deprive him of the possibility of deciding in favor of vasectomy. This does not limit the surgeon's right to decline to perform a vasectomy in individual cases.

Informed Consent. As in all other surgical procedures, informing the patient and obtaining his consent are performed at least one day prior to the operation itself. We observe the procedures generally accepted for surgery without any special modifications. Neither consent of the female partner, nor even her existence is required. Information is provided about the procedure which is almost always carried out on an outpatient basis. The chances for later refertilization are explained according to statistics in the literature with patency rates of 70–90%. **Acute complications** consisting of **bleeding** and **infections**, usually negligible, rarely occur, but are mentioned. Possible connections between vasectomy and other diseases, e.g. arteriosclerosis or prostate cancer, discussed in the past and again recently, are mentioned to the patient with reference to the relevant investigations. In cases of doubt, the physician's explanation and personal interpretation may be helpful. The need for **postoperative** semen analysis is stressed. Although other surgeons proceed differently, we do not regularly use written forms for informing the patient and we do not even insist on a written statement of consent. We do, however, note in the patient's chart that informative counselling has taken place.

Surgical Techniques of Vasectomy. Vasectomy is a good example of how simple matters may be made complicated. What is to be achieved? The goal of the operation is to occlude the ducts reliably to prevent passage by spermatozoa, permanently or as long as the patient desires it. The following procedure has been established:

> In the ambulatory patient both spermatic cords are infiltrated with an anaesthetic. The cords are digitally localized through the scrotal skin, and, if necessary, local anesthesia is supplemented by deeper infiltration. After ascertaining the effectiveness of the anesthesia, the ejaculatory duct is clamped through the skin, using a small clamp and the scrotal skin is incised over a distance 0.5–1 cm. The vas is separated from the sheath and divided over two mosquito clamps. The vas is then dissected and a piece of approximately 1 cm is excised and fixed in formalin. The vasal ends are ligated and electrocoagulated. The entrance wound is sutured with a single suture (Fig. 20.4 and 20.5). The identical procedure is performed on the contralateral side. The wounds are covered with two small dressings. After one hour the area is checked and the patient can be discharged to home care.

The following is important: the patient must be **well-informed** and not be afraid of the procedure. In dubious cases, **premedication** is highly effective. In sensitive patients placement of a venous catheter is recommended. It should not be forgotten that even in such minor surgery emergency measures may become necessary. Acute complications are rare, but when they do occur, they are extremely irritating. Even minor bleeding can spread throughout the soft tissue, resulting in scrotal hematoma up to the size of a fist.

Effectiveness. When correctly performed, vasectomy is among the safest contraceptive methods. In most larger scale studies the failure rate lies below 1% (Trussell et al. 1990). This makes vasectomy as effective as tubal ligation. Failure is due to recanalization of the divided duct, to the extremely rare occurrence of a double vas or to incomplete division of the duct. Failure rates increase with lack of experience, inferior operating techniques and difficult anatomical circumstances.

Complications. Acute postoperative complications must be distinguished from long-term complications. **He-**

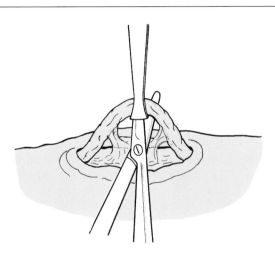

Fig. 20.4. Following a longitudinal incision of the scrotal skin along the vas deferens the vas is lifted by a small clamp

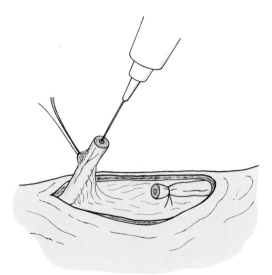

Fig. 20.5. Distal ligation of the vas deferens and cauterization of the proximal lumen

matoma of various degrees, **epididymitis** or **wound infections** up to formation of an abscess occur with a frequency of up to 5% (Alderman 1991). While this rate seems high, it should be remembered that vasectomy is a small operation performed by many surgeons with only limited experience with this procedure. Its supposed harmlessness tempts some surgeons to perform it on an outpatient basis, quickly and inattentively. The price is necessarily an increased rate of acute complications. These lead to short-term **absence from work** of an average of 2.3 days (Randall and Marcuson 1985). **Serious complications virtually never occur**; deaths during or after vasectomy have not been reported, whereas in

the USA 14 deaths/year are attributed to female sterilizations. Concerning costs, vasectomy is more economical than tubal ligation, the short-term **costs** of tubal ligation are about 3–4 times higher (Smith et al. 1985).

Long-term surgical complications are represented by **recanalization** on the one hand and the development of **sperm granuloma** on the other. Recanalization rates are reported to be about 0–3%. The actual rate depends on the surgical technique used. Resection of larger sections of the vas, burying the ends of the ducts in different planes of tissue, the use of fibrin glue or fulguration of the lumen, are all useful methods for minimizing the rate of recanalization. The use of minimal invasive techniques can on the one hand increase the chance of later refertilization but on the other hand it can also greatly increase the chance of recanalization by up to 50% (Goldstein 1983). The occurrence of sperm granuloma is likewise correlated with surgical procedures used and varies considerably. The data in the literature vary between 3 and 75%. In terms of refertilization chances, a sperm granuloma can be evaluated positively as it reduces pressure in the epididymis and epididymal tubule and so reduces the risk of a "blow-out". It is important to explain **acute complications** to the patient and particularly about the **possibility of failure**; he must be informed that in individual cases recanalization may occur even when postoperative semen analysis shows azoospermia on several occasions. If recanalization is to be completely excluded, the duct should be resected over several centimeters. Furthermore, polyorchidy and a duplex vas must be ruled out.

Vasectomy and Long-term Morbidity. Complaints of congestion, a feeling of obstruction or heaviness in the testis and epididymis as well as pain of different degrees are occasionally described by the patient, but are usually **temporary. Sperm antibodies** in the serum can be found in up to 70% of those sterilized (Heidenreich et al. 1994). Their presence is often associated with **sperm granulomas.** If refertilization is desired, we are not influenced by the presence of sperm antibodies nor by the titer, but perform refertilization in any case.

In the past, various diseases have been causally attributed to vasectomy. Based on monkey studies in 1978 it was concluded that vasectomy could enhance arteriosclerosis. Several large-scale investigations involving over 10,000 men determined that vasectomized men bore no higher risk for **arteriosclerosis, diabetes mellitus or immunological diseases** (Nieschlag 1987; Giovannucci et al. 1992). After these assumptions had been disproved, a few years ago a possibly higher incidence of prostatic carcinoma in vasectomized males was suggested by retrospective investigations (Giovannucci 1993). Follow-up studies and risk factor analyses were unable to prove a connection. Various national urological societies, including the American Urological Association

(AUA) and the German Society for Urology (DGU) have recommended informing the patient about current results and leaving the decision to him as a consenting adult. The basic problem lies in the retrospective nature of these studies. Bascically, prospective adequately controlled studies are necessary (Roth and Hertle 1994; NIH 1993; Farley et al. 1993; John et al. 1995). In the cases of prostatic cancer, these studies must additionally be designed over a 5 or, even better, a 10-year period. No connection between vasectomy and prostate cancer could be found in a large population-based case control study in men over 55 years of age (Lesko et al. 1999); further investigations were considered necessary in younger men. According to present knowledge it can be assumed that vasectomy does not increase the incidence of prostate cancer; final results from studies cannot be expected before the year 2010.

Psychosocial Effects. The history of vasectomy has already shown that psycho-sexual effects associated with vasectomy need not always be negative. On the contrary, the fact that the problem of contraception has been responsibly resolved usually has a positive effect on a relationship (Weidner and Weißbach 1992). The fear of unwanted pregnancy may disappear and sexual enjoyment may increase (Vaughn 1979). Conversely, those men who are pressured into being vasectomized (e.g. vasectomy camps!!), whose religion discourages or even forbids such procedures and whose partners are opposed to it or who are not sufficiently informed, may experience vasectomy with increased conflicts and complications. Thus the initial situation of the person is the determining factor, the expectations he places in vasectomy and how well informed he is, are key factors. Correct information, pre-surgical counselling and post-operative care and attention are important. These measures can prevent fear concerning and loss of male identity and masculinity. Long-term benefits and effectiveness of vasectomy continue to be discussed controversially (Jequier and Pryor 1998), even to the extent of spurious arguments that cryopreservation of sperm may replace refertilization or – even worse – replace information and counselling about vasectomy.

Future Developments. Both from a demographic and political point of view, as well as for the individual selecting a contraceptive method, vasectomy represents a highly safe option with few inconveniences for the patient, which can be performed rapidly at low cost. Without doubt it is superior to the equivalent female operation. It is hoped that changes in the understanding of the male role and better knowledge will bring about wider acceptance of vasectomy, especially in view of the fact that it is no longer to be considered final because in a high percentage of patients refertilization can be achieved by vasectomy reversal.

Refertilization

History of Refertilization Surgery. Single cases of vasovasostomy following accidental dissection of the vas deferens, mostly during hernia surgery, have been reported since the beginning of this century. After World War II true refertilization surgery, namely vasovasostomy and epididymovasostomy, following deliberate ligation of the ducts became more frequent and in 1948 O'Connor presented the first national survey on vasovasostomy. It is astonishing that at that early stage nationwide surveys were implemented to establish indication, frequency and success of refertilization surgery. In the USA such surveys were repeated in 1973 (Derrick et al.) and in 1979 (Wicklund and Alexander). In German-speaking countries the following situation pertains (Engelmann et al. 1990):

Along with the increase in vasectomies there is a rising number of patients who wish to reverse the procedure. Of the many reasons, three concerns emerge. First, the higher divorce rate plays an essential role; the main reason for refertilization is **divorce followed by remarriage or a new partnership.** The second most frequent request comes from couples whose family planning had been completed by vasectomy, but who now have **changed their minds** or who have suffered the **unexpected death of one of their children.** The third reason is improved economic standing and the resulting possibility of being able to afford offspring, or **psychological aspects** may prompt the desire for refertilization.

Refertilization vasovasostomy has been performed for more than 40 years; the technique has undergone major changes during that time. Initially, the macroscopical one-layer anastomosis technique, perhaps even with splinting of the small vas lumen was applied. Increasing use of the operating microscope brought with it excellent postoperative results reported mainly by Silber (1977). This prompted the development of microscopical two-layer anastomosis without splints. Improved results of surgery affected the mechanical patency of anastomosis which must be considered the real control parameter of surgical quality. However, there is a discrepancy between surgical patency of the restored vas deferens and pregnancy rates, which are distinctly lower. Today refertilization surgery is largely performed with optical devices, i.e. with loupe magnification or surgical microscopes. Patency rates of 90 % are common and are achieved by many.

Current Demand and Frequency of Refertilization. The potential demand for refertilization surgery can be roughly extrapolated from the number of sterilization vasectomies performed, from the divorce rate and from other (secondary) parameters. It has been estimated to be 250,000 to 300,000 in the USA per year (Cos et al. 1983). In German-speaking countries a survey taken in

1990 revealed that the vasectomy reversal rate was 3.5 % and requests for reversal were twice as high (Engelmann et al. 1990). It can be assumed that the number of refertilization operations will continue to increase, an unavoidable situation resulting from improved counselling.

Vasovasostomy: Indication, Counselling, Consent. The typical patient wishing refertilization contacts his doctor, usually his urologist, often the same one who had performed vasectomy. The indication is made by the patient's wishes which in turn arise from the arguments described above. As for other surgery, refertilization requires truthful counselling. Invasiveness is comparable to that of vasectomy with the exception that it requires more difficult surgical techniques. For this reason, general anaesthesia is recommended and **hospitalization of 3–4 days** should be reckoned with. As a general rule we estimate **patency rates of 80 %, pregnancy rates** are lower, i. e. **60 %**. If vasectomy was performed more **than 5 years prior**, we reduce these estimates by **a further 20 %**. The surgeon's experience with this operation (both positive and negative) should be considered. The possibility of a "blow-out" in the epididymis or even in the rete testis should be mentioned. This would then necessitate epididymovasostomy or can make surgery impossible for technical reasons.

Technique of Vasovasostomy. The patient is placed in supine position; usually a scrotal incision bilaterally or in the median of the raphe scroti is chosen. Less frequently an inguinal or infrapubic approach is used. Usually the surgeon operates while seated, avoiding interference with the operating table pillar; the operating microscope should be placed before the patient is positioned. Operating time of 2–3 hours should be anticipated, for this reason an indwelling catheter is sometimes inserted. Differing techniques have been described, initially macroscopical techniques with or without splinting of the lumen, followed by **microsurgical techniques** with loupe magnification or the operating microscope.

Macrosurgical Techniques. Initially surgical techniques without magnification and relatively coarse suturing material of 4-0 or 5-0 were used. Results were relatively poor because of complications such as sperm leakage and bad anatomical adaption of the lumen. The advantages lay in simple and rapid performance of surgery and for these reasons some surgeons prefer macroscopic techniques even today. As late as 1999 Feber and Ruiz saw advantages in shorter operating time, reduced costs and the need for fewer surgical skills (despite patency rate of 87 % and pregnancy rate of 50 %).

It is difficult to identify the vas lumen with a diameter of less than 1 mm on the nondilated side, and often it is obstructed by the suture. The technique was improved by the use of splints which were either removed at the end of surgery or, if biodegradable, were left in place (Rothman et al. 1997). Silber (1977) made a great contribution when he described the anatomical peculiarities of the severed vas with sizes differing between the dilated side proximal to the testis and the non-dilated side, and demonstrated that good operating results were best achieved with anatomically correct adaptation of the lumina.

Microsurgical Techniques. In our view, **solely macrosurgical techniques of refertilization are obsolete.** While they may be applied for vas-anastomosis, although inferior in patency, patent epididymovasostomy is achieved purely by coincidence or not at all. Whether **loupes with a 2–8fold magnification**, or an **operating microscope** with the advantage of variable magnification and increased field of vision is used depends on the personal preference of the surgeon, even if the best patency results are achieved with the operating microscope.

In the event of scrotal vasectomy, we dissect the ends of the vas deferens via a lateral scrotal incision. The scarred ends of the vas are excised. Patency of the proximal vas deferens is determined after insertion of a small flexible teflon canula by careful injection of saline solution. The liquid emerging from the distal vas end is assessed in the operating room in the operating microscope. If necessary, the epididymis is digitally massaged to obtain fluid. If no fluid is present, a "blow-out" must be assumed and the epididymis is examined. In such case we perform epididymovasostomy. Typically, whitish or yellowish fluid emerges containing viable or dead sperm. In this event, surgery is continued as vasovasostomy.

The best anatomical adaptation of the lumen is achieved using a two-layer technique by which mucosal approximation is accomplished with 6 interrupted sutures using 9-0 or 10-0 suturing material. Special vasovasostomy needles doubly armed and whose degree of curvature is adapted to the size of the vas, have proved useful. The vas ends can be aligned by using an approximator, facilitating placement of sutures. First the inner mucosal layer is sutured and should ensure a leak-proof connection. Precise positioning of the sutures will insure optimal patency rates; Goldstein et al. (1998) were able to achieve rates of 99.5 % using their "microdot marking technique" and 8 mucosa stitches. The mechanical strength of the anastomosis is achieved by the second muscular layer also using 9-0 or 10-0 sutures, however, with a single-sided and spatulated cutting needle. The short scrotal wound is closed in two layers. A well-fitting dressing supporting the scrotum is preferred by most patients and is left in place for a few days (Fig. 20.6 to 20.8).

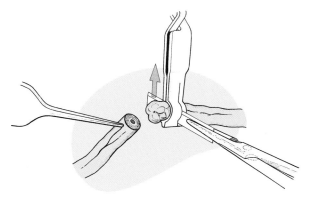

Fig. 20.6. Clean cuts of the two ends of the vas and careful bipolar hemostasis

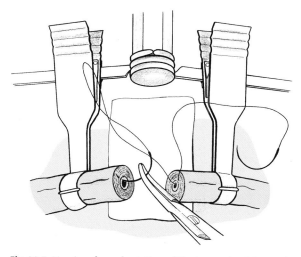

Fig. 20.7. Tension-free adaptation of the two ends of the vas by use of an approximator. Anastomosis of the mucosa is performed with nylon 10/0 double sutures

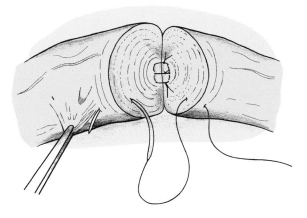

Fig. 20.8. Adaptation of the muscle layer of the vas by nylon 9/0 sutures

Results of Vasovasostomy. Results of vasovasostomy are quite variable, depending on whether one reads reports from individual authors or results from surveys; they are similarly variable depending on whether patency rates describing surgical success, or pregnancy rates which interest patients most are compared. Single authors report patency rates of 100% and pregnancy rates lying slightly below. Nationwide surveys report average results more accurately: in 1948 O'Connor had a cumulative success rate of 38–40%, in 1973 Derrick calculated a patency rate of 38% and pregnancy rate of 11–26%. In 1990, Deindl found a cumulative patency rate of 73% in German-speaking Europe and a pregnancy rate of 47%. Centers with a high operating frequency, with skillful techniques and thin sutures achieve better results. The time period between sterilization vasectomy and refertilization plays a role; even if these limits are arbitrary, the best results can be expected within the first 2 years, 10 years after vasectomy the chances for refertilization are markedly reduced (Belker et al. 1991).

Complications Following Vasovasostomy. The rate of **acute complications** is comparable with that for vasectomy or scrotal exploration, however, for differing reasons. **Specific long-term complications** result from re-obstruction after initial patency. A 3% chance of such obstruction because of scar tissue formation must be expected. If patients remain azoospermic following refertilization it is probably due to surgical failure or a more distal "blow-out" which had not been verified at the time of surgery. In these cases **re-operation** is indicated. Oligozoospermia can be the result of partial obstruction – in such cases re-operation may be successful – or due to limited testicular production. In such cases, aspiration of epididymal or testicular sperm is increasingly performed with subsequent IVF or ICSI (see Chap. 7) and additional cryopreservation (see Chap. 18).

Epididymovasostomy. If the epididymal tubule is damaged by a "blow-out", epididymovasostomy must be carried out. For technical reasons this procedure is only successful at the corpus or the cauda epididymidis. In the caput region, the diameter of the tubule is too small to accomplish fully patent anastomosis. Epididymovasostomy urgently requires microsurgical techniques, preferably using an operating microscope. We prefer to employ the end-to-side technique, others prefer side-to-side. After excising an oval window of the epididymal tunica, a single tubule containing sperm is chosen and is opened longitudinally. By placing 4 interrupted 11-0 sutures anastomosis of the tubule with the mucosa of the vas deferens is completed. The anastomosis is then finished by further interrupted sutures between the epididymal tunica and the muscularis of the vas (Figs. 20.9 to 20.13). End-to-end anastomosis is more difficult. The patency rates of microsurgical tubulovasostomy are

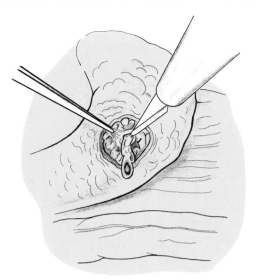

Fig. 20.9. A tubule is prepared and incised longitudinally

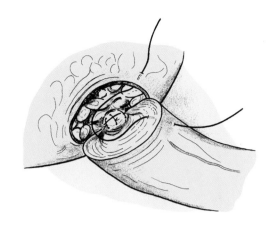

Fig. 20.12. Adaptation of the muscle layer of the vas and the tunica of the epididymis. Interrupted sutures at the anterior circumference with nylon 9/0 sutures

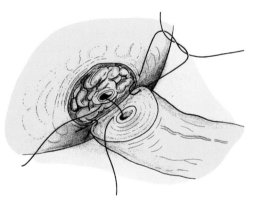

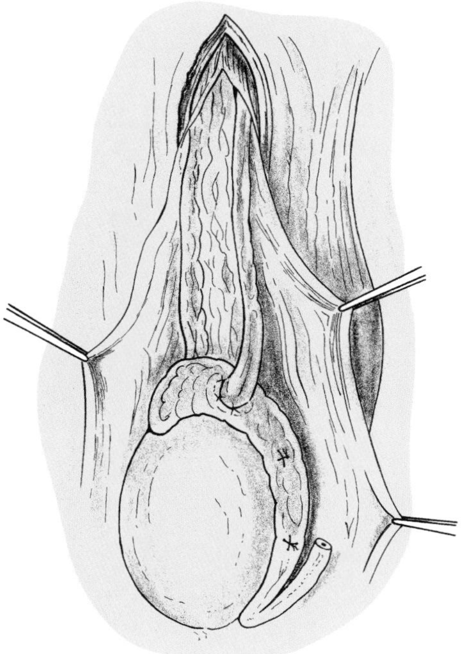

Fig. 20.10. Adaptation of the muscle layer of the vas and the tunica of the epididymis at the posterior circumference by nylon 9/0 single sutures

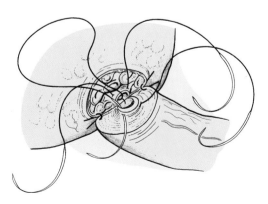

Fig. 20.11. Anastomosis between the tubule and the mucosa of the vas by nylon 10/0 doubly armed sutures

Fig. 20.13. Ligation of the epididymal tunic

between 39–100%, including single-case reports. The average patency rate is 45% and pregnancy rates are 18% (Deindl 1990).

Future Developments of Surgical Refertilization. Refertilization surgery will increase just as will sterilization vasectomy. Results, already satisfactory, will be further improved by optimization of techniques (laser suturing, fibrin glue, protein annealing) and by further solid training of surgeons in microtechniques. The very first incision must be optimal. Surgical intervention should be increasingly concerned with harvesting spermatozoa during surgery; these, following cryopreservation, will be available for ICSI – and following nonpatent anastomosis (especially in vasoepidymostomy) (Djerassi and Leibo 1994).

> We do not believe refertilization surgery is dispensible; we disagree with retrieving sperm from the testis or – even worse – from the epididymides for use in ICSI. Neither the pregnancy rates, nor costs, nor effort, nor – especially – the rate of complications are comparable with those of "conventional" refertilization surgery.

20.3 Experimental Approaches

E. Nieschlag and H.M. Behre

20.3.1 Physical Methods

Ultrasound can interrupt spermatogenesis. However, these alterations are irreversible, so that its use cannot be considered for contraception.

Heat can also influence spermatogenesis and sperm maturation negatively: increasing testicular temperature to body core temperature is sufficient to impair sperm number and function. Contraceptive approaches based on repositioning the testes from the scrotum into the inguinal canal take advantage of this effect. In this manner, the pregnancy rate of a few couples could be reduced (Mieusset and Bujan 1994). Whether wearing a special apparatus to **reposition the testes in the inguinal canal** will make this method acceptable is highly doubtful. Similarly, whether such repositioning of the testis in the inguinal canal would be connected with the same risk of malignancy as in maldescended testes needs to be resolved in largescale trials (see Sect. 8.3.2).

The proponents of this method were not able to explain the mechanism leading to suppressed spermatogenesis but considered elevated testicular temperature to almost body core temperature as the cause. Heat can influence spermatogenesis and sperm maturation in the epididymis negatively (see Sect. 13.3.9).

That increased temperature could also be reponsible for reduced spermatogenesis in repositioned testes was challenged by a study in which the scrotal testis were insulated to increase their temperature by 1°C over one year, which remained without effect on number and quality of sperm (Wang et al. 1997).

20.3.2 Plant Products and Drugs

It was long hoped that **folk medicine** based on plant products from various countries might identify substances with contraceptive effects. WHO formed a special Task Force which devoted itself to this target and investigated folk medicine in South America and Asia. A large series of substances could be identified to which contraceptive effects have been ascribed, but despite careful screening **no substance was found which was effective and without side-effects** (Farnsworth and Waller 1982).

One substance, **gossypol**, continued to interest scientists for a long period of time. Gossypol is a natural constituent of cottonseed oil which is used for cooking in some areas of China. In certain villages it induced such pronounced unwanted infertility that the effect was noticed and provoked intensive search for the cause. The results lead to comprehensive clinical studies in the Peoples' Republic of China in which over 9,000 volunteers participated (reviews in Prasad and Diczfalusy 1982; Segal 1985).

Nausea and weakness were frequent side-effects and in about 1% of volunteers hypokalemia caused paralysis which presented problems despite administration of potassium and interruption of therapy. In experimental animals gossypol caused irreversible damage to the germ cell epithelium, which is also observed in men following extended use. As gossypol occurs in two isomers which differ considerably in their toxic and fertility-suppressing characteristics, it was hoped that either by separating the isomers or by synthesis of analogs, a less toxic substance could be found that would still suppress fertility. These hopes could not be fulfilled. In the formulation tested so far the substance seems unacceptable for male fertility control (Waites et al. 1998) Nonetheless proponents of the substance continue to support its use, either disregarding its side-effects or accepting them along with its contraceptive qualities (Yu and Chan 1998).

At present another substance of plant origin is being tested for male contraception: *Tripterygium wilfordii*, which originates in traditional Chinese medicine. Here too it appeared that the toxic effects prevent clinical application (Waites 1993). No side-effect-free substance has been isolated that maintains effectiveness.

Alkylating substances can suppress spermatogenesis most effectively (see also Chap. 12 and 13). The generally irreversible damage to the germ cell epithelium and serious side-effects, which must be tolerated in chemotherapy for malignancies, however, prevent their use in contraception.

Other pharmacological agents do not interfere with spermatogenesis but rather with sperm maturation. For example, **sulfasalazine** can lead to disturbed fertility in patients taking it for e.g. inflammatory bowel disease. Toxic side-effects make the substance unsuitable for contraception (Giwercman and Skakkebaek 1986).

Nitroimidazole derivatives used as antibiotics and against protozoa can also lead to suppressed fertility by inhibiting sperm maturation in the epididymis. In general the spectrum of side-effects make long-term use, as would be required for contraception, impossible. One example is **ornidazole**, which by inhibiting glycolysis causes rapid onset of reversible infertility in rats, but whose general toxicity makes all but short-term use in humans impossible (Cooper and Yeung et al. 1999).

20.3.3 Hormonal Male Contraception

Of all the different experimental approaches and pharmacological methods tested so far for male contraception, hormonal methods come closest to fulfilling the criteria set out above (see Sect. 20.1.4). The endocrine feedback mechanism operating between hypothalamus, pituitary and testes is the basis on which hormonal approaches to male contraception rest. Its goal is to suppress spermatogenesis and to reduce sperm concentration, if possible to azoospermia.

Sperm production and secretion of testicular testosterone are so closely interwoven that it has remained impossible to interrupt spermatogenesis by hormonal means without inhibiting androgen production (see Chap. 4 and Fig. 20.14). Inhibition of FSH alone, e.g. by antibodies, leads to reduction of sperm concentration but not to azoospermia, as monkey studies have shown (Nieschlag and Behre 1986). Suppression of both FSH and LH would indeed lead to azoospermia, but would also induce symptoms of androgen deficiency which affects libido, potency, male role behavior and general metabolic processes (erythropoesis, protein, mineral and bone metabolism). For this reason inhibition of gonadotropins will always necessitate androgen administration.

> Thus the principle of hormonal male contraception is based on
> 1. The suppression of LH and FSH,
> 2. Elimination of intratesticular testosterone and
> 3. Substitution of peripheral testosterone to maintain androgenicity.

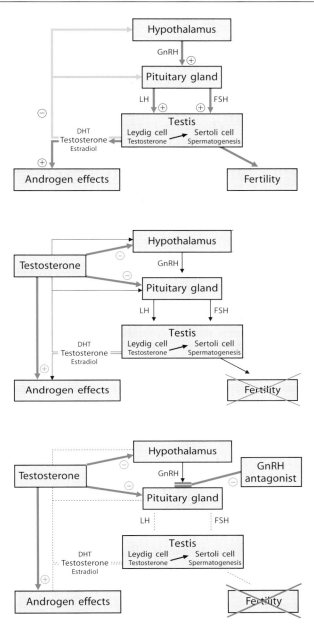

Fig. 20.14. Schematic representation of the endocrine mechanism controlling testicular function (*top*). The *middle figure* shows the principle of hormonal contraception using testosterone; the *bottom figure* shows the principle of hormonal contraception using testosterone plus GnRH antagonists

At first sight it would seem that testosterone offers the ideal substance for male hormonal contraception (Fig. 20.4). It suppresses pituitary LH and FSH secretion. Leydig cells neighboring the seminiferous tubules cease testosterone production and the intratesticular androgens necessary for spermatogenesis decrease. At the same time general masculinity is maintained by androgens supplied exogenously.

Testosterone Alone

Testosterone Enanthate. Ever since the 70s various investigations have been undertaken to **suppress spermatogenesis with testosterone**. Not until 1990 was an initial study testing this form of male contraception published by the WHO, the first study ever performed on the efficacy of hormonal male contraception. Volunteers in 10 centers on 4 continents participated and received 200 mg testosterone enanthate weekly i.m. Those volunteers developing azoospermia within the first 6 months continued to receive injections for a further year. In this period (= efficacy phase), couples refrained from using any further contraceptive methods. A total of 137 men reached the efficacy phase. During this period only one pregnancy occurred. This high rate of efficacy is well comparable to established female methods. This was a very encouraging result. However, only about two thirds of all participants developed azoospermia. The other volunteers showed strong suppression of spermatogenesis, as judged by oligozoospermia (Fig. 20.15).

In order to clarify the question whether men developing oligozoospermia can be considered infertile, a

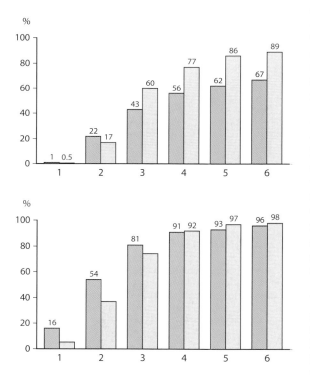

Fig. 20.15. Development of rates of oligo- and azoospermia in WHO studies on male contraception with weekly injections of testosterone enanthate with 655 men participating. The upper half shows the cumulative monthly rates of azoospermia, the lower half shows the cumulative oligozoospermia rates (<3 million/ml). The grey columns represent Caucasian males (n = 453), the red columns Eastern Asian participants (n = 202) (WHO 1995)

second worldwide multicenter study followed (WHO 1996). In this study azoospermia again proved to be a most effective prerequisite for contraception. If sperm concentrations, however, failed to drop below 3 Mio/ml, resulting pregnancy rates were higher than when using condoms. When sperm concentrations decreased below 3 Mio/ml, which was the case in 98% of the participants, then protection was not as effective as for azoospermic men, but was better than that offered by condoms (Fig. 20.15).

Even if these WHO studies represented a breakthrough by confirming a principle of action, they did not offer a practicable method. For a method requiring weekly i.m. injections is not acceptable for broad use. Moreover, several months, often up to one year, are required before sperm production reaches significant suppression. For this reason current research is concentrating on the development of long-acting testosterone preparations and on methods to hasten the onset of effectiveness.

These WHO studies revealed phenomenon important for further development: ethnic differences emerged in the suppressibility of spermatogenesis. Whereas two thirds of Caucasian men became azoospermic, 90% of Chinese participants reached this goal. Such high suppressibility was confirmed in the studies with Chinese and other east Asian men. Despite intensive research, no explanation has resulted. This phenomenon might contribute to more rapid availability of effective hormonal contraception in East Asia than in the rest of the world.

19-Nortestosterone. When searching for preparations with longer lasting effectiveness **19-nortestosterone-hexoxyphenylpropionate** was tested whose spectrum of effects is very similar to that of testosterone and which has been used as an anabolic steroid since the 1960s. The 19-nortestosterone ester injected every 3 weeks enabled azoospermia to be reached by as many men as by testosterone enanthate. Thus the 19-nortestosterone ester is as effective as testosterone enanthate but allows a longer injection interval (Knuth et al. 1992; Behre et al. 1992).

Testosterone Buciclate. Under the auspices of WHO a synthesis programme identified testosterone buciclate as a testosterone ester with long-lasting effectiveness. First tested in monkeys and then in hypogonadal patients, it showed a long effective phase of 3–4 months after a single injection (see Chap. 15). A single injection of 1,200 mg in a contraceptive study resulted in suppression of spermatogenesis comparable to that of weekly enanthate injections (Behre et al. 1995). After these encouraging beginnings progress came to a standstill as no industrial partner was willing to continue its development.

Testosterone Undecanoate. When administered orally testosterone undecanoate is not effective in suppressing spermatogenesis (Nieschlag et al. 1978). Following intramuscular injection, however, it shows a prolonged half-life and is used successfully in substitution for hypogonadism (see Chap. 15). Its long half-life makes it an interesting candidate for contraception. When administered at 6-week intervals to Caucasians the rate of suppression was at least as good as that induced by weekly injections of testosterone enanthate (Kamischke et al. 2000) and Chinese studies show it provides contraceptive protection (e.g. Zhang et al. 1999). Thus at present it seems to be a promising candidate for male contraception.

Testosterone Implants. Implants consisting of pure testosterone are used for substitution in hypogonadism in some countries (see Sect. 15.2.4). In male contraceptive studies one-time application showed efficacy comparable to weekly testosterone enanthate injections (Handelsman 1992). The disadvantage of minor surgery required for implantation under the abdominal skin is compensated for by their low price. Spontaneous extrusion may be a disadvantage. Studies with several implants are awaited.

Testosterone Combined with Gestagens. In order to accelerate the onset of testosterone effectiveness and to increase azoospermia rates, combining testosterone with other gonadotropin-suppressing substances was attempted. As for oral female contraception, gestagens were tried at first, later studies with GnRH agonists and antagonists followed.

To test gestagens various **androgen-gestagen combinations** were used. Multicenter studies were performed by WHO and by the Population Council (summary in Schearer 1978; WHO 1972–1995). Large-scale studies with depot medroxyprogesterone acetate (DMPA)

(100–150 mg i.m./month) combined with testosterone enanthate (200 mg i.m./month) were carried out. After 6 months of therapy only 53% of all volunteers reached azoospermia (Sanchez et al. 1979). Transdermal application of dihydrotestosterone combined with oral medroxyprogesterone failed to produce azoospermia in any of 6 volunteers (Soufi et al. 1983). Notable virilization of partners occurred in a similar study as intensive skin contact caused testosterone to enter the female organism (Delanoe et al. 1984).

Suppression of gonadotropins by 800 mg daily of **danazole** (a derivate of ethyl-testosterone) plus testosterone substitution was able to suppress sperm to below 5 Mio/ml in only 85% of men treated (Leonard and Paulsen 1978). We could show that the combination of **19-nortestosterone with DMPA** produced a higher rate of azoospermia than 19-nortestosterone alone (or testosterone enanthate) (Knuth et al. 1989). WHO subsequently extended these studies to 4 centers in Indonesia to investigate whether results from DMPA with testosterone enanthate (weekly) or 19-nortestosterone (3-weekly) were better. Surprisingly, both forms of therapy were not only similar, but much higher azoospermia rates were achieved than in the studies performed in Germany (WHO 1993). Obviously ethnic differences whose reasons are not understood play a role in the suppressa-

Fig. 20.16. Effectivity of various approaches to male hormonal contraception compiled from numerous single publications and shown as percentage of participants (n), different degrees of suppression of spermatogenesis. *T* testosterone; *TU* testosterone undecanoate; *TTS* trans-scrotal therapeutic system; *TE* testosterone enanthate; *LNG* levonorgestrel; *GnRH Ag* GnRH agonist; *GnRH Antag* GnRH antagonist; *DZ* danazol; *DMPA* depot medroxyprogesterone acetate; *NT* 19-nortestosterone-hexoxyphenyl benzoate; *NET* norethisterone; *CPA* cyproterone acetate

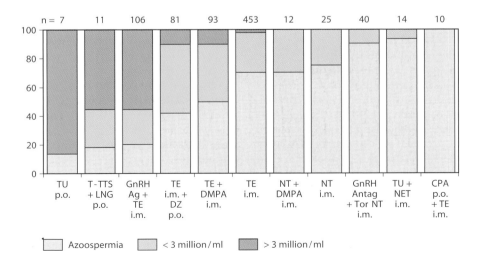

bility of spermatogenesis. Similar ethnic differences (Caucasians versus East Asians) were observed in the multicenter WHO studies with testosterone enanthate.

Combining oral testosterone enanthate i.m with levonogestrel or desogestrel induced only marginally better rates of azoospermia than giving the testosterone ester alone (Anawalt et al. 1999; Bebb et al. 1996; Wu et al. 1999).

Most recently interest has been renewed in earlier studies with **cyproterone acetate (CPA)**. Those studies used CPA alone; while it produced effective suppression of spermatogenesis, pronounced symptoms of androgen deficiency also appeared (Moltz et al. 1980; Wang and Yeung 1980); the newest studies averted androgen deficiency by simultaneous administration of testosterone enanthate. The onset of effectiveness was more rapid and efficacy was higher than when testosterone enanthate was used alone; while all participants reached azoospermia, they developed a slight anemia because of the antiandrogenic effects (Meriggiola et al. 1995). Only the combination of testosterone undecanoate with **norethisterone**, a gestagen with strong androgenic properties was similarly effective. The injections need be given only every 6 weeks and no side-effects were observed (Kamischke and Nieschlag 2000) (Fig. 20.16). **Oral cyproterone acetate** and **oral testosterone undecanoate** were combined with the intention of developing a self-applied contraceptive (Meriggiola et al. 1997). Only 1/11 volunteers became azoospermic and results were no better than with testosterone undecanoate alone (Nieschlag et al. 1978). A further step in this direction in which **transdermal testosterone** was combined with oral **levonorgestrel** resulted in azoospermia rates of only 20% (Büchter et al. 1999).

Recently oral administration of 0.5 mg levonorgestrel daily in addition to weekly injections of testosterone enanthate led to faster and more effective suppression of spermatogenesis than testosterone enanthate injections alone (Bebb et al. 1996). Recent studies with testosterone in combination with gestagens give hope for further developments using such combination regimens.

Testosterone Combined with GnRH Agonists. As gonadotropins must be suppressed in hormonal male contraception, **GnRH analogs** can be used for this purpose. Continuous administration of GnRH agonists first stimulates LH and FSH secretion, but after a certain period, blocks it by a down-regulation of the GnRH receptors. Before GnRH antagonists which directly block the GnRH receptor were available, this paradox effect was used in studies on male contraception.

Between 1979 and 1992 12 studies with a total of 106 volunteers were published using testosterone combined with GnRH agonists (review in Nieschlag et al. 1992). The agonists **decapeptyl, buselerin and nafarelin** were given at doses of 5–500 µg/d for 10–30 weeks. Only 30%

of volunteers showed decreases of sperm production under 5 Mio/ml and only 21 men suppressed to azoospermia. Altough as a whole the results were disappointing, they did confirm two important conclusions which had been generated by preclinical monkey studies:

1. After analyzing LH and testosterone levels in monkeys following injection of GnRH agonists, it was postulated that **constant infusion of agonists** must lead to better results than single injections. This assumption was proved correct by using osmotic minipumps in monkeys (Akhtar et al. 1983a). The effectiveness of this application in men was demonstrated when volunteers wore extracorporeal osmotic minipumps (Schürmeyer et al. 1984). As this principle could also be applied in patients with prostate carcinoma, the pharmaceutical industry developed depot preparations for the treatment of prostate carcinoma from which, in turn, the development of a male contraceptive profited.

2. Furthermore monkey studies showed that the simultaneous administration of testosterone and GnRH agonists attenuated the effect of each drug (Akhtar et al. 1983b). No unequivocal explanation could yet be found for this phenomenon. The diminution of effects, however, remains even when androgens alone are administered for a short time, followed by the GnRH agonist (Behre et al. 1992).

Testosterone Combined with GnRH Antagonists. In contrast to GnRH agonists, by reversible blockade of the pituitary receptor, GnRH antagonists effectively suppress LH and FSH and thus spermatogenesis from the very onset of treatment. In the monkey model we were able to show that combined administration of GnRH antagonists with testosterone, but which was delayed by two weeks, leads to azoospermia in all animals treated (Weinbauer et al. 1988; 1989). Despite the use of molecular biological methods for analyzing androgen and FSH receptors in testicular biopsies, no explanation for these phenomena has been found. The studies, however, provided the basis for clinical studies in the USA which proved the effectiveness of this principle in men. Later studies showed that simultaneous but lower doses of testosterone guaranteed the efficacy of the method (Bagatell et al. 1993; Pavlou et al. 1994). These clinical studies were performed using the **GnRH antagonist Nal-Glu**, which caused marked local side-effects after subcutaneous injection.

In the meantime a GnRH antagonist of the newest generation, synthesized by Schally and known as **cetrorelix**, has become available for use in men (Reissmann et al. 1994). After single and combined injections dose-finding studies showed effective and dose-dependent suppression of LH, FSH and testosterone in healthy men (Behre et al. 1994). The ensuing study showed that after an initial loading dose very low maintenance doses of this antagonist were sufficient to maintain effective and reversible suppression of LH and FSH (Nieschlag and Behre 1996).

Following these promising results we performed a clinical study with a combination of cetrorelix and 19-nortestosterone in healthy men. All volunteers became azoospermic. Moreover, it showed that azoospermia was achieved more rapidly than possible with testosterone alone. However, azoospermia could not be maintained with 19-nortestosterone alone once the antagonist was withdrawn. In its present formulation because of its effectiveness of only 24 hours cetrorelix must be injected subcutaneously daily. This is not practicable for a contraceptive method. Thus its further use depends on the ongoing development of a depot preparation.

In general, the combined use of GnRH antagonists and testosterone for male contraception is promising (Nieschlag and Behre 1996). The foreseeable high price of a peptidogenous GnRH antagonist may exclude its broad use in male contraception. Therefore the studies described confirm a principle whose application in practice will probably have to await the development of oral and less costly GnRH secretagogs.

20.4 Outlook

An overview of studies to date on male contraception is given in Fig. 20.16. It indicates that at least 3 approaches lead to almost complete suppression of spermatogenesis and high rates of azoospermia: the combination of testosterone with norethisterone, cyproterone acetate and GnRH antagonists.

Of the experimental approaches described, hormonal contraception offers the most promising possibility for an efficacious, practicable and acceptable male method. In order to make these approaches suitable for clinical use, further development of proven, user-friendly preparations is necessary e.g. intensified development of long-lasting testosterone preparations and depot GnRH

The Weimar Manifesto on Male Contraception

Leading researchers from all over the world met in Weimar (Germany) on June 29, 1997 for a Summit Meeting to discuss the current status and prospects for male hormonal contraception. The researchers represented academic institutions as well as international organisations such as the Population Council (New York) and the World Health Organisation (Geneva).

All agreed that contraception is an essential component of reproductive health for men and women. Without contraception, all socioeconomic progress and the future of this planet are endangered. Apart from vasectomy and condoms, no contraceptives are available for men. New forms of male contraception are required to involve men more actively in family planning and to share the benefits and burdens of contraception more equitably.

The researchers agreed that clinical research had shown that a reversible male hormonal contraceptive is feasible and effective. However, it has not yet been possible to show wide acceptability due to the inadequate funding for largescale clinical trials. There is a pressing need for product development and clinical trials of new, long-acting testosterone preparations and combinations with other agents. With adequate funding, a male hormonal contraceptive could be available in the near future.

Since any contraceptive method can only be brought to practible usage by pharmaceutical companies, the researchers urged the pharmaceutical industry to become actively involved in the development of novel male contraceptives. They also appealed in the spirit of the UN Cairo Declaration to politicians and research foundations to commit themselves to the development of male contraception for the sake of future generations.

Prof. E. Nieschlag (Chair) (University of Münster, Germany), Dr. H. M. Behre (University of Münster, Germany), Prof. W. Bremner (University of Washington, Seattle, USA), Prof. E. Diczfalusy (Karolinska Hospital, Stockholm Sweden), Prof. D. J. Handelsman (University of Sydney, Australia), Prof. I. Huhtaniemi (University of Turku, Finland), Dr. E. Johansson (Population Council, New York, USA), Prof. M.T. Mbizvo (WHO, Geneva, Switzerland), Dr. C. Meriggiola (University of Bologna, Italy), Dr. K. Sundaram (Population Council, New York, USA), Prof. R. Swerdloff (University of California, Los Angeles, USA), Prof. C. Wang (University of California, Los Angeles, USA), Dr. F. Wu (University of Manchester, UK).

antagonists or oral GnRH antagonists as well as suitable forms of gestagens. Cooperation with the pharmaceutical industry is required here for "drug development", traditionally one of their tasks.

In this vein in 1997 in the "Weimar Manifesto" leading researchers in male contraception challenged drug firms to actively support these efforts. In the meantime several firms have set up programs towards the development of a male contraceptive method, thus putting its realization within the foreseeable future.

20.5 References

Akhtar FB, Marshall GR, Wickings EJ, Nieschlag E (1983a) Reversible induction of azoospermia in rhesus monkeys by constant infusion of a GnRH agonist using osmotic minipumps. J Clin Endocrinol Metab 56:534

Akhtar FB, Marshall GR, Nieschlag E (1983b) Testosterone supplementation attenuates the antifertility effects of an LHRH agonist in male monkeys. Int J Androl 6:461

Alan Guttmacher Institute (1999) Sharing responsibility: women, society and abortion worldwide. New York

Alderman PM (1991) Complications in a series of 1224 vasectomies. J Fam Pract 33:579–584

Anawalt BD, Bebb RA, Bremner WJ, Matsumoto AM (1999) A lower dosage levonorgestrel and testosterone combination effectively suppresses spermatogenesis and circulating gonadotropin levels with fewer metabolic effects than higher dosage combinations. J Androl 20:407–414

Anderson RA, Baird DT (1997) Progress towards a male pill. IPPF Med Bull 31:3–4

April K, Köster R, Schreiner W (1993) Wie effektiv schützen Kondome vor einer HIV-Übertragung? Med Klinik 88:304–311

Bagatell CJ, Matsumoto AM, Christensen RB, Rivier JE, Bremner WJ (1993) Comparison of a gonadotropin-releasing hormone antagonist plus testosterone (T) versus T alone as a potential male contraceptive regimen. J Clin Endocrinol Metab 77:427

Bebb RA, Anawalt BD, Christensen RB, Paulsen CA, Bremner WJ, Matsumoto AM (1996) Combined administration of levornorgestrel and testosterone induces more rapid and effective suppression of spermatogenesis than testosterone alone: a promising male contraceptive approach. J Clin Endocrinol Metab 81:757–762

Behre HM, Nashan D, Hubert W, Nieschlag E (1992) Depot gonadotropin-releasing hormone agonist blunts the androgen-induced suppression of spermatogenesis in a clinical trial of male contraception. J Clin Endocrinol Metab 74:84

Behre HM, Böckers A, Schlingheider A, Nieschlag E (1994) Sustained suppression of serum LH, FSH and testosterone and increase of high-density lipoprotein cholesterol by daily injections of the GnRH antagonist cetrorelix over 8 days in normal men. Clin Endocrinol 40:241

Behre HM, Baus S, Kliesch S, Keck C, Simoni M, Nieschlag E (1995) Potential of testosterone buciclate for male contraception: endocrine differences between responders and non-responders. J Clin Endocrinol Metab 80:2394–2403

Belker AM, Thomas AJ, Fuchs EF, Konnak JW, Sharlip ID (1991) Result of 1,469 microsurgical vasectomy reversals by the vasovasostomy study group. J Urol 145:505–511

Bonnar J, Flynn A, Freundl G, Kirkman R, Royston R, Snowden R (1999) Personal hormone monitoring for contraception. Br J Fam Plann 24:128–134

Büchter D, von Eckardstein S, von Eckardstein A, Kamischke A, Simoni M, Behre HM, Nieschlag E (1999) Clinical trial of transdermal testosterone and oral levonorgestrel for male contraception. J Clin Endocrinol Metab 84:1244–1249

Cooper TG, Yeung CH (1999) Recent biochemical approaches to post-testicular, epididymal contraception. Hum Reprod Update 5:141–152

Cos LR, Valvo JR, Davis RS, Cockett ATK (1983) Vasovasostomy: current state of the art. Urology 22:567–575

Deindl F (1990) Die Refertilisationssituation in der Bundesrepublik Deutschland, der Republik Österreich und der Schweiz – eine Dreiländerumfrage. Inaugural-Dissertation, Ruhr-Universität Bochum

Delanoe D, Fougeyrollas B, Meyer L, Thonneau P (1984) Androgenisation of female partners of men on medroxyprogesterone acetate/percutaneous testosterone contraception. Lancet 1:276

Derrick FC, Yarbbrough W, Agostino JD (1973) Vasovasostomy: results of questionnaire of members of the American Urological Association. J Urol 110:556–557

Djerassi C, Leibo SP (1994) A new look at male contraception. Nature 370:11–12

De Vincenzi I for the European Study Group on Heterosexual Transmission of HIV (1994) A longitudinal study of human immunodeficiency virus transmission by heterosexual partners. N Engl J Med 331:341–346

Drake MJ, Mills IW, Cranston D (1999) On the chequered history of vasectomy. Br J Urol Int 84:475–481

Engelmann UH, Schramek P, Tomamichel G, Deindl F, Senge TH (1990) Vasectomy reversal in central Europe: results of a questionnaire of urologists in Austria, Germany and Switzerland. J Urol 143:64–67

Farley TMM; Meirik O, Mehta S, Waites GMH (1993) The safety of vasectomy: recent concerns. Bull WHO 71:413–419

Farnsworth NR, Waller DP (1982) Current status of plant products reported to inhibit sperm. Res Front Fertil Regul 2:1–16

Feber KM, Ruiz HE (1999) Vasovasostomy: macroscopic approach and retrospective review. Techniques Urol 5:8–11

Forste R, Tanfer K, Tedrow L (1995) Sterilization among currently married men in the United States, 1991. Fam Plann Perspect 27:100–107, 122

Frezieres RG, Walsh TL, Nelson AL, Clark VA, Coulson AH (1999) Evaluation of the efficacy of a polyurethane condom: results from a randomized, controlled clinical trial. Fam Plann Perspect 31:81–87

Giovanucci E, Tosteson TD, Speizer FE, Vessey MP, Colditz GA (1992) A long-term study of mortality in men who have undergone vasectomy. N Engl J Med 326:1392–1398

Giovanucci E, Ascherio A, Rimm EB, Colditz GA, Stampfer MJ, Willett WC (1993) A prospective cohort study of vasectomy and prostate cancer in US men. JAMA 269:873–877

Giwercman A, Skakkebaek NE (1986) The effect of salicylazosulphapyridine (sulphasalazine) on male fertility. A review. Int J Androl 9:38

Goebel P, Ortmann K, Blattner TH (1987) Vasektomie und Beziehungssituation – eine empirische Untersuchung an 156 Männern (Paaren). Zschr Psychosom Med 33:119–138

Goldstein M, Shihua PhL, Matthews GJ (1998) Microsurgical Vasovasostomy: The microdot technique of precision suture placement. J Urol 159:188–190

Handelsman DJ, Conway AJ, Boylan LM (1992) Suppression of human spermatogenesis by testosterone implants. J Clin Endocrinol Metab 175:1326

Heidenreich A, Bonfig R, Wilbert DM, Strohmaier WL, Engelmann UH (1994) Risk factors for antisperm antibodies in infertile men. Am J Reprod Immunol 31:69–76

Hiersche HD, Hiersche F (1995) Die Sterilisation geistig Behinderter. Gynäkologe 28:452–458

Isnardi L (1896) Die Behandlung der senilen Dysurie mit Durchschneidung und doppelseitiger Ligatur der vasa deferentia. Ther Wochenschr 111:25–36

Jequier AM, Pryor JP (1998) Is vasectomy of long term benefits? Hum Reprod 13:1757–1760

John EM, Whittemore AS, Wu AH, Kolonel LN, Hislop TG, Howe GR, West DW, Hankin J, Dreon DM, Teh CZ (1995) Vasectomy and prostate cancer: results from a multiethnic case-control study. J Natl Cancer Inst 87:662–669

Kamischke A, Nieschlag E (2000) Intramuscular testosterone undecanoate with or without oral levonorgestrel: a randomized placebo controlled clinical trial for male contraception. Clin Endocrinol 53:43–52

Knuth UA, Mühlenstedt D (1991) Kinderwunschdauer, kontrazeptives Verhalten und Rate vorausgegangener Infertilitätsbehandlung. Geburtsh Frauenheilkd 51:1–7

Knuth UA, Behre HM, Belkien L, Bents H, Nieschlag E (1985) Clinical trial of 19-nortestosterone-hexyloxyphenylpropionate (Anadur) for male fertility regulation. Fertil Steril 44:814

Knuth UA, Yeung CH, Nieschlag E (1989) Combination of 19-nortestosterone-hexyloxyphenylpropionate (Anadur) and depot-medroxyprogesterone-acetate (Clinovir) for male contraception. Fertil Steril 51:1011

Kohli KL (1973) Motivational factors and socioeconomic characteristics of vasectomized males. J Biosoc Sci 5:169–177

Leonard JM, Paulsen CA (1978) Contraceptive development studies for males: oral and parenteral steroid hormone administation. In: Pantanelli DJ (ed) Hormonal control of male fertility. Department of Health, Education and Welfare. National Institutes of Health, Bethesda, pp 223

Lesko SM, Louik C, Vezina R, Rosenberg L, Shapiro S (1999) Vasectomy and prostate cancer. J Urol 161:1848–1853

Liu X, Li S (1993) Vasal sterilization in China. Contraception 48:255–265

Martin CW, Anderson RA, Cheng L, Ho PC, van der Spuy Z, Smith KB, Glasier AF, Everington D, Baird DT (2000) Potential impact of hormonal male contraception: cross cultural implications for development of novel preparations. Hum Reprod 15:637–645

Meriggiola MC, Paulsen CA, Bremner WJ, Flamigni C (1996) A combined regimen of cyproterone acetate and testosterone enanthate as a potentially highly effective male contraceptive. J Clin Endocrinol Metab 81:3018–3023

Meriggiola MC, Bremner WJ, Constantino A, Pavani A, Capelli M, Flamigni C (1997) An oral regimen of cyproterone acetate and testosterone undecanoate for spermatogenic suppression in men. Fertil Steril 68:844–850

Mieusset R, Bujan L (1994) The potential of mild testicular heating as a safe, effective and reversible contraceptive method for men. Int J Androl 17:186–191

Miltsch B, Senn E (1999) Vasektomie: Präoperative Bedenken und postoperative Akzeptanz. Aktuel Urol 30:237–241

Moltz L, Römmler A, Post A, Schwartz U, Hammerstein J (1980) Medium dose cyproterone acetate (CPA): effects on hormone secretion and on spermatogenesis in men. Contraception 21:393

National Institutes of Health (1993) Does vasectomy cause prostate cancer? JAMA 269:2620

Nieschlag E (1986) Reasons for abandoning immunization against FSH as an approach to male fertility regulation. In:

Zatuchni GI, Goldsmith A, Spieler JM, Sciarra JJ (eds) Male contraception: advances and future prospects. Harper and Row, Philadelphia, pp 395–400

Nieschlag E (1987) Vasektomie – pro und contra. Dtsch Med Wochenschr 112:1107–1109

Nieschlag E, Behre HM, Weinbauer GF (1992) Hormonal male contraception: A real chance? In: Nieschlag E, Habenicht UF (eds) Spermatogenesis – fertilitzation – contraception. Molecular, cellular and endocrine events in male reproduction. Springer, Berlin Heidelberg New York, pp 477–501

Nieschlag E, Behre HM (1996) Hormonal male contraception: Suppression of spermatogenesis with GnRH antagonists and testosterone. In: Filicori M (ed) Treatment with GnRH analogs: controversies and perspectives. Parthenon, London, pp 243–248

Nieschlag E, Hoogen H, Bölk M, Schuster H, Wickings EJ (1978) Clinical trial with testosterone undecanoate for male fertility control. Contraception 18: 607

Nirapathpongporn A, Huber DH, Krieger JN (1990) No-scalpel vasectomy at the King's birthday vasectomy festival. Lancet 335:894–895

Ochsner AJ (1899) Surgical treatment of habitual criminals. JAMA 33:867–868

O'Connor VJ (1948) Anastomosis of the vas deferens after purposeful division for sterility. J Urol 59:229–233

Pavlou SN, Herodotou D, Curtain M, Minaretzis D (1994) Complete suppression of spermatogenesis by co-administration of a GnRH antagonist plus a physiologic dose of testosterone. 76th Meeting Endocrine Society, Abstract 1324

Prasad MR, Diczfalusy NE (1982) Gossypol. Int J Androl [Suppl] 28:53

Randall PE, Marcuson RW (1985) Absence from work following vasectomy. J Soc Occup Med 35:77–78

Reissmann T, Engel J, Kutscher B, Bernd M, Hilgard P, Peukert M, Szelenyi I, Reichert S, Gonzales-Barcena D, Nieschlag E, Comary-Schally AM, Schally AV (1994) Cetrorelix. Drugs Future 19:228–237

Reynolds RD (1994) Vas deferens occlusion during no-scalpel vasectomy. J Fam Pract 39:577–582

Rizvi SAH, Naqvi SAA, Hussain Z (1995) Ethical issues in male sterilization in developing countries. Br J Urol 76:103–105

Rosenberg MJ, Waugh MS (1997) Latex condom breakage and slippage in a controlled clinical trial. Contraception 56:17–21

Ross JA, Huber DH (1983) Acceptance and prevalence of vasectomy in developing countries. Stud Fam Plan 14:67–73

Roth S, Hertle L (1994) Verursacht die Sterilisations-Vasektomie ein Prostatakarzinom? Dt Ärztebl 91:409–410

Rothman I, Berger RE, Cummings P, Jessen J, Muller ChH, Chapman W (1997) Randomized clinical trial of an absorbable stent for vasectomy reversal. J Urol 157:1697–1700

Russell-Brown P, Piedrahita C, Foldesy R, Steiner M, Townsend J (1992) Comparison of condom breakage during human use with performance in laboratory testing. Contraception 45:429–437

Sanches FA, Brache V, Leon P, Faundes A (1979) Inhibition of spermatogenesis with monthly injections of medroxyprogesterone acetate and low dose testosterone enanthate. Int J Androl 2:136

Schearer SB (1978) The use of progestins and androgens as a male contraceptive. Int J Androl [Suppl] 2:680

Schirren C (1983) Erfahrungen mit der Vasektomie. Urologe A 22:29–34

Schürmeyer T, Knuth UA, Freischem CW, Sandow J, Akhtar FB, Nieschlag E (1984) Suppression of pituitary and testicular function in normal men by constant gonadotropin-releasing hormone agonist infusion. J Clin Endocrinol Metab 59:19

Segal SJ (1985) Gossypol: a potential contraceptive for men. Plenum, New York

Sharp HC (1902) The severing of the vasa deferentia and its relation to the neuropsychopathic constitution. NY Med J 75:411–414

Silber SJ (1977) Perfect anatomical reconstruction of vas deferens with a new microscopic surgical technique. Fertil Steril 28:72–77

Smith GL, Taylor GP, Smith KF (1985) Comparative risks and costs of male and female sterilization. Am J Pub Health 75:370–374

Soufir J-C, Jouannet P, Marson J, Soumah A (1983) Reversible inhibition of sperm production and gonadotropin secretion in men following combined oral medroxyprogesterone acetate and percutaneous testosterone treatment. Acta Endocrinol 102:625

Steiner M, Foldesy R, Cole D, Carter E (1992) Study to determine the correlation between condom breakage in human use and laboratory test results. Contraception 46:279–288

Trussell J, Hatcher RA, Cates W, Stewart FH, Kost K (1990) Contraceptive failure in the United States: an update. Stud Fam Plan 21:51–54

Vaughn R (1979) Behavioral response to vasectomy. Arch Gen Psychiatry 36:815–821

Waites GMH (1993) Male fertility regulation: the challenges for the year 2000. Br Med Bull 49:210

Waites GMH, Wang C, Griffin PD (1998) Gossypol: reasons for its failure to be accepted as a safe, reversible male antifertility drug. Int J Androl 21:8–12

Wang C, Yeung KK (1980) Use of low-dosage oral cyproterone acetate as a male contraceptive. Contraception 21:245

Wang C, McDonald V, Leung A, Superlano L, Berman N, Hull L, Swerdloff RS (1997) Effect of increased scrotal temperature on sperm production in normal men. Fertil Steril 68:334–339

Weidner W, Weißbach L (1992) Freiwillige Vasektomie in der Familienplanung – Gedanken zur Nutzen-Risiko-Analyse. Aktuel Urol 23:328–331

Weinbauer GF, Göckeler E, Nieschlag E (1988) Testosterone prevents complete suppression of spermatogenesis in the gonadotropin-releasing hormone (GnRH) antagonist-treated nun-human primate (*Macaca fascicularis*). J Clin Endocrinol Metab 67:284

Weller SC (1993) A meta-analysis of condom effectiveness in reducing sexually transmitted HIV. Soc Sci Med 36:1635–1644

WHO (1972–1998) Special programme of research, development and research training in human reproduction. Annual and biannual reports. WHO, Genf

WHO Task Force on Methods for the Regulation of Male Fertility (1990) Contraceptive efficacy of testosterone-induced azoospermia in normal men. Lancet 336:955–959

WHO Task Force on Methods for the Regulation of Male Fertility (1993) Comparison of two androgens plus depot-medroxyprogesterone acetate for suppression to azoospermia in Indonesian men. Fertil Steril 60:1062

WHO Task Force on Methods for the Regulation of Male Fertility (1995) Rate of testosterone-induced suppression to severe oligozoospermia or azoospermia in two multinational clinical studies. Int J Androl 18:157–165

WHO Task Force on Methods for the Regulation of Male Fertility (1996) Contraceptive efficacy of testosterone-induced azoospermia and oligozoospermia in normal men. Fertil Steril 65:821–829

WHO/HRP (1997) Preclinical and clinical requirements for approval to market non-latex condoms. WHO, Genf

Wicklund R, Alexander NJ (1979) Vasovasostomy: evaluation of success. Urology 13:532–534

Wolfers D, Wolfers H (1974) Vasectomy and vasectomania. Mayflower Books, London

Wright N, Johnson B, Wiggins P, Vessey M (1977) The use of sterilisation as a method of birth control among participants in the Oxford/Family Planning Association Contraceptive Study. Fertil Contracept 1:41–44

Wu FC, Balasubramanian R, Mulders TM, Coelingh-Benningk HJ (1999) Oral progestogen combined with testosterone as a potential male contraceptive: additive effects between desogestrel and testosterone enanthate in suppression of spermatogenesis, pituitary-testicular axis, and lipid metabolism. J Clin Endocrinol Metab 84:112–122

Yu Z-H, Chan HC (1998) Gossypol as a male antifertility agent – why studies should have been continued. Int J Androl 21:2–7

Zhang GY, Gu YQ, Wang XH, Cui YG, Bremner WJ (1999) A clinical trial of injectable testosterone undecanoate as a potential male contraceptive in normal Chinese men. J Clin Endocrinol Metab 84:3642–3647

CHAPTER 21

The Aging Male

C. ROLF · E. NIESCHLAG

21.1 Physiology of Aging

Demographic studies show an increasing proportion of older people in developed countries. For example, during the last 100 years in Germany the mean **life expectancy** has approximately doubled (Fig. 21.1). This development is largely due to improved hygiene, reduction of newborn mortality and more effective therapy and prevention of acute diseases in age. With larger numbers of people reaching advanced age, health problems as well as social and psychological problems of older men play an increasingly important role in clinical medicine and in research.

Specific diseases of age do not exist. However, the incidence of simultaneous occurrence of diseases increases in age. The increase of **multimorbidity** raises problems for the therapy of individual diseases. Owing to a higher number of contraindications of surgical or pharmacological treatment strategies, therapeutic options often are reduced. To what extent normal processes of aging influence the beginning and course of diseases

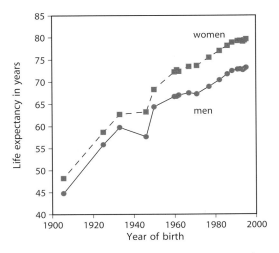

Fig. 21.1. Change in the average life expectancy of men and women in Germany from 1901 to 1992. (Statistisches Jahrbuch 1989, 1994 and 1998, Statistisches Bundesamt Wiesbaden)

and, conversely, to what extent pathological changes accelerate the physiological aging process cannot be determined reliably (DeNicola 1989).

Aging is a normal physiological process. During the process of aging, the human organism undergoes a series of morphological and functional modifications within all organs and tissues characterized by a general tendency towards reduced physiological efficiency and atrophy of various organs and systems (DeNicola 1989).

21.2 Theories of Aging

The etiology and the exact mechanism of aging are not yet completely settled. Different theories are under discussion:

According to the **program theory**, the process of aging is genetically fixed and death is a kind of predetermined self-extinction.

At the end of each chromosome several thousand copies of a certain DNA sequence consisting of six base pairs are to be found, the so-called **telomeres**. In the course of each cell division the chromosomes of somatic cells lose about 200 base pairs. According to the **telomere theory** the length of the telomere limits the lifespan of the somatic cells and thus of the entire human organism (Finkel 1998).

According to the **mutation theory** of aging, in senescence increased numbers of spontaneous mutations lead to functional and morphological changes which influence the entire organism. As an alternative to this theory, age-dependent disturbances of the DNA repair mechanisms are postulated. Mitochondrial DNA is particularly susceptible to increased mutations in advancing age (Michikawa et al. 1999).

According to the theory of **accumulation of waste products**, accumulation of certain substances (i.e. lipofuscin) damages cells and tissues and causes the changes found in age. Moreover, free oxygen radicals, which occur physiologically in oxidative metabolism and result in the damage of macromolecules may be another reason for aging.

According to the **autoimmune theory** abnormal substances are produced in age. These are recognized by the immunocompetent cells, especially by lymphocytes, plasma cells and mast cells, resulting in the formation of specific antibodies which produce irreversible cell damage.

Physiological changes of endocrine organs are also discussed as causing the process of aging.

21.3 Endocrine Changes in Senescence

Impaired performance arising in advancing age is not necessarily caused by age as such and should not be dismissed as not requiring diagnosis and therapy. Within the diagnostic workup endocrine causes for impaired performance must also be taken into consideration. Because of multimorbidity in advanced age and altered symptoms of hormone deficiency, endocrinologically determined reasons for impaired performance will often go unnoticed.

An age-dependent decrease of **growth hormone** production (hGH) is well known. Daily hGH secretion reaches its maximum at puberty and thereafter decreases continuously. hGH pulse frequency (especially during the night) and GHRH-induced hGH secretion also decrease with age. Consequently reduced hGH levels result in a decrease of general performance, reduced muscle strength and an increased tendency towards obesity (increased body mass index). Patients with manifest hGH deficiency are subject to a notably increased mortality rate caused by cardiovascular disease (Vance and Mauras 1999).

In prepubertal boys and in hypogonadal men, treatment with testosterone or hCG increases mean growth hormone levels, pulse amplitude, and **IGF-I** levels in serum. Low IGF-I levels and changes in growth hormone levels may be related to reduced testosterone levels and relative hypogonadism. This possibility has not yet been adequately explored (Swerdloff and Wang 1993).

The **cortisol** concentration in serum remains constant in age. In chronically ill, alcoholic, or obese patients, as well as in patients with hyperplasia of the prostate, no significant changes in cortisol level are detectable (Gray et al. 1991). Older men, however, with relatively high cortisol levels are characterized by reduced bone density as well as an increased rate of fractures (Dennison et al. 1999; Greendale et al. 1999).

Dehydroepiandrosterone (DHEA) and **dehydroepiandrosterone sulphate (DHEAS)** are produced in the adrenal cortex as precursors of testosterone synthesis and exhibit weak androgenic effects. Highest plasma concentrations are reached at the age of twenty to twenty-five years. Thereafter plasma levels decrease continuously, so that by the age of 60 only a third or less of DHEA(S) can be detected (Herbert 1995).

In patients with a history of coronary heart disease significantly lower DHEAS plasma levels could be observed compared with an age-matched control group. Similarly correlations between reduced DHEA(S) levels and diabetes mellitus type II, rheumatoid arthritis, some carcinomas and body fat distribution were found. Whether DHEA(S) plasma level decreases in response to chronic disease or whether increased DHEA levels have a protective function is unknown.

Melatonin is secreted from the pineal gland and is responsible for day/night rhythmicity. In senescence the melatonin concentration in serum decreases. Moreover, melatonin concentration in age is reduced in insomniac men compared to healthy men without insomnia (Garfinkel et al. 1995). To date any physiological relevance of melatonin substitution of aging men has not been demonstrated. Whether melatonin influences other endocrine functions and whether it has an inhibiting effect on aging by acting as a potential and efficient radical scavenger, as shown in vitro and in experimental animals, remains to be further elucidated (Garfinkel and Berner 1998).

The incidence of **thyroid diseases** increases with age. The typical symptoms often are no longer clearly recognizable and may lead to misdiagnosis or no diagnosis at all. Whether plasma levels of **TSH**, T_3 and T_4 show a general tendency to decrease in age is discussed controversially (Cooper 1990). Testosterone serum levels as well as SHBG levels (sex hormone-binding protein) are higher in patients with hyperthyroidism; the proportion of free bioactive testosterone remains unchanged (Ford et al. 1992). Both hyperthyroidism as well as hypothyroidism can result in reduced male fertility (Abalovich et al. 1999; Jaya Kumar et al. 1990).

Non-insulin-dependent **diabetes mellitus type II** is very often also a disease of advanced age. Usually hyperinsulinism is present, resulting in a reduction of insulin receptors in the periphery. Erectile dysfunction and retrograde ejaculations resulting from diabetes mellitus occur frequently and often independently of the duration of the disease. These symptoms are caused by diabetogenic neuropathy as well as microangiopathy. Testosterone and SHBG serum levels in diabetics tend to be lower than those in healthy men of a similar age; the incidence of diabetes is slightly elevated in men with low testosterone (Haffner et al. 1996). Comparing diabetic and age-matched, non-diabetic healthy men, increased sperm concentration, but reduced ejaculate volume and reduced motility were observed in the patient with diabetes (Ali et al. 1993). It is, however, unlikely that diabetes mellitus has a positive influence on spermatogenesis; more probably the reduced frequency of ejaculation, especially in patients with polyneuropathies, leads to an increase in sperm number accompanied by reduced motility.

21.4 Reproductive Functions of Older Men

21.4.1 Sex Hormones in Older Men

The consequences of endocrine changes in the female menopause and climacteric and the resulting influences on general well-being and health of aging women have been investigated for many years. Sex hormone replacement therapy is generally recommended for postmenopausal women. In contrast, the state of knowledge about endocrine and reproductive changes of aging in men lags far behind, and there is an absence of accepted therapeutical strategies.

A "**male climacteric**" as an abrupt age-dependent change in testicular functions, comparable to the menopause, does not exist. A sudden loss of fertility does not occur. Aging men without accompanying diseases may have testosterone levels and testicular volumes comparable to those of younger men. Independent of the state of health in aging men, a **reduced endocrine reserve capacity** of the testicular **Leydig cells** as well as the pituitary gonadotrophs is observed.

The increase of serum testosterone induced by hCG stimulation is lower in older men than in younger. Likewise the LH increase after GnRH stimulation shows a reduction in older men (Nieschlag et al. 1982; Vermeulen 1993). Whether a general decrease of **testosterone production** exists was controversial in the past (Vermeulen and Kaufman 1998). The results are contradictory owing to inconsistent selection of volunteers (reconvalescent old patients, patients from geriatric wards, men from a home for senior citizens, healthy volunteers). While decreased **testosterone serum levels** in older men were reported in the sixties, in the seventies it seemed that testosterone levels in healthy older men were not lower than in control groups of younger volunteers. In recent large scale epidemiological studies a general mean decline in serum levels of testosterone in older men was reported, but with considerable variance (Gray et al. 1991; Simon et al. 1992; Belanger et al. 1994). The greater proportion of testosterone in serum is protein-bound. In older men the proportion of **sex hormone-binding globulin** (SHBG) in serum increases; therefore the proportion of **bioactive free testosterone** decreases (Fig. 21.2). Moreover, the **circadian rhythm of testosterone serum concentration**, with highest values seen in the early morning, decreases (Vermeulen 1993). The proportion of men with testosterone concentrations falling below the normal range (<12 nmol/L) increases with age. 20% of men 60–80 years old and 33% of men over 80 years

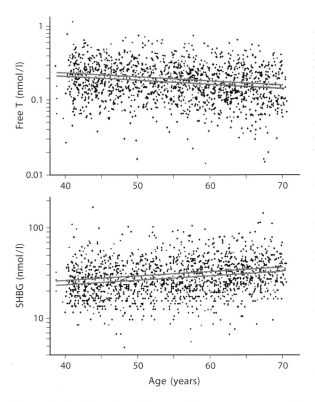

Fig. 21.2. Age-dependent changes of free testosterone and SHBG levels. Results of the Massachusetts male aging study. (From Gray et al. 1991)

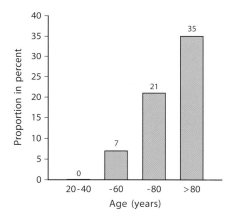

Fig. 21.3. Percentage of healthy men with hypogonadal testosterone serum levels in 300 men of different age groups. (Adapted from Vermeulen and Kaufman 1995)

have serum testosterone concentrations in the hypogonadal range (Fig. 21.3) (Vermeulen and Kaufman 1995). Nevertheless, the general impression prevails that the testosterone production and serum levels tend to remain higher in healthy older men, while a decline occurs faster in diseased aging men.

Testosterone is effective via the androgen receptor. The first exon of the androgen receptor contains a repetitive DNA sequence with a variable number of CAG triplets. With increasing age the serum testosterone level in men with relatively few (15–20) CAG triplets declines more rapidly than in men with more CAG triplets (25–30) (Krithivas et al. 1999). Whether these differences in the genotype of the androgen receptor have any clinical relevance and whether the length of the CAG triplets leads to consequences for therapy cannot be resolved at present. Routine determination of CAG triplets is not indicated at the present time.

The basal concentration of **LH** and **FSH** in serum increases slightly between 40 and 70 years of age and drastically thereafter (Nieschlag et al. 1982). The pulsatile frequency of LH secretion also declines. A mild decrease of prolactin levels is observed in aging men. The serum level of **estradiol** (E2) and **estrone** (E1) as well as of estrone sulphate remain constant in age (Gray et al. 1991). Lower testosterone levels and higher SHBG levels can intensify the influence of estrogens on the organism, which may explain the increased incidence of gynaecomastia in senescent men (Morley et al. 1990). Elevated estradiol levels relative to testosterone levels can also be found in men with benign prostate hypertrophy (Gann et al. 1995; Suzuki et al. 1995). The serum levels of the testosterone metabolite 5α-dihydrotestosterone (DHT) does not decrease with age; however, in chronically ill patients lower levels are described (Gray et al. 1991).

21.4.2 Testicular Morphology in Advanced Age

The interpretation of histological findings of testes from older men is hampered by the fact that examining testes or samples of testicular biopsies of healthy volunteers is not justifiable. Knowledge about the morphology of testes is therefore based on autopsy material or on testes removed in the course of treatment of prostatic carcinoma.

In many cases these testes of old men show no differences to those of younger men. A general decrease in **testicular volume** cannot be observed (Handelsman and Staraj 1985). In 27 of 102 testes examined from men over 90 years **testis morphology** was perfectly normal (Schlüter 1978). However, in testes of some older men alterations exist ranging from isolated anomalies to full testicular atrophy. On occasion, both normal and atrophic seminiferous tubules are seen side by side in the same testis. When signs of atrophy and hyalinization are present, in most cases **arteriosclerotic alterations** of the blood vessels can also be observed. The dimension of degenerative changes of the testes is correlated with the extent of general arteriosclerosis. In some cases abnormal variants of type A pale spermatogonia and an unusual multilayered arrangement of spermatogonia were

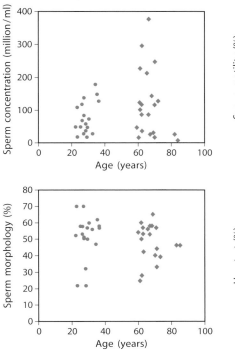

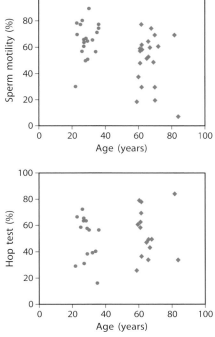

observed, a phenomenon rarely seen in younger men. Several results demonstrate that the **spermatogenetic efficiency**, i. e., the number of spermatozoa from one cell division of a single spermatogonium is reduced (it is lower in men than in most animal species) with increasing age (Johnson et al. 1990). In the testes of aging patients with prostate cancer regressive changes of the germ cells were observed, with new degenerative forms of spermatogonia, spermatocytes and spermatids appearing (Holstein 1989). Histomorphometric investigations of testes from accident victims showed that the volume of individual Leydig cells does not change. However, **a decrease in total Leydig cell number** occurs as a function of age correlating with the general decrease in testosterone production.

21.4.3 Semen Parameters in Older Men

Representative data from longitudinal studies on semen parameters of aging men are not available. The sexuality of aging men in general is still a taboo, shared both by society in general as well as by the medical profession. This may also explain why little is known about semen parameters in older men.

When investigating the semen parameters of healthy grandfathers, i. e. of men over 60 years, who had proven their fertility earlier in life, and of men over 50 years old visiting our clinic for couple infertility, the seminal parameters were in good agreement with those of the con-

Fig. 21.4. Comparison of ejaculate parameters between grandfathers and young fertile men. (Adapted from Nieschlag et al. 1982)

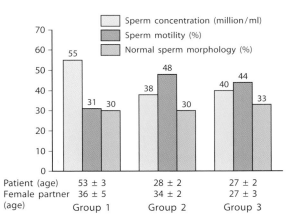

Fig. 21.5. Comparison of ejaculate parameters between older and younger men of infertile couples. (From Rolf et al. 1996)

trol group of younger fathers or younger infertile men respectively (Fig. 21.4, 21.5; Nieschlag et al. 1982; Rolf et al. 1996). **Sperm motility** was significantly lower in the older men, whereas the group of grandfathers showed higher **sperm concentrations**. These changes can be explained as a result of the lowered **ejaculatory frequency**

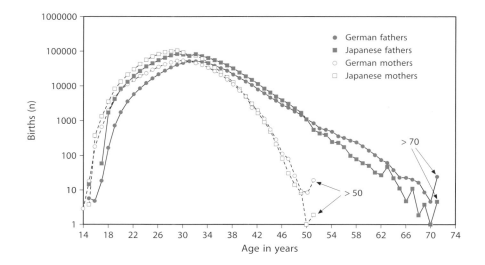

Fig. 21.6. Age distribution of parents in Germany in 1991 (Nieschlag et al. 2000)

in the older men. In **sperm function tests** (hamster-ovum-penetration test) no differences could be observed between the different age groups (Nieschlag et al. 1982).

In the group of older infertile men the **ejaculate volume** was significantly lower compared to the control groups. **Fructose concentration**, as a marker for seminal vesicle function, was lower; the others markers of accessory gland function showed no changes. Sperm production and ejaculate parameters decrease with **reduced general health** and the ability to produce an ejaculate may disappear in cases of serious diseases (Nieschlag and Michel 1986).

These observations were confirmed in middle-aged patients (52–68 years) with erectile dysfunction who still were able to deliver an ejaculate (Homonnai et al. 1982). In a further study a slight continuous decrease of sperm concentration from the age of 25 to the age of 50 years was observed but data on men over 50 years were not included (Schwartz et al. 1983).

It is unknown whether a relationship between decreased testosterone production and reduced spermatogenesis exists. In patients of our clinic presenting with couple infertility in whom manifest hypogonadism was excluded, no correlation between testosterone serum levels and ejaculate parameters could be observed (Rolf et al. 1996). This may indicate a testosterone-independent reduced productivity of testes and accessory glands in older men.

The incidence of varicocele remains constant in patients with advanced age visiting the infertility clinic (Rolf et al. 1996). Andrological diseases acquired in adulthood such as infections of the efferent ducts as well as sperm antibodies, however, are diagnosed more frequently in older patients.

Even if sperm numbers do not decrease with age, acquired infections of the efferent ducts may cause a par-

tial or even complete obstruction so that a progressive reduction of seminal parameters cannot be excluded if adequate antibiotic therapy is not initiated. This would mean that not age per se but longer exposure to infection may be responsible for deteriorating ejaculate parameters.

21.4.4 Fertility of the Aging Male

Pablo Picasso, Charlie Chaplin, Anthony Quinn and Marlon Brando are prominent examples of men who fathered children at a relatively advanced age. All these men had considerably younger female partners. Sustained fertility, however, is not a privilege of VIPs; birth statistics show that a considerable number of fathers of neonates is over 50 years, but only very few mothers in this age group are recorded. Not only in Germany, but also in Japan, a country with a completely different sociocultural and ethnic background, relatively many older men father children (Fig. 21.6).

Information on the fertility pattern of older men can also be obtained from the infertility clinic. Comparing the number of pregnancies of men over 50 years with men under 30 years, whose wives were at a comparable (advanced) age (37± vs. 34± years) at the time of conception, demonstrates that the pregnancy rates do not differ significantly. In comparison, men with younger female partners have a higher probability of fathering a child (Rolf et al. 1996; Fig. 21.7).

Often older men seeking paternity have wives whose reproductive capacity is limited because of age. In countries where IVF treatment with heterologous oocytes is

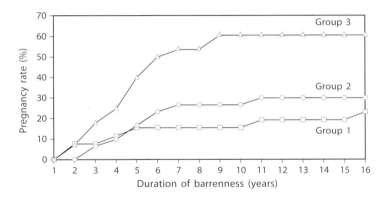

Fig. 21.7. Cumulative pregnancy rate of couples visiting the Institute of Reproductive Medicine for infertility (from Rolf et al. 1996). Mean age of patients with barrenness in group 1, men: mean 53 years, women: mean 36 years (N = 26); group 2, men: mean 28 years, women: mean 34 years (N = 30); group 3, men: mean 27 years, women: mean 27 years (N = 28)

permitted the fertilizing potential of the sperm of older men can be evaluated independent of oocyte quality. In the case of such heterologous IVF treatment, advanced age of the male causes no change in the fertilization rate or implantation rate (Gallardo et al. 1996).

> Therefore in principle older men retain their fertility. The fact of relatively rare fatherhood in men over 60 years can be explained by reduced or extinct fertility of the female partners.
> Impaired fertility in aging men should be diagnosed and treated as in younger patients.
> Age alone is no reason to eschew suitable contraception, if the female partner is of reproductive age and if there is no indication of impaired fertility.

21.5 Chromosome Abnormalities and Advanced Paternal Age

An increased incidence of chromosome abnormalities in offspring from mothers of advanced age is proven. However, the possible consequences of advanced paternal age have not been as well investigated (Nieschlag et al. 2000).

The main reason for **aneuploidy**, i.e. for **numerical chromosomal abnormality**, is a non-disjunction during the meiotic division of the gametes. In men, meiotic divisions of the spermatocytes begin in puberty. Non-disjunctions during spermatogenesis are not rare. For

example, in 4.7% of sperm of healthy men abnormal chromosome numbers were observed (Bordson and Leonardo 1991). Numeric chromosome abnormalities occur more frequently in infertile men with reduced sperm quality. In former investigations advanced paternal age was considered a risk factor for trisomy 21 (Morbus Down). However, in recent studies this could not be confirmed. In addition, no relationship could be found between the incidence of relatively frequent (and hence clinically relevant) chromosome aneuploidies characterizing trisomy 13, trisomy 18, Turner syndrome (45, XO) and Klinefelter syndrome (47, XXY) and paternal age (Bordson and Leonardo 1991).

There are indications of increasing structural chromosomal abnormalities in the sperm of older men. However, in living neonates or fetuses subject to prenatal diagnosis no increase of new structural chromosomal abnormalities was found (Hook 1986). Reciprocal translocations in children of older fathers are considered to occur at a higher frequency (Hook 1986).

Genetic mutations are the result of errors in DNA-replication. Up to the time of puberty approximately 30 cell divisions lead to a large pool of undifferentiated spermatogonia. These undergo 23 divisions per year, so that the number of divisions of a sperm in a twenty-year old man is 200, 430 for a thirty-year old and 770 divisions for a forty-five year old man (Crow 1997). At each division *de novo* mutations can take place. Thus, it is obvious that in old men increased errors of DNA transcription may occur. Late spermatids, like spermatozoa, lack their own DNA repair system. The effectiveness of anti-oxidative protective mechanisms in seminal plasma and sperm declines with increasing age; thus sperm of old men are more vulnerable to mutagens than the sperm of younger man (Tarin et al. 1998). It is now widely accepted that the incidence of autosomal dominant diseases, such as achondroplasia, polyposis coli, Marfan syndrome, Apert syndrome and basal cell naevi are associated with advanced paternal age (Bordson and Leonardo 1991; Crow 1997). The incidence of other diseases such as neurofibromatosis, retinoblastoma or the Soto syndrome increase only minimally with increased paternal age (Crow 1997). About 5% of all cardiac defects in children whose fathers are older than 35 are said to be due to advanced paternal age; this indicates that some defects are caused by newly arising dominant mutations (Crow 1997). The proportion of abortions in or after the 20th week of gestation increases continuously with increasing paternal age, independent of maternal age (Hook 1986). Hence even if offspring of older men have a slightly increased incidence of certain genetic diseases, the individual risk of such a new disease must be considered as extremely small.

> While according to the guidelines of the German Medical Board on prenatal diagnosis and predisposition to diseases, advanced age of the pregnant woman is considered as a possible justification for specific intensive prenatal diagnosis, advanced paternal age is no explicit indication for intensified prenatal diagnosis (Bundesärztekammer 1998).

21.6 Sexuality in Senescence

Generally, both women as well as men are able to maintain sexual feelings and enjoy an active sexual life in senescence.

In the aging man, however, changes in the sexual response cycle can be observed. The **excitement phase** is extended and achievement of **erection** delayed. The **plateau phase**, the time from erection to ejaculation, is often prolonged; often erections necessitate more prolonged, intense and direct stimulation. In general, although control of **ejaculation** in old men is clearly improved, the duration of the **orgasmic phase** is shorter. The intensity of semen propulsion decreases. After ejaculation the aging man experiences increasingly rapid dissipation of erection. The **refractory phase**, the period of time after orgasm in which further sexual stimulation will not produce subsequent orgasm, significantly increases for the aging man. The frequency and the duration of **nocturnal penile tumescence** in aging men is diminished, compared with that in younger men (Elliot 1990). Erectile dysfunction is increasingly present in aging men and erection problems are the most common sexual dysfunction of aging men. Diagnosis and therapy of erectile dysfunction are described in Sect. 10.2.

About 90% of men over 60 years report sexual activity; in a group of healthy men over 80 years 60% report having coitus. The presence of a female partner plays a decisive role since married men are sexually more active than single men (Morley et al. 1990).

Several pathophysiological reasons may be the cause of the **reduced frequency of sexual intercourse** with age.

The increasing incidence of multimorbidity in aging men, i.e. the high frequency of cardiovascular diseases, hypertonus, rheumatic diseases, renal diseases or diabetes mellitus, has unfavorable effects on sexuality. Also, many drugs such as antihypertensives and psychopharma-compounds may have a negative influence on sexuality. A decrease of sexual activity is often caused by psychosocial reasons such as prolonged disease or death of the spouse. Another important reason for reduced sexual activity is the negative attitude of broad parts of society towards sexuality in age. Often elderly persons are not expected to have their own sexuality; living circumstances, particularly in many homes for senior citizens with strict rules, restrict any expression of intimacy, and prohibit sexual interaction (Elliot 1990).

Inadequate or unsatisfactory sexual life may in turn also be responsible for psychosomatic diseases such as gastritis, colitis, obstipation or attacks of angina pectoris or dyspnoa in senescence.

21.7 Andrologically Relevant Diseases in Advanced Age

21.7.1 Benign Prostatic Hypertrophy

Benign prostatic hypertrophy (BPH) is a widespread disease in older men and is rarely encountered before the age of 40. It is estimated that in the USA 17% of men between the ages of 50 and 59, 27% between the ages of 60 and 69 and 35% of men between 70 and 79 show symptoms of BPH possibly requiring treatment (Jacobsen et al. 1995). Its exact etiology is not clear. Endocrine imbalance in senescence is considered a possible reason. In men castrated prior to puberty BPH is not seen. In the prostate testosterone is metabolized to dihydrotestosterone (DHT) irreversibly. Whether, however, increased DHT levels in the prostate are a reason for BPH or a consequence of the enlarged gland, is not fully settled (Pike and Ursin 1994). Statistically significant changes in testosterone levels in patients with BPH were not found. An increase of estrogen levels and decreased androgen efficiency are also discussed as a reason for BPH (Gann et al. 1995; Suzuki et al. 1995).

Possibly genetic differences in the androgen receptor also determine a disposition towards BPH. Men with a lower number of CAG triplets on the androgen receptor gene have a higher probability of developing BPH than those with more CAG triplets (Giovannucci et al. 1999).

The prostates of men with acromegaly are noticably larger than those of healthy men of equal age, despite their secondary hypogonadism (Colao et al. 1998). Normalization of growth hormone levels leads to a reduction of prostate volume. Thus growth hormone has an influence on prostate growth.

The first symptoms of BPH often are pollakisuria, dysuria and nykturia. However, in the early stage a complete emptying of the bladder is still possible (Harzmann et al. 1998). In the retentive stage complete emptying of the bladder is no longer possible, due to the slackening of the bladder's muscular system. In the stage of bladder insufficiency the muscular system and innervation adapt to this condition. Owing to obstruction in the ureter and kidneys, renal insufficiency is imminent. Furthermore it remains unclear whether BPH is a predisposing factor for prostate cancer.

The diagnosis of BPH is based on clinical history, rectal-digital palpitation, transrectal sonography, measurement of prostate-specific antigen (PSA), uroflowmetry and cystoscopy. The internationally accepted International Prostate Symptom Score (IPSS) allows patients to be categorized according to symptoms. In the diagnosis of BPH particularly prostatitis and prostate cancer must be excluded.

- Mild symptoms of BPH (**IPSS score 0–7**) require no therapy; patients should be checked regularly. Phytotherapy can be considered.
- Patients with moderate symptoms (**IPSS score 8–19**) should be treated with α-receptor blockers. Unlike α-receptor blockers the 5α-reductase blocker Finasteride reduces prostate volume. Finasteride therapy is promising when the IPSS score is between 8 and 19 and the prostate volume exceeds 40 ml (Harzmann et al. 1998).
- Severe symptoms (**IPSS score 20–35**) require transurethral resection of the prostate. In cases of very large prostate volume transvesical prostate adenoma enucleation should be performed (Harzmann er al. 1998)

21.7.2 Prostate Cancer

Nowadays prostate cancer is the most common cancer in men. Predominantly a disease of older men, peak incidence occurs in the late 60 s and early 70 s. The incidence of prostate cancer in systematically performed autopsies is significantly higher than the incidence of clinically manifested cases.

Within the recent past an increase in prostate cancer was observed, particularly in men below 60 years (Post et al. 1999). In part this can be attributed to improved regular checkups. It is not known what factors are responsible for the increase in prostate carcinoma.

The first symptoms of prostate cancer often resemble the symptoms of benign prostatic hyperplasia; however, dysuria occurs more frequently and pollakisuria less often. Hematuria is also often present. Hematogenous metastases are most frequently found in bones. Often the first symptoms are due to bone metastases with lumbar or pelvic pain. Digital rectal examination remains the most practicable method for early diagnosis. Further

screening examinations are determination of PSA and transrectal ultrasonography with prostate biopsy (Hertle and Pohl 1993; Wirth et al. 1998). Since in many cases prostate cancer is not clinically overt, the optimal intensity of adequate screening is subject to controversial discussion (Wirth et al. 1998). However, it was shown that annual PSA determination beginning at age 50 clearly reduced the mortality rate (Labrie et al. 1999). A yearly urological checkup is recommended for men from the ages of 45–50 onwards (Wirth et al. 1998).

The treatment strategy of prostate cancer depends on the stage of disease at diagnosis, on the age and the general well-being of the patient and on histological differentiation. In general radical prostatectomy, orchidectomy, radiation therapy, hormonal treatment with estrogen derivatives, antiandrogens, and today, preferably with GnRH-analogues are available modalities (Reich and Faul 1998).

21.7.3 Senescent Gynaecomastia

The incidence of gynecomastia increases with age (cf. Sect. 11.4). Gynecomastia is associated with an increase in the estrogen to androgen ratio. Moreover, several general diseases (i. e. renal insufficiency, hepatic insufficiency) as well as different drugs such as the competitive aldosterone antagonist spironolactone, digoxin, ACE inhibitors as well as cytotoxic drugs can lead to an enlargement of breast tissue (Morley et al. 1990).

Painful gynecomastia usually represents new-onset rapidly expanding breast enlargement. Differentiation of this from mammary carcinoma is also essential in male patients because cancer of the breast in males accounts for one percent of all breast cancers, and peak incidence occurs in men between the ages of 50 and 70. Moreover, a paraneoplastic, or an hCG-producing bronchial carcinoma must also be taken into consideration (Morley et al. 1990). Paraneoplastic tumors of the testes, the liver, the adrenal gland or to the gastrointestinal tract must be considered too. (See Sect. 11.4 for further details.)

21.7.4 Androgenic Alopecia

Androgenic alopecia (baldness) is the most common form of alopecia in the male. Its incidence clearly increases with age. Sect. 11.5 deals with its pathogenesis and treatment.

21.8 Hormone Substitution in Advanced Age

21.8.1 Testosterone Substitution

In general, hormone substitution, analogous to estrogen substitution in postmenopausal woman, cannot be recommended for the aging male. If clinical evidence for a latent or overt testosterone deficiency is present and serum testosterone levels in the morning are below the normal value for younger men of 12.0 nmol/L, testosterone substitution can be considered. Substitution should be performed according to the principles and dosage stated in Chap. 15. The possibility of prostate disease requires special diagnostic measures before and during testosterone substitution in this age group.

In aging men testosterone is not only essential for secondary sex characteristics, libido and potency, but causes changes in mood and cognitive function, in erythropoesis, in bone metabolism, in protein anabolism, muscle mass as well as in body fat distribution. Testosterone in the aging man is important for his sexual life as well as for several vital functions. Clinically a decline in serum levels of testosterone is associated with decreased libido and potency, as well as fatigue, reduction of muscle mass, osteoporosis and mild anaemia. In most cases isolated erectile dysfunction is caused by diseases such as arteriosclerosis or diabetes mellitus. Especially neural and vascular changes in the penis and in the small pelvis can cause erectile dysfunction.

In general, muscle mass decreases with age. In hypogonadal young patients muscularity usually is also reduced, which can be improved by testosterone substitution. In aging men short-term testosterone substitution increases lean body mass at the expense of abdominal fat (Tenover 1994). With increasing age of healthy volunteers, a gain in weight and percentage of fat mass is measured correlating to the decline in testosterone. In contrast, in hypogonadal patients receiving adequate testosterone substitution, no alteration in body weight and proportion of fat is seen because no age-dependent decrease in testosterone is present (Fig. 21.8).

Whether long-term testosterone substitution can improve age- or disease-dependent cachexia remains unclear (Liu and Handelsman 1998). Preliminary results with testosterone substitution therapy in orthopedic patients with knee protheses were promising. In some autoimmune diseases androgens may have a protective effect. The incidence of most autoimmune diseases is higher in aging men than in younger men. In women and in hypogonadal men the incidence is also higher

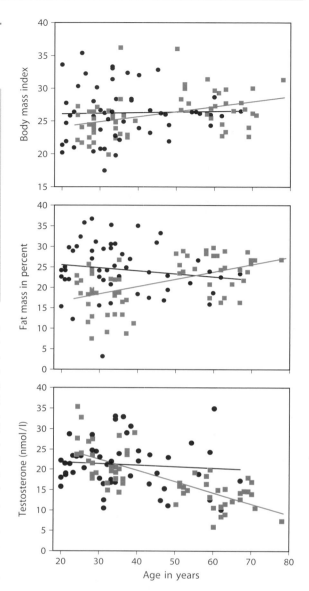

Fig 21.8. Age-dependence of body mass index, percentage of body fat mass and serum testosterone levels in healthy men (*red*) and hypogonadal men under adequate testosterone substitution therapy (*black*)

than in healthy men, therefore several autoimmune diseases may be mitigated by testosterone substitution (Tenover 1994). Only in the last few years has it been recognized that osteoporosis poses a major health problem, not only in postmenopausal women, but also in aging men. In diagnosis and therapy of both senile, as well as secondary osteoporosis, changes of androgen levels must be taken into consideration. In patients with pathological testosterone levels therapy with androgens should be considered (Francis 1999). Thus a clear improvement in bone mineral density resulted in osteoporotic patients with chronic obstructive lung diseases, who were being treated with cortisone, when they underwent additional testosterone therapy (Reich et al. 1996).

According to the results of short-term studies, testosterone treatment in patients with documented testosterone deficiency improved physical and psychic well-being in advanced age (Bagatell et al. 1994; Tenover 1994).

In the first large-scale placebo-controlled study extending over 36 months, transdermal testosterone substitution of older man led to an increase in muscle mass as well as bone mineral density (Snyder et al. 1999 a,b). The volunteers reported a subjective improvement of physical capacity. A clear increase of bone mineral density was especially noted in older men with reduced basal testosterone levels, while volunteers with normal levels prior to onset of therapy only showed a marginal increase in bone density.

There are no data indicating that testosterone substitution induces prostate cancer. The molecular processes by which androgens influence prostate growth are not yet completely understood. Androgens are essential for normal prostate growth. In the absence of androgens the prostate maintains neither its function nor its size. Exogenous testosterone substitution in hypogonadal men causes the prostate to grow until the corresponding prostate size of age-dependent healthy volunteers is reached (Behre et al. 1994). Surprisingly, in a retrospective study older men receiving testosterone over several years developed BPH symptoms less frequently than the untreated men of a control group (Hajjar et al. 1997). As androgens are known to stimulate the growth of overt prostate cancer, prostate cancer is a contraindication for androgen substitution. Case reports of prostate cancer in older patients under testosterone substitution have been published (Rolf and Nieschlag 1998).

> The prostate should be examined by digital palpation and transrectal sonography before and during substitution therapy. From the age 40 onwards the concentration of PSA (prostate-specific antigen) should be determined at six-monthly intervals during testosterone substitution.

High doses of testosterone can lead to polycythemia and elevated hematocrit values are found relatively often among older men substituted with testosterone (Hajjar et al. 1997; Sih et al. 1997); these values should be checked regularly during treatment. To avoid the complications of polycythemia, the dose must be reduced, the mode of application should be changed to transdermal testosterone or at the very least, treatment should be stopped immediately.

Table 21.1. Endocrine changes with age (related to the means of large populations, which have wide variances)

Testosterone (total)	Decrease
Free testosterone	Decrease
LH	Increase
FSH	Increase
SHBG	Increase
Estradiol (E2)	Constant
Estrone (E1)	Constant
Dihydrotestosterone (DHT)	Constant
Cortisol	Constant
Dehydroepiandrosterone (DHEA)	Decrease
Melatonin	Decrease
Prolactin	Decrease
Growth hormone (GH)	Decrease
Insulin-like growth factor (IGF-I)	Decrease

21.8.2 Other Hormone Substitution

As described above, a decrease of testosterone production is not the only endocrine change in senescence (Table 21.1). In recent years increased attention has been given to reduced secretion of **growth hormone** (GH) and **insulin-like growth-factor-I** (IGF-I). It is accepted that reduced growth hormone levels in aging man are responsible for changes in body composition. With recombinant growth hormone the possibility of substitution became available. In controlled studies it could be shown that application of growth hormone in GH-deficient men leads to anabolic metabolism with increased bone density of the lumbar spine, improved muscle strength and to reduced adipose tissue mass. Growth hormone administration in exercising elderly men does not augment muscle fibre hypertrophy or tissue GH-IGF expression, suggesting that deficits in growth hormone with aging do not inhibit the skeletal muscle tissue response to training. Reduced glucose tolerance, increased blood pressure and overhydration was observed. Therefore long-term substitution of growth hormone may induce hypertonus, diabetes mellitus or cardiomegaly (von Werder 1999; Vance and Mauras 1999). Since acromegalic patients show a markedly increased incidence of colon polyps and carcinoma, it cannot be excluded that growth hormone substitution therapy induces malignant growth. Similarly it was shown that the incidence of prostate carcinoma is elevated in men with high IGF-I serum concentration. Growth hormone substitution is not indicated in older man with physiologically decreased growth hormone levels, but regular pituitary function (von Werder 1999). Results of controlled studies of substitution with synthetic growth hormone releasing hormone analogs (GHRH) or IGF-1 have not been published so far.

> Substitution with **growth hormone**, GH releasing-hormone or IGF-1 must be considered as experimental and, on the basis of present knowledge, should be performed only in controlled studies.

In the first clinically controlled study, **DHEA substitution** induced an increase of IGF-1 levels. 70 % of the patients reported an improvement of general well-being. Further studies demonstrated an activation of the immune system with an increase of monocytes, activated T-lymphocytes and natural killer cells in older men as well as in postmenopausal women. A further large-scale placebo-controlled study, however, found no benefits of DHEA administration (Flynn et al. 1999). Further studies are needed to assess the effectiveness of DHEA therapy.

Melatonin substitution is claimed to improve the sleep quality of older men (Garfinkel et al 1995). Recently in the media, melatonin substitution was reported to prevent tumors. No human studies exist to indicate any such effect (Garfinkel and Besner 1998).

Some gynecologists advocate **estrogen substitution** of older men. Substitution with estradiol derivates is claimed to improve the symptoms of BPH and erectile dysfunction; the LDL-cholesterol level is said to decrease. Moreover, it was maintained that arthralgy, pancreas insufficiency and heart rhythm disturbances improved. These conclusions were drawn from a study without placebo control group and with an obscure study design (Umbreit 1993). Mastodynia in some patients led to termination of therapy. Physiologically plausible arguments for such substitution therapy do not exist and the observations may be explained by suggestive or auto-suggestive influences. In controlled clinical studies with high-dose estrogen preparations for the prevention of coronary heart diseases, as well as for treatment of prostate carcinoma, an increased incidence of thromboembolism as well as cardiovascular complications was noted. Moreover, estrogen serum levels favored the development of BPH in men with relatively low testosterone levels (Gann et al. 1995; Suzuki et al. 1995). Therefore, according to the present state of knowledge, estrogen substitution in men cannot be justified.

21.8.3 Outlook

Concerning reproductive as well as endocrine functions of older men, many questions are still open. Intensified investigation of the physiology of aging men is necessary. According to the present state of knowledge, uncontrolled substitution with androgens or various other hormones can be considered as irresponsible. Further studies, especially prospective placebo-controlled long-term interdisciplinary studies investigating the possible beneficial and adverse consequences of androgen substitution are urgently required.

21.9 References

Abalovich M, Levalle O, Hermes R, Scaglia H, Aranda C, Zylbersztein C, Oneto A, Aquilano D, Gutierrez S (1999) Hypothalamic-pituitary-testicular axis and seminal parameters in hyperthyroid males. Thyroid 9:857–863

Ali ST, Shaik RN, Siddiqi NA, Siddiqi PQ (1993) Semen analysis in insulin-dependent / non-insulin-dependent diabetic men with/without neuropathy. Arch Androl 30:47–54

Bagatell CJ, Heiman JR, Matsumoto AM, Rivier JE Bremner WJ (1994) Metabolic and behavioral effects of high-dose, exogenous testosterone in healthy men. J Clin Endocrin Metab 79:561–567

Behre HM, Bohmeyer J, Nieschlag E (1994) Prostate volume in testosterone-treated and untreated hypogonadal men in comparison to age-matched normal controls. Clin Endocrinol 40:341–349

Belanger A, Candas B, Dupont A, Cusan L, Diamont P, Gomez L, Labrie F (1994) Changes in serum concentrations of conjugated and unconjugated steroids in 40- to 80-year-old men. J Clin Endocrin Metab 79:1086–1090

Bordson BL, Leonardo VS (1991) The appropriate upper age limit for semen donors: a review of the genetic effects of paternal age. Fertil Steril 56:397–401

Bundesärztekammer (1998) Richtlinien zur pränatalen Diagnostik von Krankheiten und Krankheitsdispositionen (http://www.bundesärztekammer.de) Dtsch Ärztebl 95: A3236–3242

Cooper DS (1990) Thyroid disorders In: Cassel CK, Riesenberg DE, Sorensen LB, Walsh JR (eds) Geriatric medicine, 2nd edn. Springer, Berlin Heidelberg New York, pp 256–270

Colao A, Marzullo P, Ferone D, Spiezia S, Cerbone G, Marino V, Di Sarno A, Merola B, Lombardi G (1998) Prostatic hyperplasia: an unknown feature of acromegaly. J Clin Endocrinol Metab 83:775–779

Crow JF (1997) The high spontaneous mutation rate: is it a health risk? Proc Natl Acad Sci USA 94:8380–8386

DeNicola P (1989) Geriatrics: a textbook. Schwer Verlag, Stuttgart

Dennison E, Hindmarsh P, Fall C, Kellingray S, Barker D, Phillips D, Cooper C (1999) Profiles of endogenous circulating cortisol and bone mineral density in healthy elderly men. J Clin Endocrinol Metab 84:3058–3063

Elliot ML (1990) Psychological aspects of sexual dysfunction in the elderly. In: Armbrecht HJ, Coe RM, Wongsurawat N (eds) Endocrine function and age. Springer, Berlin Heidelberg New York, pp 136–146

Finkel E (1998) Telomeres: keys to senescence and cancer. Lancet 351:1186

Flynn MA, Weaver-Osterholtz D, Sharpe-Timms KL, Allen S, Krause G (1999) Dehydroepiandrosterone replacement in aging humans. J Clin Endocrinol Metab 84:1527–1533

Ford HC, Cooke RR, Keightley EA, Feek CM (1992) Serum levels of free and bound testosterone in hyperthyroidism. Clin Endocrinol 36:187–192

Francis RM (1999) The effects of testosterone on osteoporosis in men. Clin Endocrinol (Oxf) 50:411–414

Gallardo E, Simon C, Levy M, Guanes PP, Remohi J, Pellicer A (1996) Effect of age on sperm fertility potential: oocyte donation as a model. Fertil Steril 66:260–264

Gann PH, Hennekens CH, Longcope C, Verhoek-Oftedahl W, Grodstein F, Stampfer MJ (1995) A prospective study of plasma hormone levels, nonhormonal factors, and development of benign prostatic hyperplasia. Prostate 26:40–49

Garfinkel D, Laudon M, Nof D, Zisapel N (1995) Improvement of sleep quality in elderly people by controlled-release melatonin. Lancet 346:541–544

Garfinkel D, Berner YN (1998) Antioxidants and aging: is melatonin a possible, practical new hope? Nutrition 14:712–713

Giovannucci E, Platz EA, Stampfer MJ, Chan A, Krithivas K, Kawachi I, Willett WC, Kantoff PW (1999) The CAG repeat within the androgen receptor gene and benign prostatic hyperplasia. Urology 53:121–125

Gray A, Feldman HA, McKinlay JB, Longcope C (1991) Age, and changing sex hormone levels in middle-aged men: results of the Massachusetts male aging study. J Clin Endocrinol Metab 73:1016–1025

Greendale GA, Unger JB, Rowe JW, Seeman TE (1999) The relation between cortisol excretion and fractures in healthy older people: results from the MacArthur studies-Mac. J Am Geriat Soc 47:799–803

Haffner SM, Shaten J, Stern MP, Smith GD, Kuller L (1996) Low levels of sex hormone-binding globulin and testosterone predict the development of non-insulin-dependent diabetes mellitus in men. MRFIT Research Group. Multiple Risk Factor Intervention Trial. Am J Epidemiol 143:889–897

Hajjar RR, Kaiser FE, Morley JE (1997) Outcomes of long-term testosterone replacement in older hypogonadal males: a retrospective analysis. J Clin Endocrinol Metab 82:3793–3796

Handelsman DJ, Staraj S (1985) Testicular size: the effects of aging, malnutritrion, and illness. J Androl 6:144–151

Harzmann R, Weckermann D, Wawroschek F (1998) Behandlung der benignen Prostatahyperplasie. Z Ärztl Fortbild Qualitätssich 92:319–324

Herbert J (1995) The age of dehydroepiandrosterone. Lancet 345:1193–1194

Hertle L, Pohl J (1993) Urologische Therapie. Urban and Schwarzenberg, Munich

Homonnai ZT, Fainman N, David MP, Paz GF (1981) Semen quality and sex hormone pattern of 39 middle aged men. Andrologia 14:164–170

Holstein AF (1989) Morphological evidence for the involution of spermatogenesis during senescence. In: Holstein AF, Voigt KD, Grässlin D (eds) Reproductive biology and medicine. Diesbach, Berlin, pp 66–77

Hook EB (1986) Paternal age and effects on chromosomal and specific locus mutations and on other genetic outcomes in offspring. In: Mastroianni L, Paulsen CA (eds) Aging, reproduction, and the climacteric. Plenum Publishing Corporation, New York, pp 117–146

Jacobsen SJ, Girman CJ, Guess HA, Oesterling JE, Lieber MM (1995) New diagnostic and treatment guidelines for benign prostatic hyperplasia. Potential impact in the United States. Arch Intern Med 155:477–481

Jaya Kumar B, Khurana ML, Ammini AC, Karmarkar MG, Ahuja MM (1990) Reproductive endocrine functions in men with primary hypothyroidism: effect of thyroxine replacement. Horm Res 34:215–218

Johnson L, Grumbles JS, Bagheri A, Petty CS (1990) Increased germ cell degeneration during postprophase of meiosis is related to increased serum follicle-stimulating hormone concentrations and reduced daily sperm production in aged men. Biol Reprod 42:281–287

Kaufman JM, Vermeulen A (1998) Androgens in male senescence. In: Nieschlag E, Behre HM (eds) Testosterone: action, deficiency, substitution, second edition. Springer, Berlin Heidelberg New York, pp 437–471

Krithivas K, Yurgalevitch SM, Mohr BA, Wilcox CJ, Batter SJ, Brown M, Longcope C, McKinlay JB, Kantoff PW (1999) Evidence that the CAG repeat in the androgen receptor gene is associated with the age-related decline in serum androgen levels in men. J Endocrinol 162:137–142

Labrie F, Candas B, Dupont A, Cusan L, Gomez JL, Suburu RE, Diamond P, Levesque J, Belanger A (1999) Screening decreases prostate cancer death: first analysis of the 1988 Quebec prospective randomized controlled trial. Prostate 38:83–91

Liu PY, Handelsman DJ (1998) Androgen therapy in non-gonadal men. In: Nieschlag E, Behre HM (eds) Testosterone: action, deficiency, substitution, second edition. Springer, Berlin Heidelberg New York, pp 473–512

Michikawa Y, Mazzucchelli F, Bresolin N, Scarlato G, Attardi G (1999) Aging-dependent large accumulation of point mutations in the human mtDNA control region for replication. Science 286:774–779

Morley JE, Kaiser FE, Johnson LE (1990) Male sexual function. In: Cassel CK, Riesenberg DE, Sorensen LB, Walsh JR (eds) Geriatric medicine, second edition. Springer, Berlin Heidelberg New York, pp 256–270

Nieschlag E, Michel E (1986) Reproductive functions in grandfathers. In: Mastroianni L, Paulsen CA (eds) Aging, reproduction, and the climacteric. Plenum, New York, pp 59–71

Nieschlag E, Lammers U, Freischem CW, Langer K, Wickings EJ (1982) Reproductive functions in young fathers and grandfathers. J Clin Endocrinol Metab 55:676–681

Nieschlag E, Brinkworth M, Rolf C, Lerchl A (2000) Fertility and fertility related problems in the aging male. Proceedings of the 9th International Menopause Society, World Congress of the Menopause, Parthenon, London

Pike MC, Ursin G (1994) Etiology of benign prostatic hyperplasia. In: Petrovich Z, Baert L (eds) Benign prostatic hyperplasia innovations in management. Springer, Berlin Heidelberg New York, pp 1–16

Post PN, Stockton D, Davies TW, Coebergh JW (1999) Striking increase in incidence of prostate cancer in men aged < 60 years without improvement in prognosis. Br J Cancer 79:13–17

Reich OM, Faul P (1998) Aktuelle Therapie des Prostatakarzinoms. Z Arztl Fortbild Qualitatssich 92:311–318

Reid IR, Wattie DJ, Evans MC, Stapleton JP (1996) Testosterone therapy in glucocorticoid-treated men. Arch Intern Med 156:1173–1177

Rolf C, Nieschlag E (1998) Potential adverse effects of long-term testosterone therapy. Baillières Clin Endocrinol Metab 12:521–534

Rolf C, Behre HM, Nieschlag E (1996) Reproductive parameters of older compared to younger men of infertile couples. Int J Androl 19:135–142

Schlüter D (1978) Die endokrinen Organe der Über–Neunzig-jährigen. Dissertation, University of Hamburg

Schwartz D, Mayaux Mj, Spira A, Moscato ML, Jouannet P, Czy-glik F, David G (1983) Semen characteristics as a function of age in 833 fertile men. Fertil Steril 39:530–535

Sih R, Morley JE, Kaiser FE, Perry HM III, Patrick P, Ross C (1997) Testosterone replacement in older hypogonadal men: a 12-month randomized controlled trial. J Clin Endocrinol Metab 82:1661–1667

Simon D, Preziosi P, Barrett-Connor E, Roger M, Saint-Paul M, Nahoul K, Papoz L (1992) The influence of aging on plasma sex hormones in men: the Telecom study. Am J Epidem 135:783–791

Snyder PJ, Peachey H, Hannoush P, Berlin JA, Loh L, Holmes JH, Dlewati A, Staley J, Santanna J, Kapoor SC, Attie MF, Haddad JG Jr, Strom BL (1999) Effect of testosterone treatment on bone mineral density in men over 65 years of age. J Clin Endocrinol Metab 84:1966–1972

Snyder PJ, Peachey H, Hannoush P, Berlin JA, Loh L, Lenrow DA, Holmes JH, Dlewati A, Santanna J, Rosen CJ, Strom BL (1999b) Effect of testosterone treatment on body composition and muscle strength in men over 65 years of age. J Clin Endocrinol Metab 84:2647–2653

Statistische Jahrbücher 1980–1998 für die Bundesrepublik Deutschland. Statistisches Bundesamt Wiesbaden (ed) Metzler Poeschel, Stuttgart

Suzuki K, Ito K, Ichinose Y, Kurokawa K, Suzuki T, Imai K, Yamanaka H, Honma S (1995) Endocrine environment of benign prostatic hyperplasia: prostate size and volume are correlated with serum estrogen concentration. Scand J Urol Nephrol 29:65–68

Swerdloff RS, Wang C (1993) Androgen deficiency and aging in men. West J Med 159:579–585

Tarin JJ, Brines J, Cano A (1998) Long-term effects of delayed parenthood. Hum Reprod 13:2371–2376

Tenover JS (1994) Androgen administration to aging men. Endocrinol Metab Clin North Am 23:878–892

Umbreit K (1993) Ist eine Substitution mit Estradiol auch bei Männern angezeigt? Gyne 14:56–60

Vance ML, Mauras N (1999) Growth hormone therapy in adults and children. N Engl J Med 341:1206–16

Vermeulen A (1993) Environment, human reproduction, menopause, and andropause. Environ Health Perspect 101 [Suppl 2]:91–100

Vermeulen A, Kaufman JM (1995) Aging of the hypothalamo-pituitary-testicular axis in men. Horm Res 43:2528

von Werder K (1999) The somatopause is no indication for growth hormone therapy. J Endocrinol Invest 22 [Suppl 5]:137–141

Wirth MP, Spiegel T, Froschermaier SE, Mansek A (1998) Screening beim Prostatakarzinom. Z Ärztl Fortbild Qualitätssich 92:304–309

CHAPTER 22

Ethical Aspects of Reproductive Medicine*

22

K. Demmer

* Translated by T. Kopfensteiner and S. Nieschlag

22.1 Social and Cultural Context

22.1.1 A Shared Intellectual Responsibility

As an intellectual discipline, medicine is not an isolated or self-sufficient science. Medical research is not imprisoned in the ivory tower of scholars. Rather, within enlightened democratic society there is a public interest in all matters touching upon the responsible handling of human life over which, thanks to medical research, mankind has been given increasing control. Critical and constructive solidarity with all potentially affected persons is called for which lays the foundation for consentual standards; effective laws do not arise from unconcerted efforts by the legislators, but reflect the intellectual responsibility of the whole community. For the scientist this provides welcome relief. Serious decisions that have farreaching consequences in shaping the lives of others must not be made by the scientist in the solitude of his conscience for which he bears sole responsibility, even though obvious tensions between the private and public spheres will never be fully resolved.

Ethicists and moral theologians share in the efforts to form opinion in our pluralistic society; as part of the intellectual elite, they contribute solutions to problems with which society can responsibly live. This is also true for the official teachings of the **Christian churches**, regardless of whether or not the discussants share a Christian understanding of man. When the churches make a statement about medical research and its clinical application, they do so under the tacit presupposition that the content of the message can be rationally justified and thus be credible. In general Christianity has had a constructive influence on the scientific culture of the west, and will continue to do so if it succeeds in introducing into public discourse guidelines for a meaningful life which are in all respects convincing and exemplary.

22.1.2 The Structure of Interdisciplinary Dialogue

It often happens that the public has a mistaken conception of the competence of either philosophical ethicists or moral theologians so that any contribution they may make is not given its proper or due respect. Different styles of thinking which have become virtually institutionalized collide with one another, occasionally giving the impression that they have come to stand next to each other with nothing in common. This image, however, does not correspond to reality; it is better to envision underground channels developing and running here and there linking the various disciplines. In this way, the physician makes tacit assumptions which, philosophically speaking, touch on presumed concepts of the individual; the physician is not autonomous, but thinks and acts within the framework of an open system.

The same is true for the ethicist, be he philosopher or moral theologian. He does not design a self-sufficient body of thought to whose rigorous and unyielding logic every knee must bend; his thought is open to the entire range of human scientific experience and remains flexible in light of the variety of human endeavors. He is capable of learning, true to the axiom that facts cannot be argued with. And he becomes aware of his own limited competence, whenever he is confronted by the professionalism of the physician. This does not condemn the ethicist or moral theologian to silence. He is always available when the physician touches upon the implicit presuppositions with which he works, or when the physician is faced with the unavoidable ambivalence of scientific research. Is scientific research a blessing when regarded against the background of a convincing perception of humanity or can it become – by running an unconstrained course – a curse for mankind? Are the goals of research desirable? And at what price are they to be achieved? How are they to be applied in the individual case? Abstract concepts classified as good or value-neutral can change their moral qualification when put into practice. What is required then, is critical and constructive solidarity that at times swims against the tide.

22.1.3 The Dilemma of the Theologian

When the moral theologian engages in interdisciplinary dialogue, he does not propose exclusively his private opinions, regardless of how well-founded they may be. He always keeps in mind, rather, that the churches hold a privileged place for sound moral instruction and teaching; there is an initial reliance on and confidence in the church's intellectual tradition. Furthermore, as a Roman Catholic, the theologian considers his mandate in terms of partnership with the Church's authority which finds institutional expression in the offices of the pope and bishops. A precarious relationship of trust exists between official church representatives and professional theologians. Their relationship is not always an unclouded one. For the theologian, often the first to be confronted with problems, is not able to withdraw to a secure corner and leave it to others to debate and set policy. This carries unavoidable risks for his work; at times he cannot proceed beyond hypothetical answers which demand the courage to revise his position. The physician or medical researcher will understand this; they know, too, the provisional character of their knowledge. Mutual recognition of each other's limitations makes the dialogue all the more credible.

It is a different situation for the magisterium. Whoever speaks with the teaching authority of the church can take fewer risks. However, he always appeals – though in a nuanced variety of ways – to his opposite's freedom of conscience which is not abrogated. Authority has no intention of trumping plausibility. Differentiated positions will begin to emerge and patience is required on the part of all. In this process the theologian assumes the role of mediator, always pushing forward and seeking to resolve emerging difficulties in understanding, without sacrificing his own identity and integrity.

22.2 Church Statements

22.2.1 Artificial Insemination as a Springboard

The decisive condemnation of artificial insemination by Pope Pius XII (†1958) set the stage for all contemporary discussions surrounding the legitimacy of the various forms of infertility therapy. The arguments put forward can be briefly summarized as follows: what was deplored by Pope Pius XII was the artificial separation of the procreative purpose from the bodily expression of marital love; they belong essentially together. Here is a line of argumentation that will reemerge in connection with in vitro fertilization, and which continues to influence the thinking of Pope John Paul II.

Man is a bound steward, not an arbitrary creator of a given order of nature, which is interpreted as God's good creation. It does not fetter or restrain the individual, but, over the entire spectrum of its expression it protects the dignity of the person. In consistent fashion, the pope speaks out against the collection of sperm through masturbation. Although the end – the conception of new life – may be good, it does not justify the use of a means that is in itself evil.

Moreover, the underlying understanding of the institution of marriage became a matter for discussion. In heterologous protocols, for instance, the exclusivity of the community of life is apparently no longer safeguarded, insofar as a third person – via donor sperm – invades the intimate union of the couple. In purely objective terms, it was thus quite understandable to speak of adultery. It is not surprising that the pope acknowledged the emerging legal and demographic policy consequences of this problem, nor is it surprising that those issues helped confirm his negative stance. Finally, when public debate introduced the issue of a right to a child, he was persuaded to intervene; the existence of a human being is always a free and unmerited gift, never a product which is rightfully owned; in the end, that would imply a deliberate disregard for human existence.

The ethical discussion immediately following was able to introduce more precise distinctions long overdue. A first point of criticism focused on the purported interpretation of masturbation. Similar to the collection of sperm for diagnostic purposes, its underlying intention was underscored: the purpose of the act is conception and the phenomenal structure of the act itself should be interpreted in this light; neither by itself nor in the final analysis does the act itself determine its morality.

The papal understanding of the conjugal act was also subjected to question. Without wanting to detract from the fundamental unity that exists between the openness to procreation and the expression of love in the conjugal act, it should not be over-interpreted so as to excessively burden or strain practice. The fundamental dual meaning of the conjugal act is not undermined by any medical intervention but is rather borne out by the couple's primary goal; technology must not necessarily burden the spontaneity of the couple's expression of love.

In general, however, the pope and moral theologians were to a large extent in agreement in their appraisal of the population policy issues, and the legal and psychological problems associated with heterologous protocols; the dangers were seen clearly and there is no need to list them here, except perhaps to mention that sperm donation required in heterologous protocols epitomizes the tendency to trivialize human sexuality. The child falls victim, as a rule the child is denied the right to know his own father. And the father removes himself from any responsibility for the child. Should it ever be the case that he not remain anonymous, there is an enormous risk of inner conflict. Whether and to what extent the child so conceived is a lingering reminder of the absent father, thus putting pressure on the marriage or even leading to its ultimate failure, depends on a constellation of concrete factors and circumstances.

22.2.2 In Vitro Fertilization

The stage was now set for later conflicts concerning in vitro fertilization. Official teaching is unequivocally clear. The decisive texts are contained in the Instruction "Donum vitae" issued by the Congregation of the Doctrine of the Faith (1987) and Pope John Paul II's encyclical "Evangelium vitae" (1995). Corresponding exactly to the issue of artificial insemination, the hard core of the argument is the underlying anthropology of the conjugal act. With reference to Pope Paul VI's encyclical "Humanae vitae" (1968), the inseparable unity of the two meanings of the conjugal act – the expression of the couple's mutual love and the openness to new life – is affirmed as part of the continuous official church teaching. Man does not have the right to separate them artificially, as usually occurs in all technical variations of assisted fertilization. The verdict allows no exception. The fear looming in the background is obvious; it is aroused by the introduction of technology into one of the most spontaneous expressions in human life. Reproductive technologies that, as Pope John XXIII noted earlier, could be legitimately used with non-human species, cannot be transferred directly to the human situation. This judgement is definitive; the motives of those involved or concrete circumstances brook no alterations. A threshold value is established which stigmatizes any exception as recidivous; a point of reference is designated and removed from further discussion, it is a topic that is closed off to further discussion. The opinion of the Protestant Churches of Germany published under the title "On the dignity of human life" (1985) lacks this decisive clarity.

In his encyclical "Evangelium vitae" Pope John Paul II contrasts the "culture of death" present in today's society with a "culture of life". Such an emphatic choice of words may be surprising in the context of reproductive medicine which avowedly serves the transmission of life (n. 13 ff.). The expression is clarified somewhat in view of the possibility of using spare embryos as material in human experiments that are unnecessary but for the sake of socalled highranking research goals. A danger is assumed that remains to be proven in individual cases. This is in no way an exclusively Catholic concern. The opinion of the Evangelical-Lutheran Church of Germany and the German Bishops' Conference share the same fears in their joint statement "God is a friend of life" (1989).

A consensus crossing confessional boundaries can also be widely observed concerning both the ontological as well as the moral status of the embryo. Specifically human life that is owed protection begins with the syngamy or fusion of the gametes, even though this fusion does not occur at any one moment but is understood as an ongoing process. Then a new entity – distinct from the mother and with its own genetic programme – is brought forth, and begins its own course of development. That this process is subject to immanent risks does not change its basic moral status. As the most fundamental of rights, the right to life is assumed to be indivisible; its logic is equally compelling at all times. To speak of a life less worthy of protection can only be interpreted as an attack on human dignity. The concept of the individual cannot be conceived in quantitative categories; one cannot be "more" or "less" a person. At this stage of vulnerability and weakness the demands to protect human life should increase all the more, and this in terms of advocacy.

To be sure, when it speaks out in these matters it is not the role or the intention of the Catholic Church to adopt any particular philosophical system as its own. When it speaks of "person", only the transparency and lucidity of argument counts. In this regard, biological data suggest that the distinction between personal and pre-personal life that is sometimes used is an arbitrary one. While biological data do not compel a particular position to be taken, nevertheless the acceptance of personal life appears as most befitting ("Donum vitae"); this position offers the relatively most convincing alternative by affirming the legitimate desire for a maximum amount of protection for human life; it acts as a dam. The task of the philosophical discussion is to reconcile the classical categories of understanding which had been centered around prescientific conceptions of static individuated substance with the clear finality of process categories, and to introduce a dynamic concept of person: embryonic development proceeds continuously, and has the potential to gradually assume a progressively complete identity as well as autonomy.

22.3 The Coordinates of Ethical Discussion

22.3.1 The Basic Understanding of Marriage

Official church statements have the merit of providing indispensable guideposts to those engaged in public discourse. They are focal points or axes around which discussion turns regardless of the outcome. Nor is ethical reflection within the Church exempt from making further distinctions and clarifications; positions that are taken are neither specific to any one confession nor derive completely from secular world views. Morality has an autonomous character which permits universal communication.

One genuine concern in this discussion is the underlying understanding of marriage and the conjugal act. Those who believe that relevant principal issues of reproduction are fundamentally tied to the institution of marriage will apply these principles to homologous protocols. Reproductive medicine is bound by this logic; it cannot claim criteria or norms all its own. These concerns render an extension to quasi-homologous protocols meaningless. Responsibility for the social context of sexuality and reproduction fades in importance, and the dominating criterion is the care for the child conceived, in particular providing the child a home with a stable heterosexual couple, as it is of supreme importance for the formation and development of a mature and well-integrated personality as well as for the discovery of one's identity. In light of this, there arises a question for the physician: regardless of the procedures' legality, is this extension meant to be interpreted as evidence of responsible tolerance? The main goal of recent reforms in the laws of inheritance sometimes referred to in this context is to protect the illegitimately conceived child from unjust harm.

Ethical reservations multiply when the desire for a child arises quite outside the limits of such a socially supportive background. In that case it is irrelevant whether the desire for a child is on the part of a single parent or same-sex couple. In either case, the wish for offspring is fulfilled at the cost of the child. It is completely ignored that social contexts have a supportive function; the child is robbed of this protection. This is equally the case when advanced age of the woman makes long-term performance of parental duties more difficult, if not even impossible. Parents exist for the sake of the child, not vice-versa. This fundamental principle demands respect in every case.

Artificial insemination by donor will continue to cause disagreement as it presents unsurmountable difficulties. The precipitous use of the word "adultery" may be avoided because it connotes an element of unfaithfulness on the part of the individual which may not always be assumed. This limitation, however, cannot overcome the concerns mentioned earlier. They arise from the separation of genetic and legal parenthood. In terms of giving life to a child, the bodily and spiritual aspects of the relationship are separated, revealing the danger – perhaps already a burden on the couple – of a dualistic anthropology.

Certainly the child is affected to the extent that he no longer has an unambiguous and manifest genetic identity. Is there a subliminal fear here of losing one's sense of belonging? Ultimately, self-awareness of the person depends on knowledge about his origin; renouncing this legitimate expectation seems unjust, and society, too, shares in the harm that is done. The couple's wish for a child – a wish that is completely understandable – must not ignore the social responsibility they also share; the price paid to fulfill such a wish is the loss of any sense of proportion.

The concept of adoption that emerges in this context appears to be no more than a semantic trick; it reverses the original meaning of the term: no longer is a parentless child provided with parents; it becomes providing a child-less couple with a child. The couple in such a situation must ask themselves whether or not adoption in the classical sense offers an alternative. Furthermore, there is the possibility of accepting one's own fate in life with composure; this too can strengthen marital partnership and liberate energies that have an enduring effect beyond the stringently defined intimate sphere of marriage.

Reproductive medicine includes a challenge that is directed towards the Church's official teaching. This challenge revolves around the underlying **anthropology of the conjugal act**, in particular the inseparability of the act's two meanings (see 23.2.2). The ethical debate has dealt with the basic issue for a long time, although under the aspect of responsible parenthood it has already been discussed in scholarly circles within the Catholic church. The question is: does the separation of procreation from its expressive qualities through techniques of assisted fertilization that provide relief from infertility – albeit temporarily – merit such condemnation? Is the connection between the couple's expression of love and their openness to offspring understood too restrictively to the extent that the phenomenal nature of the act becomes the dominant factor in the discussion?

Ethical discussions that have taken place within scholarly circles were able to contribute distinctions long overdue. These discussions have focused on a more flexible interpretation of human action per se. The phenomenal aspect of the act is surely an important indicator, but is with certainty not the criterion determining the act's morality. The whole ensemble of factors and circumstances likewise has to be taken into account. When a couple accepts the burden of techniques accompanying assisted reproduction in order to fulfill their wish for a child this may indeed be interpreted as a valid expression of marital love. The governing intention unites both meanings of the conjugal act; technical separation will be counterbalanced by this intentional unity. Moral evaluations of reproductive technologies must take notice of this. Considering these techniques as technology's threat to one of the most spontaneous of human actions does not seem an adequate response to the actual state of affairs.

posed on the child which, even with the best intentions, cannot be fulfilled. When disillusionment sets in, repercussions will be felt throughout the marriage. A human person is never a "therapy" for a couple in a precarious relationship. Their healing must be sought at a deeper level; fulfilling the wish for a child can easily be a diversionary tactic saving the couple from the challenge of deeper emotional and psychological therapy. Emotional and psychological distress cannot be redressed through proxy.

The moral evaluation of **surrogate motherhood** in its various forms follows relatively easily, and does not require intensive scrutiny. Pregnancy is not a purely physiological process and moreover, should not be commercialized. Rather, a deep and personal bond is formed affecting both the pregnant woman as well as the child to be born. The relationship between them cannot end at the moment of birth simply on the basis of an agreement without doing violence to nature. Moreover, it cannot be ignored that resolution of conflicts possibly arising is made exceedingly more difficult. Who decides in the case of a high-risk pregnancy? Is it the surrogate mother alone who bears the responsibility or does the genetic mother have a right to speak, and if so, to what extent? Can the assumption of higher risks be settled through a contractual waiver? Could it be legally enforced? Here unresolved conflicts arise which are at the expense of the child, as the one primarily affected but having no voice at all in the matter – for this reason moral reservations need no further justification.

22.3.2 Concern for Psychosocial Health

Those facilities that offer reproductive technologies to couples aim at protecting the well-being of the child; his well-being is the foremost concern. At the same time, psychological and social factors must also be taken into account. One such consideration is the free decision of the couple; couples should not undertake therapeutic procedures under any emotional or psychological pressure from whatever source because such coercion will unquestionably affect the child negatively. It is necessary for the couple, then, to examine very carefully whether or not available alternatives offer more acceptable choices. Whoever sincerely considers all the alternatives available will achieve a greater understanding of the desire for offspring as well as a mature sense of peace.

Consultation with a trained psychologist can help in this regard. This is true especially in those situations in which the fate of childlessness proves to threaten the stability of the marriage. In such a situation, just having a child is not the solution; one risks the danger of a subliminal but real disregard for the child. Such a point of departure can have adverse effects on the child's later development; perhaps expectations are subliminally im-

22.3.3 The Bodily Inviolability of the Embryo

The logic of protecting human life hinges on regarding the **embryo as a person.** The responsibility to care for the weak and vulnerable stands or falls on this assertion. Ethical consequences are drawn from this which concern, above all, the physician involved with reproduction as well as the biologist. These consequences revolve around giving careful attention to the term "logic". It means first of all that the duty to protect life is qualitatively uniform at all stages of human existence. In principle, what is called for is the same right to life and protection from bodily harm. One cannot speak of graduated protection of life; to do so would violate the logic of the meanings of the terms used.

From this central thesis follow a series of considerations, all of which call for further development. The encyclical "Evangelium vitae" (n. 14) addresses the problem of spare embryos and sees in it the danger of human life being devalued and turned into an object to be manipulated. Now it may be argued that advancements in medical technology make such apprehensions unnecessary. The requirement that, if possible, all embryos produced through an in vitro process be transferred at one time to the woman can be fulfilled and, therefore, such misgivings are diminished. It may be self-evident that the couple must be willing to accept a multiple pregnancy if the situation arises. No one may provoke risks and then walk away from the consequences, especially if this happens at the price of evident rights being lost. No one has the right to deliberately withhold from the embryo the chance to survive. This is even valid when embryos that are produced through an "in vitro" process are to be examined for quality. In terms of the duty to support life, the same criteria hold here as much as at any other point. What level of certainty can be claimed in judging the embryo's potential for survival is a practical problem. A rule of thumb could be that the embryo should be given the benefit in case of doubt.

Within the framework of the relatively best definition, the category of "person" can be attributed to the embryo even during earliest stages. As such, the embryo is treated as a being unto itself. Consequently, this presupposition implies the rejection of experiments using human material. The individual is never exclusively a means to achieve an end independent from his own self. This variation of the categorical imperative guides the researcher who shares the anthropological premises previously mentioned. The right to intrude into the bodily integrity of the embryo in its earliest stages must be considered along similar lines. Deliberate abuse or disregard of the bodily integrity of the embryo cannot be allowed as it is the case whenever the well-being of the child – the first one to be affected – is no longer given absolute priority. The unequivocalness of this position may place strict requirements on the researcher, because one cannot speak of an assumption of risk that is not based on free and informed consent. Without doubt the embryo is in the weaker and more vulnerable position.

It then follows from this line of argument that genetic manipulation of the embryo is not admissible. At the basis of this proscription is the recognized right to unadulterated genetic patrimony. This touches on the eventual possibility of germ line therapy. The reservations emerging here envisage not only the consequences of such research, but they also seek to prevent the danger of a **eugenic mentality**. Manipulations previously performed on germ material, for example a mixture of sperm from different donors, are subject to the same apprehensions. When this is the only way to avoid the transmission of genetic defects, the couple must ask itself whether the price for progeny is not too high. That these considerations also touch upon the issue of donor gametes is obvious.

Now the objection could be raised that absolute genetic identity can never be established with certainty, and medical technology does nothing more than to hasten entirely normal processes. The objection, however, is not fully convincing, because the supposed risks are not only knowingly provoked but precipitated. It may remain an open question whether or not the same apprehensions hold in the case of sex determination because of eugenic indications; because it is difficult to agree on the disadvantages for the embryo, given that prophylactic intervention is performed. A specification of whatever kind – under strict limitations – must keep in mind the looming danger of an uncontrollable break in the dam.

Another issue is the increasing utilization of the methods of micro-injection (intracytoplasmic sperm injection; ICSI) for male infertility. Some may suspect this to be a manipulative procedure because the physician arbitrarily selects a sperm cell and injects it into the egg. Which of the many sperm cells contained in the seminal fluid would fuse with the egg is not entrusted to the natural process. This suspicion, however, appears unfounded because no selection is aimed at. And even were it possible, it would be in the service of increasing the success rate in a way completely in line with the desired goal, thus assisting the natural process. This offers the advantage of avoiding the existence of a handicapped child without resorting to illegal measures. Nor would the reproach of a naturalistic conception of the person with a corresponding eugenic mentality be applicable. Such procedures also can avoid recourse to heterologous protocols otherwise available. In the end, any possible manipulative use of these procedures does not invalidate their proper and rightful use.

Responsibility for the bodily integrity of newly conceived life entails the duty to diminish risks to life whenever possible. The medical researcher and the clinician deal with nature that is accessible empirically not only with their scientific expertise, but they also introduce into the data a projection that goes beyond it and humanizes it. The criterion for decisions is not nature as it is given, but the underlying concept of the person. This is the perspective from which to deal with the risk factors that necessarily arise. It may appear completely understandable, then, if the freezing of fertilized eggs (cryogenic preservation) – with the exception of the pronucleus stage – is rejected on account of the disproportionate risks that are entailed in such a process. Complete elimination of risks, however, is never possible; in this sense, nature is a good indicator for it is always ambivalent and constantly accompanied by risks. The moral theologian will appreciate this; his mental categories cannot and will not mask the hard facts of reality.

22.4 In Vitro Fertilization and its Moral Setting

In vitro fertilization is surrounded by an ethically explosive environment opening the door to preimplantation diagnosis and the attendant controversies. The ethical problems are polarised between status and purpose arguments: the biopsied cell is in the totipotential stage and is denied the chance to become a fully developed human being, and, in the case of a negative diagnosis, the remaining embryo is not transferred. Here selection is made purely according to genetic criteria. In this context, the word "reprogenetics" is fully justified. There is the idea that in its earliest phase life is generally replaceable. Moreover, in the background stands a genetic determinism of questionable understanding. All those involved are sucked into the vortex of technology. In view of the ever increasing costs the handicapped and their parents are threatened with becoming stigmatised. And the physician, burdened by sheer limitations of time, is pressured into making decisions; the intrinsic purpose of his activities is put to the extreme test. Whoever speaks of a lesser evil when a couple is determined to abort an embryo with forseeable handicaps remains dependent on descriptions of purely phenomenal categories.

Various cloning techniques are also made possible by in vitro procreation. It is easy to understand why reproductive cloning is generally rejected in ethical terms. It subverts the individual's rights to genetic identity and causes, as is generally believed, instrumentalisation of human life and is not compatible with the dignity of man. In addition, it contributes to biological impoverishment.

Concerning therapeutic cloning, a tension between status and purpose previously mentioned reccurs. Although there are no objections to the goals of transplantation medicine, concern arises about the means used, especially in the application of pluripotential embryonic stem cells which can only be derived from totipotenial cells. Here, medical research is faced with a real dilemma: in order to rescue future life or heal disease, present life must be sacrificed or, be denied the chance of further development. So it is the mandate of research to find a solution avoiding this conflict. The use of specialised stem cells provides no ethical problems, and can be applied under the current standards of transplantation medicine. The same would apply to the use of fetal stem cells after induced or spontaneous abortion. However, such practices would have to be examined in the light of current devotional obligations and the danger of misuse.

22.5 The Dilemma of Tolerance

Strenuous efforts to achieve a moral consensus upon which sound legal standards are built will not succeed in reconciling all conflicting points of view. There remain areas open for discussion and grey areas that become a challenge for those working in reproductive medicine, especially when, in view of their own moral convictions, unreasonable demands are made on them. Legal and moral spheres do not agree completely with each other; quick recourse to what is legally allowed cannot free one from the autonomy and burden of one's conscience. This becomes increasingly obvious in a pluralistic society which thinks in international terms and is thus subject to the pressure of international competition. Research and applied medicine are equally affected by this phenomenon. This must not necessarily result in human progress; it can also result in a levelling of standards. In this connection it should be remembered that the physician is never a living tool in the hands of the patient when he is asked for competent advice: partnership surely does not tolerate patronisation but steadfastness on the other hand does not imply hegemony; autonomy is necessarily mutual. This becomes important when judgements on behalf of others are required because the one primarily effected – namely the embryo – has no voice in the matter. There is no alternative to personal conscience. Tolerance must always be critically questioned should it contribute to possible harm that cannot be repaired. In this one postulate, self-respect and a sense of responsibility flow together. The legitimacy of a strictly circumscribed affirmation of reproductive medicine with all its opportunities and dangers depends upon this willingness.

22.6 Suggested Readings

Beier HM, Beckman JO (1991) Implications and consequences of the German Embryo Protection Act. Hum Reprod 6:607–608

Bonnicksen AL (1988) Embryo freezing: ethical issues in the clinical setting. Hastings Center Report 18:26–30

Boyle J (1991) The Roman catholic tradition and bioethics. In: Brody BA (ed) Bioethics yearbook, vol I. Theological developments in bioethics 1988–1990. The center for ethics, medicine and public issues. Kluwer, Dordrecht, pp 5–21

Cahill LS (1989) Moral traditions, ethical language and reproductive technologies. J Med Phil 14:497–522

Cahill LS (1992) Theology and bioethics: should religious traditions have a public voice? J Med Phil 17:263–272

Engelhardt HT (1973) The beginnings of personhood: philosophical considerations. Perkins J 27:20–27

Hathout H (1991) Islamic concepts on bioethics. In: Brody BA (ed) Bioethics yearbook, vol I. Theological developments in bioethics 1988–1990. The center for ethics, medical and public issues. Kluwer, Dordrecht, pp 103–117

Hildt E, Mieth D (eds) (1998) In-vitro fertilization in the 1990s. Towards a medical, social and ethical evaluation. Ashgate, Aldershot, GB

Kirby MD (1984) Bioethics of IVF – the state of debate. J Med Ethics 10:45–48

Leone S (1992) Ethical aspects of assisted reproductive technologies. Acta Eur Fert 23:141–145

Nelson P (1991) Bioethics in the Lutheran tradition. In: Brody BA (ed) Bioethics yearbook, vol I. Theological developments in bioethics 1988–1990. The center for ethics, medical and public issues. Kluwer, Dordrecht, pp 119–143

Schenker JG (1992) The rights of the pre-embryo and fetus to in-vitro and in-vivo therapy. In: Bromham DR (ed) Ethics in reproductive medicine. Springer, Berlin Heidelberg New York, pp 33–45

Sureau C, Shenfield F (eds) (1995) Ethical aspects of human reproduction. John Libbey Eurotext, Monrouge

Serra A (1988) The human embryo, science and medicine. Commentary on a recent document. In: Malherbe JF (ed) Human life, its beginnings and development. Bioethical reflections by Catholic scholars. L'Harmattan, Paris, pp 47–65

Wennegren B (1991) Human rights of an embryo. Int J Bioethics 2:46–49

22.7 Church Documents

Pope Paul VI (1969) Encyclical letter "Humanae vitae"

Congregation for the Doctrine of Faith, Instruction "Donum vitae" (1987)

Pope John Paul II (1995) Encyclical letter "Evangelium vitae"

Gemeinsame Erklärung des Rates der Evangelischen Kirche Deutschlands und der deutschen Bischofskonferenz "Gott ist ein Freund des Lebens" ("God is a friend of life") (1989)

Subject Index

D

Q

R

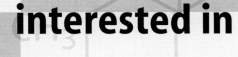